Principles of Public Health Practice

Second Edition

Principles of Public Health Practice

Second Edition

Edited by

F. Douglas Scutchfield, M.D.
Peter B. Bosomworth Professor of Health Service Research and Policy
Director, Kentucky School of Public Health
Director, Center for Health Services Management and Research
University of Kentucky Medical Center
Lexington, Kentucky

C. William Keck, M.D., M.P.H.
Director of Health
Akron Health Department
Akron, Ohio

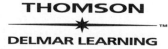
THOMSON

DELMAR LEARNING

Australia Canada Mexico Singapore Spain United Kingdom United States

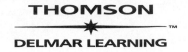

THOMSON
DELMAR LEARNING

Principles of Public Health Practice, Second Edition
F. Douglas Scutchfield and C. William Keck

Executive Director,
Health Care Business Unit:
William Brottmiller

Executive Editor:
Cathy L. Esperti

Acquisitions Editor:
Maureen Rosener

Developmental Editor:
Patricia Gaworecki

Editorial Assistant:
Matthew Thouin

Executive Marketing Manager:
Dawn F. Gerrain

Channel Manager:
Jennifer McAvey

Project Editor:
Bryan Viggiani

Production Coordinator:
Anne Sherman

Art and Design Coordinator:
Jay Purcell

For permission to use material from this text or product, contact us by
Tel (800) 730-2214
Fax (800) 730-2215
www.thomsonrights.com

Library of Congress Cataloging-in-Publication Data

Principles of public health practice / F. Douglas Scutchfield, C. William Keck [editors[.
    p. cm.
Includes bibliographical references and index.
    ISBN 0-7668-2843-3 (alk. paper)
    1. Public health administration--United States. 2. Public health.
I. Scutchfield, F. Douglas. II. Keck, C. William.
    RA445 .P67 2002
    362.1'0973--dc21   2002073640

NOTICE TO THE READER

Publisher does not warrant or guarantee any of the products described herein or perform any independent analysis in connection with any of the product information contained herein. Publisher does not assume, and expressly disclaims, any obligation to obtain and include information other than that provided to it by the manufacturer.

The reader is expressly warned to consider and adopt all safety precautions that might be indicated by the activities herein and to avoid all potential hazards. By following the instructions contained herein, the reader willingly assumes all risks in connection with such instructions.

Publisher makes no representation or warranties of any kind, including but not limited to, the warranties of fitness for particular purpose or merchantability, nor are any such representations implied with respect to the material set forth herein, and the publisher takes no responsibility with respect to such material. Publisher shall not be liable for any special, consequential, or exemplary damages resulting, in whole or part, from the readers' use of, or reliance upon, this material.

INTRODUCTION TO THE SERIES

This series in Health Services Administration is now in its second decade of providing top-quality teaching materials to the health administration/public health field. Each year has witnessed further strengthening of the market position of each of the principal books in the series, while also reflecting the continued excellence of the products. Each author, book editor, and contributor to the series has helped build what is widely recognized as the top textbook and issues collection of books available in this field today.

But we have achieved only a beginning. Everyone involved in the series is committed to further expansion of the scope, technical excellence, and usefulness of the series. Our goal is to do more for you, the reader. We will add new books in important areas, seek out more excellent authors, and improve the physical attributes of the books to make them easier for you to use.

We thank everyone, the authors and users in particular, who have made this series so successful and so widely used. And we promise that this second decade will be dedicated to further expansion of the series and to enhancement of the books it contains to provide still greater value to you, our constituency.

Stephen J. Williams
Series Editor

DELMAR SERIES IN HEALTH SERVICES ADMINISTRATION

CONTENTS

ACKNOWLEDGMENTS

There are many people who have made important contributions to the successful completion of this book. The contributing authors merit the largest share of our gratitude, of course. The field of public health is broad and ever changing, and we felt the need to call widely on the expertise of many of our colleagues. Their willingness to participate with us in this endeavor is appreciated, as is their positive response to editing suggestions we made.

We especially thank the Akron Health Commission and April Thomas at the University of Kentucky for their understanding and support of this project. In addition, our editors, Maureen Rosener and Patty Gaworecki, deserve special mention for their help and support in the preparation of this manuscript.

FOREWORD

Public health has never received the recognition it deserves. The late nineteenth and early twentieth centuries have been referred to as the "Age of Modern Medical Miracles," yet it was not "miracles" of high technology that brought this nation to the health status it now enjoys. Instead, it was public health advances that accomplished that: clean water, proper housing, immunization, eradication of smallpox, increased life expectancy and the understanding of preventive medicine as exemplified by healthy lifestyle choices.

In the past decade, we have seen two separate movements in the national and global worlds of public health. In the United States we have seen the erosion of the infrastructure of public health not because the practitioners of public health or its teachers were negligent, but because both the Congress and the Administrative Branch, with their minds on other things, contributed to the present sorry state of affairs. The Republican Party presented the nation with a *Contract with the American People,* which unlike most contracts was signed only by the government. The Administrative Branch conceived the idea of "re-inventing" government. Public health was caught in a pincers movement, both sides of which could have more honestly labeled their efforts as "downsizing" that euphemism, which frequently undermined institutions and then infrastructures, as well as reducing them in size.

The terrorist effort, mailing anthrax bacilli to prominent individuals, demonstrated our woeful inadequacy of institutions and infrastructure, which we trusted to forge the necessary alliances between health surveillance, health management and agencies of the law necessary to respond to a bio-terrorist attempt at mass destruction. Even the communication was confusing with multiple voices telling different stories. No one seemed to be in charge, in spite of the fact that the threat of bio-terrorism cannot honestly be called new.

The other great movement that affects global as well as national public health augers well, if properly harnessed, for not only the health of America but also the health of the world. Public health has been provided with a number of new tools, such as the unbelievable explosion of informatics, particularly e-mail and the Internet. This has come in a time to transmit knowledge of the tremendous growth of science, including the scientific basis of public health. The mapping of the genome and advances in genetic engineering have provided public health and medicine with knowledge hitherto almost unimaginable. And the development of new vaccines, always a welcomed advancement, comes at the very time when we need all of the expertise we can muster in this field if we are to respond adequately to bio-terrorism.

The word "globalization" has become one of our current buzzwords and although most of the popular writing on the subject has to do with the economics of globalization, it is inextricably tied up with the health of those nations to be globalized. We have truly globalized only two things and we have done them well: we have globalized the spread of infectious disease and we have seen the exportation of the cigarette into every nook and cranny of the planet. These things being true, and both being the fruits, if you will, of the industrialized world, it stands to reason that we have the obligation to globalize health. The benefits of economic globalization aside, economic globalization cannot take place if the health of developing nations is not tremendously improved. These nations are too sick to contribute to economic globalization; only the globalization of good health can change that situation.

I do not view the health status of the world with discouragement, but rather see it as an unprecedented challenge for public health, which comes at a time when we have tools recently undreamed of that can aid us in our quest. In earlier years, I worried how we could ever bring health to the developing world because it lacked a health infrastructure. But science leapfrogged over that issue, and with the cell-phone and the Internet, all it takes now is organization.

Just a few years ago representatives of the almost 150 schools of medicine and osteopathic medicine in the United States, who turn out practitioners to treat injury and illness and return people to a previous state of health without making much effort to take them beyond that, met in dialogue on several occasions with representatives of the field of public health. The early enthusiasm of both sides has faded to a lackluster substitute of what we started out to do. That situation has to be reversed. I can't think of a professional challenge presented to two interrelated but distinct groups simultaneously that carries such promise with proper guidance.

It is obvious, therefore, that there is an important role for a book that synthesizes state-of-the-art information about the problems and challenges of public health for the benefit of both students and current practitioners. I believe that Drs. Scutchfield and Keck have provided such a book. They have brought together the wisdom of many of the most knowledgeable health professionals in North America to provide the best information possible about current public health organizations and practice. For the new student, the book provides an introduction to the field of public health practice. For the current practitioner, it is a unique and vital reference. Those who make public health policy should not do so without understanding the content of this book. Only when there are enough knowledgeable and committed individuals will deplorable human suffering and unaffordable economic costs be prevented. This book is a step in that direction.

C. Everett Koop, M.D., Sc.D.

PREFACE

An interesting dichotomy has developed in the field of public health over the past several years. On one hand, the contributions made by public health measures to the improvement of health status in the United States have been documented and increasingly appreciated, and the potential for future improvement has been recognized. On the other hand, those contributions have largely been taken for granted, and public health expenditures have been slashed as part of the effort to control governmental spending at the local, state, and federal levels. This has resulted in the growing awareness in the potential improvements that can still be made to the public's health, while, at the same time the capacity of the "delivery system" in state and local health department has been diminished.

Today's public health practitioner faces a changing and somewhat ambiguous environment. There are challenging and exciting possibilities, but resources are limited. The government's role is paramount but there is public mistrust of government. Health reform is on the public's mind but the focus is on illness care rather than health promotion and disease prevention. New public health crises call for effective responses but the public is divided on priorities for action.

Successful management of health departments and other community health agencies will require enlightened and strong leadership. Public health leaders will need to understand the contributions that can be made by the application of public health principles to community health problems, to work with communities to involve them in understanding and addressing the problems that threaten them and to engineer constructive evolution of their agencies to effectively perform in a changing and uncertain environment.

There are about 500,000 individuals employed as public health workers at all levels of government in the United States. Very few of these professionals have formal public health training or even share a common academic base. There are wide variations in the capacity of local health departments across the country, and there is uncertainty about the future place of public health departments in society. Nonetheless, improvement of the public's health will require that the core functions of public health be competently executed. A cadre of public health leaders must emerge, therefore, with a clear vision of public health's place in maintaining and improving health and with the skills required to make that vision a reality. This combination of problems and opportunity suggest to us the need for *Principles of Public Health Practice, 2nd Edition*.

The second edition of this book is designed to appeal principally to two audiences. The first is the public health professional who has come to work in the public health environment without having a formal exposure to course work in public health practice, or who wishes to have on hand a review of recent developments in the field. The second audience for this text is students of the public health professions who would benefit from access to a broad text describing the organization, administration, and practice of public health.

ORGANIZATION

This new edition is organized into five major parts. The first describes the current public health environment by introducing the basic concepts and development of public health practice, determinants of health status, and the legal aspects on which public health practice is based. It also includes a new chapter on reviewing the last decade of public health information and issues.

Part two addresses the contributions made to public health at the federal, state, and local levels. Part three contains chapters that describe and discuss available tools to effectively manage a typical health department. A new chapter has been added to this section describing performance measurement and management.

Part four of this new edition describes public health practice in a number of substantive environments, including a new chapter on health promotion and disease prevention effectiveness that examines the use of new analytical tools for use in the public health arena. Part five focuses on the role of the public health department in an evolving health system, and suggests a vision of the ideal health department of the future.

ALSO NEW TO THIS EDITION

Three new appendices have been added to this new edition. They include major public health professional associations, health leadership training institutes, and core competency requirements for public health professionals.

Additionally, an instructor's guide has been created to accompany this text. It provides the instructor with discussion topics for each chapter that can be incorporated into course lectures and student writing assignments, and that can serve as study guides.

CONTRIBUTORS

Myron Allukian, Jr., D.D.S., M.P.H.
Assistant Deputy Commissioner and Director
Bureau of Community Dental Programs
Boston Department of Health and Hospitals
Boston, Massachusetts

Guadalupe X. Ayala, Ph.D. (ABD), M.P.H.
SDSU-UCSD
Joint Doctoral Program in Clinical Psychology
San Diego, California

Elizabeth A. Baker, Ph.D., M.P.H.
Associate Professor
Community Health
Saint Louis University
School of Public Health
St. Louis, Missouri

Susan P. Baker, M.P.H., Sc.D. (Hon.)
Professor
Center for Injury Research and Policy
Johns Hopkins University
Bloomberg School of Public Health
Baltimore, Maryland

Darryl B. Barnett, B.S.E.H., M.P.H., Dr. P.H.
Chair, Department of Environmental Health Science
and Clinical Laboratory Science
Eastern Kentucky University
Richmond, Kentucky

Joe E. Beck, D.A.A.S, R.S.
Associate Professor of Environmental Health Science
Eastern Kentucky University
Richmond, Kentucky

Trude Bennet, Dr. P.H., M.S.W., M.P.H.
Associate Professor
Department of Maternal and Child Health
School of Public Health
The University of North Carolina at Chapel Hill
Chapel Hill, North Carolina

Carter Blakey, B.S.
U.S. Department of Health and Human Services
Washington, D.C.

Ronald L. Cada, Dr. P.H.
Director Emeritus
Laboratory and Radiation Services
Colorado Department of Public Health & Environment
Denver, Colorado

Alan W. Cross, M.D.
Professor of Social Medicine and Pediatrics
Clinical Professor of Maternal and Child Health
Director, Center for Health Promotion and Disease Prevention
University of North Carolina at Chapel Hill
Chapel Hill, North Carolina

Suzanne Dandoy, M.D., M.P.H.
Faculty
Epidemiology Graduate Interdisciplinary Program
University of Arizona
Adjunct Professor
School of Health Administration and Policy
Arizona State University
Tucson, Arizona

Richard C. Dicker, M.D., M.Sc.
Epidemiology Program Office
Centers for Disease Control and Prevention
Atlanta, Georgia

John P. Elder, Ph.D., M.P.H.
Graduate School of Public Health
San Diego State University
San Diego, California

Michael Erickson, Sc.D.
World Health Organization
Geneva, Switzerland

Elizabeth Fee, Ph.D.
National Library of Medicine, National Institutes of Health
Bethesda, Maryland

William Foege, M.D., M.P.H.
Presidential Distinguished Professor
Department of International Health
Robert W. Woodruff Health Sciences Center
The Rollins School of Public Health
Atlanta, Georgia

Kristine M. Gebbie, Dr. P.H., R.N.
Center for Health Policy
Columbia University School of Nursing
New York City, New York

Robert M. Goodman, Ph.D., M.P.H.
Usdin Family Professor
Department of Community Health Sciences
Tulane University School of Public Health and Tropical Medicine
New Orleans, Louisiana

Pamina M. Gorbach, M.H.S., Dr. P.H.
Department of Epidemiology
School of Public Health
University of California, Los Angeles
Los Angeles, California

Lawrence W. Green, Dr. P.H.
Director, Office of Extramural Prevention Research
Public Health Practice Program Office
Centers for Disease Control and Prevention
U.S. Department of Health and Human Services
Atlanta, Georgia

Paul Halverson, M.H. S. A, Dr. P.H.
Acting Director
Division of Public Health Systems
Centers for Disease Control and Prevention
Atlanta, Georgia

Jeffrey R. Harris, M.D., M.P.H.
Health Promotion Research Center
University of Washington
Seattle, Washington

Alan R. Hinman, M.D., M.P.H.
Task Force for Child Survival & Development
Decatur, Georgia

Worley Johnson, Jr., B.S., M.P.A.
Program Coordinator
Department of Environmental Health Science
Eastern Kentucky University
Richmond, Kentucky

C. William Keck, M.D., M.P.H.
Director of Health
Akron Health Department
Akron, Ohio

R. Steven Konkel, Ph.D.
Assistant Professor
Program Coordinator
Graduate Program of Environmental Health Sciences
Eastern Kentucky University
Richmond, Kentucky

John M. Last, M.D., D.P.H.
Emeritus Professor of Epidemiology and Community Medicine
University of Ottawa
Ottawa, Canada

Joel M. Lee, Dr. P.H.
Director of Undergraduate Studies, Health Services Management
Director of Doctoral Studies
Associate Director for Academic Affairs
Kentucky School of Public Health
University of Kentucky
Lexington, Kentucky

James S. Marks, M.D., M.P.H.
Director
National Center for Chronic Disease Prevention and Health
    Promotion
Centers for Disease Control and Prevention
Atlanta, Georgia

Samuel E. Matheny, M.D., M.P.H.
Caudill Professor and Chair of the Department of Family Practice
University of Kentucky
Lexington, Kentucky

Glen P. Mays, M.P.H., Ph.D.
Department of Health Care Policy
Mathematica Research
Washington, D.C.

J. Michael McGinnis, M.D., M.A., M.P.P.
Senior Vice President
The Robert Wood Johnson Foundation
Princeton, New Jersey

David V. McQueen, Sc.D.
Associate Director for Global Health Promotion
National Center for Chronic Disease Prevention and Health
    Promotion
Centers for Disease Control and Prevention
Atlanta, Georgia

Arthur Richard Melton, M.P.H., Dr. P.H.
Deputy Director
Utah Department of Health
President
Association of State and Territorial Health Officials
    (Sept. 2000–Sept. 2001)
Salt Lake City, Utah

Thomas L. Milne, B.S. Pharm.
Executive Director
National Association of County and City Health Officials
Washington, D.C.

James F. Mosher, J.D.
Director of Alcohol Policy
Trauma Foundation
San Francisco General Hospital
San Francisco, California

Emmeline Ochiai, J.D., M.P.H.
U.S. Department of Health and Human Services
Washington, DC

Kevin A. Pearce, M.D., M.P.H.
Associate Professor
Department of Family Practice
University of Kentucky
College of Medicine
Lexington, Kentucky

K. Michael Peddecord, Dr. P.H.
Director, Institute for Public Health
Professor of Public Health
School of Public Health
San Diego State University
San Diego, California

Dennis D. Pointer, Ph.D.
Hanlon Professor of Health Services Research and Policy
Graduate School of Public Health
San Diego State University
San Diego, California

Katharine C. Rathbun, M.D., M.P.H.
Fellow
Center for Public Health Law
Kansas City, Missouri

Edward P. Richards III, J.D., M.P.H.
Professor of Law
University of Missouri Kansas City
School of Law
Executive Director
Center for Public Health Law
Kansas City, Missouri

William L. Roper, M.D., M.P.H.
Dean
School of Public Health
The University of North Carolina at Chapel Hill
Chapel Hill, North Carolina

Julianne P. Sanchez, M.A.
Graduate Student
Department of Sociology
University of Washington
Seattle, Washington

F. Douglas Scutchfield, M.D.
Peter P. Bosomworth Professor of Health Service Research
    and Policy
Director, Kentucky School of Public Health
Director, Center for Health Services Management and Research
University of Kentucky Medical Center
Lexington, Kentucky

Maria Seguí-Gómez, M.D., Sc.D.
Assistant Professor
Department of Health Policy and Management
Johns Hopkins University
Bloomberg School of Public Health
Baltimore, Maryland

Donna F. Stroup, Ph.D., M.Sc.
National Center for Chronic Disease Prevention and Health
    Promotion
Centers for Disease Control and Prevention
Atlanta, Georgia

Gregory A. Talavera, M.D., M.P.H.
Graduate School of Public Health
San Diego State University
San Diego, California

Steven M. Teutsch, M.D., M.P.H.
Senior Director
Outcomes Research and Management
Merck and Company
West Point, Pennsylvania

Stephen B. Thacker, M.D., M.Sc.
Director
Epidemiology Program Office
Centers for Disease Control and Prevention
Atlanta, Georgia

Hugh Tilson, M.D., Dr. P.H.
Clinical Professor, Epidemiology & Health Policy
University of North Carolina at Chapel Hill
Chapel Hill, North Carolina

Traci L. Toomey, Ph.D., M.P.H.
Division of Epidemiology
School of Public Health
University of Minnesota
Minneapolis, Minnesota

Carol Woltring, M.P.H.
Executive Director
Center for Health Leadership and Practice
Public Health Institute
Oakland, California

Randolph F. Wykoff, M.D., M.P.H. T.M.
Deputy Assistant Secretary for Health
U.S. Department of Health and Human Services
Washington, D.C.

Stephanie Zaza, M.D., M.P.H.
Epidemiology Program Office
Centers for Disease Control and Prevention
Atlanta, Georgia

PART
1

The Basis of Public Health

CHAPTER

1

Concepts and Definitions of Public Health Practice

F. Douglas Scutchfield, M.D.
C. William Keck, M.D., M.P.H.

The World Health Organization has defined health as ". . . a complete state of physical, mental, and social well-being and not merely the absence of disease or infirmity."[1] Societies that approach this ideal state will do so by appropriately balancing services for the diagnosis and treatment of illness with services that promote health and prevent disease.

Unfortunately, our current system of providing health services in the United States is unbalanced: it is tilted strongly toward interacting with people who are ill. This system, focused as it is on illness care, is not prepared to deal with the social issues that affect health. It is likely, for example, that health status is more closely linked to socioeconomic status and its attendant problems than to any other factor. Thus, improvement in our nation's health status will depend more on the effective application of public health techniques than on taking care of people who are ill.

This text is about public health. *Public health* is defined by John Last as

. . . one of the efforts organized by society to protect, promote, and restore the people's health. It is a combination of sciences, skills, and beliefs that is directed to the maintenance and improvement of the health of all the people through collective or social actions. The programs, services and institutions involved emphasize the prevention of disease and the health needs of the population as a whole. Public health activities change with changing technology and social values, but the goals remain the same: to reduce the amount of disease, premature death, and disease-produced discomfort and disability in the population. Public health is thus a social institution, a discipline and a practice.[2]

This chapter describes the discipline of public health and introduces concepts, problem areas, and approaches to problem solving that are part of public health practice. These issues, and others, will be referenced repeatedly and/or discussed in greater detail in subsequent chapters.

SCIENCE, SKILLS, AND BELIEFS

The scientific basis for public health rests on the study of risks to the health of populations (including risks related to the environment) and on the systems designed to deliver required services. Epidemiology and biostatistics are the scientific disciplines that underpin inquiry in all of public health. They provide the methods necessary for understanding the risks to the health of populations and individuals and for developing effective risk reduction and health promotion activities.

The skills required for effective public health practice begin with proficiency in applying the techniques required for a particular public health specialization. The most important skill, however, is the capacity to create a vision of the potential for health that exists within a community. With a clear vision comes a sense of direction and a feeling of enthusiasm that are essential if one hopes to engage a population in a process of understanding and reducing risks to its health.

Health departments are the only entities statutorily responsible for the health of their constituent populations. As a result, an underlying belief and responsibility of public health departments is that all members of the community should have access to the health promotion, disease prevention, and illness care services they need for good health. Public health is firmly grounded in the concepts of social justice, and its practitioners should be strong proponents of the ethical distribution of resources.

ASSOCIATED DISCIPLINES

Medicine played a substantial role in the development of public health. Many leaders of the public health movement during the mid to late 1800s were physicians. However, at the turn of the twentieth century the two disciplines, for a variety of reasons, began to drift apart.[3] Recent efforts have been focused on reestablishing the dialogue between public health and medicine to recognize the commonality of interest in the health of the nation's citizens.[4] In addition, recent work has showcased illustrations of effective working relations between medicine and public health.[5]

The public often has difficulty distinguishing between the practice of medicine and the practice of public health. It is important that public health practitioners are clear about the differences among them. As with medicine, the practice of public health is rooted in science and the scientific method. Medicine applies what we learn from science to the benefit of the individual patient, usually in the pursuit of the diagnosis and treatment of illness. Public health applies the knowledge gained from science to the improvement of the health status of groups of people, usually through health promotion and disease prevention activities.

Preventive medicine and **community medicine** are medical disciplines that function, to some degree, as bridges between the practice of medicine and the practice of public health. Preventive medicine physicians work to ensure the primacy and excellence of both individual and community health promotion and disease prevention efforts. Although they may interact primarily with individuals, they also deal with groups seeking to maintain and preserve their health.

Community medicine has developed as a discipline during the past 40 years, and its practitioners concentrate on the preservation of health status in communities rather than individuals. John Last defines community medicine as

> . . . the study of health and disease in the population of a specific community. Its goal is to identify the health problems and needs of defined populations, to identify means by which these needs should be met and to evaluate the extent to which health services effectively meet these needs.[2]

Public health clearly includes some elements of medical practice, preventive medicine, and community medicine. It is greater than the sum of these parts, however. It includes many other disciplines, such as nutrition, health education, and environmental health, that contribute to the improvement of the public's health status. It also concentrates on **health promotion** and **disease prevention.**

Health Promotion

Health promotion refers to

> . . . enabling people to increase control over and improve their health. It involves the population as a

whole in the context of their everyday lives, rather than focusing on people at risk for specific diseases, and is directed toward action on the determinants or causes of health.[2]

We know that prerequisites for health include a variety of factors such as shelter, food, and education among others. Good health promotion activities may involve educational, organizational, economic, and environmental interventions targeted toward specific lifestyle behaviors and environmental conditions that are harmful to health, with the intention of making health-promoting changes in those conditions.

Disease Prevention

Disease prevention techniques are usually described in one of three categories—primary prevention, secondary prevention, and tertiary prevention.

Primary Prevention

The first category, **primary prevention,** includes those activities that are intended to prevent the onset of disease in the first place. The classic example of primary prevention is immunization against infectious diseases, but the use of seat belts, the installation of air bags in automobiles, the avoidance of tobacco use, the minimal intake of alcoholic beverages, and the inspection and licensure of restaurants are all examples of common public health activities that exemplify primary prevention.

Secondary Prevention

Secondary prevention refers to techniques that find health problems early in their course so that action can be taken to minimize the risk of progression of the disease in individuals or the risk that communicable illnesses will be transmitted to others. Examples of this principle include the early diagnosis of hypertension with follow-up treatment to minimize the risk of future vascular disease, and the early diagnosis and treatment of sexually transmitted diseases to minimize the transmission potential of those conditions to others.

Tertiary Prevention

Tertiary prevention is focused on rehabilitation in an effort to prevent the worsening of an individual's health in the face of a chronic disease or injury. Learning to walk again after an orthopedic injury or cerebrovascular accident is an example.

Acute Sickness Services

Although public health focuses principally on health promotion and disease prevention, in many circumstances it has become a provider of acute sickness services to those who cannot obtain these services otherwise. Not surprisingly, sickness services are most often provided by health departments found in inner-city and rural areas of lower socioeconomic status, where access to medical care is limited. This assumption of responsibility for illness care has been controversial. Many insist it is outside the purview of traditional public health functions. Others insist that the assurance of medical services, when they cannot be obtained in any other way, is a clear public health mission, consistent with the responsibility for maintaining the public's health.

EVOLUTION OF THE DISCIPLINE

Public health departments began to appear in the United States in the middle of the nineteenth century. Since that time, public health methods and programs have evolved to meet the changing needs of the community. Many changes have been driven by scientific contributions to knowledge about risks to health and by improvements in the technology available to respond to public health issues. For more than a century, public health has moved from a period of limited scientific understanding, when infectious diseases were the major cause of death, to a period of significant and growing scientific capacity, as chronic diseases became the major killers.

INFECTIOUS DISEASE CONTROL

Scientists came to realize that the major health problems of the day were caused by microorganisms.

They also realized that understanding how the microorganisms moved from person to person could lead to strategies to prevent the transmission of disease. This realization was so revolutionary that Milton Terris has called this period the "First Epidemiological Revolution."[6] This allowed communities to develop policies and laws that would protect the public's health and to hire people to enforce them. These governmental *sanitarians* in the nation's first health departments used laws providing for quarantine, safe water, and sewage disposal to significantly reduce the toll taken by communicable disease. The later addition of vaccines and antibiotics increased the effectiveness of infectious disease control efforts. It became increasingly obvious, however, that improved socioeconomic status, decreased crowding, good nutrition, and better education had as much to do with this success story as did the newer medical interventions.[7] This reinforced the lesson that there are *determinants of health* that deserve as much attention as medical interventions when it comes to improving health status.

CHRONIC DISEASE CONTROL

Our struggles with infectious diseases continue in the present day. New organisms appear, such as the human immunodeficiency virus, or HIV, and older organisms, such as the tubercle bacillus that causes tuberculosis, return to fill new niches in our changing environment. The major causes of death and disability in the United States today, however, are chronic illnesses. Our efforts to understand and control them have led to what Terris calls the "Second Epidemiological Revolution."

We are in an era of rapidly increasing understanding of the causes of chronic disease. We have learned that heart disease, cancer, stroke, and many other chronic diseases are multifactorial in causation. A variety of genetic, environmental, and lifestyle factors interact to predispose individuals to chronic illness. In fact, up to 70 percent of premature mortality in the United States is directly related to environmental and lifestyle factors that are potentially controllable by individuals or society.[8] We describe these causes as **risk factors,** and we realize that such behaviors as the use

of tobacco, the excessive use of alcohol, unhealthful nutritional practices, and sedentary lifestyles cannot be altered without the direct, willing participation of the individuals affected in an environment that is supportive of healthful choices.

We are moving beyond an era of professionals doing things *for* others to one of professionals doing things *with* others to help them minimize risks to their health. It is a time of trying to understand the motivations of human behavior and developing constructive and ethical mechanisms to support healthful behavioral choices. It is also a time of working with governments and communities to create the most healthful living environments possible.

SOCIAL ISSUES

New problems have emerged that have public health implications and will require a new level of understanding if effective intervention methods are to be devised. They include epidemics of violence, drug abuse, teenage pregnancy, and sexually transmitted disease—problems that are not clearly understood but probably due in part to racial and ethnic prejudice, increasing numbers of single-parent families, changing cultural values, and poverty as a social norm.

Dr. Scutchfield has termed these new social/public health problems the "third public health revolution." Understanding these problems will require that we develop new scientific knowledge from disciplines not traditionally associated with public health. It will require us to develop a better understanding of human behavior, communities, their structures, and interaction among them.[9,10] Unfortunately, we are only beginning to understand the epidemiology of these problems and do not yet have robust interventions for most of them.

NEW TOOLS FOR PUBLIC HEALTH PRACTICE

A number of new tools are available to public health professionals to help them carry out public health's core functions. Frequent reference will be made to these tools throughout this textbook because of the important roles they play in the conceptualization, organization, and delivery of public health services. They are just briefly introduced here.

Report on the Future of Public Health

The contributions made by public health over the past 100 years have largely been taken for granted. In fact, public health had languished, through inattention, for many decades. Fortunately, the 1988 report titled *The Future of Public Health* by the Institute of Medicine (IOM) has focused attention on the discipline.[11] This study details the contributions made by public health while chronicling its current difficulties, and it makes very clear recommendations about how the nation's public health system should be improved to ensure that every citizen in the country has access to needed public health services.

The report defines the mission of public health as "fulfilling society's interest in assuring conditions in which people can be healthy."[11] The Study Committee of the IOM that produced the report recognized that many components of a community must work together for that mission to be successfully accomplished, but they emphasized the unique responsibility of government, at all levels, to ensure success. These governmental responsibilities are usually carried out by health departments, which are the jurisdiction's action arm to accomplish the mission articulated by the IOM. The committee suggested three core public health functions for local and state health departments: **assessment, policy development,** and **assurance.**

By assessment, the committee meant that each public health agency should

> . . . regularly and systematically collect, assemble, analyze, and make available information on the health of the community, including statistics on health status, community health needs, and epidemiologic and other studies of health problems.[11(p7)]

The committee noted that not every agency is large enough to conduct these activities in their entirety, but that each agency bears the responsibility for seeing that the assessment function is fulfilled. In essence, the committee recognized the public health department as the epidemiologic intelligence center for health in the community, providing the information necessary for effective health planning.

By policy development, the committee meant that each public health agency should

> . . . serve the public interest in the development of comprehensive public health policies by promoting use of the scientific knowledge base in decision-making about public health and by leading in developing public health policy.[11(p8)]

Policy development links science with political, organizational, and community values. It includes information sharing, citizen participation, compromise, and consensus building in a process that nurtures shared ownership of the policy decisions.

By assurance, the committee meant that each public health agency should

> . . . assure their constituents that services necessary to achieve agreed upon goals are provided, either by encouraging actions by other entities (private or public sector), by requiring such action through regulation, or by providing services directly.[11(p8)]

The committee also felt that each public health agency should work with its community to guarantee access to a basic set of health services for each citizen.[11(p8)] This is the social justice element of public health. The effective health department will work with other service providers to be sure that good quality, basic services are available to all, even if the services are provided by someone other than the health department itself.

The areas of assessment, policy development, and assurance are now considered by most to define the core functions of public health. Unfortunately, most health departments will have to improve their capacity to carry out the functions and activities associated with these responsibilities. Many health departments are too small to perform them well. They might combine with others or form alliances that will allow the sharing of expertise. Strong liaisons with academic units, where available, may also provide access to analytical and other skills. Recently, there has been the realization that the environment in which public health operates has changed. While much improvement has occurred in public health since the 1988 report, these are still turbulent times for the discipline. For that reason, the IOM has decided to revisit the issues of public health with a new committee, focused on "assuring the health of the public in the 21st century." This committee will release a report designed to reexamine issues in the 1988 report.

During the early 1990s it became apparent that the notion of assessment, policy development, and assurance did not communicate well to policy makers what public health organizations actually do. Although those in public health understood the concept, the layperson had difficulty understanding it. The U.S. Department of Health and Human Services convened a work group of stakeholders who developed a list of 10 essential health services that should be considered core components of public health practice. These 10 essential services, which were refinements and elaboration of the functions delineated in the IOM report, are:

- Monitor health status to identify community health problems
- Diagnose and investigate health problems and health hazards in the community
- Inform, educate, and empower people about health issues
- Mobilize community partnerships to identify and solve health problems
- Develop policies and plans that support individual and community health efforts
- Enforce laws and regulations that protect health and ensure safety
- Link people to needed personal health services and ensure the provision of health care when otherwise unavailable
- Ensure a competent public health and personal health care workforce
- Evaluate effectiveness, accessibility, and quality of personal and population-based health services
- Research for new insights and innovative solutions to health problems

These 10 essential public health services have been used in a variety of ways to facilitate public health activities at the federal, state, and local level. They will be a recurring theme throughout this textbook.[12]

Healthy People 2010

The process of setting national goals and objectives for the nation began in 1979 with the publication of *Healthy People: The Surgeon General's Report on Health Promotion and Disease Prevention.*[8] It was the first such report to emphasize the importance of reducing premature mortality through health promotion and disease prevention programs, and it discussed a series of age-specific goals for the nation to accomplish by 1990. Following that report, the Centers for Disease Control and Prevention (CDC) convened a series of discussions that led to a publication titled *Health Promotion/ Disease Prevention: Objectives for the Nation.*[13] This document established 226 specific health objectives to be achieved by 1990. These objectives were measurable, specific, and tied to the various priority programs listed under the rubrics of health promotion, health protection, and preventive services.

In 1987, the Public Health Service's Office of Health Promotion and Disease Prevention began a new consultative process with the nation's public health professionals to develop a set of objectives for the year 2000. The resulting *Healthy People 2000: National Health Promotion and Disease Prevention Objectives*[14], which was published in 1990, articulated three major goals:

1. Increase the span of healthy life for all Americans
2. Reduce health disparities among Americans
3. Achieve access to preventive services for all Americans

More than 300 objectives were listed within 22 priority areas and categorized as Health Status Objectives, Risk Reduction Objectives, and Service and Protection Objectives. *Healthy People 2000* has succeeded in establishing a national focus for attainable health status by the year 2000. It has been described by many as creating the destination for health promotion and disease prevention activities.

The success of these efforts has lead to the creation of the third publication of the series. *Healthy People 2010* was released in 2000. *Healthy People 2010* has two overarching goals: increasing the quality and years of a healthy life and reducing health disparities. The new version includes 467 objectives in 28 focus areas. To focus efforts in *Healthy People 2010*, ten leading health indicators were chosen for more detailed tracking. These indicators reflect the major public health concerns in the United States and were chosen based on their ability to motivate action, the availability of data to measure their progress, and their relevance as broad public health issues.

The ten indicators are:

- Physical activity
- Overweight and obesity
- Tobacco use
- Substance abuse
- Responsible sexual behavior
- Mental health
- Injury and violence
- Environmental quality
- Immunizations
- Access to health care

For each of the leading health indicators, specific objectives derived from *Healthy People 2010* will be used to track progress. This small set of measures will provide a snapshot of the health of the nation. Tracking and communicating progress on these indicators through national- and state-level report cards will spotlight achievements and challenges in the next decade. The leading health indicators serve as a link to the 467 objectives in *Healthy People 2010* and can become the basic building blocks for community health initiatives.[15]

Healthy Communities 2000

While it is extremely worthwhile to have national objectives, in the final analysis, the achievement of national objectives is dependent upon activities within each local community. The American Public Health Association (APHA), together with the CDC and other public health professional associations, devel-

oped a road map for local communities to follow to help them do their part to reach the national objectives. *Healthy Communities 2000: Model Standards. Guidelines for Community Attainment of the Year 2000 National Health Objectives*[16] is intended to help communities organize and express their local public health needs in quantifiable objectives that are consistent with the national objectives. It is likely that a similar document keyed to the new *Healthy People 2010* will be developed and published shortly.

Assessment Protocol for Excellence in Public Health

Before a community can translate its public health problems into objectives for action that are consistent, wherever possible, with national goals, those local public health problems must be identified and prioritized. We have moved beyond the time when significant progress in improved health status is possible by doing things for the community. We now realize that the community must be engaged in the process of identifying and understanding its health problems and determining the remedies to be applied. To this end, the National Association of County and City Health Officials (NACCHO), together with the CDC and other public health professional associations, developed the *Assessment Protocol for Excellence in Public Health (APEX).*[17] It guides public health agencies in the process of community assessment and public health program planning. APEX helps health departments assess their own internal strengths and weaknesses in terms of their capacity to carry out community needs assessment, to work with the community to understand its health problems and establish priorities for action, and to implement a community plan for reducing public health problems. APEX/PH has proven to be so successful that NACCHO has developed a new, more robust community health planning model called Mobilizing for Action through Planning and Partnership (MAPP). This tool is flexible and is designed to facilitate community-wide health planning efforts. Other similar programs, such as the Planned Approach to Community Health (PATCH)[18] and the Healthy Cities Project[19] are discussed later in this text.

In the future, growing numbers of local and state health departments will be using APEX, MAPP,

PATCH, or Healthy Cities as guides to developing community-based plans for identifying and addressing community health problems. Inherent in that process will be accurate assessment of risks to health and a growing capacity to communicate those risks to the public at large. Increasingly, these tools will link communities with national efforts to improve health status so that the mission of public health, "fulfilling society's interest in assuring conditions in which people can be healthy," will be realized.

References

1. Osamnczk EJ. *Encyclopedia of the United Nations and International Agreements.* Philadelphia, Pa: Taylor & Francis; 1985.

2. Last JM. *A Dictionary of Epidemiology.* 4th ed. New York, NY: Oxford University Press; 2001.

3. Starr P. *The Social Transformation of American Medicine.* New York, NY: Basic Books; 1982.

4. Reiser SJ. Topics for our times: the medicine public health initiative. *Am J Public Health.* 1997; 87(7): 1098-1099.

5. Lasker R. *Medicine and Public Health: The Power of Collaboration Health.* Chicago, Ill: Administration Press; 1997.

6. Terris M. The complex tasks of the second epidemiological revolution: the Joseph W. Mountain lecture. *J Public Health Policy.* March 1983:8-22.

7. McKinlay JB, McKinlay SM. The questionable contribution of medical measures to the decline of mortality in the United States in the twentieth century. *Milbank Q.* 1977;55(3):405-428.

8. *Healthy People: The Surgeon General's Report on Health Promotion and Disease Prevention.* Washington, DC: US Dept. of Health and Human Services, Public Health Service; 1979.

9. Scutchfield FD, Hartman K. A new preventive medicine for a new millennium. *Aviat Space and Environmental Medicine.* 1996;67(4):369-375.

10. Frumpkin H. Beyond toxicity: human health and the natural environment. *Am J Preventive Medicine* 2001;20(3):234-240.

11. Institute of Medicine, Committee for the Study of the Future of Public Health. *The Future of Public Health.* Washington, DC: National Academy Press; 1988.

12. Baker EL, Melton RJ, Strange PV, et al. Health reform and the healing of the public. Forging community health partnerships. *JAMA.* 1994;272(16):1276-1282.

13. *Health Promotion/Disease Prevention: Objectives for the Nation.* Washington, DC: US Dept of Health and Human Services, Public Health Service; 1981.

14. *Healthy People 2000: National Health Promotion and Disease Prevention Objectives.* Washington, DC: US Dept of Health and Human Services, Public Health Service; 1990.

15. *Healthy People 2010.* Washington DC: US Dept of Health and Human Services, Public Health Service; 2000.

16. *Healthy Communities 2000: Model Standards. Guidelines for Community Attainment of the Year 2000 National Health Objectives.* 3rd ed. Washington, DC: American Public Health Association; 1991.

17. *APEX/PH, Assessment Protocol for Excellence in Public Health.* Washington, DC: National Association of County and City Health Officials; 1991.

18. *Planned Approach to Community Health (PATCH): Program Descriptions.* Washington, DC: US Dept of Health and Human Services; November 1993.

19. *World Health Organizations, Five Year Planning Project.* Fadl, Copenhagen: World Health Organization, Healthy Cities Project; 1988. WHO Healthy Cities Paper, No. 2.

CHAPTER

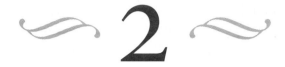

2

History and Development
of Public Health

Elizabeth Fee, Ph.D.

This chapter discusses the history and development of public health in the United States and the factors that influenced them. The first section gives an overview of public health in the United States in the eighteenth and nineteenth centuries.

PUBLIC HEALTH IN THE EIGHTEENTH AND NINETEENTH CENTURIES

In the United States, before the twentieth century, there were few formal requirements for public health positions, no established career structures, no job security for health officials, and no formalized ways of producing new knowledge. Public health positions were usually part-time appointments at nominal salary; those who devoted much effort to public health typically did so on a voluntary basis. Until the mid-nineteenth century, public health, like other governmental functions, was usually the responsibility of the social elite. The public health officer was expected to be a statesman acting in the public interest, not a politician answering to a class constituency. Men of property and wealth were believed to be independent of special interests and therefore capable of disinterested judgment.

Charles Rosenberg has eloquently described an earlier conception of both poverty and disease as consequences of moral failure at the individual and social level.[1] Disease attacked the dirty, the improvident, the intemperate, the ignorant; the clean, the pious, and the virtuous, on the other hand, tended to escape. Epidemic diseases were the consequence of a failure to obey the laws of nature and God: they were indicators of social and moral dissolution. As cleanliness was linked to godliness, virtue was an essential qualification for managing the state. The conscientious, the respectable, the educated, and the affluent were seen as naturally qualified for public office. Physicians were frequently chosen as public health officers, but lawyers or gentlemen of independent means could also be appointed.

Earliest Public Health Programs and Activities

The first public health organizations were those of the rapidly growing port cities of the eastern seaboard in the late eighteenth century. Here, the American republic intersected with the world of international trade. Local authorities tried to protect the population from the threat of potentially catastrophic epidemic diseases, such as the yellow fever epidemic that had crippled Philadelphia in 1793, while they also tried to maintain the conditions for successful economic activity.[2] Public health programs, when organized at all, were organized locally. As Robert Wiebe has argued, the United States in the nineteenth century was a society of *island communities* with considerable economic and political autonomy.[3]

Public health in this period was also largely a police function. Traditionally, port cities had dealt with epidemics by means of quarantine regulations, keeping ships suspected of carrying disease in harbor for up to 40 days. However, quarantine regulations clearly interfered with shipping, and they were energetically opposed by those whose economic interests were tied to trade.[4]

Opponents of quarantine argued that diseases were internally generated by the filthy conditions of the docks, streets, and alleys, which provided an ideal environment for *putrefactive fermentation.* City health departments attempted to regulate the worst offenders: graveyards, tallow chandleries, tanneries, sugar boilers, skin dressers, dyers, glue boilers, and slaughterhouses. They also cleaned the privies and alleys and removed dead animals and decaying vegetable matter from the streets and public spaces.[5(p50)]

Influence of Disease

The causes of disease were much in dispute by the mid-nineteenth century. The evidence available was contradictory and suggested no clear resolution to the dispute between those who believed that diseases were brought in from overseas and thus should be fought by quarantine regulations and those who believed that diseases were internally generated and thus should be fought by cleaning up the cities. Health regulations were written and revised more in response to political influence or pressure from merchants than in response to shifts in scientific thinking.

Official health agencies were sporadically moved to action by the threat of great epidemics—the devastating waves of yellow fever and cholera that periodically threatened from Europe, the Caribbean, or Latin America or were detected on ships arriving in New Orleans, Boston, or Philadelphia. These sudden, catastrophic events compelled even politicians and business leaders to devote their attention to sanitary improvements, city cleanliness, quarantines, and hospital construction.

At other times, adults and children were killed continually but in less spectacular numbers by tuberculosis, smallpox, typhus, dysentery, diphtheria, typhoid fever, measles, influenza, malaria, and scarlet fever. These diseases were met with a stolid indifference born of familiarity and a sense of helplessness. It seemed that little could be done beyond attempts to maintain general cleanliness, backed by prayer, fasting, and exhortations to virtue.[5(p87)] When free of the immediate threat of an impending epidemic, politicians tended to ignore the fate of the multitudes of immigrant poor, unless compelled to action by the insistent demands of reform groups or the fear of popular unrest.[6–8]

Early Public Health Reforms

A few cities did have active and energetic reform groups. In New York in 1864, members of the Council of Hygiene and Public Health of the Citizens' Association conducted street-by-street investigations of tenement housing congestion, slaughterhouse and stable conditions, sewage drainage, garbage heaps, and filthy habitations of many sections of the city, and correlated these with outbreaks of infectious disease and premature infant deaths.[9] Dr. Ezra R. Pulling, for example, detailed every case of typhus, typhoid fever, and smallpox found in the notorious Five Points section of Manhattan's Lower East Side. He also carefully mapped all the stables, privies (especially "privies in an extremely offensive condition"), and other *insalubrious locations* in the area, making obvious the close geographical relationship between disease and its causes.[10]

In other parts of the country, a few farsighted men and women argued for the need to collect vital statistics, register birth and death rates, and keep careful records on the health of the population. The most notable of these was Lemuel Shattuck, a school teacher, bookseller, and publisher, who was largely responsible for implementing a system of vital statistics in Massachusetts. Shattuck is especially remembered for his *Report of the Sanitary Commission of Massachusetts,* an extraordinarily comprehensive set of recommendations for public health organization.[11,12]

Shattuck's report advocated a decennial census and collection of data by age, sex, race, occupation, economic status, and locality. It discussed the need for environmental sanitation, regulation of food and drugs, and control of communicable disease. Shattuck also recommended attention to well-child care, mental health, health education, smallpox vaccination, alcoholism, town planning, and the teaching of preventive medicine in medical schools.

Shattuck's report was well received by medical reviewers but essentially ignored by the Massachusetts state legislature. Although having little direct impact at the time it was written, the report would become a central reference point for later generations of public health practitioners.

By 1860, public health activities were just beginning to move beyond the confines of local city politics. Between 1857 and 1860, quarantine and sanitary conventions were held in Philadelphia, Baltimore, New York, and Boston.[13] Although these conventions gave public health reformers an opportunity to debate the causes of disease and the most appropriate public health responses, the possibility of implementing their ideas was interrupted by the outbreak of the Civil War.

Impact of the Civil War

In its own way, the Civil War helped enforce a national consciousness of epidemic disease: two-thirds of the 360,000 Union soldiers who died were killed by infectious diseases rather than by bullets.[14,15] The ravages of dysentery, spread by inadequate or nonexistent sanitary facilities, were appalling. The United States Sanitary Commission, a voluntary organization inspired by Florence Nightingale's work in the Crimean War, promoted the health of the Union army by inspecting army camps, distributing educational materials, and providing nursing care and supplies for the wounded.

Formation of the American Public Health Association

In 1872, 10 health reformers from various parts of the country met in New York City at the home of Stephen Smith and announced the creation of the American Public Health Association (APHA). Its purpose was to advance *sanitary science* and promote the "practical application of public hygiene."[16,17] After a slow start, the new organization grew rapidly. Its members devoted themselves to the reform activities of citizens' sanitary associations and encouraged the formation and development of local and state health agencies. They organized annual meetings and presented papers on infectious diseases and on many of the practical public health issues of the day—from sewage and garbage disposal to occupational injuries and proposals for the medical inspection of prostitutes. The APHA was notable in welcoming physicians, engineers, lawyers, municipal officials, other professional groups, and lay reformers to its membership, and in this respect, it helped mold the specific character of American public health.[18,19]

First State and Local Boards of Health

In the late nineteenth century, state and local boards of health were created in many parts of the country. The first state board of health, formed in Louisiana in 1855, had largely been a paper organization. In the 1870s and 1880s, however, most states instituted their own boards of health. The first working state health board was formed in Massachusetts in 1869, followed by California (1870), the District of Columbia (1871), Virginia and Minnesota (1872), Maryland (1874), and Alabama (1875).[20] The impact of these state boards of health should not be overemphasized. By 1900, only three states (Massachusetts, Rhode Island, and Florida) spent more than two cents per capita for public health services.[21]

The Marine Hospital Service

The origins of a federal organization of public health lie in the provision of medical and hospital care for merchant seamen and sailors. In 1798, the United States Congress had passed the Act for the Relief of Sick and Disabled Seamen to finance the construction and operation of public hospitals in port cities.[22] These hospitals were poorly run and badly managed until 1871, when John Maynard Woodward became Supervising Surgeon of what was now named the Marine Hospital Service.

Woodward and other public health reformers urged the formation of a national system of quarantines and a national health board. In 1879, a disastrous yellow fever epidemic swept up the Mississippi Valley from New Orleans, prompting the United States Congress to create the National Board of Health. This consisted of seven physicians and one representative each from the army, the navy, the Marine Hospital Service, and the U.S. Department of Justice.

Responsible for formulating quarantine regulations between states, the National Board of Health soon became embroiled in fierce battles over states' rights. Many cities and states had discovered that local quarantine laws could be an excellent source of income as well as a valuable source of political patronage; they were naturally reluctant to relinquish these powers to the federal government.[7(pp157–174)] In 1883, after various battles in Congress, the National Board of Health was disbanded, and its quarantine powers reverted to the Marine Hospital Service.

Gradually, the Marine Hospital Service expanded its public health activities into public health research. In 1887, it set aside a single room as a *hygienic laboratory,* which would later be expanded into an important center for the investigation of infectious diseases.[23] In 1912, the Marine Hospital Service became the United States Public Health Service, specifically authorized to investigate the causes and spread of disease and to provide health information to the public.

PUBLIC HEALTH AS SOCIAL REFORM

The belief that epidemic diseases posed only occasional threats to an otherwise healthy social order had been shaken by the industrial transformation of the late nineteenth century. The burgeoning health problems of the industrial cities could not be ignored; almost all families lost children to diphtheria, smallpox, or other infectious diseases. Poverty and disease could not be treated simply as individual failings but were understood to be consequences of industrialization, urbanization, immigration, and exploitation.

Public Health Responses

The early efforts of city health department officials to deal with health problems were attempts to mitigate the worst effects of unplanned and unregulated growth—a kind of rearguard action against the filth and congestion created by anarchic economic and urban development.[24–29] As cities grew in size, as the flow of immigrants continued, and as public health problems became ever more obvious, pressures mounted for more effective responses to the problems.[30] New York, the largest city and the one with some of the worst health conditions, produced some of the most energetic and progressive public health leaders; Boston and Providence were also noted for their active public health programs; Baltimore and Philadelphia, however, trailed far behind.[25,31–33]

Social Reform

America no longer fit its self-image as a country of independent farmers and craftsmen. Like the countries of Europe, it displayed extremes of wealth and privilege, social misery, and deprivation. Labor and social unrest pushed awareness of the need for social and health reforms. The perceived social anarchy of the large industrial cities mocked the pretensions to social control of the traditional forces of church and state and highlighted the need for new approaches to the multiplicity of problems.[34]

Reformers and Reform Groups

An increasing number of reform groups devoted themselves to social issues and improvements of every variety. Health reformers, physicians, and engineers urged improved sanitary conditions in the industrial cities. Medical men were prominent in reform organizations, but they were not alone.[35] Barbara Rosenkrantz has contrasted public health in the late nineteenth century with the internecine battles within general medicine: ". . . the field of public hygiene exemplified a happy marriage of engineers, physicians and public spirited citizens providing a model of complementary comportment under the banner of sanitary science."[36]

Middle- and upper-class women, seizing an opportunity to escape from the narrow bounds of domestic responsibilities, joined in campaigns for improved housing, the abolition of child labor, maternal and child health, and temperance. They were active in the settlement house movement, the organization of trade unions, the suffrage movement, and municipal sanitary reform. The latter, as municipal housekeeping, was viewed as a natural extension of women's training and experience as the housekeepers of the world.[37] By the early years of the twentieth century, dozens of such voluntary health organizations were established around specific issues, thus providing the impulse and energy behind many public health reforms.[38]

The progressive reform groups in the public health movement advocated immediate change tempered by scientific knowledge and humanitarian concern. Sharing the revolutionaries' perception of the plight of the poor and the injustices of the system, they nonetheless counseled less radical solutions.[39–42] They advocated public health reforms on political, economic, humanitarian, and scientific grounds. Politically, public health reform offered a middle ground between the cutthroat principles of entrepreneurial capitalism and the revolutionary ideas of the socialists, anarchists, and utopian visionaries. As William Henry Welch, a leader of American medicine and public health, expressed it to the Charity Organization Society, sanitary improvement offered the best way of improving the lot of the poor, short of the radical restructuring of society.[43(p598)]

Economic Rewards of Reform

Economically, progressive reformers argued that public health should be viewed as a paying investment, giving higher returns than the stock market. In Germany, Max von Pettenkofer had first calculated the financial returns on public health "investments" to prove the value of sanitary improvements in reducing deaths from typhoid.[44] His argument would be repeated many times by American public health leaders. As William Henry Welch explained:

> . . . merely from a mercenary and commercial point of view it is for the interest of the community to take care of the health of the poor. Philanthropy assumes a totally different aspect in the eyes of the world when it is able to demonstrate that it pays to keep people healthy.[43(p596)]

Public health leaders argued that the demand for centralized planning and business efficiency required scientific knowledge rather than the undisciplined enthusiasms of voluntary groups.[45] Public health decisions should be made by an analysis of costs and benefits "as an up-to-date manufacturer would count the cost of a new process." The health officer, like the merchant, should learn "which line of work yields the most for the sum expended."[46]

NATIONAL AND INTERNATIONAL HEALTH

Public health was quickly becoming a national and even international issue. Although Congress was reluctant to enact federal health legislation, there were mounting pressures for U.S. attention to public health abroad. As American business was seeking enlarged foreign markets, a vocal group of intellectuals and politicians argued for an assertive foreign policy. The United States began to challenge European dominance in the Far East and Latin America, seeking trade and political influence more than territory but taking territory where it could. National defense goals included broadening control of trade routes, building a Central American canal, and establishing strategic bases in the Caribbean and Western Pacific.

Cuba and the Panama Canal

In 1898, the United States entered the Spanish-American War, expanded the army from 25,000 to 250,000 men, and sent troops to Cuba. The war showed that the United States could not afford military adventures overseas unless more attention was paid to sanitation and public health: 968 men died in battle, but 5,438 died of infectious diseases.[47,48] Nonetheless, the United States defeated Spain and installed an army of occupation in Cuba. When yellow fever threatened the troops in 1900, the response was efficient and effective. An army commission under Walter Reed was sent to Cuba to study the disease and, in a dramatic series of human experiments, it confirmed the hypothesis that yellow fever was spread by mosquitoes. Surgeon Major William Gorgas then eliminated yellow fever from Havana.[49]

This experience confirmed the importance of public health for successful U.S. efforts overseas. Earlier attempts to dig the Panama Canal had been attended by enormous mortality rates from disease.[50] But in 1904, Gorgas, now promoted to general, took control of a campaign against the malaria and yellow fever that were threatening canal operations. He was finally able to persuade the Canal Commission to institute an intensive campaign against mosquitoes. In one of the great triumphs of practical public health, yellow fever and malaria were brought under control, and the canal was successfully completed in 1914.

Bringing the Lessons Home

U.S. industrialists brought some of the lessons of Cuba and the Panama Canal home to the southern United States. The South at that time resembled an underdeveloped country within the United States, characterized by poor economic and social conditions. Northern industrialists were already investing heavily in southern education as well as in cotton mills and railroads. John D. Rockefeller had created the General Education Board to support "the general organization of rural communities for economic, social and educational purposes."[51] Charles Wardell Stiles managed to convince the secretary of the General Education Board that the real cause of misery and lack of productivity in the South was hookworm, the "germ of laziness." In 1909, Rockefeller agreed to provide $1 million to create the Rockefeller Sanitary Commission for the Eradication of Hookworm Disease, with Wickliffe Rose as director.[52] This was to be

the first installment in Rockefeller's massive national and international investment in public health.

Rose went beyond the task of attempting to control a single disease and worked to establish an effective and permanent public health organization in the southern states.[53] At the end of five years of intensive effort, the campaign had failed to eradicate hookworm but had greatly expanded the role of public health agencies. Between 1910 and 1914, county appropriations for local public health work increased from a total of $240 to $110,000.[52(pp220–221)]

Public Health at the National Level

In Washington, the Committee of One Hundred on National Health campaigned for the federal regulation of public health.[54,55] The committee was composed of such notables as Jane Addams, Andrew Carnegie, William H. Welch, and Booker T. Washington. Its president, the economist Irving Fisher, argued that a public health service would be good policy and good economics, in conserving national vitality.[56]

In 1912, the federal government made its first real commitment to public health when it expanded the responsibilities of the Public Health Service, empowering it to investigate the causes and spread of diseases and the pollution and sanitation of navigable streams and lakes.[57] The responsibilities of the Public Health Service included the medical inspection of immigrants arriving at Ellis Island, field investigations of endemic rural diseases such as trachoma, and groundbreaking research on diseases such as pellagra and Rocky Mountain spotted fever. By 1915, the Public Health Service, the United States Army, and the Rockefeller Foundation were the major agencies involved in public health activities, supplemented on a local level by a network of city and state health departments.

THE PROFESSIONALIZATION OF PUBLIC HEALTH

At the turn of the century existing health departments were often dominated more by patronage and political considerations than by economic or administrative efficiency. Progressives regretted the evils of politics and wanted to increase the pay and minimum qualifications for health officers to attract personnel on the basis of skill rather than influence. Their attempt to insulate boards of health from local political control was part of a broader movement to make all forms of public administration more rational and efficient by reducing the influence of political bosses and promoting a new group of professional administrators.[58] The goal was for a well-trained professional elite to conduct social reform on scientific lines.

These developments led to an increasing demand for people trained in public health to direct the new programs being created at the local, state, and national levels. Those attempting to develop such programs were increasingly critical of the lack of properly trained personnel; part-time public health officers were simply not adequate to staff the ambitious new programs. Public health reformers agreed that full-time practitioners, especially trained for the job, were needed. In 1913, the New York state legislature passed a law requiring public health officers to have specialized training, despite the fact that there was little agreement about what kind of specialized training was needed, much less where it could be obtained.[59,60]

Public health had been defined in terms of its aims and goals—to reduce disease and maintain the health of the population—rather than by any specific body of knowledge. Many different disciplines contributed to effective public health work: physicians diagnosed contagious diseases; sanitary engineers built water and sewage systems; epidemiologists traced the sources of disease outbreaks and their modes of transmission; vital statisticians provided quantitative measures of births and deaths; lawyers wrote sanitary codes and regulations; public health nurses provided care and advice to the sick in their homes; sanitary inspectors visited factories and markets to enforce compliance with public health ordinances; and administrators tried to organize everyone within the limits of health department budgets. Public health thus involved economics, sociology, psychology, politics, law, statistics, and engineering, as well as the biological and clinical sciences. However, in the period immediately following the brilliant experimental work of Louis Pasteur and Robert Koch, the bacteriological laboratory became the first and primary symbol of a new, scientific public health.

Bacteriology and Alternative Views of Health and Disease

The rise of bacteriology and other scientific advances in the understanding of disease contributed to the professionalization of public health.

The Rise of Bacteriology

The clarity and simplicity of bacteriological methods and discoveries gave them tremendous cultural importance: the agents of particular diseases had been made visible under the microscope. The identification of specific bacteria seemed to have cut through the misty miasmas of disease to define the enemy in unmistakable terms. Bacteriology thus became an ideological marker, sharply differentiating the *old* public health, the province of untrained amateurs, from the *new* public health, which would belong to scientifically trained professionals.

Young Americans who had studied in Germany brought back the new knowledge of laboratory methods in bacteriology and started to teach others. These young scientists were convinced that physicians should stop squabbling over medical ethics and politics and commit themselves to the purer values of laboratory research. Under their influence, the laboratory ideal soon spread throughout progressive public health circles. By the 1880s, Charles Chapin had established a public health laboratory in Providence, Rhode Island, and Victor C. Vaughan had created a state hygienic laboratory in Michigan.

In 1901, William Sedgwick reported on his bacteriological study of water supplies and sewage disposal at the Lawrence Experiment Station in Massachusetts.[61] Sedgwick demonstrated the transmission of typhoid fever by polluted water supplies, and he developed quantitative methods for measuring the presence of bacteria in the air, water, and milk. Describing the impact of bacteriological discoveries, he said, "Before 1880 we knew nothing; after 1890 we knew it all; it was a glorious ten years."[32(p57)]

The powerful new methods of identifying diseases through the microscope drew attention away from the larger and more diffuse problems of water supplies, street cleaning, housing reform, and the living conditions of the poor. The approach of locating, identifying, and isolating bacteria and their human hosts was a more elegant and efficient way of dealing with disease than environmental reform. The public health laboratory demonstrated the scientific and diagnostic power of the new public health. However, by focusing on the diagnosis of infectious diseases, it narrowed the distance between medicine and public health and brought public health into potential conflict with private medical practice. Physicians began increasingly to resent the public health officials' claim to diagnose, and often treat, infectious diseases.

Alternative Models

Although the narrow bacteriological view was dominant, there were several competing models for public health research and practice. It is worth noting the broad and comprehensive definition of public health offered by Charles-Edward A. Winslow, professor of public health at Yale University, in 1920:

> Public health is the science and art of preventing disease, prolonging life, and promoting physical health and efficiency through organized community efforts for the sanitation of the environment, the control of community infections, the education of the individual in principles of personal hygiene, the organization of medical and nursing service for the early diagnosis and preventive treatment of disease, and the development of the social machinery which will ensure to every individual in the community a standard of living adequate for the maintenance of health.[62,63]

Winslow's was not the only broad vision of public health. Alice Hamilton in Illinois conducted a survey of industrial lead poisoning and established the fact that thousands of American workers were being slowly killed by white lead.[64] Unaided by legislation, Hamilton argued, persuaded, shamed, and flattered individual employers into improving working conditions. Almost single-handedly, she created the foundations of industrial hygiene in America.

Joseph Goldberger's epidemiological studies of pellagra for the Public Health Service offer another example of a comprehensive approach to public health. In 1914, Goldberger announced that pellagra was due to dietary deficiencies and not to some unknown microorganism. He and his colleagues had cured endemic pellagra in a Mississippi orphanage by feeding the children milk, eggs, beans, and meat. He then teamed up with an economist, Edgar Sydenstricker, to survey the diets of southern wageworkers' families. They showed how the sharecropping system had impoverished tenant farmers, led to dietary deficiencies, and thus produced endemic pellagra.[65]

Alice Hamilton, Joseph Goldberger, and Edgar Sydenstricker were minority voices amid the growing majority focusing exclusively on bacteria. As most bacteriologists and epidemiologists concentrated on specific disease-causing organisms and the individuals who harbored them, only a minority continued to relate the problems of ill health and disease to the larger social environment.[66]

The Relationship between Public Health and Medicine

While the broader conceptions of public health required an understanding of economics and politics, the dominant model of public health knowledge was based almost exclusively on the biological sciences. This redefinition of public health in bioscientific terms reinforced the medical profession's claim to preeminence in the field. Physicians felt that because they were the experts in infectious diseases, they were uniquely qualified to become the ultimate authorities in the new, scientific public health.

By the second decade of the twentieth century, nonmedical public health officers were beginning to protest the dominance of public health by medical men. By this time, the sanitary engineers were the only professional group strong enough to challenge the physicians' assumption that the future of public health should be theirs. Civil and sanitary engineers had created clean city water supplies and adequate sewage systems, which were major factors in the declining death rates from infant diarrhea and other infectious diseases.[67–70]

Professional competition between the sanitary engineers and physicians became intense in the early years of the twentieth century as sanitary engineers vociferously complained about the increasing *medical monopoly* of public health. By 1912, 15 states required that all members of their boards of health be physicians, and 23 states required at least one physician member; only 10 states had no professional requirement for eligibility.[71]

With the increasing professionalization of public health, physicians came to hold a dominant but not exclusive role in the field. Leadership positions in public health departments and public health agencies were increasingly reserved for physicians. Other scientists, professionals, and nurses might be given subordinate positions. Physicians themselves were increasingly ambivalent about public health. The curious relationships between physicians and nonmedical public health practitioners would shape the subsequent development of public health practice.

PUBLIC HEALTH ORGANIZATION AND PRACTICE

The practical importance of public health was well recognized by the early decades of the twentieth century. The incidence of tuberculosis, diphtheria, and other infectious diseases was falling, apparently in response to energetic public health campaigns. School health clinics and maternal and child health centers were established in many cities with active public support. Registration for the draft in World War I revealed that a substantial proportion of young men were either physically or mentally unfit for combat, and this perception also led to increased political support for public health activities. The influenza epidemic that devastated families and communities in 1916 to 1918 underlined the continuing threat of infectious disease epidemics.

The Waning Influence of Bacteriology

After the first flush of enthusiasm for the achievements of bacteriology, many health departments were now paying more attention to community-based health activities and popular health education. In 1923, Charles-Edward A. Winslow went so far as to announce the ending of the bacteriological age and to describe popular health education as the keynote of the *new public health,* almost as far-reaching in its importance as the germ theory of disease had been some 30 years before.[63(pp53,55),72]

In the 1920s, state and municipal health departments developed new organizational units and increased their hiring of public health personnel, especially public health nurses. Although bacteriological laboratories continued to be important, divisions that were focused on tuberculosis, maternal and child health, venereal diseases, public health administration, and health education played a major role in most state and city health departments, as did divisions of sanitation and vital statistics.

Variation in Public Health Practice

Public health practice varied greatly throughout the states and cities across the country, as shown by an American Public Health Association survey of municipal public health department practice in 1923. Although some cities had extensive, progressive, and imaginative programs, others did little beyond offering a few communicable disease clinics and public health inspections.[73]

Continuing Controversy with Medicine

The relationship between the emerging profession of public health and the well-established profession of medicine continued to be problematic and controversial. The increased activity of health departments in the identification and control of infectious diseases brought health officers into conflict with private practitioners. As soon as public health left the confines of sanitary engineering and took on the battle against specific diseases, it challenged the boundaries of medical autonomy. As John Duffy has argued, the medical profession moved from a position of strong support for public health activities to a cautious and sometimes suspicious ambivalence.[74]

Major battles would be fought over the Sheppard-Towner Maternity and Infancy Act of 1921, which provided grants to states to teach prenatal and infant care to mothers.[75] Conservatives denounced the measure as socialistic, and many physicians opposed it as interfering with the proper purview of medicine. These programs were allowed to expire in 1929, showing the difficulties faced by any innovative public health or social welfare legislation in a politically conservative period.

Federal Involvement

The most important federal organization in public health continued to be the U.S. Public Health Service, an arm of the Federal Security Agency. The Public Health Service aided the development of state health departments by giving grants-in-aid, loaning expert personnel, and providing advice and consultation on specific problems.[76] For example, if a state was facing an unexplained outbreak of typhoid fever or other epidemic disease, the Public Health Service would send epidemiologists to trace the source of the disease and suggest means of preventing its spread.

Influence of the Depression

A major stimulus to the development of public health practice came in response to the depression, with the New Deal and the Social Security Act of 1935. The Social Security Act represented America's first broad-based social welfare legislation, providing old-age benefits, unemployment insurance, and public health services. Unfortunately, the attempt to include basic medical insurance within the bill was abandoned because of the determined opposition of the medical profession, pharmaceutical companies, and the insurance industry.[77–79] From the public health point of view, however, the Social Security Act was a huge leap forward. Title V of the act established a program of grants to states for maternal and child health services, administered by the Children's Bureau, and provided funds for child welfare and crippled children's programs. Title VI of the act expanded financing of the Public Health Service and allotted federal grants to states to assist them in developing their public health services.

Federal and state expenditures for public health actually doubled in the decade of the depression, fueling the expansion of local health units. In most parts of the country, efficient provision of public health services to local communities depended on county health organizations, smaller and simpler units than the larger state health departments. In 1934, only 541

counties out of the 3,070 counties in the United States had any form of local public health service, but by June 1942, 1,828 counties could boast of health units directed by a full-time public health officer.[80] Much of this gain would be lost during the war; by the end of the war only 1,322 counties had an organized health service.[81(p125),82]

Federal Funding and Training

In 1935, for the first time, the federal government provided funds, administered through the states, for public health training. Federal regulations now required states to establish minimum qualifications for public health personnel employed through new federal grants. Thus, it was no longer sufficient for state programs to employ any willing physician; some form of professional public health training was expected.

As a result of the growing demand for public health education, several state universities began new schools or divisions of public health, and existing schools of public health expanded their enrollments. By 1936, 10 schools offered public health degrees or certificates requiring at least one year of attendance.[83] By 1938, more than 4,000 individuals, including about 1,000 doctors, had received some public health training with funds provided by the federal government through the states.

The economic difficulties of maintaining a private practice during the depression had pushed some physicians into public health; others were attracted by the new availability of fellowships or by increased social awareness of the plight of the poor. In 1939, the federal government allocated over $8 million for maternal and child health programs, more than $9 million for general public health work, and over $4 million for venereal disease control.

Several important trends were stimulated by these federal funds. The first was the development of programs to control specific diseases and of services targeted to specific population groups, the *categorical* approach to public health. Second was the expansion in the number of local health departments. Third was the increased training of personnel, and fourth, the assumption of responsibility for some phases of medical care on the part of health departments.[81(pxii)]

Categorical Approach to Public Health

The categorical approach to public health proved politically popular. Members of Congress were willing to allocate funds for specific diseases or for particular groups—health and welfare services for children were especially favored—but they showed less interest in general public health or administrative expenditures. Although state health officers often felt constrained by targeted programs, they rarely refused federal grants-in-aid and thus adapted their programs to the pattern of available funds. Federal grants came in turn for maternal and child health services and crippled children (1935), venereal disease control (1938), tuberculosis (1944), mental health (1947), industrial hygiene (1947), and dental health (1947). The pattern of funding started in the 1930s would thus shape the organization of public health departments through the postwar period. As institutionalized in the National Institutes of Health, it would also shape the future patterns of biomedical research.

PUBLIC HEALTH AND THE WAR

Mobilization for war acted as another major force in the expansion and development of public health in the United States.[84] Public health was declared a national priority for the armed forces and the civilian population engaged in military production. As James Stevens Simmons, brigadier general and director of the Preventive Medicine Division of the United States Army, announced:

> A civil population that is not healthy cannot be prosperous and will lag behind in the economic competition between nations. This is even more true of a military population, for any army that has its strength sapped by disease is in no condition to withstand the attack of a virile force that has conserved its strength and is enjoying the vigor and exhilaration of health.[85]

The Need for Personnel

Health departments again suffered from a critical shortage of personnel as physicians, nurses, engineers, and other trained and experienced professionals left to join the armed services.[86] In 1940, the U.S. Public Health Service expanded its program of grants to states and local communities, sending personnel to particularly needy areas. The Community Facilities Act, for instance, provided $300 million to fund health and sanitation facilities in communities with rapidly expanding populations because of military camps and war industries.[87,88]

The Selective Service Exams

The shock of the discovery that many of the young men being called into the army were physically unfit for military service provided a powerful impetus for increased national attention to public health. The Selective Service examinations represented the most massive health survey ever undertaken, with over 16 million young men examined. Fully 40 percent of the young men examined were declared physically or mentally unfit for service, with the leading causes of rejection being defective teeth, vision problems, orthopedic impairments (from polio, for example), diseases of the cardiovascular system, nervous and mental diseases, hernia, tuberculosis, and venereal diseases.[89,90]

Mosquitoes and the Centers for Disease Control

With the war mobilization, as hundreds of thousands of workers moved to areas with defense industry plants the troops moved to Army camps.[91] Army training camps often had been placed in areas with warm climates, where the Anopheles mosquito bred in profusion and malaria was endemic. To control malaria in the South, the Public Health Service established the Center for Controlling Malaria in the War Areas. After the war, when substantial funds were made available for malaria eradication efforts, this organization was gradually transformed into the Centers for Disease Control (now the Centers for Disease Control and Prevention), which would play a major national role in the effort to control both infectious and noninfectious diseases.[92]

POSTWAR REORGANIZATION

In the immediate postwar period, considerable optimism and energy were devoted to the possible reorganization of public health and medical care. Many of the discussions of a future national medical care system posited the potential unification of preventive and curative medicine. Some public health leaders were advocating the direct administration of tax-supported medical care by health departments. Others opposed such a development, feeling that if public health and medical care administration were combined, preventive and educational efforts would be submerged by the demand for costly therapeutic services.[93]

Hospital Construction

While public health officials were debating whether they wanted to take responsibility for medical care services, the Hospital Survey and Construction Act, more popularly known as the Hill-Burton Act, was passed in 1946. Hospital construction, especially in rural areas, promised to bring everyone the benefits of medical science, without disturbing the freedoms of the medical profession or the patterns of paying for their services. The federal government would pay one-third the costs of building hospitals, setting aside $75 million for each of the first five years. No health program had ever been so generous or so popular.

Hill-Burton addressed the national demand for access to medical care without challenging the private organization of medical practice. It thus answered the desire for acute-care services while essentially ignoring preventive care and public health. The United States could have been completely covered by local health departments for a fraction of the cost of Hill-Burton, but there was no strong political constituency for public health that could compete effectively for resources with curative medicine.

Local Health Services

In 1942, the American Public Health Association provided a plan for organizing local health services across the nation.[94] Haven Emerson's report, *Local Health Units for the Nation,* found that only two-thirds of the people of the United States were covered by local public health services. It also estimated the cost of providing a modest but adequate basic health service

for each of the 1,197 additional local health units proposed. The committee noted that communities of over 50,000 should be able to provide a reasonably adequate local service at the cost of $1.00 per capita or a superior service for only $2.00 per capita.[94(p2)]

A survey of state health departments found that a multitude of agencies, state boards, and commissions were involved in public health activities, as many as 18 different agencies being involved in a single state.[95,96] The money spent for public health work also varied widely, ranging from $0.13 per capita in Ohio to $1.68 in Delaware. In most cases, the states spending the largest sums were spending most of these funds on hospital services rather than on prevention.

Changes in Disease

In the postwar years, the public health community clearly understood that the disease patterns of the country had changed: in 1900, the leading causes of death had been tuberculosis, pneumonia, diarrheal diseases, and enteritis; by 1946, the leading causes of death were heart disease, cancer, and accidents. Recognition of the importance of chronic diseases had been temporarily eclipsed by the more urgent demands of infectious disease control during the war. With the return to peace, health departments recognized that they must now come to terms with the problems and prevalence of the chronic diseases.

SOCIAL MEDICINE

In the late 1940s and early 1950s, some American public health officials welcomed the concept of social medicine as seeming to offer a fresh perspective on the problems of chronic illness. Iago Galdston, secretary of the New York Academy of Medicine, organized the Institute on Social Medicine in 1947, later publishing its papers as *Social Medicine: Its Derivations and Objectives.*[97] John A. Ryle, professor of social medicine at Oxford University, emphasized the distinctions between the new social medicine and the old public health. Public health, he said, was concerned with environmental improvement, while social medicine extended its view to "the whole of the economic, nutritional, occupational, educational, and psychological opportunity or experience of the individual or of the community."[98] Whereas public health was concerned with communicable diseases, social medicine would be concerned with all health problems—ulcers and rheumatism, heart disease and cancer, neuroses and injuries. Ryle stated that social medicine, in close alliance with clinical practice, posed the exciting challenge of the future.

The Role of Epidemiology

Ernest L. Stebbins, dean of the Johns Hopkins School of Public Health, argued that epidemiology was the essential discipline for dealing with both chronic and infectious diseases.[99] Margaret Merrell and Lowell J. Reed, statisticians from the Hopkins school, made a similar point in a brief paper that would become a classic statement on *the epidemiology of health*. They suggested a graded scale for measuring degrees of health, not simply the absence of illness:

> On such a scale people would be classified from those who are in top-notch condition with abundant energy, through the people who are well, to fairly well, down to people who are feeling rather poorly, and finally to the definitely ill.[100]

The ideas that health could be quantitatively measurable and that it could be advanced in the total absence of disease helped make connections between the new social medicine and the older public health. Epidemiology, broadening its scope to place more emphasis on the social environment, became newly fashionable as "medical ecology."[81] John E. Gordon, professor of preventive medicine and epidemiology at the Harvard School of Public Health and a prominent exponent of the "newer epidemiology," explained how the triad of "environment, host, and disease" could be applied to noncommunicable organic diseases such as pellagra, cancer, psychosomatic conditions, traumatic injuries, and accidents.[101,102] The notion of a single cause of disease (the agent) was now firmly rejected in favor of multiple causation.[99]

Troubles in Implementation

Social medicine brought considerable optimism about the possibilities for new approaches to the chronic diseases, for the integration of preventive and curative medicine, and for the extension of comprehensive health programs to the whole population.[103] In 1950, Eli Ginzberg introduced a tone of pessimism and caution, however, when he warned optimistic thinkers of an *antigovernment attitude* in the United States and the prevalent assumption that health depended on medical care, with the ever increasing provision of doctors and hospital beds. He urged public health professionals to do a more effective job of persuading the public that advances in diet, housing, and public health nursing were more important to health than the construction of hospitals. He also noted that while hospitals were being built across the country, local health officer positions stood vacant because communities refused to provide reasonable salaries.[104]

Ginzberg's prognosis proved correct in the political climate of the 1950s. The theoretical innovations of social medicine were not translated into effective health programs; acute-care facilities and biomedical research expanded dramatically in the postwar period, while public health departments struggled to maintain their programs on inadequate budgets with little political support. The postwar construction meant massive expenditures for biomedical research and hospital construction, the partial payment for medical care by expanding private insurance coverage, but the relative neglect of public health services and a complete failure to implement the more radical ideas of social medicine through attention to the social determinants of health and disease.

POLITICAL PROBLEMS OF PUBLIC HEALTH

The Committee on Medicine and the Changing Order, supported by the Commonwealth Fund, the Milbank Memorial Fund, and the Josiah Macy Jr. Foundation, recommended the extension of public health services in 1947, but it argued that the quality of public health officers must be improved by better recruitment, training, assured tenure, and adequate salaries.[105]

Harry Mustard, on the other hand, protested that the problems of public health were largely political. State health officers were of relatively low rank in the hierarchy of state officials and were limited in their freedom to introduce new proposals. Too often they accepted political constraints and bureaucratic barriers as natural and inevitable.[106] Too seldom were they willing to risk their positions by appealing to a larger constituency.

In retrospect, it also seems clear that public health failed to claim sufficient credit for controlling infectious diseases. The major scientific achievements of the war in relation to health, such as the discovery of penicillin and the use of DDT, were especially relevant to public health. In popular perception, however, scientific medicine took credit for both the specific wartime discoveries and the longer history of controlling epidemic disease. Medicine and biomedical research had essentially seized the public glory, the political interest, and the financial support given for further anticipated health improvements in the postwar world.

Public health departments needed to claim some share of the credit for declining infectious diseases and to move quickly to develop programs for the chronic diseases. Most health departments did neither of these things, but simply continued running the same programs and clinics within already established bureaucratic structures. The political atmosphere of the 1950s did not support aggressive new programs, and health department budgets were stagnant, without the funding needed to develop broad new health programs.

The Fluoridation Fiasco

Health departments did implement, or try to implement, one important new and very cost effective public health measure, the fluoridation of water supplies to protect children's teeth.[107] Despite virtually unanimous support from scientific authorities and professional organizations, however, fluoridation was denounced as a communist plot and effectively halted in many cities and towns through vocal local opposition. If such a simple and obviously effective measure could be so energetically opposed, health depart-

ments must have perceived the difficulty in instituting more adventurous or expensive interventions.

An Exception: Success with Polio

The one great triumph of the 1950s was the successful development of the polio vaccine and its implementation on a mass scale.[108–110] The success of the polio campaign was due in large part to private funding and a massive public relations campaign by the Foundation for Infantile Paralysis, which raised public awareness and developed public support, interest, and enthusiasm. The appeal for crippled children proved extremely popular, and the polio vaccination campaign, aside from some major setbacks, was a remarkable success.

DECLINE OF PUBLIC HEALTH IN THE 1950s

Despite such public success, in the 1950s the real expenditures of public health departments failed to keep pace with the increase in population.[111] Federal grants-in-aid to the states for public health programs steadily declined, falling from $45 million in 1950 to $33 million in 1959. Given inflation, the decline in purchasing power was even more dramatic. At a time when public health officials were facing a whole series of new, poorly understood health problems, they were also underbudgeted and understaffed.

Health officers were frequently limited to routine clinical responsibilities in child health stations, tuberculosis clinics, venereal disease clinics, and immunization programs, and to communicable disease diagnosis and treatment. They had little or no time for community health education, for studying new health problems, or for developing experimental programs. Indeed, in many areas health officer positions went unfilled, and local medical practitioners, working part time, provided clinical services on an hourly basis.[112]

Some state legislatures were setting up new agencies to build nursing homes, abate water pollution, or promote mental health, and they simply bypassed health departments as not active or interested in these issues. Public health officials were expressing "frustrations, disappointments, dissatisfactions, and discontentments," said John W. Knutson in his Presidential Address to the American Public Health Association in 1957.[113] Public health professionals, he said, must develop more imagination, political skills, and knowledge of human motivation and behavior. Public health students needed a better understanding of social and political forces. Instead of simply learning soon-to-be-outdated factual information, they needed an in-depth knowledge of cultural anthropology, human ecology, epidemiology, and biostatistics.[113] Even with the best possible preparation, the bureaucratic controls of state health departments tended to ensure conformity and discourage young professionals from initiating or taking responsibility for new programs or activities.[114]

In 1959, Milton Terris offered a forceful summary statement of the dilemma of public health. The communicable diseases were disappearing; their place had been taken by the noninfectious diseases that the public health profession was ill prepared to prevent or control. The public understood the fact that research was crucial, and federal expenditures for medical research had multiplied from $28 million in 1947 to $186 million 10 years later. Most of this money, however, was being spent for clinical and laboratory research; there was little understanding of the importance of epidemiological studies in addressing these problems. Schools of public health had been slow to deal with chronic illness, as had health departments, with a few notable exceptions as in the cases of New York and California. Even the small sums spent on epidemiological research had produced dramatic successes, including the discovery of the role of fluoride in preventing dental caries, the relation of cigarette smoking to lung cancer, and the suspected relation of serum cholesterol and physical exercise to coronary artery disease.[115]

In the late 1950s, public health leaders recognized and lamented the failure of their profession to assert a strong political presence or even to perceive the importance of politics to practical public health. The American Public Health Association devoted its annual meeting in 1958 to *The Politics of Public Health.*[116] The editor of the *American Journal of Public Health,* George Rosen, wrote that the education of public health workers should begin with teaching them to think politically and to understand the political process.[117] Raymond R. Tucker, mayor of St. Louis, the city hosting the APHA convention, insisted that public health officials must learn not to confuse the opposition of special interest groups with public opinion, for the general public solidly supported public health reform.[118]

THE 1960s AND THE WAR ON POVERTY

The 1960s saw the collapse of the conservative complacency of the 1950s, the growing power of the civil rights movement, riots in urban African-American ghettos, and federal support for the *war on poverty.* The antipoverty effort and other Great Society programs soon became deeply involved with medical care.[119] Growing concern over access to medical care and hospitalization, especially by the elderly population, culminated in Medicare and Medicaid legislation in 1965 to cover medical care costs for those on Social Security and for the poor. Both programs were built on the *politics of accommodation* with private providers of medical care, thus increasing the incomes of physicians and hospitals and leading to spiraling costs for medical services.[120] Other antipoverty programs, such as the neighborhood health centers that were intended to encourage community participation in providing comprehensive care to underserved populations, fared less well because they were seen as competing with the interests of private care providers.[121]

Most of the new health and social programs of the 1960s bypassed the structure of the public health agencies and set up new agencies to mediate between the federal government and local communities. Medicare and Medicaid reflected the usual priorities of the medical care system in favoring highly technical interventions and hospital care, while failing to provide adequately for preventive services. Neighborhood health centers and community-based mental health services were established without reference to public health agencies.

When environmental issues attracted public concern and political attention in the 1960s and 1970s, separate agencies were also created to respond to these concerns. At the federal level, the Environmental

Protection Agency (EPA) was created to deal with such issues as solid wastes, pesticides, and radiation. At the state level, environmental agencies were often separate from public health departments and failed to reflect specific health concerns or public health expertise. Similarly, mental health agencies were often separate from public health agencies.

Thus, the broader functions of public health were again divided among numerous agencies. Losing a clear institutional base, public health had also lost visibility and clarity of definition. For a field that depends so heavily on public understanding and support, such a loss was disastrous.

PUBLIC HEALTH IN THE SEVENTIES AND EIGHTIES

In the 1970s, public health departments became providers of last resort for uninsured patients and for Medicaid patients rejected by private practitioners. By 1988, almost three-quarters of all state and local health department expenditures went for personal health services.[122] As Harry Mustard had predicted some 40 years earlier, direct provision of medical care absorbed much of the limited resources—in personnel, money, energy, time, and attention—of public health departments, leading to a slow starvation of public health and preventive activities.[122(p52)] The problem of caring for the uninsured and the indigent loomed so large that it eclipsed the need for a basic public health infrastructure in the minds of many legislators and the general public.

In the Reagan revolution of the 1980s, federal funding for public health programs was cut. Through the mechanism of the block grants, power was returned to state health agencies, but in the context of funding cuts, this was the unpopular power to cut existing programs.[123] In the context of general budget cuts, state health departments were often left the task of managing Medicaid programs and delivering personal health services to uninsured and indigent populations. State health departments also had to deal with the adverse health consequences of reductions in other social programs; with the problems of a growing poverty population, as evidenced in drug abuse, alcoholism, teenage pregnancy, infant mortality, family violence, and homelessness; and with the health and social needs of growing populations of illegal immigrants.

The AIDS epidemic and the resurgence of tuberculosis revealed the structural contradictions and weaknesses of national and federal health policy.[124] For state and local health agencies, AIDS and tuberculosis exacerbated their existing problems but gave a new visibility and urgency to their public health efforts.[125,126] The public health community urged a major national effort in AIDS education and prevention. Much of the new funding, when it did finally come, went into research and medical care; as usual, education and prevention received much less attention. But at the same time, the mobilization of public concern provided renewed attention to public health and increased political support. The report by the Institute of Medicine, titled *The Future of Public Health,* notes:

> In a free society public activities ultimately rest on public understanding and support, not on the technical judgment of experts. Expertise is made effective only when it is combined with sufficient public support, a connection acted upon effectively by the early leaders of public health.[122(p130)]

PUBLIC HEALTH TODAY

Since the early 1990s, the whole country has been embroiled in debates over health care reform, welfare reform, drugs, violence, environmental health, and women's health issues. These are all issues of public health, yet public health as such is rarely mentioned. This is partly a failure of public health practice; we need a variety of model public health programs to demonstrate to the country what could be achieved with sufficient political will, expertise, and money. It is also in part a failure of communications. Public health professionals have not been very effective in presenting their views and accomplishments to the media, the politicians, and the public.

CONCLUSION

The growth in the technical knowledge of public health in the past 100 years has been extraordinary—and insufficiently addressed in this brief account—but our ability to implement this knowledge in health and social reform has advanced little. As we have noted, the issues of public health today include and intersect with the great social issues of modern America: health care reform and the coverage of the uninsured; environmental health and safety; welfare reform and child health; drugs and violence in the streets; women's health, reproductive freedom, abortion, and fertility control; family violence and child abuse; AIDS, tuberculosis, and emerging epidemics; the continuing problems of chronic disease; and the need for home health services and long-term care for an aging population.

Public health is a vitally important field for the future well-being of America, its citizens, and its communities. Public health professionals must learn to communicate better the vital importance of their activities, mobilize public support, build a more effective public health infrastructure, and demonstrate clearly the benefits of prevention to the public at large by finding innovative ways of responding to endemic social problems and new crises.

References

1. Rosenberg C. *The Cholera Years: The United States in 1832, 1849 and 1866*. Chicago, Ill: University of Chicago Press; 1962.

2. Powell JH. *Bring Out Your Dead. The Great Plague of Yellow Fever in Philadelphia in 1793*. Philadelphia: University of Pennsylvania Press; 1949.

3. Wiebe RH. *The Search for Order, 1877-1920*. New York, NY: Hill & Wang; 1967.

4. Ackerknecht EL. Anticontagionism between 1821 and 1867. *Bull Hist Med*. 1948;22:562-593.

5. Baltimore City Ordinance 11, approved April 7, 1797. In: Howard WT. *Public Health Administration and the Natural History of Disease in Baltimore, Maryland, 1797-1920*. Washington, DC: Carnegie Institution; 1924.

6. Rosen G. *A History of Public Health*. Expanded ed. Baltimore, Md: Johns Hopkins University Press; 1993.

7. Duffy J. *The Sanitarians: A History of American Public Health*. Urbana: University of Illinois Press; 1990.

8. Rosner D, ed. *Epidemic! Public Health Crises in New York*. New Brunswick, NJ: Rutgers University Press; 1994.

9. Citizens' Association of New York. *Report of the Council of Hygiene and Public Health of the Citizens' Association of New York upon the Sanitary Condition of the City*. New York, NY: Arno Press; 1970: xxi-xxxv.

10. Hudson A. The mapping of property and environment in Manhattan since the 1600s. *Biblion*. Spring 1993;1:47-50.

11. Shattuck L. *Report of a General Plan for the Promotion of Public and Personal Health, Devised, Prepared, and Recommended by the Commissioners Appointed under a Resolve of the Legislature of the State*. Cambridge, Mass: Harvard University Press; 1948.

12. Rosen G. *A History of Public Health*. Baltimore, MD: Johns Hopkins University Press; 1993:216-219.

13. *Proceedings and Debates of the Third National Quarantine and Sanitary Conference*. New York, NY: Edward Jones; 1859:179-180.

14. Adams GW. *Doctors in Blue*. New York, NY: Henry Schuman; 1952.

15. Woodward JJ. *Chief Camp Diseases of the United States Armies*. Philadelphia, Pa: JB Lippencott; 1863.

16. Cavins HM. The national quarantine and sanitary conventions of 1857-1858 and the beginnings of the American Public Health Association. *Bull Hist Med*. 1943;13:419-425.

17. Kramer HD. Agitation for public health reform in the 1870s. *J Hist Med Allied Sci*. 1948;3:473-488.

18. Smith S. The history of public health, 1871-1921. In: Ravenel MP, ed. *A Half Century of Public Health*. New York, NY: American Public Health Association; 1921:1-12.

19. Ravenel MP. The American Public Health Association: past, present, future. In: Ravenel MP, ed. *A Half Century of Public Health*. New York, NY: American Public Health Association; 1921:13-55.

20. Patterson RG. *Historical Directory of State Health Departments in the United States of America*. Columbus: Public Health Association; 1939.

21. Abbott SW. *The Past and Present Conditions of Public Hygiene and State Medicine in the United States*. Boston, Mass: Wright & Potter; 1900.

22. Mullan F. *Plagues and Politics: The Story of the United States Marine Hospital Service*. New York, NY: Basic Books; 1989.

23. Harden VA. *Inventing the NIH: Federal Biomedical Research Policy, 1887-1937*. Baltimore, Md: Johns Hopkins University Press; 1986.

24. Blake J. *Public Health in the Town of Boston, 1630-1822*. Cambridge, Mass: Harvard University Press; 1959.

25. Rosenkrantz B. *Public Health and the State: Changing Views in Massachusetts, 1842-1936.* Cambridge, Mass: Harvard University Press; 1972.

26. Duffy J. *A History of Public Health in New York City, 1625-1826.* New York, NY: Russell Sage Foundation; 1968.

27. Duffy J. *A History of Public Health in New York City, 1866-1966.* New York, NY: Russell Sage Foundation; 1974.

28. Galishoff S. *Safeguarding the Public Health: Newark, 1895-1918.* Westport, Conn: Greenwood Press; 1975.

29. Leavitt JW. *The Healthiest City: Milwaukee and the Politics of Health Reform.* Princeton, NJ: Princeton University Press; 1982.

30. Kraut AM. *Silent Travelers: Germs, Genes, and the Immigrant Menace.* New York, NY: Basic Books; 1994.

31. Winslow CEA. *The Life of Hermann M. Biggs: Physician and Statesman of the Public Health.* Philadelphia, Pa: Lea & Febiger; 1929.

32. Jordan EO, Whipple GC, Winslow CEA. *A Pioneer of Public Health: William Thompson Sedgwick.* New Haven, Conn: Yale University Press; 1924.

33. Cassedy JH. *Charles V. Chapin and the Public Health Movement.* Cambridge, Mass: Harvard University Press; 1962.

34. Rosenberg CE, Rosenberg CS. Pietism and the origins of the American public health movement. *J Hist Med Allied Sci.* 1968;23:16-35.

35. Shroyck RH. The early American public health movement. *Am J Public Health.* 1937;27:965-971.

36. Rosenkrantz B. Cart before horse: theory, practice and professional image in American public health. *J Hist Med Allied Sci.* 1974;29:57.

37. Ryan MP. *Womanhood in America: From Colonial Times to the Present.* New York, NY: Franklin Watts; 1975:225-234.

38. Smillie W. *Public Health: Its Promise for the Future.* New York, NY: Macmillan; 1955:450-458.

39. Wiebe RH. *The Search for Order, 1877-1920.* New York, NY: Hill & Wang; 1967.

40. Hayes SP. The politics of reform in municipal government in the progressive era. In: Hayes SP, ed. *American Political History as Social Analysis.* Knoxville: University of Tennessee Press; 1980:205-232.

41. Hayes SP. *Conservation and the Gospel of Efficiency: The Progressive Conservation Movement, 1890-1918.* Boston, Mass: Beacon Press; 1968.

42. Rogers DT. In search of progressivism. *Rev Am Hist.* 1982;10:115-132.

43. Welch WH. Sanitation in relation to the poor. An address to the Charity Organization Society of Baltimore, November 1892. In: *Papers and Addresses by William Henry Welch, Vol. 3.* Baltimore, Md: The Johns Hopkins Press; 1920.

44. von Pettenkofer M. Sigerist HE, trans. *The Value of Health to a City.* Baltimore, Md: Johns Hopkins University Press; 1941:15-52.

45. Rotch TM. The position and work of the American Pediatric Society toward public questions. *Trans Am Pediatr Soc.* 1909:21:12.

46. Chapin C. How shall we spend the health appropriation? In: Chapin CV, Gorham FP, eds. *Papers of Charles V. Chapin, M.D.: A Review of Public Health Realities.* New York, NY: The Commonwealth Fund; 1934:28-35.

47. Sternberg GM. Sanitary lessons of the war. In: Sternberg GM, ed. *Sanitary Lessons of the War and Other Papers.* Washington, DC: Byron S Adams; 1912:2.

48. Cosmas GA. *An Army for Empire: The United States Army in the Spanish-American War.* Columbia: University of Missouri Press; 1971.

49. Kelley HA. *Walter Reed and Yellow Fever.* Baltimore, Md: Medical Standard Book Co; 1906.

50. Sternberg GM. Sanitary problems connected with the construction of the Isthmian Canal. In: Sternberg GM, ed. *Sanitary Lessons of the War and Other Papers.* Washington, DC: Byron S Adams; 1912;39-40.

51. Fosdick RB. *Adventure in Giving: The Story of the General Education Board.* New York, NY: Harper & Row; 1962:57-58.

52. Ettling J. *The Germ of Laziness: Rockefeller Philanthropy and Public Health in the New South.* Cambridge, Mass: Harvard University Press; 1981.

53. Rose W. First annual report of the administrative secretary of the Rockefeller Sanitary Commission; 1910:4. In: Fosdick RB, ed. *The Story of the Rockefeller Foundation.* New York, NY: Harper & Brothers; 1952:33.

54. Rosen G. The committee of one hundred on national health and the campaign for a national health department, 1906-1912. *Am J Public Health.* 1972;62:261-263.

55. Marcus AI. Disease prevention in America: from a local to a national outlook, 1880-1910. *Bull Hist Med.* 1979;53:184-203.

56. Fisher I. *A Report on National Vitality, Its Wastes and Conservation.* Washington, DC: Committee of One Hundred on National Health; 1909. US Government Printing Office Bulletin No. 30.

57. Williams RC. *The United States Public Health Service, 1798-1950.* Washington, DC: US Government Printing Office; 1951.

58. Schiesl MJ. *The Politics of Efficiency: Municipal Administration and Reform In America, 1880-1920.* Berkeley: University of California Press; 1980.

59. Fee E. *Disease and Discovery: A History of the Johns Hopkins School of Hygiene and Public Health, 1916-1939.* Baltimore, Md: Johns Hopkins University Press; 1987.

60. Fee E, Acheson RM, eds. *A History of Education in Public Health: Health That Mocks the Doctors' Rules.* New York, NY: Oxford University Press; 1991.

61. Sedgwick WT. The origin, scope and significance of bacteriology. *Science.* 1901;13:121-128.

62. Winslow CEA. The untilled fields of public health. *Science.* 1920;51:23.

63. Winslow CEA. *The Evolution and Significance of the Modern Public Health Campaign.* New Haven, Conn: Yale University Press; 1923.

64. Sicherman B. *Alice Hamilton: A Life in Letters.* Cambridge, Mass: Harvard University Press; 1984:153-183.

65. Terris M, ed. *Goldberger on Pellagra.* Baton Rouge: Louisiana State University Press; 1964.

66. Kantor B. *The New Scientific Public Health Movement: A Case Study of Tuberculosis in Baltimore, Maryland, 1900-1910* [master's thesis]. Baltimore, Md: Johns Hopkins University; 1985.

67. Meeker E. The improving health of the United States, 1850-1915. *Explorations in Economic History.* 1972;9:353-373.

68. Haines RH. The use of model life tables to estimate mortality for the United States in the late nineteenth century. *Demography.* 1979;16:289-312.

69. Hoffman FL. The general death rate of large American cities, 1871-1904. *Publications of the American Statistical Association.* 1906-1907;10:1-75.

70. Duffy J. Social impact of disease in the late nineteenth century. *Bull NY Acad Med.* 1971;47:797-811.

71. Knowles M. Public health service not a medical monopoly. *Am J Public Health.* 1913;3:111-122.

72. Winslow CEA. Public health at the crossroads. *Am J Public Health.* 1926;16:1075-1085.

73. *Report of the Committee on Municipal Health Department Practice of the American Public Health Association, in cooperation with the United States Public Health Service.* Washington, DC: US Government Printing Office; 1923. Public Health Bulletin No. 136.

74. Duffy J. The American medical profession and public health: from support to ambivalence. *Bull Hist Med.* 1979;53:1-22.

75. Meckel RA. *Save the Babies: American Public Health Reform and the Prevention of Infant Mortality, 1850-*

1920. Baltimore, Md: Johns Hopkins University Press; 1990.

76. Mullan F. *Plagues and Politics: The Story of the United States Public Health Service.* New York, NY: Basic Books; 1989.

77. Committee on the Costs of Medical Care. *Medical Care for the American People.* Chicago, Ill: University of Chicago Press; 1932. Final report.

78. Fee E. The pleasures and perils of prophetic advocacy: socialized medicine and the politics of medical reform. In: Fee E, Brown TM, eds. *Making Medical History: The Life and Work of Henry E. Sigerist.* Baltimore, Md: Johns Hopkins University Press; 1996. In press.

79. Berkowitz ED. *America's Welfare State: From Roosevelt to Reagan.* Baltimore, Md: Johns Hopkins University Press; 1991.

80. Kratz FK. Status of full-time local health organizations at the end of the fiscal year 1941-1942. *Public Health Rep.* 1943;58:345-351.

81. Corwin EHL, ed. *Ecology of Health.* New York, NY: The Commonwealth Fund; 1949.

82. Mustard HS. *Government in Public Health.* New York, NY: The Commonwealth Fund; 1945:190.

83. Leathers WS, et al. Committee on Professional Education of the American Public Health Association. Public health degrees and certificates granted in 1936. *Am J Public Health.* 1937;27:1267-1272.

84. Mustard HS, ed. Yesterday's school children are examined for the army. *Am J Public Health.* 1941;31:1207.

85. Simmons JS. The preventive medicine program of the United States Army. *Am J Public Health.* 1943;33:931-940.

86. Mountain JW. Responsibility of local health authorities in the war effort. *Am J Public Health.* 1943;33:35-40.

87. Williams RC. *The United States Public Health Service, 1798-1950.* Washington, DC: Commissioned Officers' Association of the United States Public Health Service; 1951:612-768.

88. Furman B. *A Profile of the Public Health Service, 1798-1948.* Bethesda, Md: National Institutes of Health; 1973:418-458.

89. Perrott GStJ. Findings of selective service examinations. *Milbank Q.* 1944;22:358-366.

90. Perrott GStJ. Selective service rejection statistics and some of their implications. *Am J Public Health.* 1946;36:336-342.

91. Maxcy KF. Epidemiologic implications of wartime population shifts. *Am J Public Health.* 1942;32:1089-1096.

92. Ethridge EW. *Sentinel for Health: A History of the Centers for Disease Control.* Berkeley: University of California Press; 1992.

93. Stern BJ. *Medical Services by Government: Local, State, and Federal.* New York, NY: The Commonwealth Fund; 1946:31-32.

94. Emerson H. *Local Health Units for the Nation.* New York, NY: The Commonwealth Fund; 1945.

95. Mountain JW, Flook E. Distribution of health services in the structure of state government: the composite pattern of state health services. *Public Health Rep.* 1941;56:1676.

96. Mountain JW, Flook E. Distribution of health services in the structure of state government: state health department organization. *Public Health Rep.* 1943;58:568.

97. Galdston I, ed. *Social Medicine: Its Derivations and Objectives.* New York, NY: The Commonwealth Fund; 1949.

98. Ryle JA. Social pathology. In: Galdston I, ed. *Social Medicine: Its Derivations and Objectives.* New York, NY: The Commonwealth Fund; 1949:64.

99. Stebbins EL. Epidemiology and social medicine. In: Galdston I, ed. *Social Medicine: Its Derivations and Objectives.* New York, NY: The Commonwealth Fund; 1949:101-104.

100. Merrell M, Reed LJ. The epidemiology of health. In: Galdston I, ed. *Social Medicine: Its Derivations and Objectives.* New York, NY: The Commonwealth Fund; 1949:105-110.

101. Gordon JE. The newer epidemiology. In: *Tomorrow's Horizon in Public Health.* Transactions of the 1950 conference of the Public Health Association of New York City. New York, NY: Public Health Association; 1950:18-45.

102. Gordon JE. The world, the flesh and the devil as environment, host and agent of disease. In: Galdston I, ed. *The Epidemiology of Health.* New York, NY: Health Education Council; 1953:60-73.

103. Smillie WG. The responsibility of the state. In: *Tomorrow's Horizon in Public Health.* Transactions of the 1950 conference of the Public Health Association of New York City. New York, NY: Public Health Association; 1950:95-102.

104. Ginzberg E. Public health and the public. In: *Tomorrow's Horizon in Public Health.* Transactions of the 1950 conference of the Public Health Association of New York City. New York, NY: Public Health Association; 1950:101-109.

105. New York Academy of Medicine, Committee on Medicine in the Changing Order. *Medicine in the Changing Order.* New York, NY: The Commonwealth Fund; 1947:109.

106. Mustard HS. *Government in Public Health.* New York, NY: The Commonwealth Fund; 1945:112.

107. McNeil DR. *The Fight for Fluoridation.* New York, NY: Oxford University Press; 1957.

108. Benison S. *Tom Rivers: Reflections on a Life in Medicine and Science.* Cambridge, Mass: MIT Press; 1967.

109. Klein AE. *Trial by Fury: The Polio Vaccine Controversy.* New York, NY: Scribner's; 1972.

110. Paul JR. *A History of Poliomyelitis.* New Haven, Conn: Yale University Press; 1971.

111. Sanders BS. Local health departments: growth or illusion. *Public Health Rep.* 1959;74:13-20.

112. Aronson JB. The politics of public health—reactions and summary. *Am J Public Health.* 1959;49:311.

113. Knutson JW. Ferment in public health. *Am J Public Health.* 1957;47:1489-1491.

114. Woodcock L. Where are we going in public health? *Am J Public Health.* 1956;46:278-282.

115. Terris M. The changing face of public health. *Am J Public Health.* 1959;49:1113-1119.

116. American Public Health Association Symposium—1958. The politics of public health. *Am J Public Health.* 1959;49:300-313.

117. Rosen G. The politics of public health. *Am J Public Health.* 1959;49:364-365.

118. Tucker RR. The politics of public health. *Am J Public Health.* 1959;49:300-305.

119. Davis K, Schoen C. *Health and the War on Poverty.* Washington, DC: Brookings Institution; 1978.

120. Starr P. *The Social Transformation of American Medicine.* New York, NY: Basic Books; 1982:374-378.

121. Sardell A. *The U.S. Experiment in Social Medicine: The Community Health Center Program, 1965-1986.* Pittsburgh, Pa; University of Pittsburgh Press; 1988.

122. Institute of Medicine, Committee for the Study of the Future of Public Health. *The Future of Public Health.* Washington, DC: National Academy Press; 1988.

123. Omenn GS. What's behind those block grants in health. *New Eng J Med.* 1982;306:1057-1060.

124. Fox DM. AIDS and the American health policy: the history and prospects of a crisis of authority. In: Fee E, Fox DM, eds. *AIDS: The Burdens of History.* Berkeley: University of California Press; 1988:316-343.

125. Fee E, Fox DM, eds. *AIDS: The Making of a Chronic Disease.* Berkeley: University of California Press; 1992.

126. Krieger N, Margo G, eds. *AIDS: The Politics of Survival.* New York, NY: Baywood; 1994.

C H A P T E R

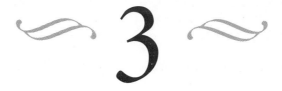

3

The Last Decade

C. William Keck, M.D., M.P.H.
F. Douglas Scutchfield, M.D.

INTRODUCTION

The seminal work done by the Institute of Medicine (IOM) in its study of the U.S. public health system is described in the 1988 IOM report *The Future of Public Health.*[1] The report is referenced repeatedly by authors throughout this book. The institute's conclusion that public health in the United States is a system in disarray acted as a wakeup call for the public health profession. The public health community was galvanized to address the shortcomings that the report described.

Former President Clinton promised comprehensive health care reform at the time of his election in 1992. This was an additional stimulus to better define the role of public health in hope that the discipline would receive appropriate attention in a national reform package. The IOM report and the president's health care initiative, coming relatively close together, acted as driving forces for the public health profession to better define its role and increase public understanding of its contributions to health. The resulting activities were far-ranging and very productive. They were characterized by a strong sense of purpose; high productivity; and unprecedented collaboration between agencies of the federal government, national public health professional organizations, academic institutions, local and state health departments, and many individuals. This collaboration and focus of effort has created a subsequent period of public health philosophic renaissance.

This chapter will describe many of the major events of the recent past that are continuing to shape the evolution of public health in this country.

INSTITUTE OF MEDICINE

The IOM report mentioned above is not gathering dust on shelves. Its documentation of the inadequate status of local public health services and recommendations for common mission and core functions got the attention of public health professionals. All public health workers should become familiar with that document and the reasons behind its damning conclusion that the U.S. public health system is a system in disarray. Among the IOM's disturbing findings were:

- There was no clear, universally accepted mission for public health.
- Tension between professional expertise and politics was present throughout the nation's public health system.
- Public health professionals had been slow to develop strategies that demonstrate the worth of their efforts to legislators and the public.
- Relationships between medicine and public health were, at best, uneasy.
- Inadequate research resources had been targeted at identifying and solving public health problems.
- Public health practice, unlike other health professions, was largely decoupled from its academic base(s).[1]

There were initially mixed reviews of these findings from the public health community. Many public health leaders objected to the characterization of their agency as being in disarray. As the report was more fully digested, however, most public health professionals came to accept the accuracy of the report's description of the public health system in the United States, and that something had to be done to reverse the reality.

Local health departments and other elements of the public health system have probably never gotten as much attention as they have received since the IOM report was published. Very real progress has been, and continues to be made in responding to the various factors critiqued by the IOM. The introspection fostered by the report has resulted in a growing clarity of the challenges that face the profession. This is helpful, but the magnitude of those challenges is also quite daunting. If there is any comfort, it lies to some degree in the growing national awareness of the needs of communities and local public health practitioners. There is a growing sense that something has to be done to improve the capacity of local health departments to do their work, and there are significant steps being taken to address that situation.

An important first step was general agreement on the mission and functions of public health. In the absence of an identifiable universal mission statement, the IOM suggested the following:

> The mission of public health is to fulfill society's interest in assuring conditions in which people can be healthy.[1(p7)]

Since the IOM was unable to identify universally accepted core functions for local health departments, they proposed the following:[1(pp7–8)]

> **Assessment** - Every public health agency should regularly and systematically collect, assemble, analyze, and make available information on the health of the community, including statistics on health status, community health needs, and epidemiologic and other studies of health problems.

> **Policy Development** - Every public health agency should exercise its responsibility to serve the public interest in the development of comprehensive public health policies by promoting the use of the scientific knowledge base in decision-making about public health and by leading in developing public health policy.

> **Assurance** - Public health agencies should assure their constituents that services necessary to achieve agreed upon goals are provided, either by encouraging actions by other entities (private or public sector), by requiring such action through regulation, or by providing services directly.

> Each public health agency should involve key policy-makers and the general public in determining a set of high-priority personal and community-wide health services that governments will guarantee to every member of the community. This guarantee should include subsidization or direct provision of high-priority personal health services for those unable to afford them.

The public health community, both practice and academic, embraced the suggested mission and the proposed core functions. They were left, then, to deal with the reality that the IOM had found the nation's public health agencies very limited in their capacity to fulfill these functions.

DEVELOPMENT OF THE TEN ESSENTIAL PUBLIC HEALTH SERVICES

The election of President Clinton in 1992 heralded the beginning of an attempt to develop health care reform. As it became clear to public health leaders that very comprehensive reform was the intent, they realized how important it would be to ensure that public health was included in a reform proposal. They also realized that public understanding of the role of public health was limited. The terms assessment, policy development, and assurance had become well accepted by the public health practice and academic communities, but they were poorly understood by the public, the medical care industry, or the policy makers who were drafting the president's reform package. The response to this realization marked the entrance of public health into a period of significant change and growth as a profession. Things had already been changing, of course, but many of those changes had been driven by external factors. Now change was being driven from within the profession, often directly responding to the findings of the IOM.

At the time of the president's inauguration, work had already begun on expanding the three core functions to a longer related list of activities or practices that more clearly defined the role of public health in the United States. The Centers for Disease Control and Prevention (CDC)[2] used the three core functions to develop an expanded list of 10 basic public health practices. A version of this list, called the "Core Functions of Public Health," appeared in Title III of the Health Security Act forwarded by President Clinton to Congress in October 1993.[3] The eventual defeat of this attempt to reform the U.S. health delivery system was a bitter blow to the Clinton presidency, but it was also a bitter blow for public health. This was the first time that a national health care reform effort recognized the importance of public health to improved health status, and included public health as an important system element. The defeat of the proposed legislation was not related to the inclusion of public health system issues in the bill.

There was value in better defining the role of public health beyond its usefulness for proposed federal legislation, however. Work to understand and describe the basic practices of public health continued, and in 1993 a list of 10 "core functions" was developed by the Washington State Department of Health as part of health care reform efforts in that state.[4] It was similar to, but not the same as, the list developed by the CDC. In 1994 another variation of the list was developed by the National Association of County Health Officials, the Association of State and Territorial Health Officials, and the federal Office of the Assistant Secretary for Health.[5] Multiple versions of public health's core functions were inherently confusing, however, and it became clear that a single list should be agreed to that could be embraced by everyone in the profession. A working group on the core functions of public health was put together in the spring of 1994, cochaired by Dr. David Satcher, director of the CDC, and Dr. J. Michael McGinnis, deputy assistant secretary for disease prevention and health promotion, and composed of representatives of the Public Health Service's (PHS) agencies and the major national public health organizations. It charged a subgroup, co-led by the CDC's Public Health Practice Program Office and the Office of Disease Prevention and Health Promotion, to develop a consensus of the "essential services of public health." The resulting statement was reviewed and revised by the Core Functions of Public Health Steering Committee, chaired by Dr. Phillip R. Lee, assistant secretary for health, and Dr. M. Joycelyn Elders, surgeon general, and composed of the heads of PHS agencies and presidents of national major public health organizations.[6]

This consensus statement provided a vision for public health in America: "Healthy People in Healthy Communities," and a mission for public health: "Promote physical and mental health and prevent disease, injury, and disability."

It also provided two brief lists. The first was intended as a description of what public health seeks to accomplish by providing essential services to the public:

- Prevent epidemics and the spread of disease
- Protect against environmental hazards
- Prevent injuries
- Promote and encourage healthy behaviors and mental health

• Respond to disasters and assist communities in recovery
• Assure the quality and accessibility of health services

The second list has been accepted as the consensus description of the 10 essential public health services:

1. Monitor health status to identify community health problems.
2. Diagnose and investigate health problems and health hazards in the community.
3. Inform, educate and empower people about health issues.
4. Mobilize community partnerships to identify and solve health problems.
5. Develop policies and plans that support individual and community health efforts.
6. Enforce laws and regulations that protect health and ensure safety.
7. Link people to needed personal health services and assure the provision of health care when otherwise unavailable.
8. Assure a competent public health and personal health care workforce.
9. Evaluate effectiveness, accessibility and quality of personal and population-based health services.

10. Research for new insights and innovative solutions to health problems.

Figure 3.1 depicts the relationship of the 10 essential services to the original three core functions.

FACULTY/AGENCY FORUM

Funded by the Health Resources and Services Administration (HRSA) and CDC, the Faculty/Agency Forum was established to address the educational and academic dimensions of the findings of the IOM. The forum's major accomplishment in 1993 was the development and publication of a compendium of competencies required for successful public health practice. They listed the skills required under the following headings: analytic, communication, policy development/program planning, cultural, financial planning and management, and basic public health science (epidemiology, biostatistics, environmental health, administration, and behavioral science).[7] The forum wanted to improve the quality of public health education and establish flourishing, permanent, broad cooperative agreements between schools of public health and major local, regional, and state public health agencies. To that end, they also proposed ways that public

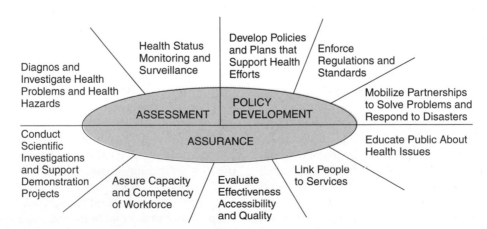

Figure 3.1. Public Health Core Functions and Essential Services
Source: Adapted from Ohio Department of Health.

agencies and institutions providing graduate education in public health could work together. After completing their work and publishing a report,[7] the forum went out of existence.

COUNCIL ON LINKAGES BETWEEN ACADEMIA AND PUBLIC HEALTH PRACTICE

The Council on Linkages was established under a cooperative agreement from HRSA through the Association of Schools of Public Health, as a sequel to the Faculty/Agency Forum. It brought representatives from national public health professional organizations and federal agencies together to "improve public health practice and education by refining and implementing recommendations of the Public Health Faculty/Agency Forum, establishing links between academia and the agencies of the public health community, and creating a process for continuing public health education throughout one's career."[8] Membership of the Council on Linkages is listed in Table 3.1.

The council's major contribution to date is its development of a modernized list of core competencies

Table 3.1. Council on Linkages Between Academia and Public Health Practice Membership Organizations

American Association of Health Plans
American College of Preventive Medicine
American Public Health Association
Association of Schools of Public Health
Association of State and Territorial Health Officials
Association of Teachers of Preventive Medicine
Association of University Programs in Health
    Administration
Centers for Disease Control and Prevention
Community-Campus Partnerships for Health
Health Resources and Services Administration
National Association of County and City Health Officials
National Association of Local Boards of Health
National Environmental Health Association
QUAD Council of Public Health Nursing Organizations
Society for Public Health Education

Source: Council on Linkages Between Academia and Public Health Practice. Available at: http://www.phr.org/Link/membership.htm.

for public health professionals. This list builds on the work of the Faculty/Agency Forum, and it represents almost 10 years of work on this subject by the council and numerous other organizations and individuals in public health academia and practice settings. Their work was compiled and cross-walked with the essential public health services to ensure that the competencies can be used to help build the skills necessary for providing these services[9] (see http://www.trainingfinder.org/competencies/list/htm and Appendix C).

This latest list of core competencies represents a set of skills, knowledge, and attitudes necessary for the broad practice of public health. The competencies are listed under the following eight domains: Analytic Assessment Skills, Basic Public Health Sciences Skills, Cultural Competency Skills, Communication Skills, Community Dimensions of Practice Skills, Financial Planning and Management Skills, Leadership and Systems Thinking Skills, and Policy Development/Program Planning Skills.

Among the council's other accomplishments are:

• Creating and distributing *The Link,* its newsletter, highlighting models of linkages between public health academic and practice settings.
• Working through the Association of Schools of Public Health (an agency member of the council) to identify practice representatives at each school of public health charged with improving their institution's linkages with practice settings.
• Beginning the process of developing Community Public Health Practice Guidelines (like the Clinical Preventive Service Guidelines), now being carried out by the CDC.
• Proposing a public health research agenda based on the 10 essential services.

PUBLIC HEALTH TRAINING PROGRAMS

When the Council on Education for Public Health (CEPH) took over public health training program accreditation from the American Public Health Association in 1974, there were 18 accredited schools of public health. The number had expanded from 10 schools in 1946 to 18 in 1974—an 80 percent increase in close to 30 years. In retrospect that seems to be a very slow expansion, but at the time it was viewed as being quite rapid. The growth responded primarily to the infusion of federal funds, including formula or capitation grants, training grants, traineeships for students, greatly expanded biomedical research funding, and even some construction monies. Most of these funds were available only to accredited schools, so it is not surprising that many of the other public health training programs faded away, leaving the independent schools of public health primarily engaged in graduate training as the nation's model of professional public health preparation.[10]

The most notable difference in the public health professional preparation landscape now and 25 years ago is the sheer number of institutions of higher education offering graduate training in public health. Today, CEPH accredits 61 schools and programs. In addition to schools of public health, in the late 1970s CEPH began to also accredit graduate community health education programs and graduate community health/preventive medicine programs.[10]

The most dramatic growth over the past 25 years has occurred in programs outside schools of public health, and much of that growth has occurred in the past 10 years. This is not at all unexpected, given that universities can assemble the resources needed to support a program much more easily than the resources needed to provide the comprehensive offerings in a school of public health. A program, for example, may offer only a generalist master of public health degree (M.P.H.) or one or two areas of specialization, whereas a school of public health must offer a full range of at least five public health concentrations, plus doctoral programs. Programs, which typically start small but often grow quite large, are the spawning ground for new schools of public health. A number of accredited programs have already made the transition to accredited schools of public health, and it is likely that more will do so.[10]

The growth in the past, however, pales in comparison to the growth that appears to be on the immediate horizon. A change from 18 to 61 institutions in 25 years is a more than 300 percent increase. It is likely that number will more than double again in the next 5 to 10 years. In addition to the more than 60 accredited schools and programs, there are currently 15 institutions in applicant status and another 60+ institutions on CEPH's "early warning list"—programs and schools that are under development, in early operational stages or just thinking about accreditation. The list grows longer every year, even as many go off this list on to the accredited list. Public health training is a growth industry and gives every sign of remaining so in the near future.[10]

CREDENTIALING OF PUBLIC HEALTH WORKERS

Among the health workforces in the United States, public health alone has no credentialing process to certify that its workforce has acquired minimal competence. To be sure, most public health workers are licensed or certified in their basic professions—nursing, medicine, environmental health, health education, counseling, laboratory technology, and so on. There is no process, however, to certify competence to practice their profession in a public health setting. This has been a controversial issue in public health for many years, but the development of accepted competencies, including a set of competencies that cut across professional boundaries, sets the stage for a certification process. The American Public Health Association and the Association of Schools of Public Health have embarked on a journey to develop such a process by 2002 for recent master of public health degree (M.P.H.) graduates.

NATIONAL ASSOCIATION OF COUNTY AND CITY HEALTH OFFICIALS (NACCHO)

The combination in 1994 of the United States Conference of Local Health Officers and the National Association of County Health Officials into a single professional association representing directors of all local health departments, named the National Association of County and City Health Officials (NACCHO), was a very significant occurrence. The organization grew in strength just as increasing attention was focused on local health departments, and it has become a very important participant in the many activities related to improving the local public health system.

In the past, the National Association of County Health Officials focused on maintaining its membership, facilitating communication, and continuing education of its members. In its new form, NACCHO is actively involved in developing public policy, its workforce, and leadership; defining and expanding the public health research agenda; developing tools to assist local health departments with community assessment; and providing technical assistance to public health practitioners. Staff and other resources have grown dramatically, and critical partnerships have been established with other public health professional organizations and key federal agencies, including participation in cooperative agreements with the CDC that provide funding for a number of the organization's expanded activities.

NATIONAL ASSOCIATION OF LOCAL BOARDS OF HEALTH

The large majority of local health departments is governed by boards of health. They consist of 3 to 15 members who, depending on the laws affecting the local jurisdiction, serve as advisors and/or policy makers (see chapter 8). Boards function as a major link between local public health agencies and the communities they serve, and board members have the potential to wield significant influence on the public health services provided and the resources made available to deliver them. Board members may be health professionals, but the majority are not; few have any training or experience in public health.

Orientation and training of local board of health members has traditionally been left to the local health department they represent, sometimes with assistance from their state health department. Additionally, boards typically focused on their local jurisdiction's needs and interacted minimally, if at all, with other boards in their own geographic area, let alone with boards from other parts of their state or other states.

It was not until the 1980s that boards of health in some states formed their own state local board of health associations. These groups sought to provide training for new board members and organize the influence of board members to address public health issues and the resources needed to deal with them. In November 1992, representatives of states with these kinds of organizations (Georgia, Illinois, North Carolina, Ohio, and Washington) came together and

formed the National Association of Local Boards of Health (NALBOH).

Since its founding, NALBOH has grown rapidly. It operates offices in Bowling Green, Ohio, and Washington, DC, and is effectively involved in a growing number of activities including training for board of health members, public health advocacy, the development of performance measurement standards, and tobacco control. It is reasonable to expect that as its membership and staff grow, NALBOH will become an increasingly important player on the local, state, and national scenes.

PUBLIC HEALTH PRACTICE PROGRAM OFFICE AT THE CDC

The establishment of the Public Health Practice Program Office at the CDC in 1988 marked a new direction for that agency. For the first time, there would be a locus in the CDC dedicated to strengthening the public health infrastructure in the United States. The Office began its work by concentrating its efforts in four areas:[11]

1. Strengthening the professional competencies of the public health workforce
2. Developing information systems that would increase access to public health knowledge
3. Building the organizational capacity of local health departments
4. Strengthening the science base for infrastructure development

Over the ensuing years, while continuing to work in these areas, the Office added to its agenda the development of science-based performance standards for public health organizations and competency standards for practitioners. It intends to use these standards and the Public Health Infrastructure objectives contained in *Healthy People 2010* as a framework for action. The Office has been very productive. Among its products are:[11]

• Health Alert Network
• Information Network for Public Health Officials
• Public Health Training Network

- Public Health Leadership Institute
  (see Appendix B)
- National Public Health Performance Standards
- Geographic Information Systems Research Center
- National Inventory of Clinical Laboratory Testing
- Electronic Laboratory Reporting
- Clinical Laboratories Improvement Amendments
- Public Health Image Library

The contribution of the Public Health Practice Programs Office to the evolution of public health has been, and is likely to continue to be, very significant. The Office has involved representatives of local and state health departments appropriately, and has proceeded with skill and sensitivity.

MEDICINE/PUBLIC HEALTH INITIATIVE

A joint effort of the American Medical Association (AMA) and the American Public Health Association (APHA), the Medicine/Public Health Initiative is an attempt to bridge the gap and develop stronger working relationships between these two disciplines. An initial National Congress in the spring of 1995, which brought national, state, and local leaders together from each discipline to explore common ground, was followed by a second gathering in 1997 at the New York Academy of Medicine. The Academy had been asked to explore and describe the current "state of the art" of collaboration between medicine and public health. Dr. Roz Lasker and the Academy's Committee on Medicine and Public Health sought out case studies demonstrating collaborative efforts, and used the meeting to highlight examples of the more than 400 case studies they collected. The nature of collaborative efforts was described in their report, *Medicine and Public Health: The Power of Collaboration*, published later in 1997.[12] In 1998, the Macy Foundation sponsored and published proceedings from a meeting in Florida titled *Education for More Synergistic Practice of Medicine and Public Health*. This conference explored the most effective way to educate and train physicians and public health professionals to enhance the synergistic practice of medicine and public health. The conference did not produce a recommended approach applicable in all situations, but it did produce agreement that the characteristics of successful collaborative practices should be extended and developed as teaching/learning centers.[13]

Some of the ongoing activities include: a 60-person national committee with representatives of AMA and APHA that meets biannually to explore ways to continue to bring medicine and public health together; over half of all states conduct state congresses to bring state-level leadership from medicine and public health together; a committee is examining curricula in schools of medicine and public health to improve awareness of each other's profession; and a research agenda around medicine/public health collaborations is under development.[14] Tangible evidence of the overlap between medicine and public health exists in both the AMA's medical journal, *Journal of the American Medical Association*, which publishes many articles of public health import, and in the AMA's policy positions on public health issues such as tobacco, substance use and abuse, sports injuries, and so forth.

MANAGED CARE

The swing to managed care after the defeat of the Clinton health care proposal could have acted as a stimulus to bring clinical care and public health into the same fold. After all, the central theme of managed care was to approach clinical care from a population perspective—that is, to understand the characteristics, epidemiologically speaking, of the managed care company's "covered lives," and to emphasize the employment of those clinical preventive services that would likely improve the length and quality of life for the enrolled population. Correctly done, this should meld with the broader population health promotion and disease prevention activities of public health services, and decrease disease and disability while helping to control medical care costs.

Unfortunately, managed care has evolved into an effort focused more on managing finances than on managing care. Many for-profit managed care companies were formed that began to compete for business by offering limited coverage plans for attractive, low prices. Prices were controlled by cutting reimbursements for providers (physicians, hospitals, etc.) and limiting access by patients to the more expensive services.[15] Patients were moved from one plan to another as employers shopped for the best prices. Many states opted to shift financial responsibility to providers by privatizing Medicaid and providing participating companies with a set amount per patient per year, allowing them to keep whatever was not spent. The trade-off was a relatively fixed and predictable state budget that was less than it previously had been. The combination of a transient "covered" population (if patients were leaving the plan before the benefit of preventive services would be seen, then money spent on prevention was wasted), and a drive to minimize costs created powerful disincentives to vigorously pursue preventive services.

The impact of managed care on health departments has been quite variable—some are affected substantially, others not at all. Certainly, those health departments that had been very involved in providing medical care to Medicaid and other underserved populations often found themselves suddenly exempted from eligibility to receive Medicaid payments in those locations where Medicaid was converted to managed care. Since the number of uninsured continued to grow as this process evolved, there was the perverse effect of diminishing resources available to the health care "safety net" as the need increased. Some health departments were able to become credentialed providers for managed care companies, and were able to receive reimbursement for some services delivered to managed care clients.[16]

The future of managed care is not clear. It is clear, however, that the current paradigm is in retreat. The restrictions on access and utilization have managed to anger both patients and providers, and support for the paradigm is diminishing steadily. No clear alternative has yet appeared, although there is a growing movement nationally for local communities to solve their access-to-care problem themselves.[17] These activities provide unique opportunities for local health departments to become leaders in the partnership development required for these local efforts to be successful.

PUBLIC HEALTH FUNCTIONS PROJECT

Organized by the federal government, this project includes representatives of federal public health agencies, national public health professional organizations, and major foundations interested in health. It has subcommittees and projects that include tracking and characterizing expenditures on public health; developing public health guidelines; training and educating the public health workforce, the public health infrastructure chapter of *Healthy People 2010;* and developing public health data for the twenty-first century, public health communications, and the essential services of public health. The project was created to help clarify the issues and develop strategies and tools to address the identified fragility of the public health infrastructure in the United States.[18]

NATIONAL PERFORMANCE STANDARDS

As noted in the thorough discussion of performance measurement in chapter 12, there was steady movement toward the development of public health performance measures during the twentieth century. The reasons for this movement are described there in detail. A recent catalyst for this evolution was the development of, and agreement about, the 10 essential services for public health. After all, if the public health profession is in general agreement about the major services required to have as healthy a population as possible, it makes sense to develop a system to measure how well the services are delivered.

The CDC, through its Public Health Practice Programs Office, launched an effort in the mid-1990s to develop a set of standards keyed to the 10 essential services that would help communities measure their capacity to deliver those services. Representatives from state and local health departments, national public health organizations, schools of public health, and federal agencies were brought together to develop performance standards for each of the 10 services. Separate standards for state and local systems were developed, and a continuum of performance levels was identified for each standard. The standard measurement tools were field tested in state and local health departments several times, and refined into workable tools now available from NACCHO and ASTHO.[19,20] In addition, a National Public Health Performance Standards Program Governance Tool intended to allow local governing bodies to evaluate themselves regarding their role in delivering the 10 services and to begin strategic planning is currently undergoing field testing.[21]

It was felt by many that these performance standards would be a mechanism to measure local health department performance. They may indeed prove helpful in that regard, but it is clear that they really measure the capacity of a *community* to deliver those services. It is clear that communities require a wide variety of services to maintain health, including, but not limited to, those services provided typically by health departments. The National Performance Standards are now proposed for use to assess the Local Public Health System (LPHS). The standards will be useful in measuring the impact of the consortium of community services required, emphasizing the notion that partnerships remain key to the improvement of health status at the local level.

COMMUNITY PREVENTIVE SERVICES GUIDELINES

In 1976, the Canadian government convened the Canadian Task Force on the Periodic Health Examination. This expert panel adopted a highly organized approach to evaluating the effectiveness of clinical preventive services. They developed explicit criteria to judge the quality of evidence from published clinical research, and uniform decision rules were used to link the strength or recommendations for or against a given preventive service to the quality of the underlying evidence. The idea was to provide the clinician with a means of selecting those preventive services supported by the strongest evidence of effectiveness. They examined evidence for preventive services for 78 conditions, and released recommendations in 1979. Revisions with coverage of new topics were created in 1984, 1986, and 1988.[22]

A similar effort was launched in the United States in 1984. The U.S. Task Force produced its first report in 1989 titled, *Guide to Clinical Preventive Services: An Assessment of the Effectiveness of 169 Interventions.*[23] In 1994, *The Clinician's Handbook of Preventive Services,* the second report of the U.S. Preventive Services Task Force, as part of the U.S. Public Health Service's Put Prevention Into Practice campaign, was published, followed by a second edition in 1998.[24] This work has successfully placed clinical preventive services on a strong science base, and identified areas of research need.

The Council on Linkages reasoned in 1993 that the same approach should be used for community-based prevention services. That is, the literature describing effectiveness of community programs and services should be scrutinized to determine which services are effective, which are not, and where the evidence is insufficient to make a judgment. The council decided to seek funding for a demonstration project to determine the value of such an approach and secured funding from the W.K. Kellogg Foundation for a pilot effort. The council set two goals for itself: to assess the desirability and feasibility of developing community preventive service guidelines, and to test the methodology for evaluating existing scientific evidence for the effectiveness of community interventions. It looked at immunization delivery, tuberculosis treatment completion, cardiovascular disease prevention, and lead poisoning prevention. The results indicated the validity of the approach.[25] The CDC was subsequently convinced the proposal was worthwhile, and established a Community Preventive Services Guidelines Project, which is currently ongoing.[26] A variety of community preventive services are currently under review, and interim reports of the project will be found in the literature. It is expected in the future that a compendium of project results will be published in a guide similar to the *Guide to Clinical Preventive Services.*

NATIONAL PUBLIC HEALTH RESEARCH AGENDA

The United States is strongly oriented to medical research and spends more money than any other country in that arena. A very small percentage of resources allocated for health-related research is spent in the domain of public health, however.[27] In a world of limited resources for public health and increasing accountability for positive health status outcomes it is increasingly important to focus attention on interventions that can be shown to be effective.

The U.S. Congress has been increasing the budget allocations for research steadily in recent years. The public health community would like to see a larger share of those dollars allocated to answer questions about community-based services. It is expected that the Community Preventive Services Guidelines Project will, among other things, create a community services research agenda by clarifying the science base for those services and noting where the science base is absent or inadequate.

Others are interested in this issue, as well. The Council on Linkages has been working to develop a research agenda based on the 10 essential services, and is working with representatives of academic institutions to bring that effort to fruition.

PUBLIC HEALTH LEADERSHIP INSTITUTES

An important response to the IOM finding in 1988 that suggested leadership in public health was suboptimal was the development of the National Public Health Leadership Institute and the subsequent development of a number of state and regional leadership institutes. These institutes have focused on identifying and training current and future public health leaders. Their development and current status are described in Appendix B.

HEALTHY PEOPLE 2010

Healthy People 2010 is the third iteration of a set of 10-year objectives for improvement in health status in the United States. *Healthy People 2010* contains a section on Public Health Infrastructure—chapter 23. The chapter contains 17 objectives: 7 in data and information systems, 3 related to workforce, 5 addressing public health organizations, and one each for resources and prevention research.[28] The addition of this subject to the document highlights the importance of improving the public health infrastructure and guarantees that progress in this area will be monitored in the best sense of the truism, "What gets measured gets done." The development of *Healthy People 2010* is described in chapter 10.

PUBLIC HEALTH CODE OF ETHICS

Public health, until recently, has been without a formal code of ethics to guide its practice. To be sure, the profession has considered itself to be inherently ethical with its activities based in an ethos of social justice, and has transferred many of the principles of medical

ethics to itself. Public health concerns are not equal to those of medicine, however. The discipline focuses more on populations than individuals, and more on prevention than cure. It includes those who are well, and for whom the risks and benefits of medical care are not particularly relevant.[29]

The Public Health Leadership Society, an outgrowth of the national Public Health Leadership Institute (see Appendix B), is leading a project to create a code of ethics for public health. A group of public health organizations is participating in the development of the code. Key principles of ethical public health practice[27] have been proposed as follows:

- Confidentiality of information
- Professional competence of employees
- Feedback from the community
- The empowerment of disenfranchised community members
- Community input on programs and policies

Key values and beliefs are proposed for each principle. It is expected that a process of open review and discussion of the proposed document will soon lead to agreement across the profession on the components that will be included in the first-ever public health code of ethics.

TERRORISM

Chemicals and communicable disease agents have been intentionally employed as weapons in human conflict for many years. Until the 1990s, their use, or contemplated use, focused principally on employment as a battlefield weapon between two opposing armed forces. The attack on the Tokyo subway system with the nerve gas sarin in 1995 brought the danger faced by civilians from chemical and biological attacks to the world's attention. The growth of terrorist attacks on civilian populations around the world created enough concern to stimulate improvement of capacity to prevent and respond to threatened or actual incidents.[30] The terrorist attacks on the World Trade Center in New York City on September 11, 2001, followed by the mailing of letters contaminated with anthrax spores to certain media outlets and national governmental figures in the United States in early October 2001, added new urgency to terrorism preparedness activities. For a discussion of these issues, please see chapter 29.

CONCLUSION

If a central theme has been emerging as public health reinvents itself, it is the importance of partnerships in practically all phases of that reinvention. Partnerships were essential for the work that led to the development of workforce competencies, and they are essential for the ongoing definition and application of those competencies. The conversion of the IOM's core public health functions into the 10 essential services required partnerships, as did the communication processes used to gain their acceptance by the profession and their inclusion in the Clinton health care reform proposal. The development of several important national public health associations and the evolution of others are examples of people working together as partners. Important work coordinated by federal agencies was and remains characterized by the many different groups and individuals that are brought to the table as meaningful participants. Public health academicians and practitioners are reconnecting and the relevance of training to practice is improving. Concentrated efforts to bring the separate cultures of medicine and public health more closely together indicate growing awareness that delivery of the 10 essential services and health status improvement are dependent on both sectors working in a coordinated fashion. Indeed, the National Performance Standards, themselves the product of working partnerships, will measure the effectiveness of Local Public Health Systems, partnerships by definition.

Public health is in a renaissance period. It has reached new levels of understanding and relevance. Its scientific base is expanding and its effectiveness is improving. Training programs are growing at an almost exponential rate, and organized efforts are focused on finding and training public health leaders. Resources do not yet match need, but innovation and change has become the norm. It is reasonable to expect this evolution to continue resulting in increasing effectiveness of the profession's organized efforts to protect the public's health.

References

1. Institute of Medicine, Committee for the Study of the Future of Public Health. *The Future of Public Health.* Washington, DC: National Academy Press; 1988.
2. Roper WL, Baker EL, Dyal WW, Nicola RM. Strengthening the public health system. *Public Health Rep.* 1993;107(6):609-615.
3. *Health Security Act, Title III-Public Health Initiatives, HR3600.* Washington, DC: 103rd Congress; 1993.
4. Washington State Department of Health. *Public Health Improvement Plan.* Olympia: Washington State Depart of Health; 1994.
5. *Blueprint for a Healthy Community: A Guide for Local Health Departments.* Washington, DC: National Association of County Health Officials; 1994.
6. Public Health in America. Available at: http://www.health.gov/phfunctions/public.htm.
7. Sorensen AA, Bialek RG. *The Public Health Faculty Agency Forum: Linking Graduate Education and Practice, Final Report.* Gainesville: University Press of Florida; 1993.
8. Council on Linkages Between Academia and Public Health Practice. Available at: http://www.phf.org/Link.htm.
9. Council on Linkages Between Academia and Public Health Practice. *Core Competencies for Public Health Practice.* Washington, DC: Council on Linkages Between Academia and Public Health Practice; 2001. Available at: http://www.trainingfinder.org/competencies/list/htm.
10. Evans P. *Council on Education for Public Health.* [personal communication]. Washington, DC; March 2001.
11. Public Health Practice Program Office. Available at: http://www.phppo.cdc.gov/.
12. Lasker RD. *Medicine and Public Health: The Power of Collaboration.* New York: The New York Academy of Medicine; 1997.
13. Hager M. *Education for More Synergistic Practice of Medicine and Public Health.* New York, NY: The Josiah Macy Jr. Foundation; 1999.

14. American Public Health Association. Available at: http://www.sph.uth.tmc.edu/mph/.

15. Robinson JC. The end of managed care. *JAMA.* 2001;285(20):2622-2628.

16. Scutchfield DS, Harris JR, Koplan JP, et al. Managed care and public health. *J Public Health Manage Pract.* 1998;4(1):1-11.

17. *Tackling the Uninsured Puzzle: Collaborating for Community Care.* Englewood, Colo: Medical Group Management Association; 2001.

18. Public Health Functions Project. Available at: http://www.health.gov/phfunctions/project.htm.

19. National Public Health Performance Standards Program Local Public Health System Performance Assessment Instrument. Available at: http://www.naccho.org/files/documents/ NPHPSP_Local_Final_11-29-01.PDF.

20. National Public Health Performance Standards Program State Public Health System Performance Assessment Instrument. Available at: http://www.astho.org/phiip/pdf/pmstate.pdf.

21. The National Public Health Performance Standards Program Governance Tool. Available at: http://www.nalboh.org/perfstds/perfstds.htm.

22. Canadian Task Force on the Periodic Health Examination. The Periodic Health Examination. *Can Med Assoc J.* 1979;121:1194-1254.

23. *Guide to Clinical Preventive Services: An Assessment of the Effectiveness of 169 Interventions.* Baltimore, Md: Williams & Wilkens; 1989.

24. *Clinician's Handbook of Preventive Services.* 2nd ed. Washington, DC: Office of Disease Prevention and Health Promotion, US Public Health Service; 1998.

25. Lloyd P, Bialek R, et al. *Practice Guidelines for Public Health: Assessment of Scientific Evidence, Feasibility and Benefits.* Washington, DC: Council on Linkages Between Academia and Public Health; 1995.

26. McGinnis MJ, Foege W. Guide to community preventive services: Harnessing the science. *Am J Prev Med.* 2000;18(1S):1-2.

27. Council on Linkages Public Health Research Project. Available at: http://www.phf.org/Link/vol13nl/ devagend-ronbialek.htm.

28. *Healthy People 2010.* 2nd ed. Washington, DC: US Depart of Health and Human Services; 2000.

29. American Public Health Association. *Code of Ethics.* 2001. Available at: http://www.apha.org/ codeofethics/.

30. *Chemical and Biological Terrorism: Research and Development to Improve Civilian Medical Response.* Institute of Medicine, National Research Council. Washington, DC: National Academy Press; 1999.

CHAPTER

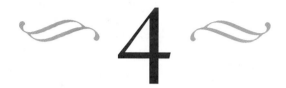

4

The Determinants of Health

John M. Last, M.D.
J. Michael McGinnis, M.D.

Determinants of health include genetic predispositions, environmental exposures (especially to pathogenic organisms), social circumstances, behavioral patterns, and medical (health) care. No single determinant is the most important: many are involved in either promoting or impairing individual and community health. Although, for a given individual, a dominant influence can be exerted by a lethal inborn error of metabolism or a disabling injury, most determinants interact, often synergistically rather than separately, with the circumstances that affect health. Sometimes the interactions are complex and nonlinear, as illustrated by disruptions of essential life-supporting ecosystems.

Use of the word *determinant* does not imply belief in determinism, which reasons that health and illness are determined by fate or some supernatural power. Other terms that convey the same meaning as *determinant* in the context of this discussion are *prerequisites for health*, and *risk (or protective) factors*. These terms are often preferable to *determinants* when talking about health and how it is affected for better or worse by the innumerable influences to which every one of us is exposed throughout the period between conception and death.

DEFINITIONS OF HEALTH

The preamble to the constitution of the World Health Organization (WHO) describes health as "a state of complete physical, mental and social well-being, not merely the absence of disease or infirmity."[1] This describes an ideal state, but is operationally limited. The word *complete* would compel an exhaustive inventory of subclassifications of the perfect, and *social well-being* is a notion with elusive boundaries. In practice, this definition cannot be used to compare personal or community health status at different times, in different places, or among different kinds of persons.

In the early 1980s when WHO initiated its health promotion programs, new dimensions were added to its definition of health to convey the important idea that individuals and groups have some control over their own health:

> Health is . . . the extent to which an individual or a group is able to realize aspirations and satisfy needs; and to change or cope with the environment. Health is . . . a resource for everyday life, not the objective of living; it is a positive concept, emphasizing social and personal resources, as well as physical capacities.[2]

Humans do not live in a vacuum but interact with each other and with many other kinds of living creatures in local, regional, and global ecosystems. A definition that takes this into account describes health as "a state of equilibrium between humans and their physical, biologic, social and cultural environment that is compatible with full functional activity."[3] If the environment is unable to sustain the population that inhabits it, then the population cannot be called healthy so a modified definition of health might read:

> Health is a sustainable state of equilibrium between humans and their physical, biological, social, and cultural environment, compatible with full functional activity of all interacting components in the ecosystem.

There are problems with this definition too. If pathogens or their vectors are part of the ecosystem, should they, too, be sustained? Experience with proliferating antibiotic-resistant pathogens and pesticide-resistant insect vectors in the second half of the twentieth century demonstrated the impossibility of winning an "arms race" against common pathogens and insect vectors. Antibiotic resistance develops more rapidly than new antibiotics can be discovered. A more realistic strategy is to find ways of living in harmony with pathogens and vectors. We do this by immunizing populations against common pathogens like the diphtheria bacillus, and by the use of bed-nets and other measures to provide protection from mosquitoes. This obviates the impossible task of eradicating all insect vectors such as mosquitoes (together with many useful insect species) by massive applications of pesticides that often have harmful effects on the environment and on animal and human health. In this context, this is a useful definition of health because it takes these determinants into account. It also cautions against taking a short-term view of health; if health is borrowed from the capital resources that future generations of humans will need for their survival, a present healthy state is an illusion.

Whether we describe them as determinants, prerequisites, or factors affecting health, we can identify six domains: inherent or genetic predispositions (including gender and age), environmental exposures (including ionizing radiation, toxic chemicals, noise), biological factors (including exposure to pathogens, immune responses), social circumstances (including income, education, social ties, levels of disparity), behavioral patterns (including diet, physical activity, sexual activity, coping, use of addictive substances), and medical care (including receipt of preventive services and treatment of acute conditions). However, simple classifications must be used with caution because they can obscure the innumerable complex interactions that commonly exist among determinants.

Genetic Predispositions

The human genome's 3 billion base pairs and 30–40,000 genes exert their influence on health in various ways. Each of us has embedded in our coding platform the assembly-line blueprint for construction of the proteins that give form to our sizes, our shapes, our personalities, even to the biological limit of our life expectancies—in theory, somewhere between 85 and 110 years, if fibroblast tissue cultures are to be believed. Eons of adaptation have given an approximate form to these instructions which are essentially similar across individuals, and sets us each on a course we call "normal"—that is, one which is not markedly disadvantaged for the environments in which we find ourselves.

In medicine and human biology, nothing is simple. Few things can be categorized in neat, clearly circumscribed compartments, and fewer still in simple binary terms. Congenital conditions may be the result of factors in the physical environment, such as chemicals or radiation, or the result of invading microorganisms, such as the rubella virus. Genetic makeup is determined by the mating patterns of one's ancestors, whose genetic makeup, in turn, was influenced by the inherent susceptibility or resistance of their ancestors to certain diseases (for example, measles, influenza, smallpox, plague, and malaria) that selectively attacked or spared particular genotypes.[4] Moreover, in virtually all settings, from primitive societies through rural agrarian states to modern industrial nations, mating tends to be more assortative than random, so patterns of gene frequency become a mosaic that is attributable to a combination of environmental, cultural, economic, social, and behavioral factors.

The *personal* qualities alluded to in the 1984 WHO definition include attributes routinely recorded in medical records and health statistics. We display health status in tables arranged according to the most important of these attributes, namely age, and sex, and sometimes according to others such as race.

Age and Sex

Age and sex are important determinants of health status. From conception through old age, mortality rates are higher for males than females, although health care utilization statistics nearly all show higher rates of utilization for females than males, even when reasons related to pregnancy and childbirth are excluded. However, females do not live longer on average than males because they use more health care services (perhaps in spite of it) but because of inherent, ill-defined biological characteristics.

Age is an obvious determinant of health. Infants, especially if they are underweight or prematurely born, are more vulnerable to many diseases than are older children. Record linkage studies have shown that premature infants are at increased risk of adult onset conditions, such as elevated serum cholesterol, hypertension, and coronary heart disease. Maternal nutritional status during pregnancy and lactation, rather than birth weight or prematurity, is probably the principal factor responsible for the apparent association of birth weight with elevated serum cholesterol, hypertension, coronary heart disease, and predisposition to diabetes in adult life.[5] The peak of fitness and good health is reached after adolescence,

and then health and physical vitality and efficiency slowly decline until the seventh or eighth decade. By the late 60s, most people are taking regular medication and can count their identified infirmities in double figures (failing eyesight and hearing, poor or no teeth, varicose veins, hernias, deteriorating genital tracts, and stiffening joints, among others). By the second half of the 80s, most people need personal care, often in a long-term-care institution.[6]

Our paleolithic hunter-gatherer ancestors had a life expectancy of 30–35 years. Procreation began in the early to mid-teens, so the generation "gap" was about 15 years—parents mostly survived long enough to nurture their offspring. Over time, populations expanded and outgrew their local ecosystems, prompting the diasporas that spread humans all over the world. The resulting gene-environment interactions fostered diversity, which evolutionary biologists regard as desirable. Despite occasional devastating epidemics, life expectancy increased over the centuries in agricultural civilizations. By the early twentieth century, it had reached 60 years in industrial nations. The gap between generations expanded to 20–25 years and is still expanding. This demographic transition led to a decline in family size. In many Western industrial nations this is below replacement level. Nuclear families, and society at large, have to shelter and sustain increasing numbers of aged and infirm dependents, likely exceeding 20 percent by the mid-twenty-first century.

These actuarial and socioeconomic facts have political implications not discussed here. They also may have long-term implications for the future of the human species. They reduce prospects for future human diversity, which relies on gene-environment interaction. Philosophers might debate whether human evolution is influenced for the better or worse by interventions such as the social, economic, and medical advances that led to the demographic and epidemiologic transitions that have yielded life expectancies in the upper 70s—and by the more deliberate interventions of new reproductive technologies and, soon, human genetic engineering. Because of the length of generations, it might be several hundred years before our descendants will be able to determine whether the actions of those now living have improved or damaged the human gene pool.

Race

Dictionaries define *race* as a major division of humankind having distinct physical characteristics. Visible diversity notwithstanding, at the molecular level of DNA, all humans are virtually identical. Social scientists have challenged the biological definition of race, arguing that the concept most often reflects social and ideological conventions. They claim that economic, social, cultural, and behavioral differences are more important than biological factors in determining differences in health status usually attributed to race.[7] While this is true, susceptibility and resistance to some conditions is unequivocally associated with the physical characteristics conventionally defined as racial. For example, pigmented skin provides better protection from solar ultraviolet radiation than skin lacking much pigment, accounting for the high incidence of all forms of skin cancer, especially malignant melanoma, among fair-skinned people who expose their skin surface to the sun. The word *race* has acquired strong emotional overtones, but classification of populations on the basis of race or ethnicity remains useful and generally valid for the analysis of social and health statistics—although the influence of confounding factors must always be borne in mind when interpreting the statistics. African Americans have higher prevalence and mortality rates from hypertension and cancer of the prostate than Americans of European origin. Native Americans (Indians) . . . and descendants of other hunter-gatherer populations in transition to Western diets and lifestyles . . . have a higher prevalence of diabetes and, among some tribal groups, of arthritis when compared to Euro-Americans. Some Orthodox Jews carry the gene for Tay-Sachs disease.

These and other conditions that are described as racially determined are either of genetic origin (such as Tay-Sachs disease) or attributable to a combination of inherited, environmental, and socially and culturally determined factors. Both African Americans and Native Americans include high proportions of persons whose traditional culture and values have been destroyed or gravely damaged. They often come from deprived socio-economic backgrounds, and the real "cause" of at least some of their high prevalence and mortality rates from the above conditions and others, such as alcohol and substance abuse, is confounded by these factors.

Physical Determinants

Physical determinants of health include first and foremost the radiant energy that reaches the earth from the sun. The sun is the giver of all life, the source of energy, the force that triggers the metabolism of carbon, nitrogen, and oxygen in plant and animal systems. However, too much sunshine is harmful: excess ultraviolet radiation causes skin cancer, and leads to cataracts.[8]

Another set of physical factors that determine health are elements essential for life, such as iron, iodine, and copper, among many others and those that harm health, such as environmental lead,[9] mercury, cadmium, and organic compounds . . . especially persistant organic pollutants (POPs). The air may be polluted with solid particulates, asbestos, or tobacco smoke. Drinking water may contain insufficient concentrations of fluoride for the manufacture of strong dental enamel, or it may contain toxic chemicals or any of innumerable pathogens.

Biological Determinants

The biological determinants of health include all the microorganisms that may cause harm, as well as biological products such as sera and vaccines that help protect against disease. Some bacteria live in symbiosis with humans in the gastrointestinal tract, manufacturing vitamins that are needed for good health. There is an uneasy truce between humans and pathogenic microorganisms for much of the time, and this truce is in the interests of both parties. If invading pathogens are too harmful, they may die if they kill their human host; if humans are totally shielded from exposure to pathogens such as common cold viruses, they lose their immunities and can then be overwhelmed when they are eventually reexposed. Many of the pathogenic microorganisms that cause ill health do so because of a combination of ecological and behavioral factors.

Another class of biological determinants of health are the essential dietary nutrients: the carbohydrates, proteins, fats, minerals, and vitamins that are derived from plant and animal sources. With these, as with many other determinants, health is optimal when the right balance is struck between deficit and excess.

Behavioral Determinants

For much of the developed world, behavioral patterns represent the single most controllable domain of influence over our health prospects. The choices we make with respect to diet, physical activity, and sex, the substance abuse and addictions to which we fall prey, our approach to safety, and our coping strategies in confronting stress, all are important determinants of health. Dietary factors have been associated with coronary heart disease, stroke, cancers of the colon, breast, and prostate, and diabetes. Physical inactivity has been associated with increased risk for heart disease, colon cancer, diabetes, and osteoporosis. Unprotected sexual intercourse is accountable not only for millions of unintended pregnancies and sexually transmitted diseases, but also for deaths from HIV, hepatitis B, cervical cancer, and excess infant mortality. Substance abuse and addiction inflict a tremendous toll on health and the lives of people throughout the world. Not only is tobacco the leading single contributor to deaths in many countries, but substance abuse as a whole represents the most prominent contributor to the constellation of preventable illnesses, health costs, and related social problems facing families and communities in the world today.

An analysis of factors underlying all deaths occurring in 1990 in the United States indicated that approximately 19 percent were attributable to tobacco, 14 percent to diet and physical inactivity, 5 percent to alcohol, and 1 percent each to firearms, sexual activity, and use of illicit drugs.[10] The impact of these behavioral factors extends far beyond the mortality tables as sources of millions of illnesses and disabilities.

As people have learned more about the impact of behavioral factors they have begun to make changes. Over the past 30 years, smoking rates have been cut in half in several developed nations, consumption of foods high in saturated fats and cholesterol have declined considerably, impressive gains have been achieved with respect to seat belt use and driving under the influence of alcohol. Still, the gap is substantial between current practices and potential gains. With increasing discoveries from gene studies on the specific and varied susceptibilities of individuals to health problems deriving from their behavioral choices, with more work to develop social signals that support patterns of behavior more conducive to health, and with enhanced understanding of neurochemical factors that shape outlooks, attitudes, tendencies, and dependencies, there is potential for moderating the impact of behavioral patterns on poor health.

We need to know and understand better the roots of these unhealthy behaviors, and we need to find ways to modify them in the interests of better health. Health education and health promotion campaigns have often failed because they send negative messages ("don't smoke, don't have casual sex, don't drink and drive," etc.) about activities that people find pleasurable and because insufficient effort has been made to understand why people behave in these health-damaging ways.

Social Determinants

In 1911, the registrar-general of England and Wales, T. H. C. Stevenson, devised an occupational classification that grouped employed persons into five *social classes.* It was immediately observed that there were striking and consistent relationships between *social class,* now usually referred to as socioeconomic status (SES), and incidence of health and sickness.

There have been many refinements of Stevenson's classification with the recognition that educational level, occupation, income, and housing conditions are interrelated and all influence health. The relationship has held true at all times since the early twentieth century and in all nations and social contexts in which it has been examined. Poverty and income disparities have been consistently associated with substantially increased risk of illness and death, independent of other risk factors. Adults, including older people, who are socially isolated have a two- to fourfold higher death rate than others, and risk of a similar magnitude is experienced by those who are poorly educated. Children who are raised in families under social stress are at greater risk of illness and injury.

The prospect for moderating the impact of these conditions is offered by the observation that home visits by trained nurses to at-risk mothers can reduce the likelihood of adverse health outcomes among their children—both risky health behaviors and criminal activity—some 15 years later.

The relationship of SES to health has several underlying causes. It is not fully explained by the fact that well-educated people have higher incomes, live in better homes where they are less exposed to environmental health risks, have better quality health care, and are more likely to avoid risk factors such as smoking, than the poorly educated. The relationship is not the same as the occupational association of health risks to dangerous trades such as underground mining. It is indirectly related, however, in that industrial and manual workers and their families tend to be financially worse off than clerical workers, to live in less salubrious housing conditions, and to have customs and habits, such as heavy use of alcohol and tobacco, that expose them to other risks.

While it is daunting to contemplate ameliorating such overwhelming influences as poverty or education, there are some hints of practical smaller scale interventions in the common ways by which social stresses act to increase health risk—through common pathways related, for example, to notions of empowerment, self-esteem, and locus of control, which might be subject to intervention.

Mind-body interactions and other intangible factors further complicate the relationship between SES and health. The subtle interaction between self-esteem, job satisfaction, and good health, for example, is influenced by levels of intelligence and insight and by one's image of one's familial and social role.[11]

Cultural Determinants

Culture is the set of values, historical traditions, customs, and intellectual, artistic, and behavioral characteristics and beliefs, including religious beliefs and associated customs, that are common to a nation or a community. They often seem to be an integral part of ethnicity and are usually maintained constantly over many generations. Medical anthropologists have identified many ways in which culture plays an important role in shaping the health and sickness experience of well-defined social groups, not only in so-called primitive societies but also in subcultures in many modern Western industrial nations. For example, variations in incidence rates of cancer of the reproductive organs (breast, cervix, and prostate) among people of different religious backgrounds seem sometimes to be related to differences in diet; sometimes to exposure, or lack of it, to sexually transmitted viruses that can cause cancer; and sometimes to culturally determined differences in reproductive behavior and breast-feeding practices.

The custom of circumcision, excision of the male prepuce, dates back to prehistory. It is embedded as a culturally determined custom in some surviving neolithic cultures (e.g., in New Guinea and Australian Aborigines where it may be related to tribal hierarchy). Jews perform ritual circumcision on the eighth day after birth, and Moslem boys undergo circumcision later in childhood. There is strong and consistent epidemiological evidence of lower rates of some types of cancer of the genital tract apparently associated with circumcision, but the true association may be with customs relating to sexual hygiene rather than circumcision.

A nation's collective attitude toward human sexuality is culturally determined and can profoundly influence several aspects of reproductive health. Particularly notable are the risks of unwanted pregnancy and sexually transmitted diseases, including HIV infection, especially among sexually active teenagers. In the United States, the pregnancy rate among 15- to 17-year-olds is more than twice that for Canada, threefold that for Sweden, and ninefold the rate for the Netherlands. Clearly the behaviors involved, including those related to the accessibility and attitudes toward contraception, are culturally derived.

Spiritual Determinants

"Spiritual determinants" here do not refer to religious beliefs but to more subtle phenomena, such as the view that individuals and communities hold of their place in nature. These views help to determine individual and community health. Reactions of individuals and families to the occurrence of life-threatening disease, for example, vary in ways that are best described as spiritual. (Do we strive so officiously to keep alive the irretrievably ill because we do not believe in an afterlife, or because we do?)

Perceptions of the relationship of humans to the natural world we inhabit can be described as "spiritual" whether or not we believe in God or the supernatural. A belief that the world was created for the benefit of humankind is sometimes associated with exploitation of natural resources and could lead to ecological catastrophe. A belief that humans are "partners" with other forms of life on earth is more compatible with long-term sustainability of essential life-supporting ecosystems. This belief is common in so-called primitive or animist religions, and to some extent Hindu and Buddhist religious philosophies.

If a healthy human species is to live forever on a healthy planet, perhaps everyone should embrace primitive or animist religions. (Of course humanity will not live *forever*. On theoretical grounds, the total longevity of the human species has been calculated to be in the range of 0.2 to 8.0 million years, with a confidence interval of 95 percent.[12] This takes no account of the possibility of extermination in a nuclear holocaust or destruction of humans and many other life forms in a slower but equally relentless ecological catastrophe.)

Medical Care

The preponderant determinants of the health status of populations fall outside the domain of medical care, but, when we fall ill our access to high-quality medical care is of vital, and increasing importance. As the population prevalence of chronic conditions increases due to greater survival rates at both ends of the life spectrum, the importance of medical care to population health will surely grow. As a result, we can anticipate that the twenty-first century will see medical care expanding its capacity for a more nurturing and supportive approach to both the psychological and emotional needs of patients. In order to accomplish this, the medical field will continue to draw upon advances in immunology, the neurosciences, molecular biology and recombinant DNA technologies, and the engineering sciences for application of new technologies in orthopedics and organ and tissue repair and replacement, vaccine development, pharmaceuticals and pharmaceutical delivery systems, human reproduction, and mood and memory function.

Interactions and Multifactoral Causation

Tuberculosis is not caused by *Mycobacterium tuberculosis* alone, but by the combination of poverty, overcrowding, poor nutrition, ignorance, and often other environmental, social, and behavioral factors that together create circumstances in which *M. tuberculosis*, the seed, finds fertile human soil in which it can grow. *M. tuberculosis* is the essential precipitating factor. The other determinants—poverty, overcrowding, poor nutrition, and so on—are predisposing, enabling, and reinforcing factors.

Many infectious microorganisms behave similarly, although the reasons for susceptibility or resistance vary. The cholera vibrio, for example, strikes hardest at those who are poorly nourished and therefore often have little or no gastric acid to kill the organism. Thus, cholera is to some extent a disease of the underprivileged. The cholera vibrio also thrives in the company of certain seasonally and climatically dependent algae,[13] which accounts for the occurrence of cholera in waves or pandemics that relate to climatic cycles.

Malaria, too, behaves in ways that make it clear there are more than mosquitoes, plasmodia, and people involved in the mathematics that determines its incidence and prevalence. Rich people mostly live further from malarial swamps than poor people do. They also tend to live in houses that are better screened against mosquitoes and to have clothing that protects more of their skin surface. As a result, they are less often the source of the blood meal that the female mosquito requires to survive. Rich (educated) people also tend to know more about the habits of mosquitoes and can take steps to reduce the risks of being bitten by them.

The relationship between infection and poverty or deprivation is strong and consistent. Throughout history, scarlet fever, measles, whooping cough, typhoid, and diphtheria have all exacted a heavier toll from the poor than from the rich.[14] The mortality rates of all these diseases declined in the nineteenth century, well before effective preventive or therapeutic measures were available. Mortality rates varied inversely with the rising standards of living as the industrial revolution advanced.[15,16]

These mortality and morbidity differentials hold true for other environmentally determined conditions, such as industrial and domestic injuries. It is understandable that workers in dangerous trades such as mining, heavy transport, deep-sea fishing, and forestry should have higher rates of occupational causes of death and injury than white-collar workers. Their homes are often unsafe, too, so domestic accidents occur more frequently than in wealthy homes, and their children have higher rates of injury because they are less likely to have a safe place to play.

There are a few exceptions to the rule about affluence and good health. Until the recent past, poliomyelitis and hepatitis A have had higher attack rates among the affluent than the poor. The explanation is that higher proportions of the poor were exposed in infancy and early childhood, when subclinical infection is more common. Among well-off people, by contrast, first exposure to these fecal-oral infections more often occurred in later childhood or adolescence, when a more severe and clinically apparent manifestation of these diseases was likely to occur. Hodgkin's disease and child leukemia follow this pattern in some degree, raising the suspicion that an infectious organism may be implicated. Breast cancer also tends to be a more common cause of death among wealthy than poor women, but this association is confounded by many other factors including breast-feeding practices and obesity, which is a risk factor for breast cancer.

PUTTING THE DETERMINANTS OF HEALTH IN CONTEXT

The necessary and sufficient causes of health and disease usually occur in specific environmental, social, occupational, and cultural contexts. In the urbanizing industrial world of the second half of the nineteenth century, horse-drawn transport was the rule. Horses had to be stabled, and they deposited large amounts of manure in these stables, which were often fairly close to the homes of even the most affluent citizens.

Horse manure is an ideal breeding ground for flies, which, the social historians report, were ubiquitous in that era.

The invention of the internal combustion engine changed all this: motor cars replaced horses, stables (and streets) full of manure became a thing of the past, and with them went most of the flies, which had been the passive vector for a great many fecal-oral pathogens that cause diarrheal diseases. Increasing affluence that provided the wherewithal for screened windows and improved kitchen hygiene also helped reduce the contamination of food by the "filthy feet of fecal-feeding flies." However, the principal determinant of reduced infant and child morbidity and mortality from diarrheal diseases in the first half of the twentieth century in the industrial world was probably the invention of the internal combustion engine, which led to this important transformation of urban ecosystems.

Ecological interactions are involved in modern public health problems in a similar manner. However, the critical links that must be broken in the causal chain have yet to be identified, even for the most common cause of premature cardiovascular death—coronary heart disease. Unsolved questions persist regarding the interaction of diet, exercise, addiction to cigarette smoking, hereditary factors, and relationships to family members and coworkers. It is not yet completely understood why coronary heart disease mortality rates in men declined by about 40 percent in the United States, Australia, and Canada between the late 1960s and the early 1990s, while the rates did not decline in the same way or at the same pace among women or decline at all (indeed, they increased for a time) in Scotland, Sweden, and Switzerland. The relationship to changes in known risk factors, such as diet, exercise, and cigarette smoking, does not follow a consistent pattern.

Even when the critical causal links have been identified, society may lack the political will to do what is required to break them. This applies to the public health problems associated with addiction to tobacco. The fact that tobacco is addictive has consistently been denied by the tobacco industry and its supporters; to admit that tobacco is addictive would place the industry in a morally untenable position. Efforts to prevent the industry from recruiting new child smokers, to replace those in older cohorts who have been killed by their addiction, are frustrated by political and ethical restraints on censorship of tobacco advertising and by a failure to find convincing ways to convey the negative message "Don't smoke" to a target population that is often inherently rebellious against parental and other adult authorities. The worldwide public health problem of tobacco addiction is more difficult to deal with because of the heavy investment of the tobacco industry in advertising and political lobbying in virtually every nation and increasingly in the developing nations.

Another prominent public health problem in the United States is intentional violence, especially homicide and particularly homicide caused by firearms among young, urban, male African Americans, many of whom belong to an alienated underclass. Most of the links in this chain of causation probably have been identified. This is a culturally determined problem. Other Western industrial nations have an urban underclass, often one that is racially distinct from the majority, but none have experienced intentional violence or homicide due to guns on a comparable scale.

The problem is usually attributed to the easy availability of handguns in the United States, which is facilitated by the constitutional *right* to bear arms and the highly successful lobbying efforts of the National Rifle Association. There is no doubt about the link between availability of handguns and homicide (as well as suicide and accidental death) caused by handguns; but it is too facile to suggest that this alone accounts for the very high mortality rates from firearm injuries experienced by young African-American males in the United States. Other cultures in which firearms are present in virtually every household, such as Switzerland, have orders of magnitude fewer deaths due to firearms,[17] as shown in Table 4.1.

The difference in mortality rates due to firearm injuries between the United States and other nations is probably due to a difference in value systems. Resorting to firearms as a way of settling disputes seems to be an almost uniquely American value. It appears to have become firmly established and further enhanced over time since early in the twentieth century. It is reinforced by the presentation in movies and on television of fictional dramas in which the heroes and villains resolve their disputes with guns. Life then imitates art.

Table 4.1. Homicide Rates per 100,000— Various Countries

Switzerland	0.1
Canada	2.2
United States	10.5

Source: World Health Organization.

There is consistent and persuasive evidence for an association, probably causal, between the portrayal of violence on television and the occurrence of violence in real life.[18] The mind-set begins early in life, when toddlers and kindergarten children watch cartoons in which the Road Runner blows up the coyote and the canary successfully thwarts the cat, always with displays of violence that are presented as though they were hilariously funny. The process continues throughout childhood and into adult life, with entertainment (now no longer necessarily funny) incessantly emphasizing violent means of settling disputes. The preferred sports of many Americans also involve displays of brute force.

Contrast this with European nations, where the television programs and cartoons that children see are generally free of violence, the most popular films and television programs are mostly about aspects of civilized behavior and variations of normal adult interactions, and the preferred sports often emphasize elegance and skill rather than brute force. These culturally determined differences are striking, and changing them will not be easy.

Human-Induced Global Ecosystem Changes

The global commons—the stratosphere, the world's climate, the oceans, the freshwater cycle, tropical and boreal wilderness forests, fertile land, stocks of biodiversity—are affected by human activities.[19] Human-induced changes in all these are important environmental determinants of health. Most important and obvious are changes in the atmosphere, briefly described here.

Stratospheric Ozone Attenuation

Chlorofluorocarbons (CFCs) are an industrially important and seemingly inert family of chemicals,

Table 4.2.   Biological and Human Health Effects of Elevated Solar Ultraviolet Radiation

Ecological Effects

- Impaired photosynthesis
- Impaired plant growth
- Impaired phytoplankton reproduction
- Viability of pollen grains reduced

Agricultural Effects

Impaired reproductive capacity of plants and animals
Possible damage to nitrogen-fixing soil bacteria
Impaired plant and animal health (e.g., cancer risk
   increased in animal herds)

Human Health Effects

- Immunodeficiency
   —Enhanced susceptibility to infections
   —Enhanced risk of cancer

- Effects on Skin
   —Sunburn
   —Loss of elasticity (premature aging)
   —Photosensitivity
- Skin Cancer
   —Rodent ulcer
   —Basal and squamous cell cancer
   —Malignant melanoma
- Effect on the Eyes
   —Cataract
   —Damage to the retina and cornea
- Effects Related to Cellular Damage

widely used as refrigerants, solvents, and aerating agents. Unfortunately they degrade to chlorine monoxide when exposed to ionizing radiation in the upper atmosphere, and chlorine monoxide destroys ozone. In 1985, observers in Antarctica reported a large region of attenuation (the "ozone hole"). The ozone layer protects the biosphere from exposure to lethal levels of solar ultraviolet radiation flux, so ozone depletion endangers many forms of life on earth—including humans. The Montreal Protocol of 1987 was an international accord to phase out production and use of CFCs. Bromine fertilizers used in rice cultivation, and nitrogen oxides produced by fossil fuel combustion, also contribute to the ozone-destroying process. CFCs have an atmospheric half-life of 50–100 years, so the stratospheric ozone layer will take many decades to recover. Surface and satellite observations show that stratospheric ozone attenuation is progressive. Since the first observations there has been a loss of 3–4 percent worldwide, and much greater seasonal losses in the circumpolar regions. This harms many organisms, ranging from ocean phytoplankton (at the base of marine food chains, and an important sink for carbon emissions) to large mammals including humans.[20]

The adverse effects on human health include increased risk of ocular cataracts, loss of skin elasticity (premature aging), and skin cancers—rodent ulcer, basal and squamous cell, and most dangerous, malignant melanoma. All have been observed with increasing frequency especially among people who do not have much protective pigment in their skin. Higher exposure can impair immunity by damaging the cells in the deep layers of the dermis that are responsible for maintaining cell-mediated immunity (Table 4.2).

Climate Change as a Determinant of Health

The Intergovernmental Panel on Climate Change (IPCC) was established in the late 1980s to assess the effects of atmospheric changes accompanying industrial development. The third assessment report of IPCC in February 2001 provided convincing evidence that climate change, that is, global warming due to accumulation of atmospheric greenhouse gases, is happening, and is caused by human activities, especially the emission products of fossil fuel combustion.[21] This could have serious effects on health, as well as on the integrity of life-supporting ecosystems[22] (Table 4.3). Several of these effects are interconnected with other human-induced alterations in the earth's life-supporting ecosystems. Destruction of tropical and boreal forests, reduced biodiversity accompanying proliferation of monoculture crops, loss of agricultural

Table 4.3.   Some Effects of Climate Change on Human Health

Impact Category	Mediating Process	Health Outcomes	Examples
Physical	Heat waves	Heat stress	Heat stroke, heart failure
Physical/chemical	Air pollution, floods, toxic waste	Respiratory disease Poisoning (acute or chronic), cancer	Obstructive lung disease, asthma
Physical/biological	Disease agents, vectors	Waterborne illness Vector-borne disease	Cholera, cryptosporidiosis, E. coli 0157
Reduced food production	Poor access	Nutritional deficits	Malaria, dengue, viral encephalitis
Allergenic weeds	Respiratory allergies	Asthma	Hemorrhagic fevers
Sociodemographic	Forced migrations, overcrowding, conflicts	Infectious diseases, emotional problems	Diarrhea, malnutrition, substance abuse, etc.

Source: Adapted from Patz, Engelberg, and Last, 2000

ecosystems to hydroelectric dam developments, irrigation systems that assume fresh water is an infinitely renewable resource, and urban and periurban sprawl that consumes agricultural land all have adverse effects, aggravated by global warming.

The direct effects of global warming, most pronounced in midlatitudes and higher, are due to warmer average ambient temperatures. Melting permafrost reduces the sustainability of Arctic wildlife and the ability of Inuit and other Northern peoples to live off the land. Summer heat waves are longer and more severe. The warming trend alters established weather patterns, and the weather is becoming unstable. There are more frequent and severe weather extremes—floods, hurricanes, severe storms, cold spells, and droughts.

The harmful effect of heat waves is aggravated by ground-level smog and high ozone concentrations in densely settled urban regions, where there is a "heat island" effect, accentuated when air laden with emissions from combusted fossil fuels, mainly from automobile exhausts, is trapped below layers of cooler air at higher altitudes. (Ground-level ozone as part of urban air pollution must not be confused with stratospheric ozone attenuation caused by ozone-destroying substances.) The frail elderly, the very young, and all with impaired respiratory or cardiovascular function can be killed by this combination of heat and pollution, especially if it is prolonged. In 1995, a two-week heat wave killed over 700 people in Chicago; the same series of heat waves killed several thousand people in India and China that summer.[23]

Urban areas are prone to severe smog episodes during heat waves. Smog is produced when emissions from fossil fuel combustion (gaseous sulfur dioxide and oxides of nitrogen) and ozone aerosol droplets and suspended solid particulate matter interact with water vapor, producing a weak atmospheric suspension of sulfuric, nitric, and nitrous acids. This inflames respiratory passages, irritates the eyes, and, if exposure is prolonged or repeated, causes permanent respiratory damage—chronic bronchitis and emphysema. Aerosol particles less than 10 microns in diameter penetrate into the bronchial tree, and particles less than about 2.5 microns in diameter reach the alveolar sacs where the air-blood exchange of oxygen and carbon dioxide takes place.

Violent storms and heavy rains are a feature of climate change. Sometimes the floods that follow severe rainstorms are aggravated by landslides from mountain slopes that have been stripped of forest cover. In 1998, Hurricane Mitch killed over 12,000 people in Honduras. Whole families drowned under layers of mud several yards deep. Droughts are also an increasing risk, and in heat waves, tinder-dry scrubland

and forests are vulnerable to fires. All such events harm habitat, forcing large numbers of people to move from their usual dwellings into temporary shelter or refugee communities. Displaced people experience several kinds of public health and social problems. Separated family members, especially children, must be reunited with their parents. Elementary personal hygiene is difficult to maintain in temporary shelters and sanitation usually is imperfect. Tuberculosis and other life-threatening infectious diseases, including diarrheal diseases, are a greater risk. Displacement into temporary shelter or refugee communities also leads to a cluster of social and emotional problems ranging from depression and delinquent adolescent conduct to substance abuse and suicide. Floods and droughts disrupt agricultural productivity and impair food security, which if prolonged may eventually be associated with nutritional deficits, and can release stored toxic chemicals from dump sites and disable sewerage systems. Floodwaters often contain drowned farm animals, so the water is dangerously polluted, and requires rigorous treatment before it is fit to drink.

Vegetation, insect pests, and microbes all flourish in warm, wet weather. Allergenic grasses and weeds proliferate and the risk of waterborne diseases increases. Insect vectors such as mosquitoes breed faster and in greater numbers, as do the pathogens they harbor, thus the risk of dangerous vector-borne diseases increases as well—malaria, dengue, viral encephalitis, rickettsial infections, viral hemorrhagic fevers, and so on. There have been several recorded cases in recent years of indigenous malaria in New York and Toronto; malaria was transmitted to residents by locally breeding anopheline mosquitoes from a person harboring the malaria parasite, to someone who has not been exposed in a malarial region. Some anopheline mosquitoes that can transmit malaria are native to northeastern North America. The risk of dangerous vector-borne diseases transmitted by culex mosquitoes, a quite different species that cannot transmit malaria, comes from a common domestic mosquito, *Culex pipiens*. It transmits West Nile fever, an ornithosis that probably entered the United States in smuggled exotic birds, and has been occurring in New York and elsewhere since 1999. Its propagation is favored by the long, hot summers. Warm, wet weather and an early spring thaw in the Rocky Mountains in 1998 favored the proliferation of wild rodents, the natural hosts of the virus responsible for hantavirus pulmonary syndrome.

The rising sea level is another climatic change affecting biological and human health. Liquids, including the oceans, expand as they get warmer. Together with increased melting of polar and alpine ice fields and glaciers, this increases the volume of the oceans. The sea level rose an estimated 4–8 inches (10–20 centimeters) throughout the twentieth century, and is predicted to rise 15–34 inches (40–88 centimeters) by 2100. This would inundate many islands and low-lying coastal regions, deltas and estuaries of many rivers, and tidal zones that are vital to marine ecosystems. The habitat and food supplies of an estimated 200–500 million people could be disrupted or destroyed in this way over the next one hundred years. This would be a more slowly progressing process of inundation and loss of habitat than occurs with severe floods, but its sociodemographic effects—enforced migration of many millions—and the associated economic and political consequences would be considerable.

There are health consequences of threats to food security. Floods, droughts, sea-level rise, altered climatic zones—all can impair food production, for instance, production of grain crops. By disrupting coastal ecosystems, sea-level rise could adversely affect coastal fisheries that are the main source of protein for many millions in southern and southeast Asia. Fisheries worldwide have been depleted already by predatory fishing practices. A tiny rise in ocean surface temperature, a consequence of global warming, can change the distribution and abundance of phytoplankton and zooplankton, and of pelagic fish such as mackerel and salmon by differentially altering growth rates and predator-prey relationships. Combined with loss of spawning grounds because of hydroelectric dam construction and pollution and silting of streams caused by logging, this threatens the long-term viability of salmon and tuna.

The movement of ocean currents is affected by global warming, as alluded to earlier. The north-south oscillations of El Niño are becoming more frequent and pronounced, in the same way as convection currents in a saucepan of water on a stove become more vigorous as the water gets warmer. This great ocean current affects climates worldwide. Its last major southern oscillation in the middle 1990s provided a good opportunity to study the effects of climate change in several regions. The warmer coastal seas off the northern Pacific coast of South America altered the balance of zooplankton and phytoplankton, increasing the former, which are symbiotic with the cholera vibrio. This pathogen was introduced into that ecosystem in bilge or ballast water on ships trading from the Bay of Bengal. The result was an epidemic of cholera with half a million cases and about 20,000 deaths.

The health consequences of sociodemographic changes could become more important in the future. As climate change displaces people from unsustainable habitats, many millions are likely to be on the move in the coming decades. Not only small island states in the Pacific and Indian Oceans, but also heavily populated regions in southern and Southeast Asia are threatened. Entire agricultural ecosystems, for example, the densely settled river deltas of the Nile and the Mississippi, could be inundated. The movement of many millions of people over brief periods of a few years, or perhaps less, could create enormous social, economic, political, and security problems for the host countries to which they migrate and for the countries through which they might pass en route. Moreover, as noted above, migratory populations and refugee communities present many public health problems. Existing public health infrastructure— might not cope with such an influx.

FUTURE CHALLENGES

By the early 1950s, many of the great infectious diseases that had scourged humans since prehistoric times were yielding to the combined onslaught of vaccines and antibiotics. Optimism was high about the ultimate conquest of all infectious diseases. All that was necessary, it was believed, was to discover more antibiotics and develop more vaccines.

The first inkling that the future would not be so rosy was the development of antibiotic-resistant strains of common pathogens, including *Staphylococcus aureus, Proteus,* and *Pseudomonas* organisms in hospitals. Optimism faded further in 1957 when a worldwide influenza pandemic took many lives. Meanwhile, malaria control was proving troublesome, as mosqui-

toes and parasites began to develop resistance. More recently, new varieties of infections, some highly lethal, have appeared: Lassa fever, Ebola virus hemorrhagic fever, legionellosis, Hantavirus diseases, Lyme disease, and others. By 1981, when the first cases of AIDS were identified, the optimism had evaporated.

By 2001, there were 40 million HIV infections worldwide. Tuberculosis has returned with new, often resistant, strains, both as a complication of HIV infection and as a public health problem in its own right among the growing numbers of homeless people in large cities in the United States and other countries. Tuberculosis remains, as it has always been, a prominent world health problem.

Compounding these problems is the fact that many people today live in parts of the world racked by low-intensity warfare, with deteriorating environments that cause them to be perpetually on the edge of famine. Undernutrition reduces further their resistance to infections of all kinds. Unprecedented numbers of people, great masses of humanity, are moving restlessly from one continent to another. Many are drawn to the seemingly affluent cities of the industrial world. Huge numbers come to the United States each year—a million or so legally, an unknown number, perhaps more than a million, illegally. The latter enter without any surveillance of their health. Increasing proportions belong to what has been called a *fourth world* of squalor and deprivation amidst the affluence all around them.

The situation worldwide is likely to worsen. Many of these people live in sprawling periurban slums in the developing world, lacking sanitation, clean water, safe food, and basic primary public health services. Add to this global warming, which is widening the range of vector-borne diseases.

All these conditions set the stage for new epidemics and pandemics of infectious diseases, perhaps due to familiar pathogens, perhaps due to entirely new ones. Even in rich nations, such as the United States, essential public health services are strained by limited resources. The cost of new epidemics and pandemics will be overwhelming. The most important determinant of good health in the next 50 years will be the successful control of infectious diseases, and the most important handbook for public health practice will remain in the future, as it has been for the past half-century, the *Control of Communicable Diseases Manual.*[24]

CONCLUSION

For several hundred years as industrial civilization has evolved, we have assumed that nature can take care of all human waste products as well as industrial toxic substances and air pollutants. Lovelock's Gaia hypothesis, E. O. Wilson's "biophilia" concept, Rachel Carson, and many others have suggested that humans and other forms of life on earth form a living entity, or are interdependent in ways that make major disruptions of life-supporting ecosystems ultimately harmful to all components. Some have provided evidence to support their advocacy, that we must find ways to live more harmoniously among the other life forms with which we share the ecosystems in the biosphere. Whether we accept these concepts or not, we must recognize that we have much to learn about the dynamics of global life-supporting ecosystems on which our survival depends. We need a new manner of thinking akin to, but with different goals from, those Albert Einstein had in mind when he stated that humans would need to come to terms with life after the development of the atom bomb.

References

1. World Health Organization. *Preamble to the Constitution.* Geneva, Switzerland: WHO; 1948.
2. *Health Promotion: A Discussion Document on the Concepts and Principles.* Copenhagen, Denmark: WHO Regional Office for Europe; 1984.
3. Last JM. *Public Health and Human Ecology.* 2nd ed. New York, NY: McGraw-Hill; 1997.
4. Cavalli-Sforza LL. *Genes, Peoples, and Language.* Berkeley, Calif: University Press; 2000.
5. Barker DJP. Rise and fall of western diseases. *Nature.* 1989;338:371-372.
6. Suzman R, Riley MW, eds. The oldest old, *Milbanic Q.* 1985;63:177-451.
7. Berkman LF, Kawachi I. *Social Epidemiology.* New York, NY: Oxford University Press; 2000.
8. Taylor HR, West SK, Rosenthal FS, et al. Effect of ultraviolet radiation on cataract formation. *N Engl J Med.* 1988;319:1429-1433.
9. McMichael AJ, Baghurst PA, Wigg NR, et al. Port Pirie cohort study: environmental exposure to lead and children's abilities at the age of four years. *N Engl J Med.* 1988;319:468-475.
10. McGinnis JM, Foege WH. Actual causes of death in the United States. *JAMA.* 1993; 270:2207-2212.
11. Marmot M, Wilkinson RG. Social organization, stress and health. In: *Social Determinants of Health.* New York, NY: Oxford University Press; 1999: 17-43.
12. Gott JR. Implications of the Copernican principle for our future prospects. *Nature.* 1993;363:315-319.
13. Epstein PR, Ford TE, Colwell RR. Marine ecosystems. *Lancet.* 1993;342:1216-1219.
14. McKeown T. *The Origins of Human Disease.* New York, NY: Blackwell; 1988;5:120-139.
15. McKeown T. *The Role of Medicine—Dream, Mirage or Nemesis?* London, England: Nuffield Provincial Hospitals Trust; 1976.
16. Black D, Morris JN, Smith C, Townsend P. *Inequalities in Health (The Black Report).* Harmondsworth, Middlesex, England: Penguin; 1982.
17. Zwerling C, McMillan D. Firearm injuries: a public health approach. *Am J Prev Med.* 1993;9(suppl):3.
18. Reel violence. *Lancet.* 1994;343:127-128. Editorial.
19. McMichael T. Footprints to the future: treading less heavily. In: *Human Frontiers, Environments and Disease.* Cambridge, England: Cambridge University Press; 2001:341-365.
20. United Nations environmental programme: stratospheric ozone depletion [annual updates]. Available at: http://www.unep.org/ozone/annualrepts.html. Accessed October 8, 2001.
21. Houghton, JT, Ding Y, Griggs DJ, Noguer M, van der Linden PJ, Xiaosu D, Maskell K, Johnson CA, eds. (2001). *Climate Change 2001: The Scientific Basis. Contribution of Working Group I to the Third Assessment Report of the Intergovernmental Panel on Climate Change.* Cambridge, England: Cambridge University Press; 896. Also available at: http://www.ipcc.ch.
22. Patz J, Engelberg D, Last JM. Effects of changing weather on health. *Annu Rev of Public Health.* 2000;21:271-307.
23. Kalkstein LS. Lessons from a very hot summer. *Lancet.* 1995;346:857-859.
24. Chin J, ed. *Control of Communicable Diseases Manual.* 17th ed. Washington, DC: American Public Health Association; 2000.

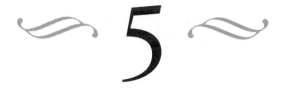

CHAPTER 5

The Legal Basis for Public Health

Edward P. Richards III, J.D., M.P.H.
Katharine C. Rathbun, M.D., M.P.H.

Public health is unique among medical specialties in being defined by law rather than physiology. While there are many public health practices that benefit affected individuals, the core of public health practice is coercive action under state authority, *the police power.* In the best of circumstances, this authority may be needed only to encourage educational efforts. At other times, however, public health authorities must seize property, close businesses, destroy animals, or involuntarily treat or even lock away individuals.

Such powers are rooted in earlier times, when the fear of pestilential disease was both powerful and well founded. In a contemporary society dominated by concern with individual rights, such draconian powers may seem unnecessary or even unconstitutional. Many public health personnel believe that the rationale for such laws is past and that public health practitioners should restrict themselves to education and empowerment. Others, looking at the resurgence of tuberculosis and an increasing inability to treat other bacterial diseases, believe that the end of the antimicrobial era is near and that traditional public health restrictions will have to be employed, requiring the sacrifice of individual rights for the common good.

This chapter has three objectives: (1) to explain the history and constitutional basis for public health law; (2) to show how public health law fits into the general rules for administrative agency law; and (3) to outline the legal issues in public health practice.

HISTORICAL PERSPECTIVE

Pestilence is one of the *Four Horsemen of the Apocalypse,* reflecting its position as a primal fear of society, yet it is difficult for individuals born after the ready availability of antimicrobial drugs and immunizations to appreciate the historic dread of deadly epidemics. In a society preoccupied with lifestyle diseases, we forget that civilizations have fallen because of communicable diseases and that pestilence has done more to eradicate indigenous cultures than has force of arms or religion.

Even in the United States, pestilence was once part of everyday life. Soon after the Constitution was ratified, for example, an epidemic of yellow fever raged in New York and Philadelphia. The flavor of that period was later captured in an argument before the Supreme Court:

> For ten years prior, the yellow-fever had raged almost annually in the city, and annual laws were passed to resist it. The wit of man was exhausted, but in vain. Never did the pestilence rage more violently than in the summer of 1798. The State was in despair. The rising hopes of the metropolis began to fade. The opinion was gaining ground, that the cause of this annual disease was indigenous, and that all precautions against its importation were useless. But the leading spirits of that day were unwilling to give up the city without a final desperate effort. The havoc in the summer of 1798 is represented as terrific. The whole country was roused. A cordon sanitaire was thrown around the city. Governor Mifflin of Pennsylvania proclaimed a non-intercourse between New York and Philadelphia.[1]

The extreme nature of the actions, including isolating the federal government, which was sitting in Philadelphia at the time, was considered an appropriate response to the threat of yellow fever. The terrifying nature of these early epidemics predisposed the courts to grant public health authorities a free hand in their attempts to prevent the spread of disease, as the following quote shows:

> Every state has acknowledged power to pass, and enforce quarantine, health, and inspection laws, to prevent the introduction of disease, pestilence, or unwholesome provisions; such laws interfere with no powers of Congress or treaty stipulations; they relate to internal police, and are subjects of domestic regulation within each state, over which no authority can be exercised by any power under the Constitution, save by requiring the consent of Congress to the imposition of duties on exports and imports, and their payment into the treasury of the United States.[2]

The American colonies adopted the English statutory and common law that recognized the right of the state to protect the health and safety of its citizens. This was called the police power, although police forces as we know them were not organized until much later. When the Constitution was written, public health power was left to the states:

> It is a well-recognized principle that it is one of the first duties of a state to take all necessary steps for the promotion and protection of the health and comfort of its inhabitants. The preservation of the public health is universally conceded to be one of the duties devolving upon the state as a sovereignty, and whatever reasonably tends to preserve the public health is a subject upon which the legislature, within its police power, may take action.[3]

The scope of the police power is broad. Defining the limits of the police power, and the rights of citizens to be protected from state actions taken pursuant to the police power, is the central legal issue in public health law.

PUBLIC HEALTH LAW AS ADMINISTRATIVE LAW

Governments act through laws passed by legislatures. These laws are of two types: criminal laws, which are intended to punish wrongdoing, and civil laws, which are intended to direct future behavior. Criminal laws are enforced by local prosecutors, state attorneys general, and the Justice Department. Civil laws are enforced by administrative agencies and through litigation by private parties. These range in size and complexity from the Internal Revenue Service and the Department of Health and Human Services, which have bigger budgets than some states, to small, specialized agencies with no full-time staff. Public health departments are among the oldest of administrative agencies, with some dating from the colonial period.

Criminal laws and regulations must be passed by the legislature, they must be specific, and they cannot be modified by the law enforcement agency based on its expertise. Persons accused of committing a crime have the right to remain silent, confront their accusers, and present witnesses, as well as the right to have counsel, a trial by jury, and certain other protections attendant on their criminal prosecution. These rights make criminal prosecutions slow and expensive, and they also limit the ability of law enforcement to respond to new problems.

Since administrative agencies do not enforce the criminal laws, they do not have to provide criminal law due process protections. Instead, they are usually given broad authority to use their expertise to develop the most effective strategies for protecting the public; they may change these strategies as conditions change or as they get better information about their effectiveness. For example, state health departments are charged with protecting the citizens from communicable diseases. Rather than the legislature deciding which diseases pose a threat to the public health, the health department is given the authority to establish regulations on communicable disease control, including the list of communicable diseases subject to reporting and other public health regulations. If individuals or businesses sue the health department to challenge these regulations, the courts will generally defer to the agency's expertise and support the regulations even when there is a controversy over the best way to solve the problem. As one court held, in a case contesting the right of the health department to close gay bathhouses to prevent the spread of HIV:

> . . . defendants and the intervening patrons challenge the soundness of the scientific judgments upon which the Health Council regulation is based . . . . They go further and argue that facilities such as St. Mark's, which attempts to educate its patrons with written materials, signed pledges, and posted notices as to the advisability of safe sexual practices, provide a positive force in combatting AIDS, and a valuable communication link between public health authorities and the homosexual community. While these arguments and proposals may have varying degrees of merit, they overlook a fundamental principle of applicable law: "It is not for the courts to determine which scientific view is correct in ruling upon whether the police power has been properly exercised. The judicial function is exhausted with the discovery that the relation between means and end is not wholly vain and fanciful, an illusory pretense."[4]

The advantages of administrative agencies are so great that legislatures sometimes pass laws that impose punishments, while claiming they are administrative laws, to avoid giving individuals full criminal law protections. While the courts generally accept the legislature's determination that a law is not a criminal law, they do examine the law and its effects as it is applied.

A law that required the permanent quarantine of persons accused of murder to protect the public's health, for example, would be a criminal law because it is based on past behavior rather than on proof of present danger to the community. Accused murderers are therefore entitled to full criminal law protections before being locked away. In contrast, if it can be that persons who commit a violent sexual assault have a high probability of committing future assaults, then it would be acceptable to lock up these persons as a threat to the public health without full criminal law protections. This is an administrative action, even though the person is locked up in a prison.[5] It is the purpose of the law that matters, not the conditions of confinement.

Public health restrictions were once carried out in prisons and jails. In one case, disease carriers were quarantined in a prison. They petitioned the court for release, claiming that they were being punished by being put in prison and treated as prisoners. The court rejected their claim and concluded the following:

> While it is true that physical facilities constituting part of the penitentiary equipment are utilized, interned persons are in no sense confined in the penitentiary, and are not subject to the peculiar obloquy which attends such confinement.[6]

The administrative rights of public health agencies are not without limit, however. Public health laws must be applied fairly. They cannot, for example, be a subterfuge for discrimination against racial or ethnic groups, who must be given equal protection under the U.S. Constitution. The courts have rejected laws that subjected the Chinese community to special health regulations without providing evidence that Chinese people were at any greater risk of contracting or spreading disease.

If a public health law's purpose and enforcement is rationally related to protecting the public's health, it will be constitutional even if it has a differential impact on different groups. Laws for controlling the spread of gonorrhea are constitutional, even if the disease is more prevalent in a specific racial or ethnic group. Laws against prostitution have been found constitutional even though they were primarily enforced against women. In the extreme case, laws requiring the testing of pregnant women for communicable diseases that affect the fetus, such as syphilis, are constitutional even though they affect only women. As the U.S. Supreme Court has pointed out in other cases involving pregnancy, the laws would also apply to pregnant men.

Public health laws also must treat state residents the same as out-of-state residents. For example, courts have struck down several laws that imposed different sanitary restrictions on out-of-state milk processors. Even if the restrictions are the same for in-state and out-of-state businesses, the courts strike down laws that unnecessarily discriminate against out-of-state businesses. For example, a requirement that milk must be processed and delivered within 24 hours would put out-of-state dairies out of business. This law would be improper if there was no evidence that the 24-hour rule was necessary to protect the public's health.

Most public health law cases were decided decades ago, and the U.S. Supreme Court gave individuals few rights. Some argue that these cases were superseded by the Supreme Court's civil liberties decisions in the 1960s and 1970s. In these rulings, the Supreme Court required criminal law protections in several cases where the legislature had said that the law was not intended to punish. In other cases, the Court recognized a right of privacy that might also apply to public health laws.

While the current Supreme Court has not directly affirmed traditional public health cases, it has upheld public health rationales in other contexts.[7] For example, it specifically rejected the Warren Court's consideration of the conditions of confinement in determining whether public safety detention is punishment. The Court rejected arguments that detainees should be held in the *least restrictive* manner necessary to en-sure their confinement. Instead, the Court allowed them to be kept with other prisoners and subjected to the same prison rules. Despite the detainees' apparent imprisonment, the Court ruled that their incarceration was not a punishment because the state's intent was merely to protect the public until the detainees could be tried.

Pretrial detention cases may prove more than is necessary to uphold public health restrictions. The difficult problem in the detention of criminally dangerous persons is determining the probability that they will endanger public safety by committing another crime. This probability is certainly less than 100 percent, perhaps substantially less. In contrast, communicable diseases can be objectively diagnosed and their risk assessed. Persons with diseases such as active tuberculosis are dangerous, irrespective of whether they intend to harm others.

INDIVIDUAL RIGHTS VERSUS PUBLIC SAFETY

There is pressure, even from some public health professionals, to give individuals more rights under public health laws than would be required by the Constitution. Indeed, this is the central legal issue in public health law, as stated above. Some states have amended their disease control laws to require court hearings before public health orders are issued against an individual. These hearings are modeled after the proceedings that are required before a mentally ill person is involuntarily committed to a psychiatric institution. Although such an expansion of individual rights seems desirable, it comes at a high price: potential paralysis of public health enforcement.

Court hearings are expensive and time consuming. No health department has a sufficiently large legal staff to have a court hearing before every enforcement action. Indeed, most health departments do not have *any* legal staff. They are at the mercy of city or county legal departments to provide attorneys when there is a hearing. Because most legal departments are understaffed, public health enforcement actions usually have low priority.

Another problem with hearings is that they take time. A hearing first must be scheduled with a judge, and then the person subject to the order must be served with notice of the hearing and given time to hire an attorney and present a defense. This prevents timely restrictions that are critical to effective disease control. Courts have recognized, in their rejection of requests for bail by persons under disease control orders, that disease carriers cannot be allowed to go free while restrictions are litigated, as the following argument shows:

> To grant release on bail to persons isolated and detained on a quarantine order because they have a contagious disease which makes them dangerous to others, or to the public in general, would render quarantine laws and regulations nugatory and of no avail.[8]

A final problem with hearings, and perhaps the most serious, is that they give the judge the opportunity to substitute her judgment for that of the public health officer. The proper role of the judge (or jury) was established in the original case ruling that involuntary immunizations are constitutionally permissible. The U.S. Supreme Court rejected the petitioner's claim that he was entitled to have a jury determine whether the state's actions were reasonable. The Court ruled that "It is no part of the function of a court or a jury to determine which of two modes was likely to be most effective for the protection of the public against disease."[9]

Despite such clear judicial support for deference to agency decision makers, many judges are swayed by the emotional appeal of the case against restriction and reject the public health authority's recommendations. Such conflicts are most common in disputes over closing unsanitary restaurants owned by friends of the local politicians. They can also arise in disease control cases when there is political pressure to not restrict individuals because they belong to a politically powerful group or because the judge does not understand the danger to others posed by the infected person.

LEGAL LIABILITY

Public health departments and public health officials are frequent targets of litigation. State and federal law provide sovereign immunity for most claims that arise from the exercise of the state's police powers to protect the public health. However, many modern health departments do more than exercise police powers, providing prenatal care, wellness clinics, and other personal health services. Health departments are also employers and must comply with state and federal employment and antidiscrimination laws, as well as laws such as the Americans with Disabilities Act. Such laws have little or no application to core police power functions, however.

Sovereign immunity is an old common law doctrine stating that the king, and later, the state and those operating on the behalf of the state, cannot be sued. If the state injures a person, the only way for the individual to get compensation under sovereign immunity is to persuade the legislature to pass a special law authorizing such compensation. In the early 1900s such laws began to clog both Congress and the state legislatures, leading to the passage of tort claims acts (TCAs) that waive sovereign immunity in certain circumstances. Congress has also passed various civil rights acts that allow suits against persons acting under the authority of state law who violate constitutional rights and certain federal laws. These laws reflect the balance between delivering cost-effective public services and holding public officials accountable for negligent or intentionally harmful actions. Since the states have only a limited duty to provide public services, allowing unlimited legal liability would encourage legislatures to reduce public services and would make it difficult to attract qualified professionals for public health service. The courts must balance the value of the service against the potential harm caused by improper actions.

Public health officials can be sued in two ways: in their official capacity or as private persons. Official capacity means the public health official is a surrogate for the government and is not personally liable if damages are awarded to the plaintiff. These lawsuits are usually brought to stop enforcement of an unconstitutional law or to stop unconstitutional or otherwise illegal behavior by the health agency, and are governed by the principle of sovereign immunity. Private capacity lawsuits assert personal wrongdoing by the official and, if they are successful, damages must be paid by the official or his or her insurer. This personal wrongdoing may be related to official duties, such as destroying a dog, or may be strictly private conduct, such as causing an accident while driving drunk. Personal liability is limited by official immunity, which seeks to protect the government's ability to act by protecting its officials.

Section 1983 Liability

Section 1983 of the Civil Rights Act of 1871 allows citizens to sue persons who, under color of state law, deprive them of their constitutional rights. Section 1983 actions can be brought against state officials in their personal capacity, but not in their official capacity. City and county and other nonstate officials can be sued in their official capacity, which allows damages to be obtained from the governmental entity, and in their personal capacity. In 1971, the U.S. Supreme Court allowed claims against federal officials who violate an individual's constitutional rights in *Bivens v. Six Unknown Named Agents of Federal Bureau of Narcotics,* 403 U.S. 388 (1971). A Bivens action is the federal equivalent of a 1983 action and would apply to employees of the Public Health Service, the CDC, and other federal agencies. Bivens actions, 1983 actions, and related actions against public health officials have similar requirements.

Section 1983 applies to anyone who acts under color of state law. It reaches everyone working under the authority of the health department, irrespective of their employment status, and can even be applied to volunteers. It does not provide for vicarious liability, so public health officials can be held personally liable only for their own actions, not those of subordinates. To prevail, the plaintiff must prove that the official's conduct violates clearly established statutory or constitutional rights that a reasonable official should have known about. If the official is mistaken about the law but had no reason to know that the actions were improper, or is acting under a law later declared unconstitutional, there is no liability. The courts also require that persons bringing 1983 actions show significant harm as well as improper conduct. This is unusual in public health restrictions because they are easily reviewed and corrected in postdeprivation proceedings before the plaintiff is harmed.

Section 1983 actions must allege that the defendant violated the plaintiff's rights under the Constitution or certain federal laws. Most public health cases allege violations of the constitutional rights of equal protection or due process. Equal protection claims arise from differential treatment that is motivated by improper discrimination, especially discrimination based on race, ethnicity, or religion. Refusing to issue a license or permit because of personal animus against the applicant could also be an equal protection violation, unless there were other rational grounds for the refusal.

Due process claims arise when the public health official does not give the party the procedural safeguards provided for in the law. If a statute required 30 days' notice and an opportunity for a hearing before destroying a dangerous building, then it could be a due process violation to destroy the building without notice. If the defendant has complied with applicable statutes, the plaintiff can claim that the Constitution requires more process than the state or local law provides. Thus, if the law provides only 24 hours' notice, the court may find that although the defendant complied, the notice period was not long enough. Claims are sometimes filed because public health officials take action without a predeprivation (prior) hearing. If the action is authorized by statute, or the court finds that waiting for a hearing would endanger the public, the court will usually dismiss the claim. Thus, a building that is partially destroyed by fire may need to be destroyed at once, without notice or hearing because of the threat it poses.

State Law Liability

State law liability is controlled by the state's constitution and the state's TCA, which differ among states. The basic principle is that state public health officials have official immunity when they are making policy decisions or performing discretionary acts, which are those that require the exercise of professional judgment. Official immunity is determined by the nature of the function and can extend to every employee of the department, although the law is not so clear that tasks done by private contractors have the same immunity as those done by government employees. Inspecting a restaurant and deciding whether it should be cited is a discretionary function. Discretionary immunity applies unless a plaintiff can show that a reasonable person in the official's position would have known that the action was unambiguously beyond the scope of the official's legal authority or was otherwise illegal. Ministerial tasks are those that do not require discretion because they either follow a predetermined plan and cannot be changed, such as following a health department checklist regulation, or they do not involve any special expertise related to public health, such as driving a car. Plaintiffs may bring ordinary negligence claims if they are injured through a ministerial function. For example, plaintiffs were allowed to recover when the government failed to follow its own regulations for approving a polio vaccine.[10]

Most states divide public health functions into government or proprietary functions. There is official immunity for discretionary governmental functions, but not for proprietary functions. These definitions vary greatly between states, with some states holding that almost all public health functions are governmental and others finding that a substantial group are proprietary. Traditional public health services such as restaurant inspection, animal control, health and safety permits and licenses, sanitation, vital statistics, and related functions are considered governmental in almost all states. Many states do not consider personal medical services, such as prenatal care clinics and general indigent health care clinics, to be governmental functions and apply ordinary medical malpractice law to them, although some states do include these under governmental immunity. However, if the medical service is related to protecting the public, rather than just helping the individual, it will be governmental. Thus, treatment and testing for tuberculosis would be a governmental function.

If the function is proprietary or ministerial, then the state TCA will determine the extent of liability and when the official is personally liable. State TCAs have differing caps on liability, varying between $100,000 and $1,000,000, and they generally prevent the recovery of punitive damages. TCAs provide that the state will defend the lawsuit and pay the claim if the official is sued personally. The TCA does not ap-

ply if the claim is for intentional wrongdoing that is outside the official's duties, such as sexual assault charges or criminal conduct. The TCA may not cover nonemployees such as contract physicians in clinics. These individuals may need to have private insurance to defend and pay claims brought against them.

LIMITATIONS ON PUBLIC HEALTH POWER

There are three types of limitations on public health power: statutory limitations, the right of habeas corpus, and political limitations.

Statutory Limitations

An administrative agency may exercise only the powers given by the law that creates it, that is, its enabling legislation. Some enabling legislation, such as the tax code, is very detailed, running thousands of pages in length. This reflects the congressional desire to exercise close control over the agency.

The enabling legislation for health departments was traditionally a general grant of authority to protect the public health and safety, with little specific legislative guidance. The details were left to the public health officers because there was little disagreement in society over the goals and methods of public health practice. As public health departments were given broader responsibilities, however, their enabling legislation grew more complicated, and their freedom of action was increasingly constrained. In several states, legislatures have greatly limited the traditional constitutional powers of health departments.

The Right of Habeas Corpus

The second major restriction on public health power is the right of habeas corpus. While courts have been willing to allow persons to be restricted without a court hearing, they require that a restricted person have access to a court to review the public health order. This review is done through a habeas corpus proceeding, which the U.S. Constitution guarantees to every imprisoned or confined person. *Habeas corpus,* roughly translated, means *"bring me the body."* It requires a judge to review the legality of a person's confinement, usually including a personal statement by the confined person.

Because a habeas corpus proceeding is held *after* the person has been confined, it does not interfere with the health department's ability to take quick action. Unlike routine court hearings, habeas corpus is used only when requested by the confined person. Many, perhaps most, people restricted by public health orders do not wish to contest the restriction. In the vast majority of cases, confinement is temporary—for a medical examination, initial treatment of a disease, or some other similarly minor inconvenience. By contrast, requiring hearings before enforcing routine or uncontested public health orders diverts limited resources from other public health agency functions.

Political Limitations

This is the most important restriction on public health authority. From the surgeon general of the United States to the health officer in the smallest town, every public health official works for politicians. In some cases they work for independent boards, rather than directly for the elected officials, but the end results are the same. Public health officers who take actions that are politically unpopular in their community will be forced out of office. Public health officers also cannot do anything that elected officials will not pay for. For example, attempts to quarantine everyone with AIDS or other communicable diseases would be impossibly expensive as well as politically suicidal. Even with the resurgence of tuberculosis, it is politically difficult to get support and resources for confinement when it is necessary to treat an individual and prevent spread of the infection.

BASIC AREAS OF PUBLIC HEALTH LAW

Public health law falls into eight basic areas: environmental health, disease and injury reporting, vital statistics, disease control, involuntary testing, contact tracing, immunizations and mandated treatment, and personal restrictions. Each of these areas is considered in turn.

Environmental Health

Food sanitation, drinking-water treatment, and wastewater disposal have been mainstays of public health since the earliest times. As health departments were given the added responsibility of guarding against toxins in the broader environment, these regulatory functions were grouped into environmental health. Most public health orders are directed at environmental health problems. Because they affect property, not persons, they do not pose the difficult issues of personal freedom that arise with the rarer communicable disease control orders.

Environmental health regulations pose two central legal questions: whether the government owes compensation to the owners of regulated property, and under what circumstances health officers can enter private premises to look for public health law violations. Both questions arise from the U.S. Constitution, which requires that property owners be paid a fair price for property taken for public purposes and prohibits *unreasonable* searches and seizures. The difficult problem is deciding if the government has searched the property unreasonably or has taken the value of the property for which the owner must be compensated.

Regulation of Property

If a city condemns a house to widen a street, for example, the city has clearly taken the house and must pay its owner. In contrast, if property is destroyed because it poses a threat to the public health, the owner is not entitled to compensation because the property is not considered to have value. In the classic food sanitation case, public health officials ordered the destruction of frozen chicken stored in a cold storage plant that had lost its refrigeration. The owners of the plant demanded a hearing to determine whether the chicken was really spoiled and compensation for the chicken that was destroyed. The court ruled that there was no right to a hearing before the destruction of property and that property that endangered the public health had no value. Thus, the owners were entitled to no compensation.[11]

This decision echoed an earlier ruling involving a compensation claim for property that had been demolished to prevent the spread of a fire in San Francisco.[12] Unlike the rotten chicken, which arguably had no value, the property owners sued for their possessions, which they claimed could have been saved before the fire reached the building, had it not been destroyed. The court rejected their claims for compensation. It held that the police power included the right to destroy property if this was necessary to protect the public safety. This destruction was not taking the property for public purpose and thus no compensation need be paid. The court rejected the claim that the authorities should have allowed the owners time to remove their property because such a delay would have increased the danger to the public.

The most controversial modern cases involve regulatory actions that do not destroy property but limit the owner's use of the property. Examples include wetlands protection laws and endangered species acts. Such environmental laws are also based on the police power to protect the public health and safety, but the threat they address is much less direct and immediate than the threat posed by rotten chicken. The courts are increasingly reluctant to defer to the agency's expertise in these cases because the harm they seek to prevent is so difficult to measure. Although the courts still rule with the agencies in most cases, property owners are given extensive rights to court hearings to contest the actions before they are finalized.

Search and Seizure

The second legal issue in environmental health is the right of the health department to enter private property to assess environmental health risks. With certain exceptions, the police may not enter private property to search for evidence of criminal activity without a search warrant approved by a judge. Such warrants are difficult and expensive to get and will be granted only when there is evidence of wrongdoing.

In contrast, most environmental health inspections are done to ensure that the owner is in compliance with the law, not because the inspector believes that the owner is violating the law. The courts do not require specific warrants for environmental health inspections, as long as there is no threat of criminal prosecution. Thus an inspection for rats does not require a search warrant based on probable cause, whereas one for toxic waste dumping in violation of criminal laws would. The courts do require that searches be related to a public health purpose. This can be satisfied by having a general plan for the inspections (called an area warrant) that describes which buildings will be searched and why.[13] Access by health inspectors can be made a condition of licensure, so that any establishment with a food handling or other public license has to admit inspectors without a warrant.

Federal Environmental Law

Since the 1960s, the federal government has passed many laws governing environmental pollution. These laws are passed under the authority of the Interstate Commerce Clause of the U.S. Constitution, which allows Congress to regulate anything that affects interstate commerce. In general, Congress has not preempted state laws governing air and water pollution and solid waste management, but has set minimum standards that the states must meet, which the states may exceed if they choose. Federal environmental laws are enforced by the Environmental Protection Agency (EPA), through private litigation when provided for in the statute, and by state agencies. While the federal government has no direct authority to force states to adopt federal clean air and water standards and enforce federal laws, it can withhold federal money from states that do not follow federal mandates. State governments almost always comply rather than forego federal funds.

Private litigation has been very important under provisions of the Superfund legislation where anyone who contributed to the pollution is liable for cleanup costs. It is not unusual for a corporation that dumped toxic substances into a landfill to sue every other business and organization that dumped into the same landfill for contributions to the cleanup costs. Such litigation can drag on for years, delaying the cleanup.

Unlike traditional state public health laws, the federal laws generally have both civil and criminal enforcement provisions. Thus the EPA can enforce the Clean Water Act through administrative law procedures, while the Department of Justice can bring criminal prosecutions against persons who violate certain provisions of the act. In these dual enforcement situations, the administrative agency cannot use its powers to circumvent the criminal due process rights of the accused. However, the EPA and state agencies can provide the Department of Justice with information filed by polluters pursuant to environmental reporting regulations or collected as part of routine agency inspections.

Disease and Injury Reporting

Basic to all public health is the reporting of communicable diseases, hazardous conditions, and injuries that are of public health significance. This information is used for tracking the course of epidemics and for intervening to protect the public health. Reporting duties transcend the patient's right to privacy and the health care provider's obligation to protect the patient's confidential information.

The constitutionality of reporting laws has been upheld in several recent U.S. Supreme Court decisions. In a case involving the reporting of controlled substance prescriptions, the Court addressed many of the concerns about public health reporting. The Court first noted that common law did not recognize the right to withhold medical information from the state. Such a right of physician-patient confidentiality arises from state or federal law and is subject to limitations such as public health reporting. The Court then held:

> Unquestionably, some individuals' concern for their own privacy may lead them to avoid or to postpone needed medical attention. Nevertheless, disclosures of private medical information to doctors, hospital personnel, insurance companies, and public health agencies are often an essential part of modern medical practice, even when the disclosure may reflect unfavorably on the character of the patient. Requiring such disclosures to representatives of the State having responsibility for the health of the community, does not automatically amount to an impermissible invasion of privacy.[14]

Every state has laws that require physicians to report certain diseases and injuries to a local or state health officer.[15] Many extend this requirement to nurses, dentists, veterinarians, laboratories, school officials, administrators of institutions, and police officials. For some diseases, health care providers are required to report only the number of cases they see. Other diseases and conditions require health care providers to give identifying information, such as name, address, occupation, and birth date, as well as information on the disease and how it might have been acquired.

While states vary somewhat in which diseases must be reported, there are about 60 diseases that are commonly reportable in all jurisdictions. The state health department can provide information on which diseases to report and to whom the reports should be directed. Most health departments will accept reports for diseases that are not on the state list of reportable diseases, although they may choose not to act on them. Health care providers have no legal liability for making a report that is not required.

HIV is the only disease where there is a significant difference in state reporting procedures. AIDS is reportable by name in all states and has been since the beginning of the epidemic. When the test for HIV was developed, many states required the reporting of HIV because it is the causal agent for AIDS and standard public health practice is to revise reporting practices when the causal agent for a disease is discovered. In several states, however, there was political opposition to HIV reporting because of the fear that public health officials would not protect the confidentiality of the reports and would use the information for improper purposes. While there is no evidence that this has ever happened, there are still states that do not require HIV reporting at the time this chapter was written.

Legally required disease control reporting is not subject to informed consent. Health care providers do not need medical records releases for disease reporting because neither they nor their patients have the right to refuse the release of the information. Although patients have no right to be informed that they are being reported to the health department, it is good practice to do so for diseases such as syphilis or measles for which the health department will contact them for additional information.

Health care providers must never knowingly report false information to public health authorities, and they are liable for any injuries, such as transmission of HIV or tuberculosis, occasioned by false reports. Although health care providers are not required to personally investigate the information that patients provide, they must truthfully report what is known to them. In reality, very few health care providers do not know their patients' correct names and addresses, because few patients pay cash for medical care or never need a prescription or other order that requires a correct identity. Health care providers who provide information in good faith are not liable if the information is incorrect.

Disease registries are a special class of reporting laws. Most disease registries are statewide and involve either cancer or occupational illness. Some, such as the CDC registry of cases of toxic shock syndrome, are national. Reporting cases to the registry may be mandatory or voluntary. Because the objective is not to control a communicable disease, there is often no penalty for failing to report to a disease registry. However, it is always desirable to have a complete registry because registries are used to determine the extent of certain problems in the community and to try to determine causes. If they are inaccurate they may give false correlations and become useless for research and prevention.

Every jurisdiction requires health care providers to report certain types of injuries to law enforcement officials or protection agencies, generally including assaults, family violence, and criminal activity. Although the victim may have a plausible explanation of the injury and be anxious to avoid reporting for fear of reprisals or because he is under investigation already, proper reports should be made despite the victim's wishes. It is not up to the health care provider to investigate the incident before reporting it; that is the job of the law enforcement agency that receives the report.

Whenever a health care provider suspects that a child has been abused or neglected, that suspicion should be reported immediately to the child protective agency.[16] Child abuse is not a diagnosis, however, but a legal finding, and medical personnel who try to investigate this crime may confuse the evidence to the point that the law enforcement agency cannot protect the child.[17] Health care providers should defer to experts in child abuse and neglect rather than attempting to make an independent determination of abuse.[18] The experts will also act as consultants to the courts and protective services.

Generally, health care providers have a responsibility to report violent or suspicious injuries to the local law enforcement agency. These include all gunshot wounds, knifings, poisonings, serious motor vehicle injuries, and any other wounds that seem suspicious. The legal assumption is that anyone who has knowledge that a crime may have been committed has a duty to report it to the police. If the patient is brought to the hospital in the custody of the police or from the scene of a police investigation, then the health care provider may safely assume that the police have been notified. In all other cases, however, the health care provider should call the police and make the report.

Vital Statistics

Vital statistics, or birth and death records, are critical to public health and are required in all states. The keeping of good vital statistics is important to society for several reasons. For one, they are a good way to monitor a population's health. The infant mortality rate is generally considered to be the single best indicator of the health of a population. Accurate vital statistics also allow for allocation of health care funds to areas of greatest need. Vital statistics are of great historical value as well, documenting a population's health through time. On the individual level, the documentation of a birth certificate establishes a person's legal existence and his or her basic legal relationships, including citizenship and parentage.

Although there have been efforts to standardize state laws on keeping vital statistics, there are still significant differences among states. The registrar of vital statistics at the state health department is the best source of information about that state's laws. It is anticipated that vital statistics records will become a more useful resource as states centralize their records and begin to correlate them with other states and with federal social security records.

The quality of death records in the United States is generally poor because physicians are not well trained in filing these reports.[19] Death certificates are problematic for several reasons.[20] Unexpected deaths frequently occur outside the hospital. The cause of death may not be immediately obvious. There may be no one to provide information on the identity of the person who died. Occasionally, there may be a question of criminal activity having been involved in the death.

The cause of death is the most important information on a death certificate, but it is generally the most inadequate. Preferably, the causes of death that are listed are codable from the International Classification of Disease. For many certificates, however, the actual cause of death is not clear, let alone codable. Cardiac arrest, for example, is a *result* of death, not a *cause*. A death certificate may list cardiac arrest as the cause of death and respiratory arrest following shock as the contributing cause, even though the patient actually died of a gunshot wound, terminal cancer, or heart disease. Ideally, the cause of death should reflect what killed the patient, not what the terminal events were.

Disease Control

Disease control is the prevention of disease in the community. While disease control specialists must be knowledgeable in the treatment of communicable diseases, the public health focus is different from that of the medical specialist who treats infectious diseases. Infectious disease specialists are concerned with the management and treatment of infected individuals. Effective public health disease control includes treatment, when indicated, but is much more comprehensive, attacking the roots of disease in the community.[21]

Disease control poses the most difficult legal questions because the rights and well-being of the individual patient are not paramount. Disease control measures frequently inconvenience a lot of people (smokers huddled in the freezing cold outside their office building are a classic example). Disease control measures also often pose a real, if small, risk of serious injury. In many cases, such as syphilis, the treatment (penicillin) that protects the public also benefits infected persons but not without some attendant risk (a possible allergic reaction to the penicillin). In some cases, such as erythromycin therapy for pertussis, the treatment makes the patient noninfectious but does not alter the course of the disease. The vaccine that prevents thousands of cases of paralytic polio may do so at the cost of an occasional case of vaccine-related polio.

Determining which disease control measures are indicated are scientific and political decisions more than legal decisions. As discussed earlier, courts generally defer to the expertise of the health officer, unless there is special legislation limiting the authority of the health officer. In most cases, however, health officers must temper good public health practice with the wishes of elected officials. Unfortunately, elected officials usually are reluctant to do anything that is opposed by a significant part of the community. For example, against the strenuous objections of most public health authorities, England stopped giving pertussis immunizations because of public outcries about the alleged dangers of the vaccine. Because pertussis had been under control for many years, most of the public had forgotten the terrible sequelae of the disease. As predicted, pertussis soon returned. Immunizations were resumed, but only at the cost of many unnecessary childhood deaths and injuries.

Involuntary Testing

One of the least intrusive disease control measures is the involuntary testing of populations at risk for communicable disease. The most common example is testing for tuberculosis in high-risk populations. Involuntary testing has three benefits. First, it allows public health officials to learn the prevalence of a disease in the community, which is difficult to accomplish with voluntary testing because of statistical problems associated with self-selected data sets. Second, involuntary testing identifies infected individuals who may benefit from treatment, and third, it identifies individuals who may need to be restricted to protect the public health.

Involuntary testing for communicable diseases is legally different from testing for personal behaviors, such as drug use or the propensity to steal from an employer. The presence or absence of a communicable disease may be objectively determined and the risk it poses easily quantified. Since there are no criminal law consequences to the diagnosis of a communicable disease, there is no need for protections against self-incrimination in disease screening. In many cases treatment will eradicate the condition. Even when treatment is not possible, only rare circumstances demand more than minimal workplace restrictions to prevent the spread of the disease. When these restrictions are required, their sole purpose is to protect others and not to punish the affected individual. Involuntary testing cannot be used to gather evidence in criminal cases without a proper search warrant. The U.S. Supreme Court has held that it is unconstitutional to prosecute pregnant women for endangering their babies when the information about their illegal drug use was collected through public health testing done with no criminal law due process protections.[22]

Contact Tracing

Contact tracing has been used for decades to control endemic contagious diseases.[23] It is done after disease reporting or involuntary testing identifies an individual as having a communicable disease. An investigator interviews the patient, family members, physicians, nurses, and anyone else who may have knowledge of the patient's contacts; anyone who might have been exposed; and anyone who might have been the source of the disease. Then the contacts are screened to see whether they have or ever have had the disease.

Many persons object to contact tracing as an invasion of privacy. It may be, but only in a very limited sense. Contact-tracing interviews are always voluntary; there is no legal coercion to divulge the names of contacts.[24] A more serious objection, especially with venereal diseases, is the risk of breaches of confidentiality. As a matter of law, the courts do not consider the risk of such breaches of confidentiality to be sufficient reason to restrict contact tracing. As a matter of public health practice, there have been no significant breaches of the confidentiality of public health records.[25] When suspected breaches of confidentiality have been investigated, they are usually traced back to the patient's own disclosures or to those of people whom the patient has told of the condition.

It has also been argued that contact tracing is not legally justified because it is too expensive or because it is ineffective. The courts have rejected these arguments because contact tracing is indeed highly efficient in finding infected persons.[26] This was best demonstrated in the campaign to eradicate smallpox, which was controlled not by universal immunization but by extensive contact tracing to find infected individuals.[27] Fellow villagers and tribal members were encouraged in various ways to identify infected persons. When people with smallpox were identified, they were quarantined and everyone in the surrounding community or village vaccinated. In this way, smallpox was eventually reduced to isolated outbreaks and then eradicated.

Immunizations and Mandated Treatment

The police power to protect the public health and safety extends to involuntary treatment of persons who pose a threat to the community. The most common examples of involuntary treatment are state-mandated immunizations for childhood diseases. In the only immunization case ever decided by the U.S. Supreme Court, the Court held that it was constitutionally permissible to force an individual to be vaccinated for smallpox by arguing:

> We are not prepared to hold that a minority, residing or remaining in any city or town where smallpox is prevalent, and enjoying the general protection afforded by an organized local government, may thus defy the will of its constituted authorities, acting in good faith for all, under the legislative sanction of the state. If such be the privilege of a minority, then a like privilege would belong to each individual of the community, and the spectacle would be presented of the welfare and safety of an entire population being subordinated to the notions of a single individual who chooses to remain a part of that population.[9]

A patient who refuses to accept treatment for a contagious disease may be ordered to accept the treatment by a health officer or, depending on the jurisdiction, by a court. A common practice is to incarcerate a recalcitrant patient until the patient consents to the treatment. This coerced consent is not obtained as a sham of an informed consent, but as a way to obviate the need for physically forcing the treatment on the patient. It also gives the patient an opportunity to contest the treatment through a habeas corpus proceeding.

Most mandatory immunization laws contain exemptions for individuals who have a high probability of being injured by the immunization. Many of these laws also exempt persons who have religious objections to immunization. Although the U.S. Constitution allows mandatory immunization of religious objectors, most states do not take advantage of this power. The effectiveness of immunization laws depends on compliance by health care providers and parents. If health care providers give medical exemptions to a large percentage of their patients, the level of immunity in their school system might drop low enough to support a disease epidemic. If a child is improperly exempted from immunization, the health care provider could be held liable should the child contract the disease and suffer any permanent sequelae.

The most difficult political problem in immunization law is the compensation of persons injured by vaccines. (This same issue arises when a person is injured by mandatory treatment for a communicable disease.) Just as persons inducted into the armed forces have no right to sue the government either for deprivation of liberty or for injuries suffered in the line of duty, so persons injured by disease control measures have no constitutional right to compensation. In many cases, however, the government has chosen to allow compensation through laws such as the National Vaccine Injury/Compensation Act.

Personal Restrictions

The most intrusive public health measures are ongoing restrictions of an individual's liberty. A classic example is the case of *Typhoid Mary*. Some people who are infected with typhoid become chronic carriers. If they work in food handling or preparation or in child care, they can spread the disease to others. If they work at other jobs, they pose no risk of disease transmission to their casual contacts. Typhoid Mary was a real person who was a typhoid carrier. She was a threat because she worked as a cook and refused to stop this work. Every time the health department located her, usually through a new outbreak of typhoid, she would move and change her name, but not her occupation. Typhoid Mary infected more than a hundred people, and several of them died of the disease. She was finally placed under house arrest to keep her from cooking and infecting others.

A 1941 case, also involving a typhoid carrier, is a good example of the court's view of the appropriateness of personal restrictions to control disease. The case concerned the issue of whether the identity of typhoid carriers could be disclosed if necessary to prevent them from handling food and thus exposing others to disease. It was argued:

> The Sanitary Code which has the force of law . . . requires local health officers to keep the state department of health informed of the names, ages and addresses of known or suspected typhoid carriers, to furnish to the state health department necessary specimens for laboratory examination in such cases, to inform the carrier and members of his household of the situation and to exercise certain controls over the activities of the carriers, including a prohibition against any handling by the carrier of food which is to be consumed by persons other than members of his own household. . . . Why should the record of compliance by the county health officer with these salutary requirements be kept confidential? Hidden in the files of the health offices, it serves no public purpose except a bare statistical one. Made available to those with a legitimate ground for inquiry, it is effective to check the spread of the dread disease. It would be worse than useless to keep secret an order by a public officer that a certain typhoid carrier must not handle foods which are served to the public.[28]

The most extreme public health restriction is quarantine, or isolation. The word "quarantine" derives from *quadraginta*, meaning 40. It was first used between 1377 and 1403 when Venice and the other chief maritime cities of the Mediterranean adopted and enforced a 40-day detention of all vessels entering their ports.[29] Quarantine was widely used until the 1950s. For self-limited diseases such as measles, the infected person was required to stay home without visitors. For chronic diseases, such as infectious tuberculosis before anti-tubercular agents were available, the infected person might be required to stay at a sanitarium with other infected patients.

With the advent of antibiotics and effective immunizations, quarantine was seldom necessary to prevent the spread of communicable disease. It was still used by tuberculosis control programs when dealing with recalcitrant tuberculosis carriers, but it was usually the homeless and alcoholics who were held because this was the only way to ensure that they got their medicine.

When it was discovered that AIDS was a communicable disease, there was some discussion of using quarantine to prevent its spread. Although it was never considered seriously, the resulting hysteria made public health authorities reluctant to consider quarantine and isolation in any circumstances. Several states, bowing to public pressure, rewrote their disease control laws to make it very difficult to restrict disease carriers. These limitations on the use of restrictive measures are not mandated by the Constitution, and the U.S. Supreme Court has never ruled that public health restrictions of individuals are improper.

The repercussions of these policies were evident in the growing number of reports of the spread of tuberculosis and other diseases from known carriers to health care providers and members of the general population.[30] These were cases that could have been prevented but were not because of limits on the use of effective isolation.[31]

With the reemergence of tuberculosis in the early 1990s and the increase in cases of pan-drug-resistant tuberculosis, public health authorities in many states were facing a deadly, untreatable disease without the legal tools necessary to control its spread. Public health officials had to go to their legislatures and ask the legislators to restore powers they had taken away in the 1980s, including the right to use isolation and mandatory treatment without crippling legal process requirements. Many states, such as New York, restored adequate legal authority and public health officials were able to mount a successful campaign to control the reemergence of tuberculosis. Some states, however, were unwilling to revise their laws and still put substantial hurdles in the way of effective management of communicable disease, including drug-resistant tuberculosis. In the future, public health professionals should be wary of giving up powers through legislation, even if they do not feel they need those powers. Nothing requires health departments to use their full constitutional authority, but once this authority is surrendered, it can be very difficult to regain when necessary to manage an unforeseen future outbreak.

THE FUTURE OF PUBLIC HEALTH LAW

Public health faces several challenges: (1) an increasing threat of communicable diseases, both untreatable viral diseases, such as HIV, and bacterial illnesses, such as tuberculosis, that have become relatively resistant to antimicrobial drugs; (2) increasing public distrust of governmental programs, such as disease control measures, that interfere with private interests; and (3) increasing pressure to divert limited public health funds into acute medical care and lifestyle-related chronic diseases.

The key to understanding public health practice and policy is the realization that the mission of public health is to protect the population. Ideally, the interests of the population and the interests of affected individuals will be the same. When they are not, the U.S. Constitution allows individuals to be restricted for the public interest. This power should never be abused, and it should not be used unless necessary. Public health professionals must understand the law, however, and must defend their right to act in the public's interest. This is often politically unpopular, but it is critical to preserving public health authority. The greatest threats to the public's health are public health professionals who do not understand their legal duties and are guided instead by political expediency.

References

1. *Smith v Turner,* 48 US (7 How) 283, 340-341 (1849).
2. *Holmes v Jennison,* 39 US (14 Pet) 540, 616 (1840).
3. In re Halko, 246 Cal 2d 553, 556 (1966).
4. *City of New York v New St. Mark's Baths,* 497 NYS 2d 979, 983 (1986).
5. *Allen v Illinois,* 478 US 364 (1986).
6. *Ex Parte McGee,* 185 P 14, 16 (Kan 1919).
7. Richards EP, Rathbun KC. *Law and the Physician, A Practical Guide.* Boston, Mass: Little Brown & Co; 1993.
8. *Varholy v Sweat,* 15 So 2d 267, 270 (Fla 1943).
9. *Jacobson v Massachusetts,* 197 US 11 358, 363 (1905).
10. *Berkovitz by Berkovitz v US,* 486 US531 (1988).
11. *North Am. Cold Storage Co. v City of Chicago,* 211 US 306 (1908).
12. *Surocco v Geary,* 3 Cal 69 (1853).
13. *Camara v Municipal Court of City and County of San Francisco,* 387 US 523 (1967).
14. *Whalen v Roe,* 429 US 589, 602 (1977).
15. Chorba TL, Berkelman RL, Safford SK, Gibbs NP, Hull HF. Mandatory reporting of infectious diseases by clinicians. *JAMA.* 1989;262:3018-3026.
16. Gaus SM. Reporting child abuse. "Whistle blower protection" and physician responsibility. *Mich Med.* 1988;87(4):191-193.
17. Johnson CF, Showers J. Injury variables in child abuse. *Child Abuse Negl.* 1985;9(2):207-215.
18. Morris JL, Johnson CF, Clasen M. To report or not to report. Physicians' attitudes toward discipline and child abuse. *Am J Dis Child.* February 1985;139(2):194-197.
19. Cole SK. Accuracy of death certificates in neonatal deaths. *Community Med.* February 1989;11(1):1-8.
20. Davis BR, Curb JD, Tung B, et al. Standardized physician preparation of death certificates. *Control Clin Trials.* June 1987;8(2):110-120.
21. Richards EP. The jurisprudence of prevention: society's right of self-defense against dangerous individuals. *Hastings Const Law Q.* 1989;329:16.
22. *Ferguson v City of Charleston.* 532 US67 121 SCt 1281, 149 LEd2d 205 (2001).
23. Hothcote HW, Yorke JA. *Gonorrhea Transmission Dynamics and Control.* New York, NY: Springer-Verlag; 1984.
24. Woodhouse DE, Muth JB, Potterat JJ, Riffe LD. Restricting personal behaviour: case studies on legal measures to prevent the spread of HIV. *Int J STD AIDS.* March/April 1993;4(2):114-117.
25. *Guide to Public Heath Practice: Principles to Protect HIV-Related Confidentiality and Prevent Discrimination.* Washington, DC: Association of State and Territorial Health Officers; 1988.
26. Potterat JJ, Spencer NE, Woodhouse DE, Muth JB. Partner notification in the control of human immunodeficiency virus infection. *Am J Public Health.* 1989;79(7):874(3).
27. Carrell S, Zoler ML. Defiant diseases: hard-won gains erode. *Med World News.* 1990;31(12):20(7).
28. *Thomas v Morris,* 36 NE2d 141, 142 (NY 1941).
29. Bolduan C, Bolduan N. *Public Health and Hygiene.* Philadelphia, Pa: WB Saunders; 1941.
30. Haley CE, McDonald RC, Rossi L, et al. Tuberculosis epidemic among hospital personnel. *Infect Control Hosp Epidemiol.* 1989;204:10.
31. Dooley SW, Villarino ME, Lawrence M, et al. Nosocomial transmission of tuberculosis in a hospital unit for HIV-infected patients. *JAMA.* 1992;267:2632.

PART
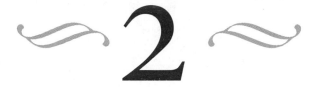
2

Settings for Public Health Practice

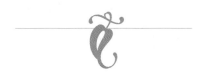

CHAPTER

6

The Federal Contribution to Public Health

William L. Roper, M.D., M.P.H.
Glen P. Mays, M.P.H., Ph.D.

The federal government has a profound influence on the structure and content of population-based efforts to protect and improve health within the United States. Tracking the federal influence on public health policy and practice can be difficult, however, because this influence is achieved through numerous policy and regulatory instruments, and it is shaped by a complex array of legal, political, financial, and institutional structures. Nonetheless, a complete understanding of the practice of public health in the United States requires a critical examination of the federal government's many roles and responsibilities. This chapter reviews the legal and political basis for the federal government's contributions to public health activities, and examines the primary institutional and policy instruments through which it makes these contributions.

HISTORY OF FEDERAL INVOLVEMENT IN PUBLIC HEALTH

The federal government assumed relatively minor roles in protecting and improving public health throughout much of the nation's history. As scientific knowledge about the causes of disease expanded during the eighteenth and nineteenth centuries, individual cities and states within the United States were the first to respond with public facilities, programs, and regulatory provisions designed to prevent and control diseases within the population.[1] Governmental institutions devoted to health and disease existed almost exclusively at the local and state levels. Meanwhile, federal involvement was limited to the Marine Hospital Service, a system of public hospitals established in 1798 to care for merchant seamen. The federal government's role in health began to expand slowly during the early twentieth century when the Marine Hospital Service was transformed into the United States Public Health Service and the position of surgeon general was created to lead the institution.[2] By 1918 this institution had received the authority to administer medical examinations to aliens, to experiment with projects to expand health care in rural areas, and to implement programs that prevent and control sexually transmitted diseases.[1] Also during this period, the United States Congress began to explore the use of federal regulatory powers in preventing and controlling diseases. The 1906 passage of the Food and Drug Act created the nation's first federal regulations covering the manufacture, labeling, and sale of food products.

Federal health activities expanded dramatically during the 1920s and 1930s through the creation of numerous governmental programs designed to increase access to personal health services. The Sheppard-Towner Act of 1922 established the first federal grant-in-aid program supporting the delivery of personal health services. This act created the Federal Board of Maternal and Infant Hygiene and authorized it to administer funding to states for maternal and child health services such as home nursing and obstetrical care.[1] The program soon became a widely replicated model for other federal health programs, wherein the federal government provides funding and oversight to state agencies, which in turn design and implement the programs.[3] Similar programs were created to fund the development of local public health clinics (1935), the training of public health workers (1935), the prevention and control of sexually transmitted diseases (1938), and the creation of community mental health centers (1946).

The federal government's involvement in biomedical research and disease control also expanded dramatically during this period. The National Institutes of Health (NIH) was created in 1930 from a former laboratory within the Marine Hospital Service, expanding rapidly to investigate a broad range of diseases and treatments. Specialized research institutes were soon added to NIH to investigate topics such as cancer, neurological diseases, environmental health issues, and mental health disorders. The federal Center for Disease Control (CDC) was established in 1946, initially to control malaria and other vector-borne diseases during World War II. The CDC's scope of activity expanded dramatically over the years to cover all communicable disease control efforts and, eventually, a broad range of prevention activities involving chronic diseases, injuries, and environmental health risks.[4] The agency was eventually renamed the Centers for Disease Control and Prevention to reflect this larger scope of activity.

The federal government's dominant role in health care financing was solidified in 1965 with the passage of Titles 18 and 19 of the Social Security Act. Title 18 created the federally funded and federally administered Medicare program that financed medical care for the nation's elderly and, eventually, the nation's permanently disabled populations and those with end-stage renal disease. Title 19 established Medicaid, a federal program jointly funded and administered by the states that financed health services for a variety of low-income populations. Numerous other grant-in-aid programs were established during the 1960s and 1970s to fund specific types of health services and programs, such as community health centers, family planning services, dental services, tuberculosis diagnosis and treatment, home health care, childhood developmental and screening services, and health professions training programs.[3]

The financial consequences of an expanding federal role in health care and public health became apparent in the 1970s with spiraling national health care expenditures. In response, the federal government assumed another important role within the nation's health system—that of health resources management and cost containment.[5] Prominent congressional action during the 1970s included: the Health Maintenance Organization Act of 1973, which created incentives for the development of health care delivery and financing systems that would later become known as managed care; and the National Health Planning and

Resources Development Act of 1974, which established review and certification requirements for the development of new health facilities and services.

A number of federal health initiatives were reorganized and, in some cases, scaled back during the 1980s as overall federal health expenditures continued to escalate. Clusters of related federal grant-in-aid programs supporting health and social services were combined into large block grants that gave states more flexibility over how federal funds could be spent. This federal strategy was used in part to stimulate efforts by states and local governments to develop further their health and social service systems.[6] Critics, however, charged that block grants were also used to mask overall reductions in federal funding for these services.[7] Block grants established specifically for public health activities included the Maternal and Child Health Block Grant, the Family Planning Block Grant, and the Preventive Health and Health Services Block Grant.[8] Also during this period, the federal Health Care Financing Administration (HCFA), now known as the Centers for Medicare & Medicaid Services (CMS), implemented bold changes in health care payment policies within the Medicare program to encourage greater efficiency in health care delivery, including a prospective payment system for hospital care in 1984 and a resource-based payment scale for physician services in 1992. HCFA also began large-scale experiments with managed care plans in both the Medicare and Medicaid programs.

Another notable expansion in federal health activity occurred during the 1990s as public concerns turned toward issues of health care quality, patient protection, and health care choice. Historically, individual states had wielded the authority to regulate the practices of health professionals and health insurance plans.[9] Federal involvement in these issues had been limited to the providers and plans that participate in federal health programs such as Medicare, Medicaid, and the Federal Employee Health Benefits Program (FEHBP). The rapid growth of managed care during the 1990s, however, stimulated public concerns about health care quality and choice within private health insurance plans. The legislative response to these concerns has been an unprecedented expansion in federal involvement on issues related to clinical practice and health insurance practices.[10–12] Examples include the 1996 congressional legislation establishing a mandatory 48-hour minimum hospital stay for patients after childbirth; and regulations established as part of the Health Insurance Portability and Accountability Act of 1996 requiring health plans to provide guaranteed renewable insurance coverage to patients with preexisting medical conditions.

In addition to these regulatory activities, the federal government has increasingly turned toward informal and indirect ways of influencing clinical practice and quality of care at the population level.[12] One strategy has been to establish standards and systems for measuring quality within federal health care programs such as Medicare and Medicaid. Because large numbers of health care providers and health plans are involved in these programs, these standards and measures are likely to have important spillover effects on quality and clinical practice in private health care markets.[13] Another strategy has been to use the federal government's convening power to bring together health plans, providers, and other health care stakeholders to reach voluntary, collective agreements on issues of appropriate care and systems for ensuring health care quality. Examples include the federal government's involvement in efforts to develop and expand the Health Plan Employer Data and Information Set (HEDIS) system for monitoring the performance of health plans, and more recently the federal government's roles in developing measures of health care quality as part of the collaborative National Forum for Health Care Quality Measurement and Reporting.[14]

As yet another strategy for addressing public concerns about health care quality, the federal government has steadily strengthened its support for health services research, outcomes research, and prevention research during the 1990s. Spearheaded by federal agencies such as the Agency for Healthcare Research and Quality, or AHRQ (formerly the Agency for Health Care Policy and Research, or AHCPR), along with HCFA (now CMS) and CDC, these federally sponsored research initiatives have sought to uncover ways of applying existing health knowledge, resources, and technologies to realize improvements health care quality and outcomes.[15] Increasingly, these initiatives have also focused on disseminating such evidence broadly among health professionals to improve the practice of health care and public health on a populationwide basis. In the contemporary era of health care and public health, the federal government's purchasing power, convening power, and research power have proven to be powerful instruments in shaping the nation's public health and medical care systems.

POWERS AND ACTIONS OF THE FEDERAL GOVERNMENT IN PUBLIC HEALTH

The federal government's authority in the realm of public health originates with the U.S. Constitution, which divides governmental power between the state and federal levels. The strongest and most visible sources of federal power in public health flow from the constitutional authority to tax, spend, and regulate interstate commerce.[16] The most direct way in which the federal government uses its taxation and spending powers to benefit public health is through the allocation of federal resources to public health programs and services. Federal taxing and spending authority enables the federal government to exist as the nation's single largest purchaser of health services. Similarly, this authority allows the federal government to fund a broad array of categorical-grant

and block-grant programs that support public health programs and services delivered at state and local levels. Total federal health spending has increased dramatically over the past 35 years, from $4.8 billion in 1965 to nearly $400 billion in 1999 (Figure 6.1).[17] Correspondingly, the federal share of all health expenditures in the United States has risen from 12 percent in 1965 to almost 33 percent in 1999 (Figure 6.2). By comparison, state and local government spending on health has remained relatively stable at 13 to 14 percent of all U.S. health expenditures. Federal health expenditures are projected to climb to $713 billion by 2008, continuing to account for nearly 33 percent of all health spending.

Personal health services account for the vast majority of federal spending in health. In 1999, 91 percent of the $400 billion in federal health expenditures was dedicated to federal programs that finance the delivery of personal health services.[17] These programs include

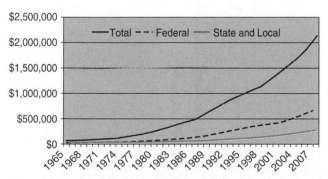

Figure 6.1. Annual Governmental Expenditures in Health, 1965–2008 (in $ millions)

Note: Data before 1999 are actual; data on and after 1999 are projected.

Source: Authors' analysis of data from: US Health Care Financing Administration. *National Health Expenditures by Type of Service and Source of Funds. Calendar Years 1960–99.* Washington, DC: US Department of Health and Human Services; 2000.

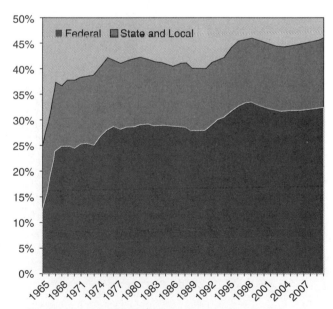

Figure 6.2. Proportion of National Health Expenditures Contributed by Government Spending, 1965–2008

Note: Data before 1999 are actual; data on and after 1999 are projected.

Source: Authors' analysis of data from: US Health Care Financing Administration. *National Health Expenditures by Type of Service and Source of Funds: Calendar Years 1960–99.* Washington, DC: US Department of Health and Human Services; 2000.

Medicare, Medicaid, FEHBP, the Department of Defense and Department of Veteran's Affairs' health care systems that provide health care to active-duty military personnel and veterans, the Civilian Health and Medical Program for the Uniformed Services (CHAMPUS) that covers health care for family members of military personnel, and the State Children's Health Insurance Program (SCHIP) that covers health care for low-income uninsured children. Because state governments participate in funding both Medicaid and SCHIP, federal expenditures account for only part of the program costs associated with these programs.

Approximately $4.7 billion in federal funds were allocated to public health programs in 1999, such as the Maternal and Child Health Block Grant and the Preventive Health and Health Services Block Grant (Figure 6.3).[17] Consequently, federal public health spending comprised only 1.1 percent of all federal

health spending in 1999, down from 4.4 percent in 1965 (Figure 6.4). This trend results from the fact that federal spending on personal health services has dramatically outpaced spending on public health programs over the past 35 years. By comparison, state and local government spending on public health programs reached almost $42 billion in 1999 (Figure 6.3), accounting for 26 percent of all state and local health expenditures (Figure 6.4) and 90 percent of all governmental expenditures on public health programs.

In addition to resource allocation authority, the federal government uses its taxation and spending powers in several other ways to influence public health. First, the federal taxation power is often used to discourage private activities and behaviors that threaten the public's health, and to encourage activities that enhance public health and well-being.[16] For example, the federal government imposes taxes on cigarettes and alcohol that help to discourage con-

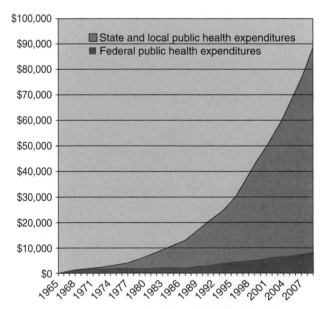

Figure 6.3. Governmental Expenditures on Public Health Programs, 1965–2008 (in $ millions)

Note: Data before 1999 are actual; data on and after 1999 are projected.

Source: Authors' analysis of data from: US Health Care Financing Administration. *National Health Expenditures by Type of Service and Source of Funds: Calendar Years 1960–99.* Washington, DC: US Department of Health and Human Services; 2000.

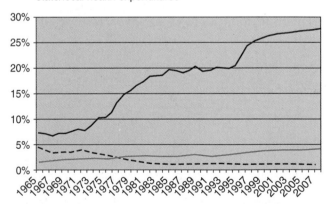

Figure 6.4. Proportion of Governmental Health Expenditures Devoted to Public Health Programs, 1965–2008

Note: Data before 1999 are actual; data on and after 1999 are projected.

Source: Authors' analysis of data from: US Health Care Financing Administration. *National Health Expenditures by Type of Service and Source of Funds: Calendar Years 1960–99.* Washington, DC: US Department of Health and Human Services; 2000.

sumption of these harmful products by raising the total prices that consumers must pay. Similarly, federal fuel taxes can be viewed as instruments for discouraging excessive fuel consumption that is harmful to air quality. The use of governmental taxation powers for purposes of behavior modification raises some important ethical issues because this strategy could be perceived as governmental endorsement of harmful activities, and because this strategy could lead government to become financially dependent on the tax revenue generated by harmful activities. Such ethical issues are less apparent when federal taxation powers are used to encourage behaviors that benefit public health. For example, the federal government provides tax exemptions to employers that provide health insurance coverage for their workers.[18]

Second, the federal government uses its spending authority to influence the actions of state governments that receive federal funds.[16] The federal government may establish a variety of conditions that states must meet to receive funds through various federal grant-in-aid programs. For example, the federal government requires state Medicaid programs to establish a minimum set of program benefits and to conform with federal program eligibility criteria to receive federal Medicaid funds. The federal government also uses its spending on nonhealth programs to induce states to undertake activities that benefit public health. For example, federal highway construction programs frequently include provisions that encourage states to adopt policies that promote highway safety, such as seatbelt campaigns and speed-limit regulations.

Third, the federal government frequently uses its spending authority to create new information and technologies that improve the practice of public health and medicine. The federal government is by far the largest funding agency for biomedical and behavioral research concerning health. By supporting the work of federal researchers as well as university-based scientists, the federal government engages in the discovery of new health interventions and new ways of organizing, delivering, and financing these interventions. These discoveries shape the scope and content of work carried out by health professionals and health care facilities across the nation as well as globally. Frequently, federally funded research pro-

vides the scientific foundation for the development and marketing of new drugs, devices, and other technologies produced by the pharmaceutical and health technology industries. In many cases, these discoveries also inform the design and implementation of health policies and regulations carried out by federal, state, and local governments. In 1999, the federal government spent $15.2 billion for health-related research through agencies such as NIH, CDC, HCFA (now CMS), and AHRQ (formerly AHCPR).[17]

While the power to tax and spend is substantial, the federal government's authority to regulate interstate commerce is often regarded as its most important instrument for influencing public health.[16] This authority provides the legal basis for federal involvement in public health issues that historically have fallen within the exclusive domain of state and local governments, including water and air quality, food and drug safety, occupational health, and health care quality and patient protection. Under this authority, the U.S. Congress has passed legislation regulating industrial and commercial activities that introduce toxins into the air, water, and soil; the manufacture, labeling, and sale of pharmaceuticals and food products; the working conditions that employers maintain for their personnel; and most recently the practices of health insurance plans and their affiliated health care providers. The constitutional provisions protecting state sovereignty, however, impose strict limits on the federal government's commerce power. The U. S. Supreme Court has ruled against a variety of federal legislative and executive actions that were perceived to interfere in purely intrastate issues, including federal restrictions on the possession of handguns and the disposal of hazardous waste. The federal government's public health authority related to interstate commerce is therefore heavily dependent upon judicial interpretations of constitutional law. These interpretations evolve over time as case law develops and as legal, social, and political values change.

In addition to its official constitutional powers, the federal government also uses a variety of informal mechanisms for influencing public health. Both elected and appointed officials within the federal government frequently use the visibility and stature of their federal offices to advance public health causes and address public health issues.[19] These mechanisms may include: raising public awareness about important public health topics through speeches, conferences, publications, and public education campaigns; convening major stakeholders in public health to identify important public health problems and potential solutions; and communicating and negotiating with relevant organizations and/or governments to achieve voluntary participation in and compliance with public health initiatives. In some cases, these activities may be undertaken to create broad-based political support for specific legislation under consideration by the U.S. Congress. In other cases, these activities are undertaken exclusively to influence the behavior of individuals and organizations through informal mechanisms, and are therefore unrelated to legislative agendas within the federal government. The U.S. surgeon general often leads federal government efforts to inform and influence health-related decision making among individuals, health professionals, health care organizations, and other stakeholders. A variety of other government officials may also provide federal leadership on specific health policy issues, including the president and vice president, the administrators of key federal agencies such as the U.S. Department of Health and Human Services and the CDC, and individual members of Congress that have a strong knowledge of and interest in public health issues.

ORGANIZATION OF THE FEDERAL GOVERNMENT

The federal government's roles in public health are carried out through all three branches of government. The legislative branch occupied by the U.S. Congress holds constitutional authority for creating federal programs, policies, and regulations that influence public health, and for appropriating the federal funds that allow them to be implemented. The executive branch holds the authority for implementing public health programs and enforcing health-related policies and regulations through its many administrative agencies. The executive office also has responsibility for informing the budgetary and legislative processes of Congress. The judicial branch occupied by the federal courts carries out the critical responsibility of interpreting and adjudicating the federal government's public health authority in view of constitutional law, legislative action, and legal precedent.

Organization of the Legislative Branch

Most legislative action involving federal health programs and policies can originate in either house of Congress. Constitutional provisions, however, require that legislation involving the levying of taxes begin in the U.S. House of Representatives. Two basic forms of legislative action are undertaken by Congress: (1) *authorization* legislation is used to create or modify federal programs and policies; and (2) *appropriations* legislation is used to allocate federal funding to authorized programs. Authorization legislation begins when a member of Congress submits a bill that proposes to create or alter the structure and operation of a federal program, policy, or agency. Often this bill includes specifications for the program's maximum expenditure amount and duration.

The process through which an authorization bill becomes a law includes the familiar steps of (1) assignment to a legislative committee for review and consideration; (2) committee hearings to facilitate legislative deliberation on the bill; (3) committee markups during which committee members offer amendments; (4) committee reporting of the bill to the full legislative body (House or Senate) for further amendments and approval; (5) House and Senate joint conferencing on the bill once versions are approved by each house of Congress; (6) final approval of the conference bill in both houses; and (7) approval (or veto) by the president. Voting majorities of two-thirds in each house are required to overturn a presidential veto.

Health-related authorization bills are reviewed and considered by numerous legislative committees within the House and Senate, but four committees process the majority of such legislation.[7] In the Senate, the Finance Committee holds jurisdiction over all proposals involving Medicare and Medicaid, whereas the Health, Education, Labor, and Pensions Committee (formerly the Labor and Human Resources Committee) considers legislation involving public health programs, health workforce and medical education issues, health regulatory issues (e.g., food and drug regulations or medical privacy regulations), and health research initiatives (e.g., NIH programs). In the House, Medicare legislation falls under the jurisdiction of the Ways and Means Committee; however, bills involving Medicare Part B (physician services and ancillary services) also fall under the purview of the Commerce Committee. Additionally, the House Commerce Committee considers most legislation involving Medicaid, public health programs, health workforce issues, health regulatory issues, and health research initiatives.

Appropriations bills are handled as part of the congressional budget process. This process makes a key distinction between entitlement programs and discretionary programs. Entitlement programs are those for which the authorizing legislation requires the federal government to pay benefits to all individuals, governments, or other entities that meet program eligibility criteria. Spending on entitlement programs currently makes up more than half of all federal spending.[7] The largest health related federal entitlement programs include Medicare and Medicaid. For these programs, federal expenditures are determined largely by the number of individuals that meet the eligibility criteria, rather than by explicit legislative action. By contrast, discretionary programs are subject to Congress' annual appropriations process. This process involves congressional consideration of 13 different bills that fund discretionary programs. Each body of Congress has an appropriations committee to oversee this process, with subcommittees providing the detailed review and consideration of individual appropriations bills. Appropriations for most public health programs are included in a bill that funds the departments of labor, health and human services, and education. Appropriations for Department of Veteran's Affairs health programs are included in a separate bill considered by the Subcommittee on Veterans Affairs and Housing and Urban Development in each house of Congress.

Congress maintains several established mechanisms for obtaining information about the health issues, policies, and programs under its consideration.[20] The General Accounting Office (GAO), often considered the watchdog arm of Congress, is charged with monitoring the financial and operational performance of federal agencies and programs, and with investigating policy issues of significant congressional interest. The GAO maintains an analytical division devoted to issues of public health and health services delivery, which wields substantial influence over federal public health policy by informing Congress about the performance of federal public health programs and about the need for policy and programmatic changes. Much of the GAO's work is undertaken in response to requests from individual members of Congress. Another legislative institution, the Congressional Budget Office (CBO), provides the legislature with information about the current and potential cost of federal programs and policies. In the domain of federal health policy, the CBO is active in producing estimates of future federal health care expenditures resulting from current and proposed health programs, as well as estimates of the costs incurred by health care purchasers and providers in complying with current and proposed health care regulations. These estimates are often profoundly influential, and occasionally controversial, in congressional policy debates. A third congressional institution that is active in the federal health policy arena is the Congressional Research Service (CRS), which analyzes and syntheses information from a variety of sources to inform legislative decision making. The CRS produces systematic reviews of the scientific literature that are relevant to federal health policy decisions, as well as descriptive analyses of existing federal and state laws that may inform these decisions.

Organization of the Executive Branch

The executive branch of federal government comprises the executive office of the president, 15 cabinet-level departments, and several independent agencies. The majority of health-related programs and policies are administered by the U.S. Department of Health and Human Services; however, a number of other executive departments administer such programs, including the Department of Education, Department of Labor, Department of Veterans Affairs, Department of Defense, Department of Agriculture, and Department of Transportation (Figure 6.5). Additionally, several

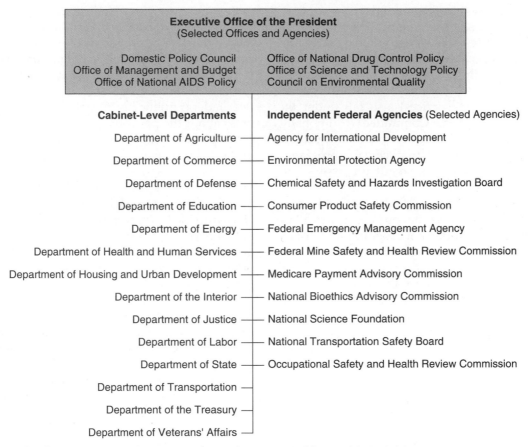

Figure 6.5. Federal Executive Branch Agencies Contributing to Public Health Activities

Source: Authors' analysis.

administrative units within the executive office of the president play important roles in the development, coordination, and management of public health policies and programs. These governmental agencies and their contributions to public health are detailed below.

Department of Health and Human Services

Most of the federal agencies that administer public health programs and services are organized within the U.S. Department of Health and Human Services (DHHS) (Figure 6.6). This cabinet-level department administers programs involving public health services, medical care financing and delivery, mental health and substance abuse services, and social services including income support and child welfare programs. Eight of the agencies within DHHS comprise the U.S. Public Health Service, a functional division of DHHS devoted to public health activities. Each of these agencies is described below.

Centers for Disease Control and Prevention

The Centers for Disease Control and Prevention (CDC) operates 11 administrative units devoted to preventing and controlling specific disease, injury, and disability risks on a national level through research, epidemiological surveillance and investigation, and program development and dissemination

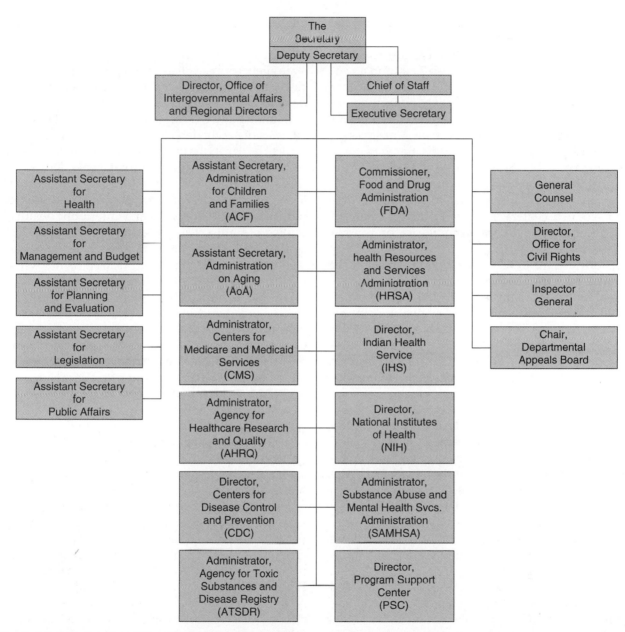

Figure 6.6. Organization of the U.S. Department of Health and Human Services

Source: U.S. Department of Health and Human Services (http://www.hhs.gov/); 2001.

activities. Because of this broad scope of activity, the CDC has become known worldwide as the nation's leading public health agency. The CDC carries out its mission through a staff of more than 7,500 and an annual budget that totaled $2.6 billion in fiscal year 1999. The CDC maintains a strong intramural research program that utilizes advanced laboratory and field resources to examine disease risks, transmission routes, and prevention and control strategies for a wide range of public health threats. Additionally, the CDC maintains an extensive extramural research program that involves a broad network of university-based research centers in scientific investigation of public health risks and opportunities for prevention and control.

Historically, the CDC's research and development initiatives have emphasized laboratory and epidemiological methods for investigating disease transmission and control mechanisms and evaluating prevention interventions. In recent decades, the CDC's scientific agenda in public health has expanded to include the application of behavioral and social sciences for the study of public health issues such as the adoption and diffusion of prevention practices among health professionals and populations at risk, and the cost-effectiveness of community-level interventions such as health education campaigns. As evidence of this new emphasis, the CDC created a Program for Prevention Effectiveness Research in 1991 to foster the development and application of social science methods for the study of public health intervention performance in real-world settings. Six of the functional units within the CDC are organized around specific disease processes, populations, and intervention opportunities. The remaining 5 units address national public health resource and infrastructure needs that cut across specific disease areas and populations. The 11 operating units of the CDC are described in Table 6.1.

Among all the federal health agencies, the CDC is undoubtedly the most heavily invested in intergovernmental relationships with state and local public health organizations. Many of the CDC's initiatives in disease surveillance and control depend upon activities carried out by state public health agencies and their affiliated local health departments. For ex-ample, the National Notifiable Diseases Surveillance System and the Behavioral Risk Factor Surveillance System depend upon data collected and reported by state agencies (as well as local agencies in the former case). Likewise, state and local agencies frequently depend on the specialized expertise and technology maintained at CDC for activities such as laboratory analysis of newly detected unknown pathogens and control of particularly potent infectious disease outbreaks. To address these mutual dependencies, the CDC maintains a series of efforts to equip state and local public health workforces with the necessary expertise and technology to carry out public health activities of national importance. For example, CDC assigns trained staff to work in each of the nation's state public health agencies, as well as many local health departments, carrying out disease surveillance and control activities as well as special research and demonstration initiatives. Perhaps the oldest and largest of these initiatives, the CDC's Epidemic Intelligence Service (EIS), has placed health professionals in state health departments around the nation since 1951 to carry out two-year fellowships devoted to epidemiological investigation.[4] The CDC also maintains a number of workforce development initiatives that range from training and continuing education programs to staff exchange programs—all designed to strengthen state and local public health agency capacities for implementing core public health activities.

Finally, the CDC routinely develops cooperative agreements with state and local agencies as well as professional associations for the development of specific programs and tools to enhance public health capacity. For example, the CDC's Public Health Practice Program Office has worked collaboratively with the National Association of County and City Health Officials (NACCHO) for nearly a decade in developing self-assessment tools for local public health organizations, including the widely used *Assessment Protocol for Excellence in Public Health* (described in chapter 1). Moreover, this CDC office is currently developing a national performance measurement system for public health organizations in collaboration with state and local health agencies.[21]

Table 6.1. Operational Units of the U.S. Centers for Disease Control and Prevention

Units for Disease-Specific and Population-Specific Health Issues

National Center for Chronic Disease Prevention and Health Promotion	Fields research and development activities involving chronic disease prevention and early intervention for health conditions such as cancer; cardiovascular disease; diabetes; arthritis; and the special health concerns of maternal, infant, and adolescent populations. Among other activities, this center fields the Behavioral Risk Factor Surveillance System that collects periodic national and state-level data on adult health risk factors.
National Center for HIV, STD, and TB Prevention	Administers surveillance and disease prevention and control programs that target the transmission of the serious and often-interrelated communicable diseases of human immunodeficiency virus (HIV); other sexually transmitted diseases; and tuberculosis.
National Center for Infectious Diseases	Sponsors research and program development activities designed to prevent and control a wide array of existing, emerging, and resurgent infectious diseases—including those that pose unique health threats due to drug resistance or intentional transmission through bioterrorist acts.
National Center for Injury Prevention and Control	Designs and fields research and intervention programs that focus on the prevention of both unintentional and intentional injuries occurring outside the workplace.
National Institute for Occupational Safety and Health	Supports scientific investigations of workplace health threats and designs preventionand control programs to improve safety and wellness and reduce health risks within occupational settings.
National Center for Environmental Health	Fields research and intervention efforts designed to forestall illness, disability, and death due to human interaction with harmful environmental substances such as indoor and outdoor air pollutants; hazardous wastes; waterborne pathogens and pollutants; food-borne pathogens; and lead exposure.

Units for Cross-Cutting Resources and Infrastructure

National Center for Health Statistics	Functions as the nation's public health data repository by fielding national surveys of health status, health behavior, and health care practices and by maintaining vital and health statistics databases. Among the periodic national surveys and surveillance systems fielded by the center are: the National Health Care Survey, the National Immunization Survey, the National Health Interview Survey, and the National Health and Nutrition Examination Survey. The center also maintains efforts for tracking national statistics on prenatal care, births, deaths through the National Vital Statistics System.
Public Health Practice Program Office	Performs research, technical assistance, program development, and evaluative activities designed to strengthen the nation's public health infrastructure and improve the organization and operation of state and local public health systems. This office sponsors initiatives that target the development of state and local public health agencies and administrators, public health laboratories, public health information systems, and global public health workforce and infrastructure capacities.

(continues)

Table 6.1. *(continued)*

Units for Cross-Cutting Resources and Infrastructure	
Epidemiology Program Office	Supports the development and use of epidemiological surveillance systems, analytical methods, and tools throughout the CDC and the public health organizations with which it interacts. Among other activities, this office maintains the National Notifiable Diseases Surveillance System, which tracks the incidence of 52 high-priority infectious diseases among U.S. residents.
National Immunization Program	Oversees national and state-based efforts to expand age-appropriate vaccination coverage rates for children, adolescents, and adults. This agency has been heavily involved in the development of immunization registries and tracking systems at the provider level, the community level, and the state level.
Office of the Director	Provides management, oversight, and coordination for all CDC activities. This office also houses administrative units devoted to cross-cutting public health issues of high importance, including offices for women's health, minority health, global health, vaccine programs, and technology transfer.

SOURCE: Authors' analysis.

Other Agencies of the U.S. Public Health Service

The CDC effectively functions as the federal government's lead agency for both scientific and practice-based public health activities. Nevertheless, a number of other federal agencies within DHHS carry out critical public health functions that complement those of the CDC. Key among these agencies are the seven additional entities that comprise the U.S. Public Health Service.

The *Health Resources and Services Administration* (HRSA) administers nearly $4 billion annually through federal programs designed to expand public access to health care professionals and facilities, particularly in underserved areas. The largest of these programs are organized within four main bureaus, and a variety of smaller programs and policy development initiatives are administered by separate offices and centers within HRSA. The Maternal and Child Health Bureau within HRSA administers an array of services and programs designed to increase the timely delivery and uptake of prenatal, infant, and child health services to ensure the health of children and their families. This bureau administers grants to states through the Maternal and Child Health Services Block Grant, which supports programs designed to reduce infant mortality; provide compre-

hensive care for women before, during, and after pregnancy and childbirth; reduce adolescent pregnancy; improve childhood vaccination coverage; and meet the nutritional and developmental needs of children and their families. The bureau also administers categorical grant programs that support the provision of emergency medical services for children and the delivery of abstinence education services to children and adolescents.

The Bureau of Primary Health Care within HRSA provides funding and technical assistance to agencies that provide comprehensive primary care services in medically underserved areas, including local health departments as well as nonprofit community health centers. HRSA's Bureau of Health Professions maintains programs for monitoring and improving the accessibility of health professionals within the United States, including the National Health Services Corps, which sponsors professionals to practice in medically underserved communities. Other initiatives sponsored by this bureau are designed to address training needs and potential workforce shortages and surpluses of health professionals in various fields of specialization and practice settings. A Bureau of HIV/AIDS Services administers funding and technical assistance to programs that provide primary medical care and support services to individuals with HIV and AIDS, and to programs that conduct clinical research on HIV services.

A special programs division within HRSA manages a variety of health resource initiatives. These include the Hill-Burton program, which ensures that health facilities funded through the federal Hill-Burton Act meet their obligations to provide adequate levels of free and reduced-fee care to low-income populations. Also administered through this office is the federal Organ Procurement and Transplantation Network that coordinates organ and tissue donation activities. A number of independent offices and centers within HRSA administer smaller and more focused programs, including those devoted to rural health policy, minority health, telehealth, managed care, and public health practice.

The *National Institutes of Health* (NIH), also organized within the U.S. Public Health Service, is the nation's leading agency for biomedical research. The NIH sponsors both intramural and extramural research activities on many different issues of public health importance. Comprised of 25 separate research institutes and centers, the NIH emphasizes both laboratory research and, to a lesser but growing extent, clinical research. Medical schools and academic health centers across the country depend on NIH for most of their research funding, as NIH operates with a budget that totaled nearly $16 billion in fiscal year 1999. The single largest NIH research effort, the Human Genome Project, endeavors to characterize the human genome through a complete mapping and sequencing of the human DNA—an initiative that could have profound public health applications through disease prevention and early detection strategies. Other NIH units with a specific public health focus include the National Cancer Institute, the National Institute of Allergy and Infectious Diseases, the National Institute of Child Health and Human Development, the National Heart, Lung, and Blood Institute, and the National Institute of Environmental Health Sciences.

The *Agency for Healthcare Research and Quality*, or AHRQ, (formerly the Agency for Health Care Policy and Research) administers a smaller and more focused health research enterprise in comparison to NIH. The agency's sponsored research generally focuses on the organization, delivery, and financing of health services—which includes preventive and public health services but often emphasizes medical care services. Issues of health care quality and accessibility are additional research areas with particular relevance to public health activities. The agency is particularly active in the development of clinical practice guidelines and strategies for evidence-based clinical practice grounded in sound scientific research. The agency is also increasingly focused on initiatives to disseminate information on health care quality to health care consumers, providers, and purchasers to improve the effectiveness and efficiency of health care delivery.

The *Food and Drug Administration* (FDA) functions as the nation's largest consumer protection agency by administering regulatory programs to ensure the safety of food, cosmetics, medicines, medical devices, and radiation-emitting products. Veterinary food and medications also fall under the regulatory purview of the FDA. As specified in the federal Food, Drug and Cosmetics Act of 1962 and the FDA Modernization Act of 1997, the FDA's responsibility in drug and device regulation involves ensuring the safety as well as the efficacy of these products. For all of the products monitored by the FDA, the agency ensures accurate labeling, marketing, and consumer information. In carrying out these activities, the FDA inspects food and drug manufacturing facilities, tests products, reviews scientific evidence in support of safety and efficacy claims, and monitors labeling and marketing practices. The FDA enforces its regulatory authority through both governmental influence and legal sanction. The agency frequently encourages manufacturers of products to undertake voluntary corrections or institute voluntary product recalls when problems are identified. When necessary, the agency can obtain court orders to prohibit the manufacture and sale of products or to seize and destroy existing products. The agency can also pursue criminal penalties against manufacturers and distributors.

The *Indian Health Service* (IHS) administers programs that provide health services to federally recognized American Indian and Alaska Native tribes. This unit of the U.S. Public Health Service provides health services directly through IHS-operated facilities, and by contract with tribal organizations. Federally operated facilities consist of 37 hospitals, 64 health centers, 50 health stations, and 5 school-based health clinics. The health organizations supported through IHS funds provide both medical and public health services to native populations.

The *Agency for Toxic Substances and Disease Registry* (ATSDR) operates programs to prevent and control exposure to hazardous substances. With strong administrative ties to the CDC, the agency performs public health assessments of waste sites; maintains health surveillance systems and registries for hazardous substances; provides consultation to governments and corporations regarding the use, transport, and storage of hazardous substances; responds to emergency releases of hazardous substances; and conducts applied research in hazardous substance assessment and containment. The agency also maintains a series of education and training initiatives concerning hazardous substances that target health professionals, industrial and environmental workers, and the general public.

The *Substance Abuse and Mental Health Services Administration* (SAMHSA) administers programs for the prevention, treatment, and rehabilitation of substance abuse and mental illness. The agency manages two large federal block grant programs that provide states with funds to implement an array of prevention and treatment programs: the Mental Health Services Block Grant; and the Substance Abuse Prevention and Treatment Block Grant. The agency also maintains an extensive surveillance and research portfolio concerning the quality, cost, accessibility, and outcomes of mental health and substance abuse services. Finally, the agency is actively involved in providing technical assistance and consultation to mental health and substance abuse service providers.

Other Agencies of the U.S. Department of Health and Human Services

Several other agencies within the U.S. Department of Health and Human Services play important roles in public health activities even though their primary areas of operation lie outside the functional domain of the U.S. Public Health Service. Prime among these

agencies is the Health Care Financing Administration (HCFA), which was renamed the Centers for Medicare & Medicaid Services (CMS) in July 2001. CMS administers the federal government's largest medical care financing programs, including: Medicare, which covers elderly and disabled individuals; Medicaid, which covers low-income families and children; and the State Child Health Insurance Program (SCHIP), which covers low- and moderate-income uninsured children. The Medicaid and SCHIP programs are particularly important funding sources not only for mainstream medical care providers, but also for public health providers that serve vulnerable and underserved populations. CMS exercises only partial control over the design and operation of these two programs because individual states have flexibility to modify eligibility standards, program benefits, and delivery and payment mechanisms under these programs. Moreover, many states have secured federal waivers to institute Medicaid managed care programs that deviate from federal program requirements—such as waivers that allow states to impose limits on a recipient's choice of providers.

Because CMS controls a substantial proportion of the nation's health care financing resources through Medicare, Medicaid, and SCHIP, the agency is able to use its influence and purchasing power to effect changes in clinical and administrative practice across the entire U.S. health system. For example, CMS creates incentives for managed care plans to participate in the quality measurement initiatives maintained by the National Committee for Quality Assurance, and to field periodic consumer satisfaction surveys using a common measurement instrument developed by AHRQ. CMS also carries out periodic inspections and surveys of health care facilities that participate in the Medicare and Medicaid programs, to ensure quality of care in these facilities. These activities are likely to affect the quality of care not just for beneficiaries of federal health programs, but also for the millions of other health care consumers that are served by these providers.

Other agencies within the Department of Health and Human Services that contribute to public health activities include the Administration on Aging, which administers social and health services programs for older Americans; and the Administration for Children and Families, which operates programs for the social and economic support of children and families. The Administration on Aging programs that are relevant to public health include those that address the health information and health education needs of the elderly; the nutritional, social support, and long-term-care needs of the elderly; the health and social support needs of formal and informal caregivers for the elderly; and the safety, injury prevention, and violence prevention needs of the elderly. By comparison, the Administration for Children and Families' programs relevant to public health include the federal Head Start program that provides early educational opportunities and nutritional support to young impoverished children; the Family and Youth Services program that, among other activities, provides health education and counseling services to homeless and runaway youth; programs to prevent and treat sexual abuse among children; and programs that provide health and support services to children and adults with developmental disabilities and mental retardation.

DHHS maintains several offices at the departmental level that are designed to coordinate public health activities across the major agencies and units within the department. These offices help the department as a whole to realize opportunities for cross-agency collaboration in addressing major public health issues that span multiple areas of operation and expertise. These offices also help the department to achieve a unified voice in communicating public health issues to the public and other major constituencies in health. The Office of the Surgeon General, perhaps the most widely known departmental office, serves as the nation's leading spokesperson for public health issues. The surgeon general also oversees the Commissioned Corps of the U.S. Public Health Service, a collection of more than six thousand federal health professionals that provide first-response intervention in the event of national public health emergencies.

The Office of Disease Prevention and Health Promotion works to coordinate federal preventive health programs across the department, including the effort to develop and monitor national health promotion and disease prevention objectives for the nation through the *Healthy People 2000* and *Healthy People 2010* programs. The Office of Emergency Preparedness coordinates health-related disaster preparedness and response activities for the department, while the Office of International and Refugee Health serves as the department's coordinating agency for global health initiatives. Several other department-level offices develop policy, public awareness strategies, and research initiatives for major national health priorities, including the Office of HIV/AIDS Policy, the Office of Minority Health, the Office on Women's Health, the Office of Family Planning, the Office of Adolescent Pregnancy Programs, and the President's Council on Physical Fitness and Sports.

Other Federal Agencies with Public Health Responsibilities

A number of other federal agencies are not part of the U.S. DHHS but nonetheless contribute substantially to federal public health activities. Many of these agencies carry out their public health activities in close collaboration with administrative units of DHHS. Key among these agencies is the U.S. Department of Agriculture (USDA), which sponsors an array of health-related programs involving nutritional support, food safety, and farm-worker and rural health. Among the best-known public health programs administered by this department is the Special Supplemental Food Program for Women, Infants, and Children, commonly known as WIC, which provides food assistance and nutritional education for pregnant women, postpartum and breastfeeding women, infants, and young children in low-income households. Another large nutrition program administered by the department is the Food Stamp Program, which provides low-income individuals and families with assistance in purchasing food products to reduce hunger and improve diet among disadvantaged populations.

Several other nutritional programs are administered by the USDA for low-income populations, including a food commodity distribution program and the National School Lunch and School Breakfast Programs. The USDA's Food Safety and Inspection Service works to ensure the safety of meat and poultry products through the routine inspection and evaluation of product production, content, and labeling. The department's Office of Public Health and Science works closely with the FDA and CDC to evaluate food-borne disease risks within the population and to develop policies, plans, and regulations to prevent and control these risks. The department also operates a consumer education program on food-borne illnesses jointly with the FDA, which strives to expand the use of safe food handling and preparation practices among consumers. Finally, the USDA contributes to public health activities through a broad range of rural development programs, including initiatives to improve access to health care in rural areas through telemedicine projects and through efforts to attract and retain health professionals in underserved areas.

Though not a cabinet-level department, the Environmental Protection Agency (EPA) makes substantial contributions to federal public health activities through its role in developing and enforcing a wide array of environmental health and safety regulations. The EPA's regulatory authority extends to air quality, water quality, radiation exposure, solid waste disposal, pesticides and toxic substances, and issues of environmental justice. In addition to enforcing federal environmental laws and developing regulations authorized by these laws, the EPA maintains an array of partnerships with businesses and community organizations designed to foster voluntary efforts to improve environmental health conditions. These partnerships include efforts to reduce the production of greenhouse gasses, to promote energy conservation within businesses and communities, and to prevent environmental pollution associated with pesticide use. The EPA also administers a variety of public education and information dissemination programs designed to encourage environmentally sound practices among consumers and businesses.

The U.S. Department of Housing and Urban Development (HUD) engages in public health issues through a variety of federal programs to address the health risks associated with housing and homelessness, and to address the health needs of populations residing in public housing facilities and shelters. HUD maintains a large program to reduce lead poisoning risks in housing units that are supported through federal housing assistance programs, and to educate citizens about lead hazards and optimal prevention and abatement practices. The department also administers the federal Lead-Based Paint Hazard Control Grant Program, which funds state and local governments to implement initiatives that control and abate lead hazards in privately owned low-income housing units and in areas near Superfund cleanup sites. Similarly, HUD administers programs to promote safety and prevent injuries in low-income housing facilities, and it cooperates with HRSA in administering federal grant programs to support the provision of health education and primary health care services to homeless populations (through the Health Care for the Homeless Program and the Outreach and Primary Health Services for Homeless Children Program) and to residents of public housing facilities (through the Public Housing Primary Health Care Program). HUD also maintains several programs that promote access to quality health care facilities by offering low-cost mortgage insurance to hospitals, nursing homes, assisted-living facilities, and nonprofit group medical practices for use in construction or rehabilitation of these facilities. The largest federal programs administered by HUD—such as the Operating Subsidy for Public Housing Program, the Section 8 Rental Certificate and Voucher Program, the Federal Housing Administration mortgage insurance programs, and the Community Development Block Grant Program—do not address health issues directly, but they nonetheless influence health indirectly by reducing homelessness, improving housing quality and affordability for low- and moderate-income populations, and enhancing community facilities and services.

The U.S. Department of Education plays an important role in federal public health activities through its programs to address the health education and health services needs of students. The department administers the Safe and Drug-Free Schools Program, which is the federal government's primary instrument for preventing and reducing violence and drug, alcohol and tobacco use in and around the nation's schools through education and outreach interventions. This program funds state and local education agencies and state governor's offices to implement a variety of education and prevention programs, and involves close collaboration with other federal agencies within the CDC, the NIH, the Administration on Children and Families, and the Office of National Drug Control Policy. In cooperation with CMS, the department administers the Insure Kids Now Through Schools Campaign, a school-based initiative to enroll eligible low-income uninsured children in SCHIP programs. Similarly, the department provides administrative assistance and support for the Healthy Schools Healthy Communities Initiative, a federal program administered by HRSA to fund the development of school-based health centers that provide comprehensive primary care, health promotion, and disease prevention services to at-risk children. Finally, the department assists state, local, and private educational institutions in developing health education and health promotion curricula for students through its Office of Educational Research and Improvement. This office funds the development, evaluation, and dissemination of a wide range of educational initiatives, including those devoted to educating students about health issues and practices for disease prevention and health promotion.

The U.S. Department of Labor contributes to the federal government's public health agenda through its programs and policies to promote health and safety in the workplace. The department's Occupational Safety and Health Administration (OSHA) develops and enforces federal regulations regarding workplace safety and health conditions, as authorized under the federal Occupational Safety and Health Act. These regulations include those related to indoor air quality, noise exposure, hazardous materials exposure, protection from hazardous equipment and facilities, and employee training regarding safety practices. OSHA also develops partnerships with employers to encourage voluntary compliance with beneficial health and safety practices.

Other health-related programs administered by the department include the Safe Work/Safe Kids Initiative, which involves efforts to educate employers, parents, and schools about the health and safety issues faced by youth workers, and efforts to enforce state and federal child labor laws. The Labor Department is also charged with enforcing and adjudicating provisions of the federal Family and Medical Leave Act, which allows eligible employees to take unpaid leave from jobs to care for family members. The department's Pension and Welfare Benefits Administration is actively involved in enforcing federal regulations covering employer-provided health insurance benefits. These regulations include provisions of the Newborns' and Mothers' Health Protection Act of 1996, which mandates minimum hospital stay benefits for women after childbirth; provisions of the Health Insurance Portability and Accountability Act of 1996, which requires employer-provided health insurance benefits to be more portable and renewable for employees; and provisions of the Employee Retirement and Income Security Act of 1974 (ERISA) which, among other things, creates standards for employer self-insured health plans. The Department of Labor also oversees worker compensation benefits provided to federal employees and workers covered under the federal Black Lung Benefits Program (for mine workers) and the federal Longshore and Harbor Workers Compensation Program (for workers employed on or near U.S. navigable waters).

The U.S. Department of Transportation maintains an array of federal public health programs involving the safety of public and private transportation systems. The department's Federal Highway Administration operates programs to improve pedestrian and bicycle safety, encourage safe driving practices, and enhance highway construction and maintenance to prevent roadway-related injuries and fatalities. These programs include both educational initiatives and infrastructure improvements. Another division within the department, the National Highway Traffic Safety Administration, is charged with developing and enforcing safety standards for motor vehicles, and with providing discretionary grants to state and local governments for local highway safety initiatives. This agency also contains an active research unit that investigates trends in driving behavior and in motor vehicle crashes, and that evaluates the effectiveness of traffic safety programs. Other divisions within the Department of Transportation administer safety policies and regulations for commercial motor vehicles, aviation, railroads, public transit agencies, and maritime transportation.

Two cabinet-level departments contribute substantially to federal public health efforts primarily through the large health care systems that they operate. The U.S. Department of Defense operates a health care system for the nation's military personnel and their family members that includes nearly one hundred hospitals and more than five hundred ambulatory clinics that serve more than 8.2 million individuals worldwide.[22] The department oversees a managed care system known as TRICARE, consisting of a health maintenance organization (HMO) type plan, a preferred-provider plan, and a managed indemnity plan, to improve the quality and efficiency of care delivered to these populations. The department is also actively engaged in research and development activities to identify more effective and efficient ways of delivering health care to its populations. Findings from these activities often inform the design and operation of other public and private health care systems.

Similarly, the U.S. Department of Veterans Affairs (VA) operates a health care system for the nation's military veterans, consisting of 173 medical centers, 391 outpatient centers, and 131 nursing facilities organized within 22 regional networks. The department's Veterans Health Administration oversees this system, which focuses its services on a priority population of low-income veterans with service-connected health problems. The VA health system includes Veteran Outreach Centers that provide readjustment counseling services for veterans of armed hostilities including and following the Vietnam War. The VA also maintains a variety of outreach programs for homeless veterans and for those with alcohol and drug abuse problems. A substantial biomedical and health services research program also exists within the VA system, which makes valuable contributions to the existing body of scientific knowledge about health, disease, and health services delivery.

Many other federal agencies maintain relatively limited and targeted contributions to public health activities. For example, the U.S. Department of Justice oversees a large federal initiative to develop the nation's public health systems for detecting and responding to acts of bioterrorism. This department also pursues federal health objectives through legal action, such as the federal government's efforts to obtain remuneration from the tobacco industry for cigarette-related illnesses experienced by Medicare beneficiaries and Medicaid recipients, and its efforts to protect health care consumers by enforcing federal antitrust policy against health care institutions (in cooperation with the Federal Trade Commission). Likewise, the U.S. Department of Commerce sponsors a variety of research and development projects that focus on the use of telemedicine applications for en-

hancing health care accessibility, efficiency, and quality. Finally, the Federal Emergency Management Agency (FEMA) oversees federal activities in preparing for and responding to natural and human-made disasters.

Additionally, several administrative units within the executive office of the president play important roles in the development, coordination, and management of federal public health policies and programs (Figure 6.5). Key among these units is the Office of Management and Budget (OMB), which is responsible for preparation of the president's budget proposal to Congress and for the overall financial management of federal programs and services. The OMB is also responsible for implementing provisions of the 1993 Government Performance and Results Act, which requires federal agencies to develop and measure specific performance objectives for the programs and policies they administer.[23] Under this initiative, public health organizations that receive federal funding are developing outcome objectives and performance measures in an effort to demonstrate accountability for these federal funds.[24] Another unit within the executive office, the Domestic Policy Council, is charged with developing coordinated federal policies to address broad-based health and social issues. Created in 1989, the council consists of the administrators of major health and social services agencies within the federal government, and has developed policies in areas such as tobacco control, children's health insurance, gun safety, patient's rights, and Medicare policies. The executive office also includes offices that conduct policy development and coordination activities on important public health issues such as environmental quality, AIDS policy, science and technology policy, and drug prevention and control.

Organization of the Judicial Branch

Federal courts also play important roles in shaping public health policy and practice, primarily through their authority to interpret federal public health powers in view of constitutional provisions and federal laws passed by Congress. Federal courts have jurisdiction over issues that involve federal laws, such as when citizens, corporations, or governments dispute federal public health regulations and programs on the constitutional grounds of state sovereignty. Federal courts also have jurisdiction over disputes that arise between citizens, corporations, or governments of different states. Thus, interstate conflicts involving environmental issues such as water quality, air pollution, or hazardous waste disposal fall within the domain of federal courts.

The federal judiciary is organized in a three-tier structure, with U.S. district courts serving as the trial courts where most federal cases begin. There are 94 federal court districts in the United States, with at least 1 district existing within each state. The second tier of the federal judiciary comprises the 12 U.S. courts of appeals. These courts hear cases that are appealed from the district court level, as well as cases that are appealed from decisions made by federal regulatory agencies. The U.S. Supreme Court is the third tier of the judiciary, consisting of the chief justice and eight associate justices. The Supreme Court hears a limited number of cases that involve the Constitution or federal law. These cases may originate either in lower federal courts or in state courts.

The Supreme Court has been profoundly influential in clarifying the division between federal and state public health authority in recent years. An increasingly prevalent interpretation of constitutional law, often referred to as the concept of new federalism, holds that governmental police powers are largely reserved for the states under constitutional law, and are therefore restricted at the federal level.[16,25] In keeping with this concept, the U.S. Supreme Court has overturned a number of federal public health laws that sought to assert federal regulatory authority over that of the states. Recent examples include the 1997 court decision to overturn provisions of the Brady Handgun Violence Prevention Act requiring background checks on handgun purchasers,[26] and the 2000 decision to overturn civil rights provisions of the Violence Against Women Act of 1994.[27]

THE FEDERAL LEGISLATIVE PROCESS

The process of federal policy making in public health derives not only from the established congressional committee structure and system of legislative rules described earlier, but also from the complex and changing array of individuals and organizations outside the legislative branch of government that engage in the federal political process. These entities contribute information, advice, and in some cases campaign funds in an effort to inform and influence congressional decision making on public health issues.[19,28] Such contributions may be made informally through communication and interaction with individual members of Congress and their staffs, or formally through testimony given at congressional hearings, study commissions, and task forces. Some of these entities also attempt to influence congressional decision making by appealing directly to members of the public, including the constituents of key members of Congress, through public education efforts and mass media campaigns.

The nonfederal entities involved in informing and influencing federal legislative decisions in health policy are many and varied, and have grown over time in tandem with the federal government's expanding involvement in health-related programs and regulations. These entities fall into one of six general categories: professional and trade associations; issue-oriented interest groups; political action committees; individual corporations and labor unions; policy think tanks; and nonpartisan research firms.[29] The latter two types of organizations generally contribute information, research and policy recommendations only, and do not engage directly in lobbying members of Congress nor in contributing to congressional campaign funds (federal law prohibits tax-exempt nonprofit organizations from engaging in these activities). Political action committees, by contrast, are formed primarily to participate in electoral politics through campaigning and contributing to campaign funds. In addition to these nongovernmental groups, federal health agencies in the executive branch of government play important roles in informing and influencing congressional decision making, often in tandem with groups outside the federal government. These agencies wield considerable influence in the legislative policy-making process because members of Congress often rely on them as key sources of information about federal health programs and policy needs, and because these agencies are often directly involved in the annual process of preparing the president's budget proposal to Congress. As a consequence, interest groups in public health often attempt to inform and shape congressional decision making indirectly through their relationships with federal health agencies.

Some of the most active interest groups in federal public health policy making represent public health professionals and public health organizations at local and state levels. The nation's oldest and largest professional association, the American Public Health Association (APHA), plays an influential role in advocating for federal programs and policies that address public health issues. Representing more than 50,000 members from over 50 occupational settings in public health, the APHA maintains a 125-year history of involvement in federal policy advocacy. The APHA's legislative activities include developing policy statements about key public health issues that are disseminated to members of Congress; testifying in congressional hearings about public health issues and programs; and informing APHA members, affiliated organizations, and members of the public about public health issues and federal public health policy deliberations. Other public health professional associations that carry out similar advocacy activities include the National Association of County and City Health Officials (NACCHO), which represents a majority of the nation's 2,900 local governmental public health agencies; and the Association of State and Territorial Health Officials (ASTHO), which represents the nation's 51 state public health agencies as well as their counterparts in the U.S. territories. All of these organizations carry out a broad scope of activities in addition to their federal policy advocacy responsibilities.

Other professional and trade associations frequently engage in advocacy activities on behalf of federal health policy issues. Among the most influential professional associations in the health policy domain is the American Medical Association (AMA), which plays a substantial role in shaping virtually every major piece of federal health care legislation through its advocacy and lobbying activities.[30,31] Additionally, there are national professional physician associations that represent most specialty areas of medicine—such as the American Academy of Pediatrics, the American

College of Preventive Medicine, and the American College of Obstetricians and Gynecologists—and these entities are also active in federal public health policy issues. A variety of provider-based associations are likewise heavily involved in advocacy and lobbying activities concerning federal health policy issues, including the American Hospital Association, the American Medical Group Association, and the National Association of Community Health Centers among others. Powerful advocacy groups also exist for specific health issues, such as the American Cancer Society, the American Lung Association, the American Heart Association, and the National Alliance for the Mentally Ill. Interest groups also represent the legislative interests of key health care consumers, including the American Association of Retired Persons, Families USA, and various labor unions. Educational and scientific organizations engage in the federal health policy process through their own advocacy associations, including the American Association of Medical Colleges, the Association of Schools of Public Health, and the Coalition for Health Services Research. Additionally, governmental associations hold substantial influence in the federal health policy arena, including the National Governor's Association and its affiliated institutions, the National Conference of State Legislatures, the National Association of Counties, and the National League of Cities.

Industry-based trade associations are among the most powerful interest groups involved in the federal health policy arena because of the resources they bring to the tasks of advocacy and lobbying. In some cases these associations support policy positions that are directly opposed to those of the public health interest groups, such as the tobacco industry's opposition to federal tobacco control policies, or the firearms industry's opposition to federal gun control proposals. In other cases, public health associations cooperate with major industry associations to advocate for policies of mutual interest. For example, the Pharmaceutical Research and Manufacturers of America often advocate for federal policies supporting childhood and adult immunization in partnership with public health organizations. Other frequently involved health care industry associations include the American Association of Health Plans, the Health Insurance Association of America, and the Washington Business Group on Health (a nonprofit policy think tank for employer-related health policy issues). In recent years, several health advocacy associations have formed that bring professional, governmental, and industry organizations together to pursue shared interests in public health policy issues. Perhaps the best example of this type of association is the Partnership for Prevention, which includes members from public health organizations, health plans, hospital systems, employers, governmental health agencies, and consumer groups.

The federal legislative process is informed not only by organized interest groups, advocacy associations, and executive-branch federal agencies, but also by recognized nonpartisan experts in science and policy. Congress uses a number of mechanisms for obtaining outside expertise relevant to policy deliberations, and these mechanisms are particularly important when complex issues of public health and biomedical science are involved. One formal mechanism for obtaining this advice is to invite testimony from leading experts as part of congressional hearings and study commissions. These experts are often drawn from academic institutions and independent research institutes. Another important mechanism is the creation of a standing federal advisory commission by congressional legislation. An example of such a commission is the Medicare Payment Advisory Commission (MedPAC) established by the Balanced Budget Act of 1997 to advise Congress on policy issues affecting the Medicare program. Like its predecessors the Prospective Payment Assessment Commission and the Physician Payment Review Commission, MedPAC consists of a panel of experts from academia, the health professions, and government that produces regular reports and briefings on the performance of the Medicare program for Congress, and recommends policies and regulations for legislative consideration.

Another institution that serves as a nonpartisan source of information and advice for the Congress is the Institute of Medicine (IOM) within the National Academy of Sciences. The National Academy of Sciences was chartered by Congress in 1863 to serve as an external source of research, investigation, and advice for Congress and any federal agency. The Institute of Medicine was added to the Academy in 1970.

Though organizationally independent from Congress and the federal government, the institute plays critical roles in informing legislative decision making. Organized as a nonprofit organization that convenes the nation's leading scholars and professionals to examine important issues in public health and medicine, the institute initiates studies in response to requests from Congress and from federal agencies. It has produced a large number of influential studies and reports on public health issues, including topics in infectious disease control and prevention, vaccine safety, bioterrorism, medical errors and health care quality, and public health infrastructure.

The numerous nonfederal experts and interest groups active in federal public health policy are far from unified in their policy interests and advocacy strategies. Nonetheless, their collective impact on the federal policy-making process is substantial, both as sources of information and as agents of political influence. Some elements of the contemporary policy-making process remain controversial and subject to change, particularly in view of concerns that existing campaign financing laws allow political contributions to play a growing role in this process.[32] Despite such concerns, the federal legislative process remains a pluralistic approach to governmental decision making in the allocation of public health resources and in the regulation of personal and commercial actions influencing health.

THE FEDERAL REGULATORY PROCESS

The federal government's influence on public health derives not only from legislative activity, but also from the actions of executive-branch federal agencies in developing and enforcing regulations on personal, professional, and commercial behavior. A federal agency's authority to develop and enforce regulations originates from one or more of three sources: the enabling legislation for the agency; the authorizing legislation for programs and policies administered by the agency; and the authorizing legislation that modifies the functions of the agency or its programs.[7,33] Most agencies develop regulations using the notice-and-comment procedure established by the federal Administrative Procedure Act. Under this procedure, agencies develop regulations pursuant to the relevant legislative directives, publish drafts of these regulations in the Federal Register, solicit and consider comments from interested individuals and organizations, and modify regulations in response to these comments. Final regulations are codified by publication in the Code of Federal Regulations. Additionally, some federal agencies are required to use formal adjudication mechanisms as part of their regulation development process, including the use of cross-examination and rebuttal witnesses. These agencies include the Federal Trade Commission, the Consumer Product Safety Commission, and the Occupational Safety and Health Administration.

In many cases, the legislative authority to promulgate regulations is distributed across multiple federal agencies. For example, authority over health insurance benefits regulation is distributed across the U.S. Department of Labor (for employer-provided insurance), CMS (for Medicare, Medicaid, and SCHIP), the U.S. Department of Defense (for military personnel and families), and the U.S. Office of Personnel Management (for federal employees and families). For this reason, effective regulatory development and enforcement at the federal level often requires interagency coordination. In some cases, presidential executive orders are used to ensure coordination and consistency in the regulatory policies developed by multiple federal agencies. This approach was used by President Clinton in 1998 to implement regulatory provisions of the Patient's Bill of Rights initiative uniformly across all health plans participating in federal programs. In other cases, federal agency coordination is achieved through informal interaction among relevant agencies during the regulatory development process.

The notice-and-comment procedure used for federal regulation development provides interest groups with an important avenue for influencing federal public health policy outside the federal legislative process. Groups that represent the institutions and individuals affected by federal regulations are typically the most active participants in this procedure. Once regulations are finalized and encoded, the federal judicial system becomes the primary venue for affected entities to pursue claims about federal regulatory authority and enforcement. The federal courts adjudicate three primary types of claims regarding federal regulations: claims that a regulation exceeds the authority granted to the federal government under the Constitution; claims that a regulation exceeds the authority granted to the federal agency by congressional legislation; and claims that a regulation is enforced improperly or inequitably by the federal agency.[34] Claims of the latter type typically begin with adjudication by the federal agency involved, and can be appealed directly to the U.S. appellate courts. Other types of claims most often originate in U.S. district courts.

Just as Congress uses outside advisory groups to inform legislative decision making, many federal agencies rely on advisory groups to propose and review regulatory decision making. For example, MedPAC, which was established by congressional legislation in 1997, frequently provides comments and feedback to the U.S. Department of Health and Human Services concerning proposed and current regulations developed for the Medicare Program by CMS. In other cases, presidential executive orders are used to empanel advisory commissions that assist federal agencies developing health-related regulations. For example, the National Bioethics Advisory Commission was established by executive order in 1995 to advise executive agencies regarding the development and enforcement of federal policies and regulations governing research involving human subjects. In other cases, regulatory advisory bodies are created through the initiatives of federal agencies themselves, such as the EPA's Common Sense Initiative, which involves representatives from industry, environmental justice organizations, labor organizations, and state and local governments in a consensus-based regulatory development process.[35]

INTERGOVERNMENTAL RELATIONSHIPS

Federal public health activities achieve their impact on population health largely by influencing the activities undertaken by public health institutions at other levels of government and the private sector. Federal public health grant-in-aid programs shape the types of activities carried out by state health agencies and their counterparts operating at the local level. Federal regulatory actions also exert a strong influence on state and local public health activities, because public health agencies operating at these levels are often responsible for monitoring and enforcing compliance with federal regulations. Clearly, this strong federal influence enables state and local public health agencies to undertake a much broader scope and scale of activity than would be possible otherwise. This influence may also pose challenges for states and localities. One frequent criticism is that federal spending policies induce state and local government agencies to develop policies and programs in response to federal revenue streams rather than in response to community needs and priorities.[36] Another criticism is that the federal government's regulatory authority often creates unfunded mandates, which oblige state and local governments to undertake activities without providing the federal funds to cover the costs of these activities.[37] For these reasons, determining the desirability and appropriateness of federal action in public health is not always straightforward. Federal actions can have unintended effects on public health practice at state and local levels.

Federal agencies shape state and local public health activities in ways other than through spending and regulatory authority. These agencies frequently lend technical assistance and scientific expertise to states, counties, and municipalities seeking to implement public health programs and policies within their jurisdictions. The CDC is perhaps the best-known federal agency for undertaking such activities, which include: regular consultation with state and local health officials regarding disease prevention, detection, and control strategies; development of information and communication systems to facilitate state and local interaction with CDC officials; development of model programs and standards for implementation at state and local levels; and assignment of CDC officials to work in state and local public health agencies to facilitate the exchange of knowledge and expertise. Most other federal health agencies are involved to some extent in efforts to support state and local public health activities through information dissemination and technical assistance.

Federal agencies are involved to a lesser extent in the direct provision of public health services at the state and local level. Federal agencies engage in direct service provision most often in response to emergencies and disasters that have the potential to exceed state and local public health capacities.[38] Examples include outbreaks of unusual or particularly harmful infectious diseases, and natural disasters such as floods, earthquakes, and hurricanes. In rare cases, federal agencies may engage in direct service provision as part of public health research and demonstration initiatives, such as the testing of a new immunization delivery program or the development of a new disease surveillance method. A 1998 study of public health activities performed in the nation's largest local public health jurisdictions (at least 100,000 residents) found that direct federal involvement in performing public health activities occurred in less than half of these jurisdictions.[20] Where such involvement did occur, the activities most commonly performed by federal agencies included investigating adverse health events, providing access to laboratory services needed for public health surveillance and investigation, and developing support and communication systems among health-related organizations (Table 6.2).

The federal government also plays important roles in shaping global public health policy and practice through relationships with public health institutions in other countries. Many of these activities are carried out through participation in the World Health Organization (WHO), a specialized unit of the United Nations founded in 1948 to foster international cooperation in addressing public health issues and in strengthening national health systems. Through its participation in WHO, the federal government helps establish international standards and policies on issues such as disease detection, surveillance and reporting; health technology purchasing and dissemination; vaccine and pharmaceutical products utilization; environmental health conditions; and the accessibility and quality of health care services. The CDC is often the federal government's lead agency for carrying out WHO-sponsored initiatives in global disease prevention, control, and eradication. The CDC also maintains an array of related activities in global public health surveillance and capacity-building, including training programs for public health workers from foreign countries. Another federal agency that frequently engages in international cooperative efforts around health issues is the United States Agency for International Development. This agency assists impoverished and recovering foreign countries develop programs for family planning and reproductive health, infectious disease prevention and control

Table 6.2. Federal Agency Participation in Public Health Activities in U.S. Local Public Health Jurisdictions with at Least 100,000 Residents, 1998

Activity	Percent of Jurisdictions with Federal Agency Participation
Any Public Health Activity	**44.2%**
Specific Types of Activities	
1. Community health needs assessment	6.8%
2. Behavioral risk factor surveillance	4.6%
3. Adverse health events investigation	21.9%
4. Access to laboratory services	15.7%
5. Analysis of health determinants	5.2%
6. Analysis of preventive services use	2.6%
7. Support and communication networks	10.6%
8. Information provision for elected officials	3.4%
9. Prioritization of health needs	5.7%
10. Implementation of public health initiatives	9.7%
11. Community health improvement planning	4.6%
12. Resource allocation planning	2.3%
13. Resource deployment for priority needs	5.7%
14. Assessment of local health department	0.6%
15. Provision of and linkage to health services	8.3%
16. Evaluation of public health services	4.3%
17. Use of process/outcomes measures	4.0%
18. Public information dissemination	10.0%
19. Media information dissemination	5.4%
Average: Assessment Activities (1–6)	46.6%
Average: Policy Development Activities (7–12)	6.0%
Average: Assurance Activities (13–19)	5.5%
Average: All Activities	7.0%

SOURCE: Authors' analysis of data from: Mays GP, Halverson PK, Stevens R. The contributions of managed care plans to public health practice: lessons from the nation's largest local health departments. *Public Health Reports.* 2001;114:49-61.

(particularly HIV/AIDS), child survival, and maternal health. These types of international initiatives strengthen the nation's defenses against global health risks while simultaneously helping to achieve global improvements in health and well-being.

THE FUTURE OF FEDERAL CONTRIBUTIONS TO PUBLIC HEALTH

The federal government's efforts to protect and promote health at the population level derive principally from its authority to allocate resources to public health programs and to regulate activities that have

important effects on health. Undoubtedly, these federal roles will remain powerfully influential forces in the public health system of the future, even as shifts in political power and public priorities alter the specific forms and functions of federal public health initiatives. Emerging trends within the nation's public health system, however, suggest that the federal government may rely more heavily than previously on its ability to shape public health policy and practice through informal leadership, particularly its power to convene major stakeholders in public health and mobilize collaborative, multi-institutional responses to public health issues.

Among the new developments that are placing increased emphasis on federal public health leadership is the expanding collection of stakeholders that contribute to population health. A growing number of institutions and professionals outside the realm of governmental public health are using population-based approaches for identifying health needs and risks, preventing disease and injury, and improving the effectiveness and efficiency of health services delivery.[39–42] Consequently, public health professionals face unprecedented opportunities to align the interests and actions of these diverse stakeholders to improve population health. Federal health agencies are uniquely positioned to bring together these entities on a national level for purposes such as reaching consensus about priority health needs and risks; pooling resources and expertise; identifying optimal intervention strategies; coordinating programs and services; and negotiating organizational roles and responsibilities in public health.

Public health's expanding array of stakeholders include managed care plans and medical care providers, which are increasingly exploring population-based approaches for disease prevention and disease management to meet market demands for lower health care costs and improved health outcomes.[42–44] Other important stakeholders in public health include employers and health care purchasers, which face growing incentives to invest in population-based initiatives to promote workforce wellness, productivity, and retention and to ensure value in their health care purchases.[45–47] Community-based organizations such as churches, civic groups, human service providers, educational institutions, and philanthropies are also assuming larger roles in public health activities, particularly as these institutions gain an enhanced understanding of the relationships between population health status and other social and economic problems.[43,48,49] In the private sector, pharmaceutical companies and health information technology firms are expanding their involvement in population-based disease management interventions and health education campaigns, particularly as they recognize the social and economic gains to be realized from more appropriate utilization of preventive and therapeutic interventions.[50,51] Given this expanding array of stakeholders, a key federal leadership challenge lies in using its visibility and influence within the health system to mobilize multi-institutional responses to national public health priorities.[52,53]

A second, related development in the nation's public health system is the growing recognition that many of the nation's most pressing public health problems cannot be addressed through governmental action alone, nor through public health action alone. Prime among these problems are the persistent disparities in health experienced by population groups defined by race and ethnicity, gender, education and income, disability, geographic area, and sexual orientation.[54] Although the nation as a whole has realized substantial gains in population health in recent decades, the nation's minority and disadvantaged populations bear a disproportionate burden of disease, injury, and mortality—particularly African Americans, Hispanics, Native Americans, and Pacific Islanders. Prominent examples of these disparities include elevated rates of infant mortality, low-birthweight infants, mortality due to cancer and cardiovascular disease, diabetes, HIV/AIDS, exposure to environmental toxins, and injuries.[55,56] Minority and disadvantaged populations also face substantial disparities in accessing needed health services due to financial, geographic, linguistic, and cultural barriers to care. Left unchecked, these disparities are likely to grow in magnitude as the nation's minority and disadvantaged populations grow in size.

In 1998 the federal government's *Health Disparities Initiative* established the goal of eliminating racial and ethnic disparities for six common health issues by the year 2010. Moreover, eliminating health disparities has been identified as one of two overarching goals for the year 2010 national health objectives established in *Healthy People 2010*.[54] Addressing the unmet health needs of minority and disadvantaged populations over the next 10 years is likely to require concerted, sustained action from the full complement of health, social, economic, and cultural institutions that affect these populations. Accomplishing these urgent goals over the next 10 years will require strong, and perhaps unprecedented, leadership at the national level to mobilize and coordinate responses to persistent population-based disparities in health.

A third emerging development in the nation's public health system involves the complex and evolving dynamics of disease transmission. The resurgence of well-known diseases such as tuberculosis and pneumonia, combined with the emergence of new diseases caused by agents as varied as hantavirus and pfiesteria, has demonstrated the continuing threats to population health posed by infectious agents and environmental toxins.[57–59] New scientific evidence suggests that infectious agents and environmental toxins may be important contributors to many common chronic diseases, including peptic ulcer disease, atherosclerosis, heart disease, cancer, and arthritis.[60–62] The emergence of drug-resistant strains of infectious diseases such as tuberculosis and *Staphylococcus aureus* raises concerns that the nation's armamentarium of antimicrobial interventions may be losing its effectiveness due to overuse and inappropriate use in clinical applications.[63] The nation's public health organizations are further challenged by the variety of mechanisms through which new and previously unobserved diseases are introduced within populations. Increasingly, disease transmission is a global process facilitated by the ease and speed with which humans, animals, agricultural products, and pollutants move between countries and regions of the world.[57,59] Moreover, the environmental and climatic changes occurring in many regions of the world potentially create opportunities for disease transmission cycles to extend into previously unaffected areas (for example, the 1999 West Nile Virus outbreak in New York City). These multiple, global transmission routes make it impossible for health professionals practicing at the community level to keep apprised of all possible disease risks facing a population of interest. Moreover, disease outbreaks due to acts of bioterrorism remain a constant threat to population health in the modern geopolitical environment.[57]

In view of the complex and changing patterns of disease epidemiology, the federal government faces new imperatives to mobilize international partnerships for disease surveillance and control. At the same time, the federal government faces imperatives to strengthen communication and information-sharing mechanisms among the variety of domestic health care providers and public health institutions involved in disease prevention, identification, monitoring, and control. Ensuring the full cooperation of international and domestic stakeholders in disease control efforts is unlikely to be achieved through federal regulatory and financing initiatives alone. Consequently, the federal government's informal powers in public agenda-setting, consensus development, and coalition-building are likely to become increasingly important in addressing the nation's emerging disease risks.

These emerging developments in the nation's public health system demand that the federal government continue to exert a major influence on public health practice and policy in the years to come. This influence is essential for addressing health issues and disease risks that are too broad in scope and scale for individual states and localities to resolve effectively on their own. The federal government's formal authority to influence public health is necessarily restrained by the constitutionally guaranteed powers of states to construct their own public health programs and policies in response to local priorities and needs. This formal authority is also subject to the federal political processes that shape congressional legislation in public health. The federal government's informal mechanisms for influencing public health policy and practice, which collectively can be described as public health leadership strategies, are less dependent on legal and political structures. Strong leadership is an increasingly important power in the contemporary public health environment comprised of diverse institutional stakeholders, persistent health disparities, and global disease processes.

References

1. Hanlon G, Pickett J. *Public Health Administration and Practice.* New York, NY: Mosby; 1984.
2. Institute of Medicine, National Academy of Science. *The Future of Public Health.* Washington, DC: National Academy Press; 1984.
3. Shonick W. *Government and Health Services: Government's Role in the Development of the U.S. Health Services 1930-1980.* New York, NY: Oxford University Press; 1995.
4. Centers for Disease Control and Prevention. History of CDC. *MMWR.* 1996;45:526-528.

5. Anderson OW. *Health Services in the United States: A Growth Enterprise Since 1875.* Ann Arbor, Mich: Health Administration Press; 1985.

6. Omenn GS. What's behind those block grants in health? *N Engl J Med.* 1982;306(17):1057-1060.

7. Kennan SA. Legislative relations in public health. In: Novick LF, Mays GP, eds. *Public Health Administration: Principles for Population-Based Management.* Gaithersburg, Md: Aspen Publishers; 2000;539-566.

8. Leviss PS. Financing the public's health. In: Novick LF, Mays GP, eds. *Public Health Administration: Principles for Population-Based Management.* Gaithersburg, Md: Aspen Publishers; 2000:413-430.

9. Brennan TA, Berwick DM. *New Rules: Regulation, Markets, and the Quality of American Health Care.* San Francisco, Calif: Jossey-Bass; 1996.

10. Moran DW. Federal regulation of managed care: an impulse in search of a theory. *Health Aff.* 1997;16(6):7-33.

11. Fuchs BC. Managed Health Care: Federal and State Regulation. Washington, DC: Congressional Research Service; 1997.

12. Roper WL. Regulating quality and clinical practice. In: Altman SH, Reinhardt UE, and Shactman D, eds. *Regulating Managed Care: Theory, Practice, and Future Options.* San Francisco, Calif: Jossey-Bass; 1999:145-159.

13. Scheffler RM, Clement DG, Sullivan SD, Hu TW, Sung HY. The hospital response to Medicare's Prospective Payment System: an econometric model of Blue Cross and Blue Shield plans. *Med Care.* 1994:32(5):471-485.

14. Miller T, Leatherman S. The National Quality Forum: a 'me-too' or a breakthrough in quality measurement and reporting? *Health Aff.* 1999; 18(6):233-237.

15. Eisenberg JM. Health services research in a market-oriented health care system. *Health Aff.* 1998;17(1):98-108.

16. Gostin LO. Public health law in a new century: part II, public health powers and limits. *JAMA.* 2000; 283(22):2979-2984.

17. US Health Care Financing Administration. *National Health Expenditures by Type of Service and Source of Funds: Calendar Years 1960-99.* Washington, DC: US Department of Health and Human Services; 2000.

18. Pauly MV. Health Benefits at Work: An Economic and Political Analysis of Employment-Based Health Insurance. Ann Arbor: University of Michigan Press; 1999.

19. Litman TJ. The politics of health: establishing policies and setting priorities. In: Lee PR and Estes CL, eds. *The Nation's Health.* 4th ed. Boston, Mass: Jones and Bartlett. 1994:107-120.

20. Mays GP. Organization of the public health delivery system. In: Novick LF, Mays GP, eds. *Public Health Administration: Principles for Population-Based Management.* Gaithersburg, Md. Aspen Publishers, 2000.63-116.

21. Halverson PK, Nicola RM, Baker EL. Performance measurement and accreditation of public health organizations: a call to action. *J Public Health Manage & Pract.* 1998;4(4):5-7.

22. De Leon R, Bailey S. *Military Health System: A Joint Overview Statement.* Washington, DC: US House of Representatives, Committee on Appropriations, Defense Subcommittee; 2000.

23. General Accounting Office. *Performance Budgeting: Past Initiatives Offer Insights for GPRA.* Washington, DC: GAO; March 1997.

24. National Research Council, Panel on Performance Measures and Data for Public Health Performance Partnership Grants. *Assessment of Performance Measures for Public Health, Substance Abuse, and Mental Health.* Washington, DC: National Academy Press; 1997.

25. Ferejohn JA, Weingast BR. *The New Federalism: Can the States Be Trusted?* Palo Alto, Calif: Hoover Institution Press, Stanford University; 1997.

26. Wing KR. *The Law and the Public's Health.* Ann Arbor, Mich: Health Administration Press; 1999.

27. Gostin LO. *Public Health Law: Power, Duty, Restraint.* San Francisco: University of California Press; 2001.

28. Rochefort DA, Cobb RW. *The Politics of Problem Definition: Shaping the Policy Agenda.* Lawrence: University of Kansas Press; 1997.

29. Berry JM. *The Interest Group Society.* New York, NY: Little Brown & Co; 1984.

30. Moran M. *Governing the Health Care State: A Comparative Study of the United Kingdom, the United States, and Germany.* London, England: Manchester University Press; 1999.

31. Starr P. *The Social Transformation of American Medicine.* New York, NY: Basic Books; 1983.

32. Gais T. *Improper Influence: Campaign Finance Law, Political Interest Groups, and the Problem of Equality.* Ann Arbor: University of Michigan Press; 1996.

33. Schick A. *The Federal Budget: Politics, Policy, Process.* 2nd ed. Washington, DC: Brookings Institute; 2000.

34. Federal Judicial Center. *The Federal Courts and What They Do.* Washington, DC: Government Printing Office; 1997.

35. Environmental Protection Agency. *Consensus Decision-Making Principles and Applications in the EPA Common Sense Initiative.* Washington, DC: Government Printing Office; 1997.

36. Conlan TJ. *From New Federalism to Devolution: Twenty-five Years of Intergovernmental Reform.* Washington, DC: Brookings Institute; 1998.

37. Posner PL. *The Politics of Unfunded Mandates: Whither Federalism?* Washington, DC: Georgetown University Press; 1998.

38. Turnock BJ. *Public Health: What It Is and How It Works.* Gaithersburg, Md: Aspen Publishers; 2000.

39. Roper WL, Koplan JP, Stinnet AA. 1994. Public health in the new American health system. *Frontiers of Health Serv Manage.* 1994;10(4):32-36.

40. Baker EL, Melton RJ, Stange PV, Fields ML, Koplan JP, Guerra FA, Satcher D. Health reform and the health of the public. *JAMA.* 1994;272:1276-1282.

41. Showstack J, Lurie N, Leatherman S, Fisher E, Inui T. Health of the public: the private-sector challenge. *JAMA* 1996;276(13):1071-1074.

42. Roper WL, Mays GP. The changing managed care—public health interface. *JAMA.* 1998;280(20):1739-1740.

43. Lasker, RD. *Medicine and Public Health: The Power of Collaboration.* New York: NY: Academy of Medicine; 1997.

44. Halverson PK, Mays GP, Kaluzny AD, Richards TB. Not-so-strange bedfellows: models of interaction between managed care plans and public health agencies. *Milbank Quarterly.* 1997;75:113-138.

45. Christianson JB. The role of employers in community health care systems. *Health Aff.* 1998;17(4):158-164.

46. Lee D, Lopez L. An invitational workshop on collaboration between quality improvement organizations and business coalitions. *Joint Commission J on Quality Improvement in Health Care.* 1997;23(6):334-341.

47. McLaughlin CP. Balancing collaboration and competition: the Kingsport, Tennessee experience. *Joint Commission J on Quality Improvement.* 1995;21(11):646-655.

48. Bruce TA, McKane SU. The community-based public health initiative: lessons learned. In: Mays GP, Miller CA, and Halverson PK, eds. *Local Public Health Practice: Trends and Models.* Washington, DC: American Public Health Association; 2000.

49. Mays GP, Miller CA, Halverson PK. *Local Public Health Practice: Trends and Models.* Washington, DC: American Public Health Association; 2000.

50. Keys IR. Take it to heart: a national health screening and education project in African-American communities. A joint project of the NMA and Bayer Corporation. *J of the Nat Med Assoc.* 1999; 91(12):649-652.

51. Hirano D. Partnering to improve infant immunizations: The Arizona Partnership for Infant Immunization (TAPII). *Am J Prev Med.* 1998;14(3 suppl):22-25.

52. Marcus L. *Renegotiating Health Care: Resolving Conflict to Build Collaboration.* San Francisco, Calif: Jossey-Bass; 1999.

53. Hatcher MT, Niccola RM. Building constituencies for public health. In: Novick LF, Mays GP, eds. *Public Health Administration: Principles for Population-Based Management.* Gaithersburg, Md: Aspen Publishers; 2000;510-520.

54. US Department of Health and Human Services. *Healthy People 2010: Understanding and Improving Health.* Washington, DC: Government Printing Office; 2000.

55. Smith DB. *Health Care Divided: Race and a Healing Nation.* Ann Arbor: University of Michigan Press; 1999.

56. Hogue CJR, Hargrave MA. *Minority Health in America: Findings and Policy Implications from the Commonwealth Fund Minority Health Survey.* Baltimore, Md: Johns Hopkins University Press; 2000.

57. Centers for Disease Control and Prevention. *Preventing Emerging Infectious Diseases: A Strategy for the 21st Century.* Atlanta, Ga: CDC; 1998.

58. Binder S, Levitt AM, Sacks JJ, Hughes JM. Emerging infectious diseases: public health issues for the 21st century. *Science.* 1999;284(5418):1311-1313.

59. Mayer JD. Geography, ecology and emerging infectious diseases. *Soc Sci & Med.* 2000;50(7-8):937-952.

60. Gupta S et al. Elevated Chlamydia pneumoniae antibodies, cardiovascular events, and azithromycin in male survivors of myocardial infarction. *Circulation.* 1997;96:404-407.

61. Baseman JB, Tully JG. Mycoplasmas: sophisticated, reemerging, and burdened by their notoriety. *Emerging Infect Dis.* 1997;3:21-32.

62. Muhlestein JB, Anderson JL, Hammond EH, Zhao L, Trehan S, Schwobe EP, Carlquist JF. Infection with Chlamydia pneumoniae accelerates the development of atherosclerosis and treatment with azithromycin prevents it in a rabbit model. *Circulation.* 1998;97:633-636.

63. Vermund SH, Fawal H. Emerging infectious diseases and professional integrity: thoughts for the new millennium. *Am J Infect Control.* 1999;27(6):497-499.

CHAPTER

7

The State Public Health Department

Suzanne Dandoy, M.D., M.P.H.
A. Richard Melton, M.P.H., Dr. P.H.

Massachusetts was the first state to take responsibility for the health of its people by creating a board of health in 1869. By 1909, all states had health departments whose tasks focused primarily on the recording of births and deaths and the control of communicable diseases. Today, state health departments have expanded their activities to include improving the health of children and pregnant women, controlling chronic diseases, preventing injuries, regulating health care facilities, developing emergency medical services and other health care resources, and protecting the environment.

In its 1988 report, the Institute of Medicine's Committee for the Study of the Future of Public Health (IOM Committee) noted that states are close enough to the people to maintain a sense of their needs and preferences, yet large enough, in most cases, to command the resources necessary to get the important jobs done.[1] In fact, because state health departments were created to meet the differing needs and prefer-

ences of the people in each state, their functions and activities show wide variation. Departments also vary in organizational structure, per capita expenditures, staffing patterns, responsibility for local health services, political influence, and relationships with other agencies.

Each of these topics is explored in this chapter, which focuses on trends over time and current issues. IOM Committee recommendations regarding specific topics are included as a yardstick for comparison with actual conditions.

FUNCTIONS OF STATE HEALTH DEPARTMENTS

Government responsibility in public health includes the *agenda-setting function*.[2] Each state health department must identify goals and strategies to improve the health of its citizens. To set and implement this agenda, the state health department assesses the health status and needs of the population; plans strategies and health programs to address unmet needs; obtains financial assistance to support these plans; sets and enforces standards; provides technical assistance to local health departments and other governmental and nongovernmental agencies; and, in limited circumstances, delivers health services directly (in most states, local health departments are the primary government entity providing public health services directly to individuals).

Traditional versus Newer Functions

Until the 1940s, state health departments focused almost solely on six basic public health services: collection of vital records and statistics; control of communicable diseases; environmental sanitation; laboratory services; public health education; and maternal and child health.

As antibiotics and vaccines became available to control the spread of communicable diseases, citizens voiced their desire for government to give attention to other health problems. In the late 1950s, the U.S. Congress began offering states federal funds to support specific new services for certain groups of people or for particular diseases. These *categorical* programs addressed areas in which state health departments traditionally had not been involved, such as heart disease, diabetes, migrant labor, mental retardation, and the construction of new hospitals and clinics.

This expansion of state health department activity has continued, stimulated by the availability of federal funds, the necessity of meeting federally enacted mandates, and the growth of state health laws. For example, in the past decade state health departments have expanded activities aimed at reducing tobacco use, responding to possible acts of bioterrorism, and addressing asthma as a public health problem.

In 1997, 33 states reported substantial use of the *Healthy People 2000* national objectives in setting state objectives and program priorities.[3] The availability of baseline data often determined the selection of health objectives. Many states are developing new data systems to track progress toward meeting state objectives in the public health programs and now are using the national health objectives for 2010 as part of their state health planning process.[4]

Typical Responsibilities

Typical responsibilities of a state health department are presented in Table 7.1. Many of these activities are expansions and variations on the original six basic functions, particularly health information (vital records and statistics), disease and disability prevention (communicable disease control and laboratory services), health protection (environmental sanitation), health promotion (public health education), and maternal and child health services.

Health Information

The collection and preservation of vital records, and the analysis and use of information from such records, are major functions of state health departments. Now states also gather and analyze data on the health of the population and the characteristics of the medical care delivery system. State health departments are the legal repositories for birth and death records in most states, and they may also keep records of marriages, divorces, and terminations of pregnancy.

Data from these vital records, along with data from disease registries, surveys of health care providers and facilities, disease case reports, screening programs, and laboratory analyses, are used for several purposes: to influence the creation, continuation, or modification of programs; to identify disease patterns or outbreaks; to identify racial and ethnic health disparities; to determine priorities for resource allocation; and to assist in planning health care delivery sites and facilities.

Disease and Disability Prevention

Preventing disease and disability, particularly communicable disease, is a unique function of health departments in every state; no other state agency is given the lead responsibility for this function. As pertussis, measles, and other communicable diseases have been brought under control, state health department attention and resources have shifted to other health problems, such as AIDS, hepatitis, breast cancer, injuries, and cardiovascular disease. State activities in these areas include screening programs, labo-

Table 7.1.   Typical Responsibilities of a State Health Department

Health Information

- Recording and issuing certified copies of birth and death certificates
- Publishing health statistics
- Birth defects registry
- Cancer registry

Disease and Disability Prevention

- Screening newborns for inborn errors of metabolism
- Immunization programs
- AIDS screening, counseling, and partner notification
- Tuberculosis control
- Screening children for lead
- Investigating disease outbreaks
- Laboratory testing for infectious diseases
- Medical care for children with handicapping conditions
- Education on use of occupant restraints in vehicles

Health Protection

- Testing waters in which shellfish are grown
- Issuing permits for sewage disposal systems
- Monitoring drinking water systems
- Inspecting dairies
- License hospitals, nursing homes, and home health agencies
- Examining and certifying emergency medical personnel
- Inspecting clinical laboratories

Health Promotion

- Food vouchers for pregnant women, infants, and children (WIC)
- Prenatal care for low-income women
- Dental care for low-income children and adults
- School health education
- Family planning services
- Cholesterol and high blood pressure education programs
- Tobacco use cessation programs

Improving the Health Care Delivery System

- Scholarships for medical and nursing students
- Certificates of need for construction of health facilities
- Development of rural health policies and services
- Collecting and analyzing data on health care costs
- Quality assurance for managed care plans

ratory testing, health education, technical advice, issuance of isolation and quarantine orders, immunizations, public information, and chemotherapy.

Health Protection

Citizens' concern with the general cleanliness of the environment has expanded, requiring state oversight of public drinking water, ambient air, food service facilities, sewage systems, and sources of radiation. State health departments have also been asked to regulate the medical care delivery system. Initially, this was to ensure the hygiene, proper staffing, and safety of health facilities. However, anxiety over the increasing costs of health care led policy makers to give state health departments responsibility for regulating facility charges, bed capacity, and service enhancement; gathering data on health care costs; and, more recently, monitoring the availability and quality of medical care provided to the population. To improve access to care, health departments recruit physicians for medically underserved areas and provide scholarships and loans for medical and nursing students. Thus, state health departments have been charged with protecting not only the public's health, but also the public's access to quality medical care.

Health Promotion

Going beyond educating the population on how to avoid infectious diseases, health promotion efforts in state health departments now focus on lifestyle issues, maintenance of health, and prevention of injury. Health education programs at schools and workplaces address diet, exercise, tobacco use, and stress reduction, with emphasis on reducing risk factors for cancer and cardiovascular diseases.

Health Care Delivery

The involvement of state health departments in direct delivery of care began with clinics for pregnant women and children. As federal and state funds have become available, direct services have expanded to include family planning, cancer screening, dental health, treatment for tuberculosis and sexually transmitted diseases, and, most recently, primary medical care. In each of these undertakings, the state's role centers on program planning, setting and enforcing standards, developing procedures, and providing technical assistance and funding, while the clinical care is actually delivered at the local level, through either the private or public health delivery system.

ORGANIZATIONAL ISSUES

Before 1960, almost all public health functions provided by states were located in state health departments. As programs became more complex and as demands for new types of services increased, many public health activities were assigned to other state agencies. Table 7.2 shows this for Virginia. Lewis-Idema and Falik maintain that, although public needs are ever changing, public agencies tend to be static, with institutionalized perspectives and responsibilities.[5] Thus, new problems tend to generate new programs that are assigned to new agencies rather than to generate changes in existing agencies. Public health leaders may be perceived as having no interest in new ideas or as not having the political skills needed to lead and direct a particular program. Often, special interest groups want separate administration for their particular programs so they can exert more control over their operation.

Major governmental health functions that are assigned to other agencies include mental health, financing of medical care for the indigent, and environmental protection. The IOM Committee analyzed this fragmentation of public health functions and made specific recommendations regarding closer linkages between programs that now exist in separate agencies.[1]

Mental Health

In only five states are health departments also the state mental health authority, reflecting a long trend in segregating physical and mental health problems.[6] This division of leadership at the state level results in separate service delivery systems at the local level, with little coordinated planning around client needs. The IOM Committee recommended that public health and mental health leaders devote efforts to strengthening the linkages between the two fields, particularly to inte-

Table 7.2. Health Responsibilities in State Agencies Other than the State Health Department: Virginia

Department of Agriculture
- Inspects grocery stores
- Inspects food processing plants

Department of Education
- Supervises health teaching in schools
- Supervises delivery of health services in schools

Department of Environmental Quality
- Controls air pollution
- Controls water pollution
- Oversees solid and hazardous waste disposal

Department of Health Professions
- Licenses 12 categories of health professionals

Department of Labor and Industry
- Regulates occupational health and safety

Department of Medical Assistance Services (Medicaid)
- Finances medical care to the indigent and categorically needy
- Funds a health status screening program for children
- Provides case management services for newborns

Department of Mental Health, Mental Retardation, and Substance Abuse Services
- Operates mental hospitals
- Directs community mental health and substance abuse services

Department of Motor Vehicles
- Educates the public on occupant safety and seatbelt use

Joint Commission on Health Care
- Develops legislative proposals for improving access to medical care

grating these functions at the service delivery level. Yet, little has been done to implement this recommendation. Mental health agencies have strong advocacy groups that lobby state legislatures for money and facilities, sometimes at the expense of public health programs.

Financing Medical Care

The state's participation in financing medical care usually resides outside the state health department. When the federal Medicaid program started in 1965, states had to select a single state agency to manage the program. Initially, some states assigned this role to health departments. As the Medicaid program grew, both in dollars and in numbers of people receiving care, responsibility for operating the program shifted either to a separate state agency or to the social services/welfare agency. Only five state health departments manage their state's Medicaid program.[6]

Coordination and Control of Services

When a state health department retains responsibility for the Medicaid program, there is greater integration of Medicaid-financed services with other public health services, using the same delivery system. Thus, both federal Medicaid and state public health funds are coordinated to provide services to eligible clients. When public health and Medicaid are administered separately, on the other hand, the state health department loses some of its control, particularly over programs for pregnant women and children—the largest constituency served by Medicaid.

As Medicaid eligibility has been expanded by Congress to cover more pregnant women, children, and adolescents, every state's Medicaid budget far exceeds its public health budget. State funds allocated to Medicaid bring federal dollars to each state, on a matching basis, while state funds appropriated for public health often stand alone. Therefore, Medicaid and public health compete for state funds, with public health usually losing the battle.

IOM Committee Recommendations

Although the IOM Committee report recommended that each state health agency include responsibility for Medicaid, most state health officers opposed any attempt to take back this function.[7] They believed it would detract from, rather than enhance, their public health activities, by linking them too closely to *welfare* programs.

Environmental Protection

Although mental health has never been a significant part of state health departments and medical care financing has moved to separate agencies without much protest from state health officials, the removal of environmental health programs from state health departments has been viewed as a significant loss to public health. Many environmental monitoring and control activities previously handled by state health departments, in areas such as air pollution, groundwater contamination, and solid and hazardous waste disposal, have been transferred to separate environmental protection agencies.

Background

These programs grew from the health department's original work in sanitation, but became increasingly complex as technology advanced and more potential pollutants were identified. Citizens demanded more protection of and from the environment, businesses became concerned about the costs of compliance with environmental health standards, and regulatory decisions became more complicated. Directors of state health departments frequently had no expertise in new environmental issues. Governors and legislators, wanting to give greater visibility to environmental issues, created new environmental agencies, following the example of the federal Environmental Protection Agency.

IOM Committee Recommendations

The IOM Committee noted that this separation of environmental health functions has led to a lack of coordination of efforts and an inadequate analysis of the health effects of environmental problems. Environmental protection agencies are more likely to focus on regulatory requirements and engineering technology than on risk to human health. Therefore, the IOM Committee recommended that state and local health agencies strengthen their capacities for identifying, understanding, and controlling environmental problems as health hazards. In some states, even after environmental programs were transferred, expertise in environmental health risk assessment has been retained within the state health department as a resource for the environmental agency.

Recent Trends

The number of state health agencies that are the lead environmental agencies has shown a steady decrease, from 19 in 1978 to 8 in 2000.[8] However, most state health departments have lead responsibility for at least one environmental health function, usually food sanitation, safe drinking water, radiation control, risk assessment, and/or toxic substance investigation. Recently, the federal government has provided funding to state health departments to improve states' surveillance, laboratory capacity, and response functions for biological and chemical agents used in bioterrorism.[9]

CURRENT ORGANIZATION OF STATE HEALTH DEPARTMENTS

In the United States there are 57 state health agencies (1 in each of the 50 states, the District of Columbia, American Samoa, Guam, Puerto Rico, the Federated States of Micronesia, Northern Mariana Islands, and the U.S. Virgin Islands), each of which may be a freestanding, independent department or a component of a larger state agency. Because some of these agencies are not truly "departments" of state government, the Association of State and Territorial Health Officials adopted the term *state health agency* to signify that agency of state government that is vested with primary responsibility for public health within the state.[10]

Superagencies and Umbrella Agencies

Beginning in the 1960s, state health departments were merged with other departments, usually social services or welfare departments, to form *superagencies,* or they were placed under a cabinet secretary in an *umbrella agency,* following the pattern of the federal Department of Health and Human Services. The main difference between these two types of consolidation is that a state health agency usually retains more autonomy under the umbrella arrangement.

In 1952, only Maine and Missouri had state public health functions in an umbrella or superagency. By 1969, there were 8 states with such arrangements, by 1972, 16 states, and by 1980, 22 states.[11–13] State health agencies in 20 states plus the District of Columbia

were part of such agencies in 2000, indicating that some states had reversed this consolidation.[6]

Rationale

The stated purpose of bringing together several separate departments under one roof was to increase coordination between programs serving the same population groups and to provide more political control over policy decisions. These superagencies most often bring together health and social services for the aged, children and adolescents, families, the developmentally disabled, those needing income assistance, and those with substance abuse problems. A typical organizational chart of an umbrella agency is presented in Figure 7.1. In addition to the state health functions, this large secretariat includes Medicaid, employment services, mental health, mental retardation, and social (welfare) services. The director or secretary of such an agency is usually a political appointee, frequently with little or no health expertise.

Public Health Opposition

Public health leaders have generally opposed such mergers because the superagencies focus more on services for the poor or families with problems, rather than on protecting or improving the health of the total population.[1] Unless service delivery at the local level has also been merged or colocated, there may be little benefit to clients from such mergers of agencies at the state level. In 1990, the Wyoming superagency was divided into separate health and welfare departments. One of the main reasons for the separation was the perception that the state health agency had difficulty obtaining funds from the legislature because the welfare services represented such a large portion of the budget.[14] The IOM Committee recommended that each state have a department of health that groups all primarily health-related functions under professional direction and separate from income maintenance functions of state government.[1]

Name of the State Health Agency

If it is an independent entity or part of an umbrella agency, or secretariat, the state health agency is titled

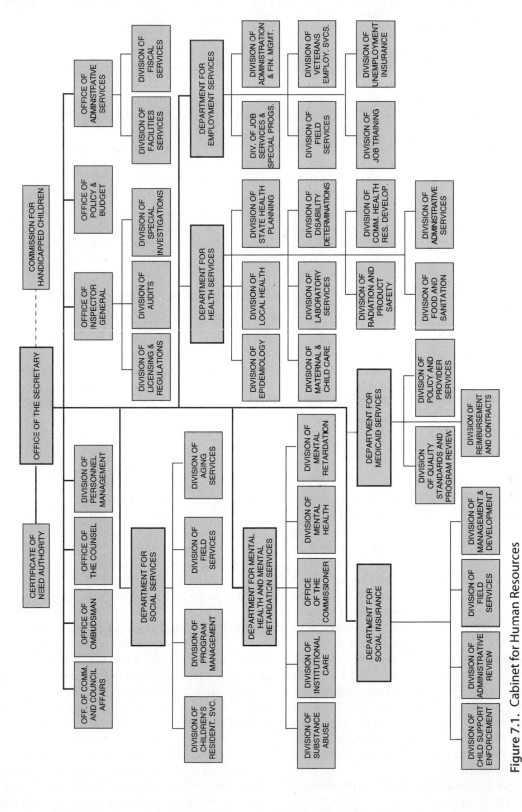

Figure 7.1. Cabinet for Human Resources

Source: Public Health Foundation. *State Health: Agency Organization Charts*. Washington, DC: Public Health Foundation; 1992.

the Department of Health, Department of Public Health, or Department of Health Services.[15] If it is combined with another agency, the public health unit is usually called a Division of Health or Public Health.

When public health functions have been combined with environmental functions, *health* is more likely to appear in the agency title, for example, Department of Health and Environment, than when public health is combined with social services agencies. The latter are frequently named the Department of Human Resources or Human Services, supporting the assertion that public health's visibility is lost when such a merger occurs.

STATE BOARDS OF HEALTH

In the late 1800s, state governments created boards of health even before state departments of health to make rules to prevent the spread of diseases and improve general sanitary conditions in the states. As these boards hired employees to enforce the rules, departments of health were organized. In 1972, all but four states had a state board of health in some form.[13]

Role of Boards of Health

Thirty-seven (80 percent) of the 46 boards in 1972 were policy making, that is, responsible for making, adopting, promulgating, and enforcing rules and regulations pursuant to state health codes.[13] The remaining nine boards were advisory only and usually located in states where public health functions had been consolidated into a superagency or an umbrella agency.

From 1971 to 1980, major structural changes took place in state health departments. In addition to those that were consolidated with other departments of state government, 13 state boards of health were disestablished in this time period.[16] By 2000, only 21 states had boards still making policy, and 14 others just had advisory boards or committees at the department level.[6] While 80 percent of states with freestanding departments of health retained a board of health, only half the states in which public health was located in a superagency or an umbrella agency had a board. From 1972 to 1992, the number of boards of health responsible for hiring the state health director also decreased—from 15 to 4.[17,18]

The functions previously assigned to boards of health have been assumed by the executive branches of state governments, with policy decisions being made by political appointees instead of citizens' groups. As governors seek more control over health policy, they want the authority to select health directors who will carry out political platforms.

Even when state boards of health had a stronger role, they were never representative of the state's population. The majority of board members were appointed by governors and represented various medical and health interests. Consumers held only 11 to 12 percent of seats on state boards of health.[16]

Specialized Boards and Committees

Replacing or supplementing the board of health in many states are specialized boards or committees established by state statute to oversee particular programs. Many of these boards are technical, bringing to the state health agency particular expertise not found in the staff, for example, in genetics or rural health. Other special boards are established to make decisions on a particular function in the state health department, such as rules regarding the practice of emergency medical technicians, licensure of hearing aid dispensers, or expansion of health facilities. Special interest groups have lobbied state legislatures to establish these committees, with defined membership representing the regulated community and the public, in preference to having policies made by a board of health or the state health director.

IOM Committee Recommendation

The IOM Committee recommended that each state have a health council that reports regularly on the health of the state's residents, makes health policy recommendations to the governor and legislature, promulgates public health regulations, reviews the work of the state health department, and recommends candidates for director of the department.[1] The committee proposed that the purpose of the council should not be the control of health matters by health professionals but the making of policy judgments on public health by lay citizens. In reality, however, most states appear headed in a different direction, with less power given to such a representative group and more control residing in the elected and appointed officials of the executive branch of state government.

STATE HEALTH DIRECTORS

The title of the chief executive of the state health agency is usually director or commissioner; in a few states the position is called state health officer or secretary. The important factor is not the title but who makes the appointment. Whether the director of the department is appointed by the governor, a board, or the head of an umbrella agency or superagency is crucial in determining the health director's level of authority, access to state policy makers, and participation in health policy decisions.

The director of the state health agency is appointed by the governor to a cabinet level position in 36 states and the territories, by the head of a superagency in 14 states, by the state board of health in 4 states, and by the mayor in the District of Columbia.[18] Where there is direct access to the governor, the health director has a greater opportunity to influence health policy in both the executive and legislative branches.

Qualifications of State Health Directors

Traditionally, a physician held the position of state health officer, with medical requirements being part of state law. At first, most of these physicians had no training in public health. As schools of public health were created, however, physicians trained specifically for positions in public health administration directed most state health departments. In 1977, all but six states had physician health directors.[17] Twenty-three of the 44 physicians were specialists in public health and preventive medicine, and 30 had a public health degree.

Changes with Reorganization

Concomitant with the consolidation of some state health departments into superagencies or umbrella agencies in the 1970s, states began removing the medical criteria for appointment. Even after the trend to merge health departments with other state agencies

declined, states continued to repeal the requirements for physician directors. By 2000, only 25 states required a medical degree for their state health official, and the number of state health officials who were physicians was down to 33.[6,15] In 1997, only 17 state health directors had public health degrees.[19]

These changes in qualifications of state health directors related to the transition occurring in the responsibilities of state health agencies. As health departments became more involved in issues of environmental protection and regulation of the delivery of medical care, governors and state legislatures concluded that health directors should have more political and administrative skills. As a result, legislatures either combined the health department with other agencies, under a politically appointed secretary or executive, or changed the qualifications for the health director, to allow nonphysicians to serve in this capacity.

As salaries for government service lagged behind the earnings of physicians in other specialties, the pool of public health-trained physicians, particularly those with education or interest in administration, also declined. Today, even in those states requiring the state health director to have a medical degree, the physicians selected often have not had training or prior experience in public health or management.

Tenure of State Health Directors

Increased turnover in state health directors and changes in their qualifications have occurred as the positions have become more political. In the first half of this century, many state health officers served from 20 to 35 years. They were respected leaders in health affairs in their communities and also were frequently leaders in state medical societies. For example, the terms of the first two state health officers in Virginia covered a total period of 48 years, from 1908 to 1956.

By contrast, the tenure of state health directors has decreased markedly in the past 20 years. In 1997, the average tenure for *former* state health officials from all 50 states was four years.[19] Of the 57 health officials in states and territories in 1989, only 3 remained in those same positions 10 years later.[20] By 1999, the states of California, Florida, Kansas, and Minnesota each had 9–10 state health directors in the previous 15 years.

Those state health directors appointed by boards of health generally have longer tenure in office than those appointed by governors, because governors want to appoint department heads who will carry out their policies and initiatives. The largest number of changes in state health officials occurs in election years.[20]

IOM Committee Recommendations

The IOM Committee recommended that the director of each department of health be a cabinet level officer, with doctorate-level education as a physician or other health professional, education in public health, and extensive public sector administrative experience.[1] Provisions for tenure in office, such as specific terms of appointment, should be enacted, the committee said, to promote needed continuity of professional leadership. In recent years, only four states have had specific terms of appointment for their state health directors.

INTERNAL ORGANIZATIONAL STRUCTURE AND STAFFING

There is an old expression that form should follow function. One would thus expect state health departments to be organized around the functions they perform. Because many functions are the same in each state, similar organizational structures might be assumed. That assumption is only partially true. Each state health department's internal organizational arrangement has developed over time and represents unique attributes of that state's government, processes, and prevailing culture. In states where the health department is responsible for local services, the structure is more complicated because there are both centralized and decentralized components.

Two Examples: Rhode Island and Washington State

Organizational charts for two state health departments are presented in Figures 7.2 and 7.3. The chart for the Rhode Island Department of Health shows a characteristic set of public health functions, plus two components not frequently seen in health departments: the medical examiner and licensure of health professionals. Because of its small size, Rhode Island has no local health departments, so all services are provided by the state health agency. State law requires that the Director of Health be a physician. The Washington State Department of Health, shown in Figure 7.3, was separated from a merged health and welfare agency in the late 1980s. The state health official, who is called a secretary, reports directly to the governor. Because the secretary is not required to have medical credentials, there is a separate health officer position held by a physician. Washington also has a policy-making board of health.

The Need for Flexibility

As little as possible of the organization's structure should be codified in statutes so that the department may respond to new needs, such as genetic diseases or injury prevention. Ideally, the state health director can restructure the organization and adjust resources to address emerging problems.

Staffing

The numbers and kinds of staff needed at the state level will depend on the responsibilities assigned to each state health department; distances between population centers; types of medical care facilities to be regulated; density and economic status of populations served; degree of responsibility for direct delivery of services; and the number, size, autonomy, and sophistication of local health departments. State and territorial health departments employ approximately one-third of the public health work force in the United States.[21]

Occupational Groups

Two-thirds of state health agency staff are in the professional, technical, and administrative areas; the remaining one-third are in clerical and other support areas. Registered nurses are the largest single professional group, followed by environmental health personnel and nutritionists.

Over time, there have been changes in specific occupational categories. The number of dentists in

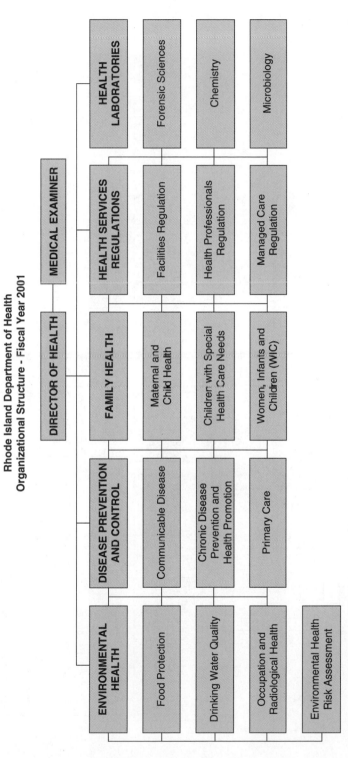

Rhode Island Department of Health
Organizational Structure - Fiscal Year 2001

DIRECTOR OF HEALTH

MEDICAL EXAMINER

ENVIRONMENTAL HEALTH
- Food Protection
- Drinking Water Quality
- Occupation and Radiological Health
- Environmental Health Risk Assessment

DISEASE PREVENTION AND CONTROL
- Communicable Disease
- Chronic Disease Prevention and Health Promotion
- Primary Care

FAMILY HEALTH
- Maternal and Child Health
- Children with Special Health Care Needs
- Women, Infants and Children (WIC)

HEALTH SERVICES REGULATIONS
- Facilities Regulation
- Health Professionals Regulation
- Managed Care Regulation

HEALTH LABORATORIES
- Forensic Sciences
- Chemistry
- Microbiology

Figure 7.2. Rhode Island Department of Health Organizational Structure—Fiscal Year 2001

Source: Reprinted with permission of the Rhode Island Department of Health.

115

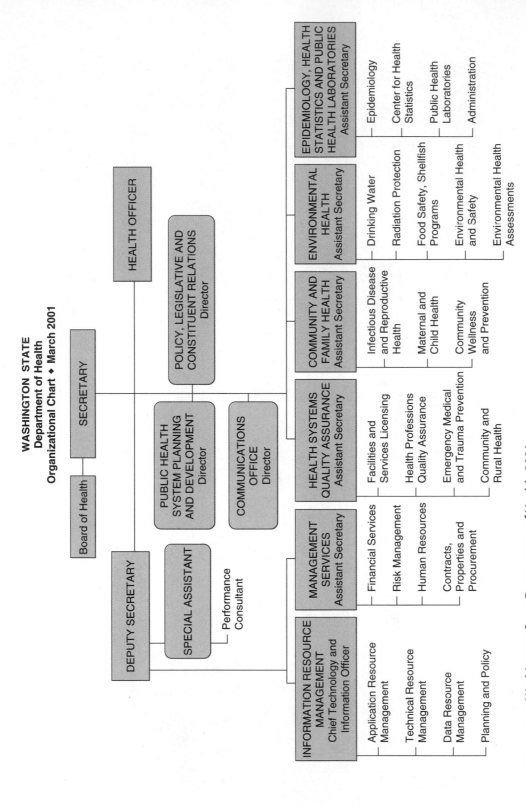

Figure 7.3. Washington State Department of Health, 2001

Source: Reprinted with permission of the Washington State Department of Health.

state health agencies decreased by 40 percent from 1979 to 1989 while nutritionists and dieticians almost doubled in number.[22] The decline in dentists reflects a shift in priorities and a reduction in financial support for dental health programs in state health departments. Expansion of the WIC program and increased emphasis on lifestyle changes, particularly those related to diet, have increased the need for nutrition staff.

FUNDING

As with staffing patterns, the expenditures of state health departments are difficult to compare across states because the responsibilities of these departments vary so widely. For almost 20 years, the Public Health Foundation collected data on public health expenditures by categorical program. In 1991 (the last year for which data are available) state health departments spent $11.2 billion on public health programs. Three-quarters of these expenditures were for personal health services, including $1.5 billion for the operation of institutions.[23] Most of these personal health funds were used at the local level, either through local health departments, subunits of the state health department, or contracts with other service providers.

In the 1990s, the focus of data collection changed from categorical program expenditures, such as dollars for tuberculosis control, to funds spent on the 10 essential public health services[24] (see chapter 3 for a listing of the services). The Public Health Foundation surveyed nine states as a sample of nationwide expenditures. These states reported spending $8.8 billion on the essential public health services in 1995.[25] Expenditures were not limited to state health departments, but also included local public health and state substance abuse, mental health, and environmental agencies. Sixty-nine percent of the funds were spent on personal health services such as direct care services provided to individuals (under category 6b of the 10 essential services). The remaining 31 percent of expenditures were for population-based services, which are those interventions directed to the entire population. The population-based services averaged

$42 per capita across the nine states. The money was spent by the following agencies:

State health departments	44%
State environmental agencies	23%
Local health departments	20%
State substance abuse and mental health agencies	13%

These data emphasize that public health activities are carried out by a variety of state and local agencies, not just health departments. The survey report also concluded that obtaining comparable data across all states for such expenditures would be very difficult.

SOURCES OF FUNDS

In 1990 (the last year of data specific to all states), state health agencies received 50 percent of their funding from state legislatures, 37 percent from federal grants and contracts, 7 percent from fees and third-party reimbursements (excluding Medicaid), 3 percent from local sources, and 3 percent from other sources, such as grants from private foundations.[23] The single largest source of federal funds was the U.S. Department of Agriculture, which oversees the Supplemental Food Program for Women, Infants, and Children (WIC program). This program accounted for 20 percent of all funds spent by state health departments, with 40 percent of these funds used for vouchers for the direct purchase of food. The Centers for Disease Control and Prevention (CDC) and the Health Resources and Services Administration (HRSA) are the other major sources of federal funds used by state health departments. Beginning in the late 1980s, the expansion of Medicaid to cover more pregnant women and children provided an additional source of funding for services to these population groups.

Categorical and Block Grants

Federal funds come to states both as categorical grants, which focus on a particular health problem or population group, and as block grants, which have a broader public health focus. In general, categorical grant programs are controlled by extensive federal regulations and lengthy reporting requirements. They may lack flexibility to meet differing state needs.

Block grants were created in the early 1980s "to achieve greater flexibility in the use of funds, meaning more efficient use of tax dollars and more cost-effective service to recipients."[26] Initially, the block grants specified no priorities, objectives, or required outcomes. Decisions on how to use the funds were left entirely to state legislatures and governors, who frequently used the grants to fund programs the state was unwilling or unable to support with state revenues. States favored block grants because they provided more opportunities to meet state priorities or fill gaps in state funding. Twenty-one previously separate programs were consolidated into these four blocks. Left as categorical programs were childhood immunization, tuberculosis control, family planning, migrant health centers, and sexually transmitted disease control. The maternal/child health and prevention block grants are major sources of financial support for all state health departments.

Prevention Block Grant

The prevention block grant is used by state health departments to support chronic disease prevention, health education and risk reduction, emergency medical services, laboratory testing for communicable diseases and environmental toxins, rodent control, dental health, and a variety of other services. Since its inception, this grant has provided the most flexibility of all funding sources used by state health departments. However, the multiplicity of uses of these grant dollars state by state made it hard for Congress to identify exactly which services were being funded with the prevention block. As a result, Congress failed to increase funding for this grant at the same rate it did for categorical grants.

In 1992, Congress modified the prevention grant, linking it to the National Health Objectives for the year 2000. Beginning in 1993, all expenditures from the grant had to be directed toward specific national objectives, as selected by each state. A state level advisory group was required to hold public hearings on proposed uses of the grant.[27] In turn, the federal gov-

ernment required more accountability from states in the use of the funds and removed the decisions from the legislative process.

The preceding chapter describes the changing climate in the federal government regarding block grants. It is likely that there will be substantial efforts to decrease federal funds, put them in block grants, and hold states accountable for how the funds are spent. The pendulum is clearly swinging toward decreased categorical spending, more block grants (though with lower funding), and greater accountability.

Newer Sources of Funds

State and federal funding for communicable disease control programs increased markedly during the 1980s and 1990s, primarily to prevent and treat HIV/AIDS. Expenditures also increased for the control of tuberculosis, sexually transmitted diseases, and vaccine-preventable diseases. During this period, expenditures on chronic disease programs remained stable. This disparity reflects the willingness of appropriating bodies to allocate money to prevent diseases that spread person-to-person, but their relative lack of interest in reducing diseases influenced by lifestyle and behavior, even though the latter are responsible for more morbidity and mortality in the population.

In response to perceived threats from bioterrorism and emerging infections, the federal government invested funds, beginning in 1999, to improve the public health infrastructure in states. Through cooperative agreements with CDC, states received funds to develop better information and communication systems, improve employee skills in surveillance and epidemiology, enhance laboratory capacity for chemical and biological agents, and increase the organizational capacity for response.[9]

Tobacco settlement dollars have provided an additional new source of funding for state health departments. In 1998, 46 states and the tobacco industry settled the states' lawsuits for recovery of their tobacco-related disease costs in Medicaid recipients. State legislatures had the authority to allocate the settlement funds given to each state. By 2000, 15 states had made substantial commitments and others had made lesser commitments to fund tobacco use prevention and cessation programs with this money.[79] The tobacco settlement dollars have also been used to fund general public health programs, Medicaid expansion, health research, and a wide variety of non-health-related programs in the states.

PERFORMANCE STANDARDS

State health departments have joined a nationwide effort to focus on performance accountability for the functions assigned or expected of such agencies. In partnership, CDC and the Association of State and Territorial Health Officials have developed a set of performance standards for public health practice in state health departments.[29] The standards are organized around the 10 essential public health services. States will collect and analyze data on their achievement of these standards, using a comprehensive performance assessment instrument. The overall goal is to improve the quality and increase the scientific base for public health.

STATE-LOCAL RELATIONSHIPS

A former state health officer once said, "The federal government has most of the money, the state government has most of the legal authority, and the local government has most of the responsibility for protecting the health of the people."[30] To protect the health of citizens, state health departments must have a mechanism for delivering services to people where they live and work. The relationship between state and local health departments reflects the geography, politics, and funding patterns of each state.[31]

Organizational Relationships

One type of state-local organizational relationship is centralized, with either no local health departments or local agencies that are operated by the state health department.[18,32] Of the 11 centralized state health systems, 4 are in very small states (Delaware, Hawaii, Rhode Island, and Vermont) that do not have local health departments. In 7 states, organizational control over local health departments is shared between state and local governments.

Sixteen states have a completely decentralized organization, in which local government (city, township, county, or some combination) directly operates health departments. This decentralized pattern is more common in the West, where distances between towns are great and local control is popular. An additional 16 states have some mix of centralized and decentralized control, with local health services provided by the state health department in some jurisdictions, usually rural areas, and by local governments in other jurisdictions, primarily cities and counties with large populations.

Where organizational control is centralized, the state government supplies most of the funds for local health work, so state priorities determine which services are provided at the local level.[18,32] In decentralized situations, local health departments derive a greater percentage of their budgets from local government and tend to be more responsive to local needs.

STATE RESPONSIBILITIES FOR LOCAL SERVICES

Whatever the state-local organizational relationship, state health departments are responsible for establishing standards for local public health functions and holding local agencies accountable to those standards.[1] States may develop requirements for specific services to be offered locally, data to be collected and reported, and minimum staffing requirements to be met. Services inappropriate for smaller units, such as the provision of reference laboratories, or for which there must be statewide consistency, such as the inspection of health care facilities, are usually organized at the state level. The state health department has the additional responsibility of representing the needs of local health units with other state agencies, within both executive and legislative branches of government. In developing policy and allocating resources, state and local public health officials must communicate and collaborate.[33] Formerly they often viewed their relationship as a "we/they" situation, but are now more likely to see state and local health agencies as part of a total public health system that requires cooperation to succeed.

STATE-PRIVATE RELATIONSHIPS

Medical Profession

In the early years of this century, the medical profession was strongly supportive of the creation of state health departments, and members of the medical community often sat on boards of health and served as state health officers. As state health departments have become increasingly involved in the direct delivery of care to persons who cannot afford care in the private sector, however, the relationship between the state health department and the state medical society has frequently deteriorated. Whereas earlier physician health officers were invited to participate in medical society meetings, today's nonphysician health officers are viewed with suspicion by the medical community, and they often do not have the same access to medical colleagues that their predecessors did. Nonphysician administrators are also frequently criticized for not seeking medical advice or not informing the medical society of their plans.[1]

State health departments need the support of the medical profession to help pass key legislation through state legislatures and to provide medical expertise on many public health issues. Strengthening their relationship with state medical organizations is therefore an important challenge for today's state health departments.

Managed Care

Public health agencies and managed care plans have a similar goal: to keep the population they serve as healthy as possible. As managed care became a major form of health care delivery in the United States, state health departments sought opportunities to work with the managed care plans in their states. To assist states in this effort, the Association of State and Territorial Health Officials published, in 1995, a collection of issue briefs on managed care.[34]

Roper and Mays note that the interaction between managed care plans and public health agencies can be grouped into three types: delivery of personal health services, exchange of health data and information, and development and implementation of community interventions and policies.[35] While local health departments interact with managed care plans to deliver personal health services, state health agencies emphasize information exchange and community interventions. State agencies want managed care data for surveillance of communicable diseases and identification of trends in key health indicators. However, most initial collaboration between state health departments and managed care plans focused on the delivery of medical services to Medicaid-eligible individuals.[36] Few states reported collaboration around population-based projects. Only four states reported that managed care organizations shared disease incidence data with the health departments. Chief among concerns expressed by managed care plans were the difficulties in matching data systems, proprietary concerns for releasing data, and privacy issues over sharing medical information. The report noted that financial resources were needed to coordinate the data systems of state governments and managed care plans.

In some states, the health department has been assigned oversight of the quality of care delivered by managed care plans. Such a regulatory role for the state health department may reduce the willingness of managed care plans to share information and to embark on community interventions with the state agency.

CONCLUSION

Although state health departments retain ultimate responsibility for protecting the health of their citizens, their roles, significance, and visibility are frequently overlooked. More attention is focused on national and local health agencies. The federal government supplies the majority of government funds for health services through the Medicaid and Medicare programs and through categorical and block grants. Local health departments are where citizens actually seek public health services. The state health department is viewed as just a pass-through agency, passing funds and regulations from the federal and state to the local level, but not contributing significantly to the planning, development, and implementation of health services.

To obtain the legal authority and fiscal resources necessary to carry out its mission, a state health department must work with the governor and the state legislature. As noted earlier, the nature of this relationship will depend on where health functions are located in the executive branch and how accessible policy makers are to the state health director. The IOM Committee found that many state health departments did not have the influence necessary to acquire needed resources.[1] Without strong state boards of health or other public health advocacy groups, such as state public health associations, state health departments frequently have been left powerless and impoverished in the competition over state assets.

The roles and functions of state health departments will continue to evolve as they have in the past. The public increasingly needs protection from new causes of morbidity and mortality, such as violence, drugs, emerging infectious diseases, and toxic substances in the environment, while old challenges, including health disparities between ethnic groups and excess infant mortality, remain. The public also expects more regulation of health facilities and services that may cause harm. State health departments of tomorrow will be required to meet these expectations with new approaches and new policies.

References

1. Institute of Medicine, Committee for the Study of the Future of Public Health. *The Future of Public Health.* Washington, DC: National Academy Press; 1988.
2. McGinnis JM, Harrell JA, Artz LM, Files AA, Maiese DR. Objectives-based strategies for disease prevention. In: Detels R, Holland WW, McEwen J, Omenn GS, eds. *Oxford Textbook of Public Health.* 3rd ed. New York, NY: Oxford University Press; 1997.
3. *Measuring Health Objectives and Indicators: 1997 State and Local Capacity Survey.* Washington, DC: Public Health Foundation; 1998.
4. *Healthy People 2010: Understanding and Improving Health.* 2nd ed. Washington, DC: US Department of Health and Human Services; 2000. US Government Publication No. 017-001-00550-9.
5. Lewis-Idema D, Falik M. Health departments and Medicaid agencies: is the cold war really over? In: *Collaborative Strategies to Improve State and Local Public Health Systems or Is the Cold War Really Over?* Portland, Me: National Academy of State Health Policy; 1990.
6. Association of State and Territorial Health Officials. Fact sheets regarding state health information. *State Health Agency Profile Database.* Washington, DC. Available at. http://www.statepublichealth.org/. Accessed March 8, 2001 from ASTHO database.
7. *Responses to the IOM Report: The Future of Public Health.* Washington, DC: Association of State and Territorial Health Officials; 1990.
8. Burke TA, Shalauta NM, Tran NL, Stern BS. The environmental web: a national profile of the state infrastructure for environmental health and protection. *J Public Health Manage Pract.* 1997;3(2):1-12.

9. Emergency preparedness and response for bioterrorism. Draft program announcement. Atlanta, Ga: Centers for Disease Control and Prevention; January 22, 1999. Available at: http://www.astho.org/phiip/pdf/012299bioterrorismRFAdraft.pdf. Accessed March 8, 2001.
10. Association of State and Territorial Health Officials. By-laws. Washington, DC.
11. Williams SJ, Torrens PR. *Introduction to Health Services.* 6th ed. Albany, NY: Delmar Thomson Learning.
12. *Public Health Agencies 1980. A Report on Their Expenditures and Activities.* Washington, DC: Public Health Foundation; 1981.
13. Gossert DJ, Miller CA. State boards of health, their members and commitments. *Am J Public Health.* 1973;63(6): 486-493.
14. SHAs-freestanding agencies v. superagencies. *Public Health Macroview.* Washington, DC: Public Health Foundation; 1995;7(1):1.
15. *Directory of State and Territorial Health Agencies, 2000-2001.* Washington, DC: Association of State and Territorial Health Officials; 2000.
16. Gilbert B, Moos MK, Miller CA. State level decision making for public health: the status of boards of health. *J Public Health Policy.* 1982;3(1):51-61.
17. Terris M. Letter to all state health officials on results of questionnaire on training and experience. New York Medical College; December 2, 1977.
18. *Profile of State and Territorial Public Health Systems: United States, 1990.* Atlanta, Ga: Public Health Practice Program Office, Division of Public Health Systems, Centers for Disease Control; 1991.

19. Shon K. SHO tenure study. Internal memo. Washington, DC: Public Health Foundation; September 17, 1999.

20. *Study of State Health Official Turnover.* Internal document. Washington, DC: Association of State and Territorial Health Officials; 2000.

21. Gebbie K. The public health work force: enumeration 2000. New York, NY: Columbia University School of Nursing; December 2000. Available at: http://www.columbia.edu/dept/nursing/publications. Accessed February 15, 2001.

22. *State Health Agency Staffs, 1989.* Washington, DC: Public Health Foundation; 1992.

23. *Public Health Agencies 1991: An Inventory of Programs and Block Grant Expenditures.* Washington, DC: Public Health Foundation; 1991.

24. Public Health Functions Steering Committee. *Public Health in America.* US Public Health Service; 1994.

25. Eilbert KW, Barry M, Bialek R, Garufi M, Maiese D, Gebbie K, Fox CE. Public health expenditures: developing estimates for improved policy making. *J Public Health Manage Prac.* 1997;3(3):1-9.

26. *Health and Human Services Department Block Grants.* Washington, DC: US Department of Health and Human Services; 1981. HHS Fact Sheet.

27. Public Law 102-531; 1992.

28. *Show Us the Money: An Update on the States' Allocation of the Tobacco Settlement Dollars.* A report by the Campaign for Tobacco Free Kids, American Cancer Society, American Heart Association, American Lung Association; October 1, 2000.

29. *Draft State Assessment Tool.* US Department of Health and Human Services. Centers for Disease Control and Prevention; May 2000. Available at: http://www.phppo.cdc.gov//nphpsp/. Accessed April 21, 2001.

30. Nitzkin, J. Quoted by: Cundiff D. The future of state-local relationships in public health. *Bull Am Assoc Public Health Phys.* 1993;39(2):1-2.

31. Mullan F, Smith J. *Characteristics of State and Local Health Agencies.* Baltimore, Md: The Johns Hopkins University School of Hygiene and Public Health. Health Program Alliance; 1988.

32. DeFriese GH, Hetherington JS, Brooks EF, et al. The program implications of administrative relationships between local health departments and state and local government. *Am J Public Health.* 1981;71(10):1109-1115.

33. Joint Council of State and Local Health Officials. *Principles of Collaboration Between State and Local Public Health Officials.* Washington, DC: Association of State and Territorial Health Officials and National Association of County and City Health Officials; February 2000.

34. *Managed Care Monograph Series.* Washington, DC: Association of State and Territorial Health Officials; November 1995.

35. Roper WL, Mays GP. The changing managed care-public health interface. *JAMA.* 1998;280(20): 1739-1740.

36. *Public Health and Managed Care. Inspection Report.* Office of Inspector General; July 1999. US Department of Health and Human Services. Publication No. OEI-01-98-00170. Available at: http://www.dhhs.gov/progorg/oei/reports/a385.pdf. Accessed March 4, 2001.

CHAPTER

8

The Local Health Department

Thomas L. Milne, B.S. Pharm.

The first local health department in the country was formed by the City of Baltimore in 1798. Several large cities formed health departments in the early 1800s, and counties followed suit in the late 1800s and during the first half of the twentieth century. By 1953, there were a reported 1,239 health departments serving local jurisdictions.[1] As stated in the 1988 report from the Institute of Medicine (IOM), "New ideas about causes of disease and about social responsibility stimulated the development of public health agencies and institutions. As environmental and social causes of diseases were identified, social action appeared to be an effective way to control diseases. When health was no longer simply an individual responsibility, it became necessary to form public boards, agencies, and institutions to protect the health of citizens. Sanitary and social reform provided the basis for the formation of public health organizations."[2]

MISSION OF LOCAL HEALTH DEPARTMENTS

Specifically, the mission of local health departments is to protect, promote, and maintain the health of the entire population of their jurisdiction. They fulfill several functions in pursuit of that mission, including assessment, policy development, and assurance, the "core functions of public health." While specific services vary widely between health departments, those more commonly found include: completing community assessments to determine community strengths and needs; collecting and analyzing vital statistics; monitoring for and controlling outbreaks of infectious diseases; diminishing environmental health risks; providing limited "personal health" services including childhood and adult immunizations; providing health education; advocating for and referring people without health care resources; and developing local ordinances to protect the health of jurisdictions served. Additionally, local health departments are responsible for enforcement of public health statutes enacted by federal and state governments.

Importance of Local Health Departments

The national public health system includes a complex array of federal, state, local, and voluntary agencies. It is in local communities, however, that public health services actually reach the citizens of this country. A 1988 IOM report stressed the importance of local public health departments, stating:

> . . . no citizen from any community, no matter how small or remote, should be without identifiable and realistic access to the benefits of public health protection, which is possible only through a local component of the public health delivery system.[2]

Current Status of Local Health Departments

For the purposes of this chapter, *local health department* is defined as "an administrative or service unit of local or state government concerned with health and carrying some responsibility for the health of a jurisdiction smaller than the state.[3] That definition accommodates a broad range of organizations without regard to service or operational status. Using this definition, in 2001 there were nearly three thousand local governmental agencies fulfilling public health responsibilities at some level in most areas of the country.[4] Every state either has local health departments, which are entities of city, county, town, and/or district government, or it has divisions of the state health department that operate at the local level. Local health departments employ approximately 135,000 full-time and part-time employees, providing direct personal health services to an estimated 50 million people annually and carrying out core public health functions in their jurisdictions. The total cost of these activities nationwide is about $13 billion annually.

At the start of the new century, the roles and functions of local health departments are changing significantly. Contributing factors include shifts in the organization of medical care services; increasing numbers of uninsured citizens; increasing demands

for public accountability; and heightened public awareness of issues with public health implications such as environmental health, violence, emerging infectious diseases, and bioterrorism. Moreover, increasing demands from other sectors compete for resource streams that have traditionally supported local public health services.

To anticipate the changes—and to appreciate their impact on the whole health care system and the nation's health status—it is important to examine the history of local health departments as well as their current roles and capacities. This chapter provides a historical overview and a current survey of local health departments. It then discusses ways in which changes might occur and the potential impact of those changes.

HISTORICAL PERSPECTIVE

The necessity for a governmental agency at the local level to protect, promote, and maintain a community's health has not only been reiterated over the past decade, but it has also been confirmed time and again over the past century. For example, a major recommendation of President Hoover's 1931 White House Conference on Child Health and Protection was:

> To make everywhere available these minimum protections of the health and welfare of children, there should be a district, county or community organization for health, education and welfare, with full-time officials, coordinating with a statewide program which will be responsive to a nationwide service of general information, statistics and scientific research. This should include: (a) Trained, full-time public health officials, with public health nurses, sanitary inspection, and laboratory workers.[5]

Then, in 1945, Haven Emerson, M.D., described the six basic functions of a local health department as follows:[5]

1. Vital statistics, or the recording, tabulation, interpretation, and publication of the essential facts of births, deaths, and reportable diseases

2. Control of communicable diseases, including tuberculosis, venereal diseases, malaria, and hookworm disease

3. Environmental sanitation, including supervision of milk and milk products, food processing, and public eating places, and maintenance of sanitary conditions of employment

4. Public health laboratory services

5. Hygiene of maternity, infancy, and childhood, including supervision of the health of the school child

6. Health education of the general public so far as this is not covered by the functions of departments of education

The primary responsibilities of early health departments were communicable disease control and sanitation. They developed and expanded their scope of service over time in response to the particular needs and characteristics of the community in which they were established. Most of the services developed were of a primary or secondary prevention nature, but many departments also moved to fill gaps left by providers of clinical services. Consequently, there is now a core of personal health programs and services that are common to most local health departments, but there is also wide variation in the type and extent of additional activities that local health departments carry out.

Specifically, the widely disparate needs of urban and rural settings and significant differences in the structure of state and local government services has resulted in wide variation in type and number of services, organizational structure, per capita expenditures, and staffing patterns of local health departments.

CHANGING CONTEXT

Through the late 1980s and 1990s, a great deal of work was done at the national level to strengthen local health departments and systems. The IOM report identified three "core functions" of public health: assessment, policy development, and assurance.[2] In 1994, a national work group produced a set of "essential services" that are needed to carry out basic public health responsibilities at all levels of the national public health system.[6] The 10 essential public health services include the following:

1. Monitor health status to identify community health problems

2. Diagnose and investigate health problems and health hazards in the community

3. Inform, educate, and empower people about health issues

4. Mobilize community partnerships to identify and solve health problems

5. Develop policies and plans that support individual and community health efforts

6. Enforce laws and regulations that protect health and ensure safety

7. Link people to needed personal health services and assure the provision of health care when otherwise unavailable

8. Assure a competent public health and personal health care workforce

9. Evaluate effectiveness, accessibility, and quality of personal and population-based health services

10. Research for new insights and innovative solutions to health problems

The delineation of the essential services has, in turn, provided the basis for the development of national public health performance standards, for studies of national public health expenditures, and for the design of local public health assessment tools (including *APEXPH* and MAPP). Together with activities under way in the field to strengthen local systems, including Turning Point, public health leadership institutes, and various demonstration projects, the groundwork is being laid for significant improvement in local public health practice.

CHARACTERISTICS OF LOCAL HEALTH DEPARTMENTS

Local health departments vary widely with regard to several important characteristics. These include organizational issues such as jurisdictional type, their size and staffing patterns, the services they provide, and the functions they fulfill.

Organizational Issues

Organizational issues of local health departments include jurisdictional type, authority to operate, relationship to their state health department, and governance structure. There are significant variations among departments in all of these factors.

Jurisdictional Type

Local health departments are governmental entities serving jurisdictions of towns, cities, counties, and/or districts (see Figure 8.1). A sizeable number, 15 percent, are agencies of a town or township jurisdiction. Only 10 percent are single city health departments. 60 percent are run by a single county government, and another 7 percent are city-county entities, in which case, the local health department may report either to a

Type Health Department	1992	2001
Other	2%	0%
City/County	13%	7%
Multi-County	11%	8%
City	7%	19%
Town/Township	11%	15%
County	56%	60%

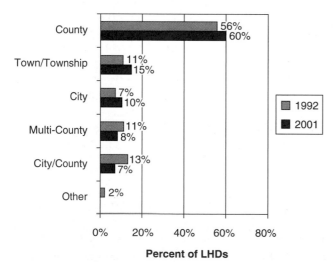

Health Department Types: 1992–2001

Figure 8.1. United States Local Health Departments by Type of Jurisdiction, 1992–1993 vs. 2001[7,8]

joint council or commission made up of county and city elected officials or to both county and city boards of health.

Eight percent of local health departments serve districts, which are jurisdictions made up of several independent counties that have joined together.[7] In Idaho, for example, 44 counties were organized into seven district health departments, each comprising 4 to 8 counties. This created a larger population and tax base for the new health departments, which allowed them to expand staff numbers and skills and provide a broader and more consistent range of services throughout the state.

Authority to Operate and State-Local Relationships

Typically, local health departments derive their authority from their state health department and from the county or city government of which they are a part. Organizational relationships between local health departments and their state health department vary widely from state to state.

Independent Departments

In most states, including Washington, Minnesota, and New York, for example, local health departments operate independently from their respective state health departments. In these states, the governing bodies for most local health departments develop and/or approve their budgets, set priorities, develop local health ordinances, and hire their directors/health officers.

An important advantage of this model is that the priorities of local government and the community can be integrated easily into the health department's services. Disadvantages can include a lack of communication among departments, noninvolvement of local health departments in state planning and decision making, and uneven service delivery across the state.

Interdependent Departments

In other states, local health departments are entities of the state, or else they work in an interdependent fashion with their state health department. In Florida, for example, local health departments are entities of state government and also have a direct reporting relationship to county government. The state health department approves the county health department budget, sets priorities, and determines the programmatic emphasis. The county usually contributes tax dollars to the state health department budget and, after developing the county budget, contracts with the state for service. The county makes only limited policy and programmatic decisions. The selection of a county health official is begun by the state health department, with review and appointment made by the county board of commissioners. County health department staff are also state employees. Variations on this model are found in Virginia, Louisiana, and Georgia.

Advantages of this model are that services can be provided uniformly within the state, and priorities can be addressed statewide. Disadvantages include the need for county health departments to "serve two masters" and the limited ability of a county health department to focus on locally determined priorities, programs, and policies.

A small number of states, including Tennessee, Oklahoma, and Pennsylvania, use a combination of the independent and interdependent models. In these states, the larger cities and/or counties typically organize their own independent health department (e.g., Nashville-Davidson County, Tennessee), while local or regional offices of the state health department serve the remaining cities or counties in the state, often organized into regions.

Advantages of this variation include ensuring the availability of state-run public health services in smaller communities that have few resources, while giving broader authority and local control to the health departments serving larger communities. Disadvantages may include inconsistency in policy development, and significant variation in services.

Importance of Communication

Regardless of the administrative relationship between state and local health departments, efforts must be made by both parties to ensure open channels of communication and maximum effectiveness of the system. Problems in these areas are reported by both parties, and a number of efforts have begun in recent years in some states to further the collaboration between them.

Development of and regular revisits to the Washington State Public Health Improvement Plan[9] and the Illinois "I-Plan"[10] are two early examples of concerted efforts between state and local health officials to collaborate on goals and public health systems. The Joint Council of State and Local Public Health Officials has produced and distributed to all state and local health departments a set of principles on collaboration between these two levels of the national public health system.[11] In at least two instances—the Health Alert Network funding, begun in 1998, and the Public Health Threats and Emergencies Act of 2001—Congress has required that states include local health departments in state planning, and that local priorities and needs directly benefit from specific federal program funds sent to the states. All these efforts are being undertaken to improve the level of communication, decision making concerning resource allocation and policies, and the provision of technical assistance from state to local health departments.

The Special Case of City Health Departments

The responsibilities of city health departments operating in charter cities differ somewhat from the authorities and responsibilities of other local health departments because cities generally have broader discretionary powers than other entities of local government. A city charter "empowers them to do almost anything the state does not prohibit them from doing, whereas counties generally can only do the things for which they are specifically empowered."[12]

City health departments differ from county health departments in other ways as well. Many county functions are required by the state, and counties must act as agents of the state in carrying them out. By contrast, cities usually can modify their health department services more readily and, in some states, can choose whether to even have a health department. For revenue, cities usually can rely on more types of taxes, including property, sales, and in some cases, income taxes, whereas counties generally can rely only on property taxes. As described in the next section, the source of these differences may lie with how and when city and county health departments were formed.

Governance Structures: Local Boards of Health

Boards of health were first established in the eighteenth century, when local citizens were appointed by city governments to deal with important diseases and conditions of the time. Today, boards of health govern three out of four health departments in the country.[8] The composition of boards of health varies according to state law. In some states, including California and Florida, a local governmental body (e.g., county board of commissioners) serves as the local board of health, while in others, state law mandates that health professionals and/or other members of the community be included on the board of health. The size of local boards of health varies widely, usually ranging between 3 and 15 members.

Roles of Boards of Health

Many local boards of health have policy-making authority, including budget approval and ordinance adoption, while other boards serve principally in an advisory capacity. As shown in Figure 8.2, almost all boards of health, 88 percent nationwide, have statutory authority to establish local health policies, fees, ordinances, and regulations. About 60 to 65 percent also approve the budget and/or hire the agency head, and 60 to 65 percent establish community health priorities.[8]

Most local boards of health also serve as a link between local public health agencies and the community they serve. In this capacity, the board of health represents the community's interest in adopting priorities and establishing needed services, while also communicating with the community about health department goals and services available. Members of boards of health who are not elected officials may also be able to lobby legislators more directly than is possible for local health officials.

The Role of Jurisdiction Size

Nationwide, boards of health in smaller jurisdictions (those with populations of fewer than 100,000) tend to have greater statutory authority than those in juris-

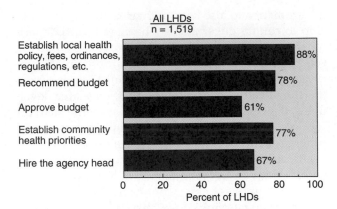

	0 to 24,999 n=650	25,000 to 49,999 n=360	50,000 to 99,999 n=263	100,000 to 499,999 n=203	500,000 + n=43
Establish local health policy, fees, ordinances, regulations, etc.	89%	90%	89%	77%	74%
Recommend budget	82%	82%	75%	69%	58%
Approve budget	63%	66%	64%	48%	35%
Establish community health priorities	77%	79%	81%	72%	58%
Hire the agency head	63%	74%	73%	66%	56%

Figure 8.2. Statutory Authority of United States Boards of Health in Jurisdictions with a Board of Health, 1992–1993[8]

dictions with larger populations. The size of the population served may also be correlated with the presence or absence of a board of health. Of health departments serving the smallest population, 76 percent are governed by boards of health. Of those serving populations between 25,000 and 50,000, 80 percent are governed by boards of health. Of health departments serving populations over 500,000, only 59 percent are governed by them.[8]

The reason for the higher prevalence and greater role of boards of health in smaller jurisdictions may be historical. In the early twentieth century, most of the existing local health departments had been developed in larger cities; health departments serving small populations were rarely found. As state health departments developed, legislation often followed to ensure that all areas of the state were covered by a governmental public health presence at the local level. In many low-population areas, boards of health were created and given that responsibility.

Sources of Funding

Most health departments receive funding from several sources including local taxes; state grants; federal grants, either directly or through the state; foundation grants; reimbursement for personal health care; and fees for licensures, inspections, and certifications. The largest source of funding is from local government, comprising 44 percent of health department budgets. The other principal sources of funding, in order of size, are state funding (including federal pass-through dollars) at 30 percent, service reimbursement (including Medicaid, Medicare, insurance, licenses, permits, etc.) at 19 percent and direct federal grants, accounting for 3 percent of budgets. Another 4 percent comes from a variety of other sources, including foundations and donations.[7] As is shown in Figure 8.3, there has been a significant shift in funding sources since 1992, with local funding replacing state and federal pass-through as the principal source of support.[7,8] This probably reflects, in large part, the flattening of support from federal categorical grants during this period. (See Figure 8.3)

The Medicaid Question

During the first half of the 1990s, most local health departments provided personal health services to Medicaid-covered clients. In 1990, 76 percent of health departments billed Medicaid.[3] Data from a 1992–1993 survey found that Medicaid revenues accounted for 7 percent of total health department revenues.[8] By the mid-1990s many states restructured their Medicaid programs, moving their programs from fee-for-service to capitated payment systems and attracting managed care organizations (MCOs). In those states, some local health departments successfully worked to retain their Medicaid revenue base by contracting with MCOs, by becoming Federally Qualified Health Centers, or by using other strategies. Most, however, found their Medicaid revenues sharply reduced.

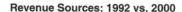

Funding Source	1992	2000
Local	0.34	0.44
State	0.4	0.3
Federal	0.06	0.03
Service Reimbursement	0.17	0.19
Other	0.03	0.04

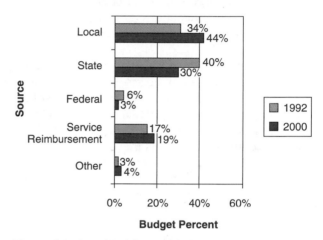

Figure 8.3. Local Public Health Departments: Shifts in Sources of Funds, 1992–2000[7,8]

Fees

Another important source of revenue, particularly for environmental health programs, is the collection of fees for licenses, certifications, and inspections. Although in many communities fees are not charged for personal health services (because many of the patients are low income), it is usually considered acceptable to charge for the provision of environmental services. Fees are charged for the licensing of such facilities as restaurants, barber shops, health-related facilities, recreational facilities, sewage treatment operations, and tanning salons, among others.

Size of Local Health Departments

The size of local health departments can be characterized by the size of the population of the jurisdiction served, the size of the department's staff, or its total annual expenditures. Variation in each of these factors is considered next.

Population of Jurisdiction Served

Populations served by local health departments can range from very large—approximately nine million for Los Angeles County and eight million for New York City—to communities of between one and two hundred people.

Most local health departments serve jurisdictions with relatively small populations. Jurisdictions with fewer than 50,000 residents account for 69 percent of the nation's health departments; 50 percent of all health departments serve jurisdictions with fewer than 25,000 residents.[7] Health departments that serve small populations are likely to have a small tax base, few staff, and a relatively limited configuration of services. For example, for local health departments serving fewer than 25,000 people, the median annual budget is only $214,658, and the median number of staff is just 8.5. For local health departments that serve populations between 25,000 and 50,000, the median annual budget is $600,000, and the median number of staff is 18.[7]

At the other end of the spectrum, 4 percent of local health departments serve populations of 500,000 or more; 14 percent serve populations between 100,000 and 499,999; and 13 percent serve populations between 50,000 and 99,999. These health departments tend to provide a greater number of services, have larger budgets, and employ more staff. For example, for health departments serving between 100,000 and 499,999, the median budget is $5,100,000 and the median number of staff is 110. The largest health departments, serving over 500,000, have a median budget of $27,000,000 and 437 staff.[7]

Staffing Size

As indicated in the preceding section, the staffing size varies widely among local health departments. Data from 1992–1993 studies showed that 42 percent employed fewer than 10 staff.[8] More recent data show that health departments nationally employ an average of 67 full-time equivalent (FTE) staff, with a median of 13 FTEs.[7] This indicates a trend toward declining staff sizes overall when compared to 1997 data which showed an average of 72 FTEs and a median of 16 FTEs.[13] The difference in staff sizes between health departments is striking. Those serving the smallest populations, fewer than 25,000 residents, employ an average of 13.9 and a median of 8.5 FTEs, while those serving the largest populations, greater than 500,000, employ an average of 612 and a median of 437 FTEs.[7]

The number of health departments with very small staffs is of great concern to many health professionals. Staffing size is directly related to a department's ability to provide the essential services listed earlier in this chapter.

Total Annual Expenditures

Total annual health department budgets have increased over the past eight years, growing from a median of $500,000 in 1993 to $621,100 in 2001, or about 3 percent per year.[7,8] The average expenditure in 2001 was $4,505,096, a figure that is greatly skewed by the largest health departments. The mean and median total annual expenditures by population size are shown in Table 8.1.[7] Detailed information comparing the use of annual budgets is not available.

Services and Functions

Local health departments provide a wide range of services that affect nearly all persons residing in or visiting the United States. When public health services are working well and preventing the occurrence, or reducing the spread, of disease, the public is virtually unaware of their existence. Epidemics are avoided, water quality remains safe, and healthy behaviors are adopted with little fanfare. This relative invisibility of local health departments belies the existence of a wide range of public health activities.

What follows is a broad summary of the major services provided by local health departments. Although data are available on over 50 different services provided by local health departments, descriptions of all of them are not possible here.

Table 8.1. U.S. Local Health Departments: Average and Median Annual Expenditure by Size of Jurisdiction Served, 2001[7]

Jurisdiction Size	Average Expenditure	Median Expenditure
0 to 24,999	$ 437,637	$ 214,658
25,000 to 49,999	$ 1,227,538	$ 600,000
50,000 to 99,999	$ 2,552,669	$ 1,827,526
100,000 to 499,999	$ 7,671,500	$ 5,100,000
500,000 or more	$66,200,000	$27,000,000

Environmental Health

Although in many states the lead responsibility for environmental health lies with an agency other than the health department, 85 percent of local health departments are responsible for at least some environmental health services.[7]

Most health departments (85 percent) continue to fulfill the long-standing tradition of providing food safety services, including such activities as restaurant licensure and inspection, and training of food handlers.[7]

Other traditional environmental health services include assurance of the safety of public and private water supplies, solid waste management, management of sewage disposal systems, and vector and animal control.

In response to growing awareness of environmental contamination and the links between human health and the environment, many local health departments have taken a leading role in the assurance of indoor air quality, tobacco and secondhand smoke regulation, pollution prevention, emergency response, and management of hazardous materials. Local health departments are increasingly becoming the source of information for the community about environmental risks, and many have initiated programs in occupational health and safety. The emergence of the West Nile Virus in the eastern United States at the turn of this century was a classic example of an emerging vector-borne disease that required a hastily assembled response from local and state health departments with little in the way of new resources.

Table 8.2 shows the percent of local health departments that provide selected environmental services, by size of the population served. As the size of population increases, more environmental services tend to be provided.

Primary Care and Personal Health Care Services

Notwithstanding the trends related to Medicaid reimbursement described earlier, local health departments continue to provide personal health services. Each year, 40 million people receive some type of personal health care from local health departments, including immunizations, Early and Periodic Screening, Diagnosis, and Treatment (EPSDT) services, prenatal care, tuberculosis screening and treatment, treatment of sexually transmitted diseases, and other discrete services aimed at restoring and maintaining health and preventing transmission of disease. Figure 8.4 shows the percentage of local health departments that provide selected personal health services.[7]

In most states, state or local governments are required to provide at least some health care services to the indigent and to others who have no other means of accessing care.[14] Many counties throughout the nation are designated as providers of last resort, often providing more services than they are legally obligated to provide.

Trends in Personal Health Care Services

In general, the level of personal health care services provided by local health departments is directly

Table 8.2. U.S. Local Health Departments: Selected Environmental Health Services Provided, Directly or by Contract, by Size of Population Served, 2001[7]

Service	All LHDs	0 to 24,999	25,000 to 49,999	50,000 to 99,999	100,000 to 499,999	500,000 +
Food Safety	85%	80%	89%	88%	92%	93%
Sewage Disposal	74%	71%	77%	78%	79%	69%
Lead Screening & Abatement	74%	70%	78%	83%	79%	85%
Private Drinking Water	72%	70%	70%	74%	82%	63%
Emergency Response	61%	56%	67%	64%	65%	72%
Vectors	61%	54%	66%	72%	68%	76%
Indoor Air Quality	44%	37%	51%	51%	52%	62%
Surface Water Pollution	43%	45%	41%	37%	43%	43%

related to their size. Fewer than one-fifth of all local health departments provide primary care, which is defined as comprehensive care available 24 hours per day.[7]

In the late 1990s, many local health departments chose to eliminate or significantly curtail personal health services to focus on population-level public health activities. In some cases, that decision was also related to declining Medicaid revenues, as discussed earlier. Regardless of the rationale, the availability of primary care and personal health services from local health departments declined significantly between 1992 and 2001 (see Figure 8.5).[7,8] By the end of the 1990s, however, managed care organizations (MCOs) were finding the provision of services to Medicaid enrollees less attractive and began dropping their state contracts. Although in some locations health departments were prepared to resume services to larger numbers of Medicaid clients, in others the capacity to provide personal health services had been lost. At this writing, it is too early to determine the long-term impact on medical care access for Medicaid enrollees and other disenfranchised populations as a result of the MCO experience. It is clear that once primary care capacity is reduced or eliminated in local health departments, that capacity is difficult to rebuild. (See Figure 8.5 following)

The role of local health departments in the delivery of personal health care services is currently in a state of flux. The cost of these services, their availability elsewhere in the community, and the concern that such services might overshadow a health department's core functions are questions that must be considered and resolved in each community.

In communities where local health departments do not provide primary care services, the health departments still have the responsibility of ensuring that needed personal health care services are available and accessible to everyone in the jurisdiction. Indeed, over 80 percent of local health departments report that they assess the extent to which clinical preventive services, such as screening, immunization, and counseling services, are provided in the community by others. Local health departments may collect information on a wide variety of indicators of availability of services, including the number of practicing physicians, the existence of ambulatory care centers, the types of community agencies, the number of providers that accept Medicaid reimbursement or have translation services, and others.[7]

In many jurisdictions, local health officials have worked closely with other providers to try to ensure that adequate services are accessible to vulnerable populations. Most local health departments collaborate with hospitals and independent providers (90 percent of LHDs), with community health centers (54 percent), and with managed care and health maintenance organizations (50 percent) to ensure health care access.[5] Examples of partnerships and linkages that have been developed include subcontracting with

Service	Percentage
Primary Care	18%
HIV Treatment	25%
Dental Care	30%
Prenatal Care	41%
WIC	55%
Family Planning	58%
EPSDT	59%
HIV Testing & Counseling	64%
STD Testing & Counseling	65%
Tuberculosis Testing	88%
Childhood Immunizations	89%
Adult Immunizations	91%

Service	1992	2001
EPSDT	79%	59%
WIC	78%	55%
Family Planning	68%	58%
Prenatal Care	64%	41%
Dental Health	45%	30%
Primary Care	30%	18%

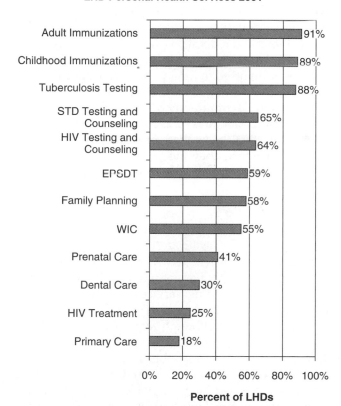

Figure 8.4. Percent of Local Public Health Departments Providing Selected Personal Health Services, 2001[7]

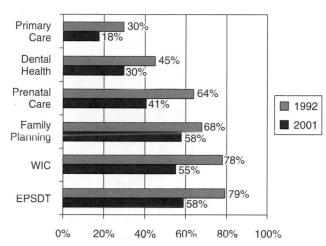

Figure 8.5. Comparison of Primary Care and Personal Health Services Provided by LHDs, 1992–2000[7]

hospitals for obstetric services, assisting in the application for federal grants, and working with private providers to accept patients unable to pay for health care services. These are just a few examples of the approaches used by local health officials to try to ensure that the people they serve actually get the care they need.

Population-Level Services

The traditional core responsibility of local health departments is to ensure that the overall population of the jurisdiction it serves enjoys the highest level of health status possible. Primary care and personal health services discussed in the previous section have evolved in more recent years, principally to address gaps in health care coverage. Just as these services are in flux, population-focused services continue to evolve. Such services in the contemporary local health department include community assessment and involvement, policy development, and health assurance activities.

Community Assessment and Involvement

Local health departments have conducted assessment activities for many years, collecting data descriptive of various aspects of community demographics, local provider system capacities, and local morbidity and mortality. Comprehensive community assessments are a relatively recent phenomenon, inspired in large part by the 1988 IOM report[2] and facilitated by the development of several assessment tools. Examples of assessment tools include *APEXPH* (Assessment Protocol for Excellence in Public Health),[15] PATCH (Planned Approach to Community Health),[16] and Healthy Communities 2000: Model Standards,[17] all developed in the early 1990s, and MAPP (Mobilizing for Action through Planning and Partnerships).[18] The latter tool, released in 2000, is Web based (www.naccho.org/) and includes a community process for strategic planning based on the findings of the comprehensive assessment. The tool also links with the national performance standards tool.[19]

Conducting community assessments has become a fairly standard activity in communities. Eighty percent of local health departments conduct or contract for assessments, and another 10 percent report that another organization in the community performs this function.[7] Most assessments incorporate a variety of data sources, including census demographics, vital records, state disease databases, hospital discharge information, special epidemiologic studies, and the results of focus group interviews reflecting the community's perceived beliefs, perceptions, and values about health and health status conditions.

Most local health departments use the result of assessments to develop plans that address the most pressing needs within their community. Increasingly, health departments are involving their communities in the assessment and planning processes. This trend reflects the understanding that issues with relevance to health status easily exceed the capacity, resources,

and authority of local public health agencies. Improvements in community health status depend upon community understanding of, participation in, and where possible, ownership of plans and community action to achieve those improvements.

Policy Development

As the second of the three core public health functions, policy development has been performed by local health departments since their inception. Much of the policy developed, however, has been a reflection of budget and service decisions, many of which, in turn, were made for local health departments by state policy and through the acceptance of categorically funded state and federal programs. Increasingly, however, contemporary local health departments are paying closer attention to local policy needs, particularly as they are driven by community assessments and the development of community plans. Health department leaders and policy makers are paying more attention to ensuring that the services provided, as well as the manner in which they are provided, are consistent with community interests, preferences, and needs.

Health Assurance

The IOM's definition of *assurance*, the third of the core functions of public health, is "to make sure that necessary services are provided to reach agreed upon goals, either by encouraging private sector action, by requiring it, or by providing services directly."[2] Primary care and more limited personal health services were discussed earlier. Although such services do have population-level impacts, they are not generally considered population-level public health services. Many health departments have decreased their provision of personally directed health services to focus more on assessment, policy development, and population-level assurance services.

Clearly, environmental health services, described earlier, constitute population-level services. Most health departments provide one or more environmental health service, with food safety, sewage disposal, and drinking water services most frequently provided directly or contracted. In many communi-

Service	Percent
Occupational Safety and Health	13%
Violence Prevention	22%
Injury Control	37%
Cardiovascular Disease Screening	50%
Diabetes Screening	53%
Cancer Screening	58%
Tobacco Use Reduction	68%
High Blood Pressure Screening	81%
Epidemiology & Surveillance	84%
Health Education/Risk Reduction	87%
Communicable Disease Control	94%

LHD Assurance Services, 2001

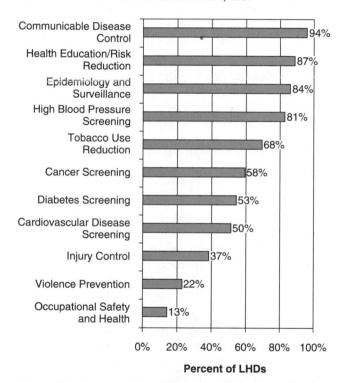

Figure 8.6. Selected Population-Level Assurance Services Provided by LHDs, 2001[7]

ties, however, environmental health services are either provided by another organization or aren't provided at all. Surface water pollution (57 percent), indoor air quality (55 percent), emergency response (39 percent), and vectors (39 percent) are the leading examples.[7]

Other population-level public health assurance services provided are summarized in Figure 8.6. As in years past, communicable disease control and health surveillance are frequently provided. Increasingly, local health departments are providing risk reduction services. The growing number providing tobacco use reduction services may reflect the increase in resources resulting from the Master Settlement Agreement negotiated between the tobacco industry and the states.

Staffing Patterns

Local health departments currently employ a total of about 135,000 people. These include over 30 distinct professional types. Figure 8.7 shows the findings of a 1989 study of registered professions employed in local health departments nationwide. Clerical/secretarial staff and registered nurses were most frequently found, with over 90 percent of local health departments employing people in such positions. Other positions found but not shown in the figure included planners/analysts and public information specialists.

A more recent study demonstrated that the composition of the workforce has changed somewhat, although administrative and clerical staff, environmental specialists/scientists, and nurses remain the most frequently employed professionals in local health departments. Frequently mentioned occupations not mentioned in the 1990 study include health information systems specialists, public health policy analysts, public health dental workers (nondentists), and laboratory workers.[7]

As the population of the jurisdiction increases in size, there tends to be more variety in staff composition. As is the case in state health departments, the number of staff in local health departments varies considerably, depending on the scope of services provided and the level of funding in each department.

PROFILE OF AGENCY TOP EXECUTIVES

The characteristics, qualifications, and tenure of agency top executives show considerable variation. Unfortunately, however, no recent studies describing local public health executives have been conducted. All of the data in the following three sections reflect a study conducted in 1992.[7]

Service	Percent
Epidemiologist	11%
Dentist	17%
Toxicologist/Environmental Specialist	18%
Social Worker	27%
Licensed Practical Nurse	33%
Health Educator	37%
Nutritionist/Dietician	51%
Physician	62%
Engineer/Sanitarian	77%
Registered Nurse	90%
Clerical/Secretarial	94%

Professions Employed in LHDs 1989

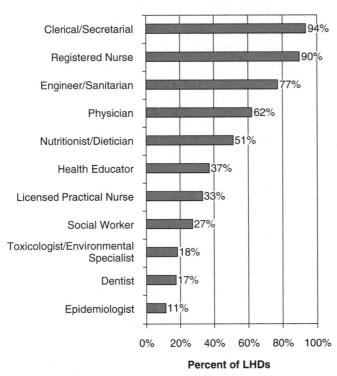

Figure 8.7. Percent of LHDs Reporting Full and/or Part-Time Staff, 1989[20]

Characteristics of Agency Top Executive

The chief executive officer (CEO) of the local health department usually is also the health official, but in some departments these responsibilities reside in two different individuals. CEOs bear responsibility for administrative issues and management of their agen-cies, and if they lack public health or medical training, they may rely on appropriately trained and licensed health officials or medical advisors to make health or medical decisions.

Most health departments (79 percent) are served by a full-time agency executive. Not surprisingly, as the population of the jurisdiction served increases, the likelihood that the job of agency executive will be a full-time position also increases, from 69 percent in the smallest agencies to 96 percent in the largest.

The majority, or 60 percent, of local health directors are male, and over 96% of local health directors are Euro-American. Only 2 percent are African American and another 2 percent are Hispanic. The majority of both groups are executives for the largest jurisdictions.

Qualifications of Agency Top Executives

In 1992 to 1993, approximately 37 percent of agency top executives held some type of medical doctoral degree (e.g., M.D., D.V.M., D.O.). Of these, 77 percent required the medical degree for the job. Agency top executives in jurisdictions serving populations over 500,000 are much more likely to hold a medical degree than their counterparts in all other jurisdictions—63 percent in the largest areas, as compared with 29 to 40 percent in the smaller jurisdictions. Seventeen percent of all agency heads have graduate public health degrees. In some jurisdictions, there are statutory requirements that the chief health official must have both medical and public health degrees.

It appears that the number of agency top executives with medical degrees is declining somewhat, a change that has been reported anecdotally for several years. It may be due to a move toward professional managers as agency heads.

Tenure of Local Health Directors

Although studies have not been done in recent years, anecdotal evidence suggests that the tenure of local health directors changed little since the 1990 NACCHO survey of local health departments. That study showed 16 percent had been in their positions for fewer than two years, 27 percent for two to five years, 25 percent for five to nine years, 25 percent for ten to nineteen years, and 7 percent for twenty years or more. The majority of the agency top executives (57 percent) had been in their positions for more than five years.

That same study showed that the tenure of health directors serving jurisdictions with large populations was shorter than that of health directors serving smaller populations. In jurisdictions of over 500,000 people, 55 percent of the health directors had held their positions for less than five years, and only 17 percent had held their positions for more than ten years. By contrast, in jurisdictions of under 50,000 people, 43 percent had been in their positions for less than four years, and 29 percent had been in their positions for more than ten years.

The tenure of local health agency heads contrasts sharply with the shorter tenure of state health officials. In 2000, the average tenure of state health department directors was two years.[20] Many attribute the difference in tenure to a lesser degree of politicization of health officer positions at the local level.

DISCUSSION

Local health departments experienced significant change during the decade of the 1990s and in the early years of the new century. The Institute of Medicine study published in 1988 created a new framework for public health, and has contributed to significant changes in the practice. Information technology, somewhat late in coming to public health, has also made a significant impact on practice. By 2000, over 80 percent of local health departments had access to the Internet, were using e-mail to speed communication, and were gaining experience rapidly with high-speed electronic access to information.[21] Local health department experiences with Medicaid, managed care, and primary care access issues during the period also tended to result in expanded relationships with the medical care community. Initiation of community assessment and other local activities tended to result in increased partnerships with businesses, the faith community, and other nonprofit organizations.[7]

At the national level, work was nearly completed on the development of performance standards for state and local public health departments and boards of health,[19] and a national strategic plan for public health workforce development was published.[22] Due in large part to national attention paid to consequences of potential bioterrorism events, Congress requested and received from CDC a study of national, state and local public health capacity,[23] and passed legislation to identify and address significant infrastructure gaps and to improve public health preparedness for such events.[24]

All of these events and changes, taken together, offer great promise to both future public health department success and to improved health outcomes for communities. The potential exists, if these changes become trends, for increased and more timely access to information, improved targeting of federal funding for local public health core capacity development, improvements in the availability of public health services, increased competence of the public health workforce, and greater involvement of community partners in public health issues.

It is perhaps this latter factor—community involvement—that holds the greatest promise for improved community health status. Experience from both the Turning Point Program of 1997–2001[25] and the healthy communities movement have shown that the involvement of social service organizations, businesses, churches, and others in addressing public health and quality of life issues has resulted in expanded resources, innovation, and broader ownership of planning and problem resolution. Broader involvement also increases the likelihood that the root causes of population-level health issues, including poverty, poor educational attainment, racism, and other social injustices, are addressed.

Local public health departments will continue to play a critically important role, even in an environment of highly interactive and successful community partnering. No other organization, private or governmental, has the responsibility for ensuring that the health interests and needs of the public are addressed. In keeping with that responsibility, it is the obligation of local health departments to be accountable to their communities, carrying out the core public health functions and periodically reporting to the community about health status and system problems.

Clearly, those responsibilities cannot be carried out effectively and completely by microsized health departments that have few resources and little support of elected officials. A concerted effort involving federal, state, and local leadership over the next several years will be required to build the necessary infrastructure to ensure that all communities enjoy the protection of the essential public health services.

References

1. Mountin J, Flook E. *Guide to Health Organizations in the United States.* Washington, DC: US Public Health Service; 1953.
2. Institute of Medicine, Committee for the Study of the Future of Public Health. *The Future of Public Health.* Washington, DC: National Academy Press; 1988.
3. *National Profile of Local Health Departments.* Washington, DC: National Association of County and City Health Officials; 1990.
4. Unpublished database of local health departments. Washington, DC: National Association of County and City Health Officials; August 2001.
5. *The Children's Charter.* President Hoover's White House Conference on Child Health and Protection. Washington, DC; 1931.
6. *Public Health in America.* Washington, DC: Public Health Functions Steering Committee; Fall 1994.
7. *Local Public Health Agency Infrastructure: A Chartbook.* Washington, DC: National Association of County and City Health Officials; 2001.
8. *1992-1993 National Profile of Local Health Departments.* Washington, DC: National Association of County and City Health Officials; 1995.
9. *Public Health Improvement Plan.* Olympia: Washington State Department of Health; 1994.
10. *Project Health: The Reengineering of Public Health in Illinois.* Springfield: Illinois Department of Public Health; 1999:9, 12.
11. *Principles of Collaboration between State and Local Public Health Officials.* Washington, DC: Joint Council of State and Local Public Health Officials; February 2000.
12. Turnock BJ. Testimony presented at public hearing on "County Governments and Health Care Reform" held by the National Association of Counties; October 19, 1992.
13. *1997 Profile of Local Health Departments.* Washington, DC: Unpublished data from the National Association of County and City Health Officials; 1997.
14. *Too Poor to Be Sick: Access to Medical Care for the Uninsured.* Washington, DC: American Public Health Association; 1988:39.
15. *Assessment Protocol for Excellence in Public Health (APEXPH).* Washington, DC: National Association of County and City Health Officials; 1991.
16. *Planned Approach to Community Health (PATCH).* Atlanta, Ga: Centers for Disease Control and Prevention; 1993.
17. *Healthy Communities 2000: Model Standards.* Washington, DC: American Public Health Association, 1991.
18. *Mobilizing for Action through Planning and Partnerships.* Washington, DC: National Association of County and City Health Officials; 2000.
19. *National Public Health Performance Standards Program.* Atlanta, Ga: Public Health Practice Program Office/ Centers for Disease Control and Prevention; 2000.
20. *Study of State Health Official Turnover.* Washington, DC: Association of State and Territorial Health Officials; 2000.
21. *Research Brief: Information Technology Capacity and Local Public Health Agencies.* Washington, DC: National Association of County and City Health Officials; July 1999.
22. *A Global and National Implementation Plan for Public Health Workforce Development.* Atlanta, Ga: Public Health Practice Program Office/Centers for Disease Control and Prevention; 2001.
23. *Public Health's Infrastructure.* Report to the Appropriations Committee of the United States Senate. Atlanta, Ga: Centers for Disease Control and Prevention; 2000.
24. *Public Health Threats and Emergencies Act of 2000.* Authored by Senators William Frist and Edward Kennedy. Washington, DC: US Government Printing Office; 2000.
25. *Advancing Community Public Health Systems in the 21st Century: Emerging Strategies and Innovations from the Turning Point Experience.* Washington, DC: National Association of County and City Health Officials; January 2001.

PART

3

Tools for Public Health Practice

CHAPTER

9

Leadership in Public Health Practice

Dennis D. Pointer, Ph.D.
Julianne P. Sanchez, M.A.

Think like a person of action,
Act like a person of thought.
Aristotle

This chapter will help you gain an understanding of *leadership,* one of the most important organizational and management concepts. The chapter first explores the concept of leadership. Then it summarizes what is known about the factors related to leadership effectiveness and posits an integrative model that blends different perspectives on leadership. The chapter concludes with suggestions for improving leadership knowledge and skills.

Before proceeding, think about these questions.

- What is leadership? What is the essence of the concept?
- Is leadership synonymous with management, or is leading just one of many things a manager does? In what ways are they different, or how are they the same?

- Think of several individuals you feel are exceptional leaders. What, if anything, do they have in common?
- Think of several individuals who are truly poor leaders. What, if anything, do they have in common?
- How does leadership affect the performance of a group or organization?
- Have you ever known people who were successful leaders in one situation and failures in others? Why is this the case?

WHAT IS LEADERSHIP?

Leadership is the means by which things get done in organizations. A manager can establish goals, strategize, relate to others, communicate, collect information, make decisions, plan, organize, monitor, and control; but without leadership, nothing happens.

Leadership is one of the most valued management abilities. Public health agencies and their divisions, departments, units, and programs can thrive under superior leadership. They can face considerable difficulty or even fail when it is poor. Managers who have the ability to lead are therefore in demand.

Defining Leadership

As important as leadership is, however, it is difficult to conceptualize vigorously. Here is a definition of leadership that includes only the essential attributes about which most scholars working in the field would have little disagreement:

> Leadership is the process through which an individual attempts to intentionally influence another individual or group in order to accomplish a goal.

- Leadership is a *process.* It is a verb, an action word, not a noun. Leadership manifests itself in doing; it is a performing art.
- Only individuals lead. The *locus* of leadership is a person. Inanimate objects do not lead, groups do not lead, organizations do not lead; only people do.
- The *focus* of leadership is other individuals and groups. A leader cannot exist without followers. Followers might be individuals, groups, members of an organization, or the population of a nation.
- Leadership entails *influencing* followers—their thoughts (the cognitive target), their feelings (the affective target), and/or their actions (the behavioral target). Influence is leadership's center of gravity and most critical element.
- The objective of leadership is *goal accomplishment.* Leadership is instrumental; it is done for a purpose.
- Leadership is *intentional,* not accidental. All of us *unknowingly* influence others hundreds of times each day, but these are not acts of leadership.

Leadership is exercised in a lot of different places and in a wide variety of situations, not just by managers in the workplace. Persuading a friend to have dinner at one's favorite restaurant, for example, requires leadership. All the key elements are there: a locus of leadership, a follower, and an act of intentional influence undertaken to accomplish a goal.

ORGANIZATIONAL LEADERSHIP

All organizations exist to accomplish tasks that are too large and/or complex to be undertaken by individuals or small groups working alone. Organizations do this by subdividing work, over and over again until tasks are small enough and simple enough to be performed by an individual. In the process, the organizations are partitioned into a series of departments, divisions, sections, or programs, all of which must be managed.

Leadership in a Public Health Agency

The provision of public health services in a community is a task so large and complex that an organization must undertake it. A public health agency assumes this task and proceeds to subdivide it: a department of environmental health does some parts; maternal and child health does other parts; laboratory services does other parts; and so on. The provision of services in environmental health, to cite just one example, in turn, is so large and complex a task that it, too, must be subdivided. It is parceled out among different divisions (for example, water and air).

Figure 9.1 presents a schematic organizational chart of a typical public health agency. The figure focuses on just one of four segments of a much larger organizational structure. In each component there is a managerial office, associated with which are sets of expectations called **roles.** Roles are constellations of things the manager is expected to do.[1] Roles are attached to the office, not the particular person occupying it. Office holders may come and go, but roles remain the same.

Leadership versus Management

There are many different managerial roles, and leadership is only one of them. Leadership and management are not synonyms. A manager is an individual who holds an office to which roles are attached, whereas leadership is one of the roles attached to the office of manager. This is a point that causes considerable confusion.

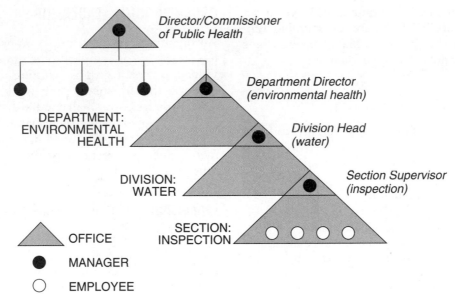

Director/Commissioner
of Public Health

Department Director
(environmental health)

DEPARTMENT:
ENVIRONMENTAL
HEALTH

Division Head
(water)

DIVISION:
WATER

Section Supervisor
(inspection)

SECTION:
INSPECTION

△ OFFICE

● MANAGER

○ EMPLOYEE

Figure 9.1. Public Health Organizations: Components and Managerial Offices

Performance of the leadership role is how managers get things done; without leadership or with poor leadership, the organization is impaired. Although leadership is not the only role of the manager, it is certainly the central one. All of the other roles of the manager, such as formulating goals, developing strategies, communicating, making decisions, and resolving conflicts, are converted into results through leadership.

Leadership Role of the Manager

Put Figure 9.1 under a magnifying glass and you have Figure 9.2. It focuses on one managerial office in the public health agency's chain of command. The manager is a subordinate of the director and a peer of other department directors having the same reporting relationship. Simultaneously, the manager holds a superordinate position within the department of environment health services.

There are several key points that can be illustrated by focusing on the leadership role of the manager in Figure 9.2.

Multidirectionality

Leadership is **multidirectional.** The department director leads subordinates, but also leads peers, superiors, and individuals and groups outside the agency.

Only when leadership is conceptualized as intentional influence is the proper distinction between managing and leadership made. The director of the department of environmental health services intentionally influences or leads but does not manage peers, for example, in chairing a committee to implement Assessment Protocol for Excellence in Public Health (APEX*PH*) standards. The director also may lead a superior by providing direction prior to an upcoming budget review meeting with the governor, county supervisors, or city council. Additionally, the director might engage in the leadership role when working with other units of government and community organizations. The department director leads in all directions simultaneously. Thus, leadership's arrows of influence point in several directions.

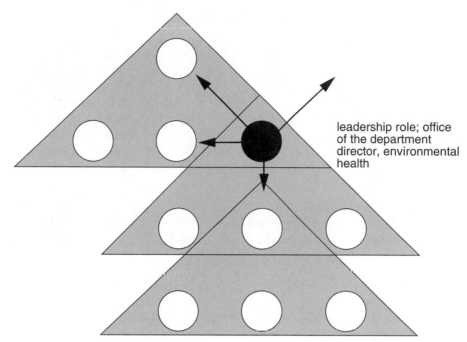

leadership role; office of the department director, environmental health

Figure 9.2. Directionality of the Manager's Leadership Role

The Focus Downward

Although leadership is multidirectional, the **downward focus** has received the greatest amount of attention and study. When thinking of leadership, what first comes to mind is the relationship between managers and their subordinates. The vast majority of leadership research has this focus. Most acts of leadership are pointed downward, primarily toward direct subordinates but secondarily towards subordinates in lower and lower layers of the agency.

Leading Other Managers

When engaging in leadership, irrespective of the direction of influence, the focus is generally other managers. For the most part, managers lead other managers.

Power

The extent to which leadership attempts are successful depends on the amount of *power* associated with a particular managerial office and the person holding it. Power can be defined as the potential to influence. The more power managers possess, the greater the potential they will be able to influence other individuals and groups. Leadership is the use of power to exert influence.

Power can come from many sources. An important source of power in organizations is the office held, where power is the result of formal authority. Some other sources of power include:

- information, knowledge, skills, abilities, and experience (expert power)
- connections with other individuals and groups who possess influence (referent power)
- control of incentives (reward/coercive power)
- one's own persona (charismatic power)

LEADERSHIP EFFECTIVENESS

All managers are not equally effective or successful as leaders. It is important to understand why in order to select good leaders and improve leadership skills.

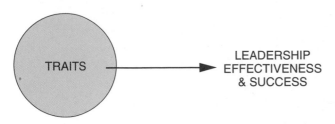

Figure 9.3. The Nature Argument

What Influences Leadership Effectiveness?

There has been a raging debate for the last 50 years regarding what makes a successful leader, and there are three very different points of view: nature, nurture, and situational.

Nature

According to this view, which is illustrated by Figure 9.3, leadership effectiveness is primarily a result of traits and dispositions that individuals are endowed with at birth or develop very early in life. By the time a person assumes a management position, these characteristics are set and nearly impossible to change in any significant way. Some people have traits that predispose them to be successful leaders, whereas others do not.

Nurture

According to this view, shown in Figure 9.4, leadership effectiveness is primarily due to skills and behaviors that can be learned. Personal traits and dispositions provide the foundation upon which abilities are acquired and behaviors are developed, but they are only the foundation. Individuals who are exceptional leaders make themselves, they are not born.

Situational Factor

Figure 9.5 illustrates the argument that leadership effectiveness is primarily due to the characteristics of the situation in which managers find themselves. Inborn traits, abilities, and behaviors are important, but they are very situation specific. In one situation, certain traits, abilities, and behaviors may predispose a manager to be an effective leader; in a different situation, the result could be ineffectiveness and failure.

Discussion

To underscore the practical importance of these different perspectives, consider the following questions:

- If you agree with the nature argument, which personal traits and dispositions do you think are most associated with leadership effectiveness and success?
- If you agree with the nurture argument, which abilities and behaviors affect leadership effectiveness and success? What are the best ways to acquire these abilities and develop these behaviors?
- If you agree with the situational argument, which factors are most important?
- Do you think that nature, nurture, and situational factors work together to influence leadership effectiveness? If so, why?

The importance of this issue is further underscored by two questions that scholars have been trying to help practicing managers answer for almost half a century:

- If you wanted to select an effective and potentially successful leader, what traits, abilities, and behaviors would you look for?

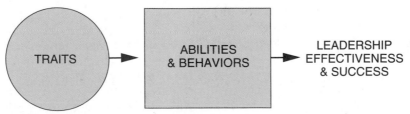

Figure 9.4. The Nurture Argument

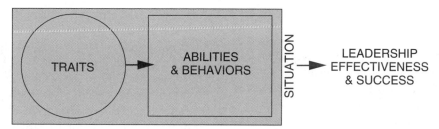

Figure 9.5. The Situational Argument

- If you wanted to improve your own leadership effectiveness, what traits, abilities, and behaviors would you focus on developing or improving?

Review of the Research

What follows is not a thorough review of the literature; the objective is to provide an introduction only. To explore the area further, consult the key references provided. It is interesting to note that none of the basic work in this area has been conducted in public health organizations.

The vast majority of theorizing and research on leadership effectiveness can be classified into three different perspectives: **trait, behavioral,** and **contingency.**[2] In the next sections, these perspectives are described, some of their major studies reviewed, and key findings highlighted. Additionally, several emerging leadership theories and concepts are introduced.

The Trait Perspective

Because it is individuals who lead, it is natural and reasonable to look for those characteristics of individuals that might separate effective leaders from ineffective ones. Indeed, this is where early research began.

In the late 1930s, psychologists became interested in leadership and began investigating relationships between individual characteristics and leadership effectiveness in organizations. Even though as early as the 1940s it was suggested that these relationships were weak and not generalizable across different situations,[3] the research continued. Just about every attribute imaginable has been studied.[4]

The most comprehensive review of this literature was conducted by Roger Stodgill in his classic work *Handbook of Leadership.*[5] Stodgill examined 287 studies undertaken from 1904 through 1970. Stodgill's review, and the earlier review of Sartle[6] identified a small number of traits that seemed to be present in leaders (as compared to followers) and in good leaders (as compared to poor ones). These included intelligence, dominance, self-confidence, high energy level, and task-relevant knowledge. However, the findings were inconsistent and the relationships were very weak, suggesting that there are no individual traits that consistently predict leadership effectiveness or always differentiate those who lead from those who follow.[7]

It is difficult to argue individual traits have no effect whatsoever on leadership effectiveness. Such a conclusion runs counter to experience, logic, and common sense. Researchers began to appreciate that traits had an impact, but not in the way originally imagined. Instead, they concluded:

- Traits are best thought of as predispositions. A particular trait or set of traits to predispose (though not cause) an individual to engage in certain behaviors that may or may not result in leadership effectiveness.
- Multiple traits can be associated with a given behavior, and more than one behavior can be linked to an individual trait.
- It is behavior, and not traits per se, that is most closely related to leadership effectiveness.

These three observations help explain why a set of universal leadership traits has yet to be discovered. Nonetheless, research in this area continues.[8]

The Behavioral Perspective

Interest in leadership behaviors emerged as it became apparent that individual traits were inadequate to explain variations in leadership effectiveness. Researchers reasoned that if trait variation could not explain such differences, perhaps the behaviors that flowed from them could. Most of this research has focused on:

- Identifying dimensions that can be used to describe and categorize different leadership behaviors
- Developing models of leadership style, where a style is defined by a combination of behaviors
- Examining how specific leadership styles are related to effectiveness
- Developing more rigorous ways to conceptualize and measure leadership effectiveness

Early Work

The first study employing a behavioral perspective was conducted by Kurt Lewin and his associates at the University of Iowa in the 1930s.[9] These researchers compared three styles of leadership—autocratic, democratic, and laissez-faire—in groups of preteen boys. Leaders of the groups were confederates of the researchers and were instructed on how to perform the various styles.

Democratic leaders coordinated activities of the group and facilitated majority rule and decision making on important matters. Autocratic leaders directed the activities of the group and made important decisions without input from members. Laissez-faire leaders, who accidentally emerged during the course of the study, provided neither facilitation nor direction. This work was significant because it focused on behavior rather than traits, identified and described different leadership styles, and found that variations in style had an impact on followers.

Ohio Studies

Several major studies of leadership were undertaken immediately after World War II. One of the most widely cited was conducted by a group of investigators at Ohio State University.[10] These researchers addressed the question of how behavior of a leader impacts on work, group performance, and satisfaction. Instruments were designed to measure leadership behavior as perceived by managers themselves, as well as by their peers, superiors, and subordinates.

Two dimensions of leadership behavior were identified: *initiating structure*, or the degree to which a manager defined and organized the work that was to be done and the extent to which attention was focused on accomplishing objectives established by the manager; and *consideration*, or the extent to which the manager exhibited concern for the welfare of the group and its members, stressed the importance of job satisfaction, expressed appreciation, and sought input from subordinates on major decisions.

Initiating structure and consideration were not conceptualized as opposite ends of the same continuum, but rather as separate and independent dimensions. A manager's behavior could range from high to low on both dimensions. As depicted in Figure 9.6, the two dimensions combine to form four distinct leadership styles.

Researchers hypothesized that group performance would be maximized when a manager had a leadership style that was high in both consideration and initiating structure. However, numerous follow-up studies have found little consistency between these leadership styles and group satisfaction or performance.[11,12] As with the trait research, it appeared that other factors were confounding results.

Michigan Studies

In related work, Rensis Likert and his colleagues at the University of Michigan specified two leadership behaviors: job centered and employee centered.[13] They were defined similarly to consideration and initiating structure in the Ohio studies. Investigations conducted in a wide variety of industries found that effective supervisors were employee centered. They focused on needs of the group and also established high-performance goals that were determined jointly with their followers.[14,15]

The Managerial Grid

While the Ohio and Michigan studies provided the theoretical underpinnings for the behavioral per-

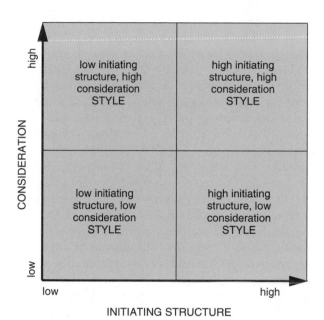

Figure 9.6. Ohio Leadership Study: Behaviors and Styles

2. *high production and high people orientation* leadership behavior is goal/task centered but seeks a high degree of subordinate involvement
3. *low production and high people orientation* leadership behavior focuses on creating fulfilling relationships even if goal/task accomplishment and productivity suffer
4. *low production and low people orientation* leadership behavior is focused on neither goal/task accomplishment nor fulfilling the needs of subordinates, and minimal energy is expended on execution of the leadership role
5. *moderate production and moderate people orientation* leadership behavior focuses on balancing goal/task accomplishment with subordinate need fulfillment

Blake and Mouton contended that the high production- and high people-oriented style was most effective and resulted in the best outcomes in terms of group productivity and satisfaction, irrespective of the situation faced. Little research supports their assertion, but there is some evidence that this style is preferred by managers and perceived by them to be most effective.[17]

Bipolar Model

Robert Tannebaum and Warren Schmidt portrayed leadership behavior as a continuum that ranged from manager centered to follower centered.[18] In the manager-centered style, considerable authority is exercised and followers have little opportunity to participate in making decisions that affect them. Leadership behavior is autocratic and directive. In the follower-centered style, by contrast, the manager exercises a minimum of authority, and followers have considerable freedom to set their own goals and determine how tasks should be executed. Leadership behavior is democratic and participatory.

Contrary to previous models, Tannebaum and Schmidt conceptualized leadership behavior as bipolar. One was either manager centered, follower centered, or somewhere in between. The authors explicitly stated that there was no one style that would be equally effective in all situations. Additionally, they noted that the effectiveness of a particular style

spective, several other works are frequently referred to in most reviews of this literature. Blake and Mouton, for example, formulated the managerial grid, which they popularized in their book of the same name.[16] Their model, originally developed as a consulting tool, was extensively employed in leadership development programs during the 1960s and 1970s. The grid has two dimensions: *production orientation* and *people orientation*.

In production orientation, leadership behaviors are directive and focused on accomplishing assigned objectives or tasks. In a people orientation, by contrast, leadership behaviors are focused on enhancing the quality of manager-follower and follower-follower interactions. A manager's behavior can range from low to high in both dimensions, resulting in five different leadership styles:

1. *high production and low people orientation* leadership behavior focuses exclusively on goal/task accomplishment and maximizing productivity through explicit direction and tight control

depended upon three factors: characteristics of the manager (such as their traits/dispositions, skills, and values); characteristics of followers (such as their skills/knowledge/experience, readiness to assume responsibility, understanding of goals and tasks); and characteristics of the situation (such as time availability, nature of the problem). This model underscored the point that leadership effectiveness depended on contingencies, and they suggested some important ones. However, the model did not specifically indicate how a manager should select the most effective style in specific circumstances.

The Contingency Perspective

Beginning in the early 1960s, it became increasingly apparent that variations in leadership effectiveness and success could not be adequately explained by either traits or behaviors. Attention turned to incorporating situational characteristics, or contingencies, into leadership models. Recall that this notion was first introduced in the 1940s. A number of leadership contingency models have been developed, but only three are discussed here: leadership match, path-goal, and leadership effectiveness and adaptability (LEAD). The first two models have been the subject of considerable empirical research, and the last has been extensively employed as a teaching and leadership development tool. The section concludes with a discussion of attribution theory, which deals with the manager as a contingency.

Leadership Match Model

The first comprehensive contingency model of leadership was developed by Fred Fiedler.[19–21] His model is complex, and only a highly simplified description of it is provided here. The underlying notion is that managers are unable to alter their style to any appreciable degree. Leadership effectiveness thus depends not on fitting one's style to the situation, but rather on selecting a situation that is conducive to one's style.[22]

Based on previous behavioral studies, two leadership styles were specified: task oriented and employee oriented. Fiedler developed a unique and controversial way to measure them. After completing a 20-item questionnaire, subjects were assigned a least-preferred coworker (LPC) score. The LPC score reflected the degree of regard a respondent held for the coworker whom he or she preferred least. Managers with low LPC scores (disregard for the least-preferred worker) were classified as having a task-oriented leadership style. Managers with a high LPC score (favorable evaluations of the coworker who was least preferred) were classified as possessing an employee-oriented style.

Fiedler also identified three situational factors: manager-follower relationship, which could be good or poor; task structure, which could be either high or low; and manager position power, which could range from strong to weak. The combined effect of these three factors is to produce situations that are favorable, moderately favorable, or unfavorable to the manager.

Based upon studies conducted with hundreds of groups in a variety of organizations, it was determined that managers with a task-oriented leadership style were most effective in situations that were either favorable or unfavorable. Managers with an employee-oriented leadership style, on the other hand, did better in situations that were moderately favorable. It is important to note that there have been several criticisms of this work, including questions regarding the validity of the LPC questionnaire and concerns that situational factors and leadership style may not be independent of one another.[23,24]

Path-Goal Model

The path-goal leadership model is based on the expectancy theory of motivation,[25,26] which addresses why someone is motivated to do one thing rather than another. Expectancy theory focuses on effort, performance, rewards, and the relationships between them, which are referred to as expectancies, instrumentalities, and valences.

An **expectancy** is the relationship between effort and performance. Sometimes a given amount of effort results in a high level of performance, at other times it does not. **Instrumentality** is the degree to which a person perceives that performance will lead to rewards. Finally, a **valence** is the strength of a person's preference for different types of rewards. According to expectancy theory, a person will be highly moti-

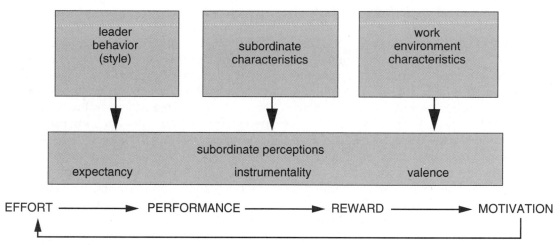

Figure 9.7. The Path-Goal Model

vated when effort results in performance (high expectancy) and when performance leads to rewards (high instrumentality) that are valued (high valence).

Whereas expectancy theory describes these relationships, the path-goal model of leadership is interested in the factors affecting them. This model was formulated initially by Martin Evans[27,28] in the early 1970s and then refined by Robert House and Terrance Mitchell.[29,30] It has undergone constant revision over the years.

According to the path-goal model, the manager exercises influence to increase the motivation of a follower attempting to accomplish a specific goal, in a particular context, during a finite period of time. As depicted in Figure 9.7, a follower's level of motivation is a result of his or her perceptions of expectancies, instrumentalities, and valences. Such perceptions are affected by three sets of contingencies: leadership behavior/style, features of the work environment, and characteristics of the follower.

In most leadership situations, follower characteristics and features of the work environment are not under the direct control of the manager; in the short run they are fixed. Follower characteristics include such things as:

- Needs and motives (for example, the degree to which they value achievement, power, and affiliation)

- Ability to perform the task (their knowledge, skills, and experience)
- The extent to which they feel they have control over critical contingencies that affect their performance in a given situation

Features of the work environment include, among others, the extent to which the task is structured or unstructured, the amount of time available to complete the task, the nature and degree of interdependence among work group members, and a host of organizational characteristics.

The contingency most under a manager's control is his or her own leadership style. The dimensions that define leadership style are presently conceptualized as instrumental behavior (defining objectives and specifying the task to be performed), participatory behavior (seeking follower input on decisions that affect them), and achievement-oriented behavior (establishing goals and setting expectations that challenge followers).

Some of the implications of the path-goal theory of leadership include the following:[31]

- One of the most important aspects of leadership behavior is stimulating the release of follower effort and motivation.

- Often the path between effort, performance, and rewards is unclear. The manager must do everything possible to establish clear connections.
- In leading, the manager should appreciate that individuals' valences are varied, that is, people value various rewards differently. The manager should understand what a follower values and construct rewards accordingly.
- Leadership behavior should help followers define expectancies. Issues that need to be addressed include how a follower directs his or her effort so that it results in adequate, if not exemplary, performance and what additional knowledge, skills, and experiences a follower needs to perform assigned tasks.
- Leadership behavior should focus on clarifying instrumentalities. It is important followers understand the specific type and amount of reward that will flow from a given level of performance.
- The manager should be mindful of how work environment characteristics affect follower expectancies, instrumentalities, and valences and the implications of these effects for the selection of a leadership style. For example, when a task is very unstructured, a follower may not know how to perform the job successfully (instrumentality is low). In such instances, a higher level of instrumental leadership behavior may be required.

The LEAD Model

The leadership effectiveness and adaptability (LEAD) model was developed by Paul Hershey and Kenneth Blanchard while they were affiliated with the Center for Leadership Studies at Ohio University.[32] According to this model, differing degrees of task- and relationship-oriented behavior (defined in a way similar to the Ohio and Michigan studies) produce four different leadership styles:

1. *high task, low relationship*
2. *high task, high relationship*
3. *low task, high relationship*
4. *low task, low relationship*

Hershey and Blanchard argued that the single most important contingency in selecting an effective leadership style is the follower's task-relevant maturity. Maturity is a function of three traits: motivation, or energy to expend assigned task; responsibility and ability to plan, organize, and complete the task; and competence, or the necessary knowledge, skills, and/or experience, to perform the task proficiently.

A mature follower is highly motivated, is willing and able to assume responsibility, and possesses the necessary competencies. An immature follower lacks motivation, is not willing or is unable to assume responsibility for the task, and does not have the necessary competencies. It is important to note that maturity is situational and task specific; a follower may be very mature performing one task and quite immature performing another.

Hershey and Blanchard provide suggestions regarding which styles are most effective with followers having varying degrees of task-relevant maturity. If the maturity of the follower is very low, the model suggests using a style that is high task- and low relationship-oriented. In this case, the follower is unmotivated, is not willing or able to assume responsibility, and does not possess the competencies necessary to perform the task. Therefore, to get the task done, leadership must be very directive. A low degree of relationship-oriented behavior is recommended so as not to reinforce the follower's state of immaturity.

If the maturity of the follower is exceedingly high, the model suggests using a low task- and relationship-oriented leadership style. Here the follower is extremely motivated, is very responsible, and possesses all the competencies necessary to perform the task. The follower does not need (and, in fact, would likely not appreciate) task directiveness; he or she knows what to do and how to do it. High relationship-oriented behavior is not needed because the follower gets reinforcement from colleagues and performance of the task itself. In this case, task and relationship responsibilities are totally delegated to the follower.

This is a highly abbreviated and simplified description of a model that has many more features than can be discussed here. For example, the authors provide a dynamic interpretation that focuses on sequences of leadership behaviors to enhance follower maturity. They have designed a package of questionnaires that provide feedback regarding the extent to which leaders perceive themselves employing the four different leadership styles; how others (subordinates, peers, superiors) perceive their leadership styles; and how selection of different leadership behaviors aligns with the most appropriate style suggested by the model.

Attribution Theory

One important leadership contingency factor is a manager's personal frame of reference. Attribution (sometimes referred to as perceptual or cognitive) theory[33,34] holds that a manager's selection of a leadership style depends on the way follower behavior is perceived and interpreted.

Managers notice some things and are totally unaware of others. Furthermore, what is noticed is always filtered through the manager's distinctive cognitive frame and reshaped by it. Based on such perceptions, a manager attributes effects to the follower's behavior. There are two general types of attributions: internal (such as lack of follower effort and/or ability) and external (such as bad luck, inadequate task design by others, and poor supervision).

According to attribution theory, a manager's choice of leadership behavior is significantly influenced by such attributions. For example, a manager might employ one leadership style if a follower's poor performance is attributed to task overload but a different one if the cause is laziness.

Attribution theorists argue that in many cases, a manager's choice of leadership style may be due more to the perceptual and cognitive frame than the "reality" of the situation itself. Indeed, reality is only what one perceives it to be. To reiterate, the basic notion of attribution theory is a simple one: an important determinant of leadership style is the manager's perceptions and attributions.[35] The resulting admonition is important: managers need to be aware of these inherent biases and develop ways to minimize them.[36]

Implications of the Contingency Perspective

There are several implications that transcend the specific models of leadership described in this section but arise from a general contingency perspective. First, the contingency perspective underscores the fact that leadership effectiveness is situational. Leadership behaviors and styles focus on influencing specific followers (whether individuals or groups), in a specific context, performing a particular task in order to accomplish an objective at a particular point in time. All of these contingencies vary from one situation to another. Thus, the most effective leadership style in one situation is unlikely to be optimally effective in another. Three sets of contingencies seem to be most closely related to leadership effectiveness: (1) characteristics of the manager; (2) characteristics of the followers; and (3) characteristics of the immediate context in which the manager and followers interact.

Much of leadership behavior has to do with stimulating and then focusing follower motivation. Leadership effectiveness, in turn, depends on a manager having a diverse repertoire of styles and being able to move flexibly among them. A manager must also possess the ability to diagnose the most critical contingencies of a given situation and select an effective leadership style for that situation. The way a specific leadership situation is diagnosed depends on the manager's perceptions and attribution of causes to follower behavior. Finally, to be an effective leader, a manager must have ability to execute the chosen style effectively.

Taken to the extreme, contingency-driven leadership may appear erratic and arbitrary because the leader behaves differently toward the same followers in different situations or differently toward followers in the same situation. This can be confusing and frustrating for followers unless the manager is very explicit about the reasons for behaving in a particular way.

A final implication from the contingency perspective relates to the theory itself. Given the large number of contingency factors and the complex ways in which they are interrelated, it is highly unlikely that a general theory of leadership effectiveness will be formulated anytime soon.

Emerging Theories and Concepts

The trait, behavioral, and contingency perspectives form the basis for most leadership theory, research, and practice. However, in the past decade, some new perspectives have been developed. In this section the transactional/transformational and charismatic theories of leadership are described. A collection of concepts that broaden thinking regarding leadership effectiveness are also introduced.

Transactional and Transformational Leadership

James McGregor Burns, in his classic work *Leadership*, identified two types of politicians—*transactional* and *transformational*.[37] There is a growing body of literature that draws a distinction between these two leadership orientations in organizations.[38] Whereas transactional leadership attempts to preserve the status quo, transformational leadership seeks to upset and replace it.

Models of leader behavior examined up to this point view managers as involved in exchange relationships with followers. The defining characteristic of these relationships is transactional: "I'll provide what you want if you'll give me what I want." Transactional leadership entails recognizing what followers want and giving it to them if their performance warrants it. As Kuhnert and Lewis note, "In these exchanges transactional leaders clarify the roles followers must play and the tasks they must complete in order to reach their personal goals while fulfilling the mission of the organization."[39]

This sounds very much like the path-goal model of leadership, in which the manager attempts to influence follower expectancies, instrumentalities, and valences. The objective of leadership is to get followers to comply with the rules of the game as it is currently being played. The result of such transactions, proponents of the theory contend, is ordinary levels of performance.[40] Performance improvements, if they occur at all, are marginal and achieved incrementally over a long period of time.

Transformational leaders, on the other hand, are concerned with changes rather than exchanges. Seeking to alter both the objective and the nature of manager-follower interactions, they motivate followers to take on difficult goals they normally would not pursue and to adopt the value that work is far more than the performance of specific duties for specific rewards. The relationship between transformational managers and their followers is not contractual but empowering. Advocates of the transformational orientation suggest that it produces extraordinary levels of performance that flow from enrollment in a cause rather than compliance with a set of rules.[41]

Transactional and transformational modes of leadership are distinguished by the type of goals pursued, the nature of manager-follower relations, and the values to which managers and followers adhere. Table 9.1 compares the two modes of leadership with regard to these and other characteristics.

Charismatic Leadership

Charisma is derived from a Greek word meaning "divinely inspired gift" or "state of grace." It is a characteristic that has been attributed to those with truly exceptional leadership abilities. The concept was first introduced into the organizational literature by Max Weber who defined charismatic authority as being based on "devotion to the specific and exceptional sanctity, heroism, or exemplary character of an individual person."[42] The concept has received renewed interest by scholars who have focused on a small sub-

Table 9.1. Transactional and Transformational Leadership

Dimension	Transactional	Transformational
Goal	maintain status quo	upset status quo
Activity	play within the rules	change the rules
Locus of reward	self (maximize personal benefits)	system (optimize systemic benefits)
Nature of incentives	tit for tat	the greater good
Manager-follower interaction	mutual dependence	interdependence
Needs fulfilled	lower level (physical, economic, and safety)	higher level (social- and self-actualization)
Performance	ordinary	extraordinary

set of individuals able to exercise extraordinary levels of influence.[41, 43] Charismatic leadership is

> a distinct social relationship between the leader and follower, in which the leader presents a revolutionary idea, a transcendent image . . . the follower accepts this course of action not because of its rational likelihood of success, but because of an effective belief in the extraordinary qualities of the leader.[44(p3:5)]

It has been increasingly recognized that charisma is not a characteristic of the manager per se, but rather a result of the interaction of many factors: manager and follower traits; manager and follower behaviors; the relationship between the manager and followers; situational dynamics; and the nature of the goal being sought. Table 9.2 shows a list of characteristics that have been identified in the literature.

It is clear that the present notion of charisma weaves together concepts from the trait, behavioral and situational perspectives. Because charisma is, by definition, rare as well as complex, it is exceedingly difficult to study. As a result there has been little empirical research in this area.[45]

Toward a Broader Conceptualization of Leadership Effectiveness

There has been a trend over the last decade to reconceptualize what constitutes leadership effectiveness and the factors that account for it.[46] The contention, although not always explicitly stated, is that past theorizing and research, in its quest for methodological rigor and empirically testable relationships, has been far too narrow. Writers such as Warren Bennis,[47] James Kouzes and Barry Posner,[48] Gareth Morgan,[49] Tom Peters,[50] Peter Senge,[51] and Peter Vail[52] suggest that high-performance leadership depends on such things as systems thinking, visioning, facilitation of learning, and follower empowerment.

Systems Thinking

Managers lead in systems, and all of them have a number of attributes in common, even though their surface features may vary. Effective leaders possess a highly refined understanding of systems—their form,

Table 9.2. Characteristics of a Charismatic Leader

Nature of the goal manager traits	• revolutionary/transformational • self-confidence • dominance • need for influence/power • strong conviction in beliefs • creativity • high energy level • enthusiasm
Leadership behaviors	• ability to conceptualize and convey transcendent vision/ideology • ability to inspire and build confidence • use of unconventional means • rhetorical fluency
Follower traits	• dependence • need to transcend self and situation
Follower behaviors	• dedication • commitment
Manager-follower interaction	• projection of idealized traits/behaviors on the leader by followers • identification (psychological fusion) of followers with leader • empowerment of followers by leader
Nature of the context	• crisis • uncertainty • transformation • deprivation

Sources: Dow TE. The theory of charisma. *Social Q.* 1969;10: 306–318. Shils EA. Charisma, order and status. *Am Sociol Rev.* 1965; 30:199–213. Wilner AR. *The Spellbinders: Charismatic and Political Leadership.* New Haven, CT: Yale University Press; 1984.

operating dynamics, and the way they achieve stability and undergo change.

It is difficult to think systemically. As Peter Senge notes, "since we are part of the lacework ourselves, it's doubly hard to see the whole pattern. . . . Instead we tend to focus on snapshots of isolated parts of the system and wonder why our deepest problems never get solved."[51(p7)] Systems thinking requires mastering a conceptual framework and associated set of analytical tools and techniques that enhance understanding of patterns and how they can be changed.

Visioning

In order to lead, one must be going somewhere and accomplishing something that is worthy of follower effort. A vision is the target that beckons so that the most effective manager can lead by pulling, not pushing. Effective managers have the ability to formulate rich images of future states that are both possible to achieve and highly desirable. Ideas for the images, ranging from general dreams to specific goals, may be the product of the manager, the followers, or both.

When communicated powerfully (often through symbols and metaphors) and shared by all members of a system, a vision releases and focuses energy. It fosters genuine commitment and enrollment and not simply compliance.

Facilitating Learning

Organizations and the environments in which they operate are not static but constantly undergo change. Increasingly such change is revolutionary rather than evolutionary. Change of the revolutionary variety has been characteristic of health services, both public and private, during the last decade.

In periods of revolutionary change, ways of thinking and doing that have been very successful in the past rapidly lose much of their value. In such instances, organizations face two challenges if they are to thrive. First, they must unlearn what is no longer relevant. Second, they must develop new mental maps, acquire new knowledge, and develop new sets of skills. Effective leaders facilitate this follower unlearning and relearning.

Empowering Followers

Rosabeth Kanter observes, "Powerlessness corrupts. Absolute powerlessness corrupts absolutely."[53(p285)] The essence of leadership is getting things done, yet there is pitifully little that managers can do by themselves.

Followership is the reciprocal of leadership. Effective and successful leadership is dependent upon effective, successful, and empowered followers. For example, team-oriented approaches to continuously improve quality, such as total quality management (TQM) and continuous quality improvement (CQI), have attracted increasing attention; both require high levels of follower empowerment to be successful.

The effective leader views followers as the primary source of organizational creativity, energy, and value added. The effective leader creates a climate that empowers followers, so they are willing and able to make their maximum potential contribution.

An Integrative Framework

Over half a century of research has identified a number of factors that seem to be related to leadership effectiveness. Figure 9.8 shows an integrative framework that summarizes and interprets these findings. Given the concepts that have been covered in this chapter, the model should be relatively self-explanatory. Accordingly, only selected aspects of it are highlighted here.

Leadership Style

A manager's leadership style is the pattern of behavior in which he or she engages to intentionally influence followers to accomplish a goal in a particular situation. Leadership style can be specified by three sets of behavioral dimensions: focus, objective, and approach.

Focus

Focus is the direction of a manager's influence. External leadership is directed outward, outside the boundary of the organizational component for which the manager is responsible (that is, toward superiors, peers, and/or individuals and groups outside the organization). Internal leadership is directed downward, toward subordinates within the manager's organizational component.

Objective

Objective is what a manager hopes to accomplish in exercising influence. A transformational leader

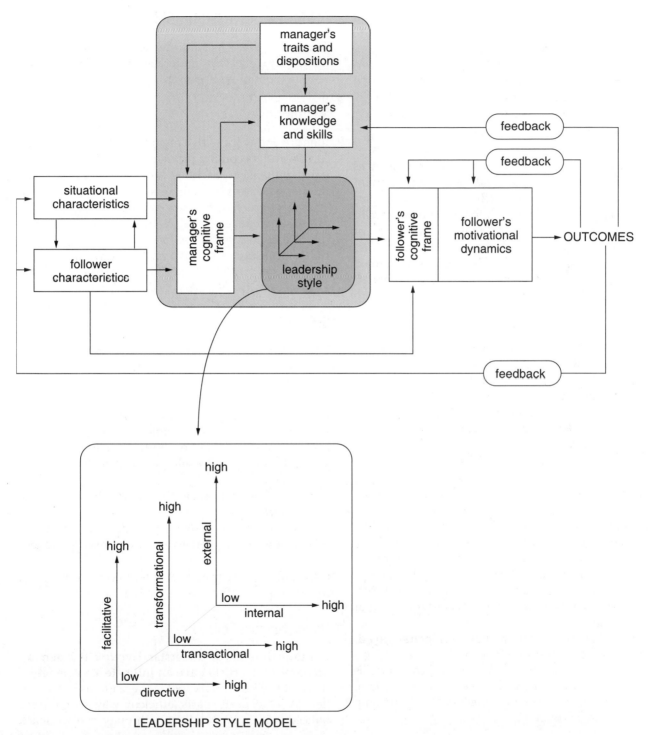

LEADERSHIP STYLE MODEL

Figure 9.8. Leadership: An Integrative Framework

seeks to alter the nature of both the goals sought and manager-follower interactions; the objective is to change the status quo. A transactional leader, by contrast, attempts to optimize the outcome of manager-follower exchange relationships by achieving stated goals in the most efficient manner within the "rules" as presently defined.

Approach

Approach is the way in which a manager influences followers. In exercising *directive* leadership, a manager defines the task and specifies how it is to be performed. The focus is on goal accomplishment, and little attention is paid to manager-follower or follower-follower relationships. In exercising *facilitative* leadership, a manager involves followers in making decisions that affect them, and considerable attention is paid to fulfilling their needs.

Style

A manager's behavior can vary between high and low on each of these three sets of dimensions, the specific combination of which defines one's leadership style in a given situation. This is influenced by two sets of factors: the manager's traits and dispositions, knowledge and skills; and the characteristics of the followers and the situation, which are filtered through the manager's distinctive cognitive frame.

The manager's leadership style, in turn, affects the motivational dynamics (expectations, instrumentalities, and valences) of followers, who are mediated by their own cognitive frame. Leadership style affects follower efficiency, effectiveness, creativity, satisfaction, turnover, and absenteeism. The feedback loops depicted in Figure 9.8 can be either positive (reinforcing a given characteristic) or negative (dampening or extinguishing it).

All models leave out more than they include, in addition to overly simplifying complex relationships and dynamics. This one is no exception. The model is admittedly crude and incomplete. Its purpose is to stimulate thinking about how pieces of the leadership jigsaw puzzle fit together.

DEVELOPING LEADERSHIP SKILLS

There are several ways to develop leadership skills: mentoring, reflecting, understanding self and followers, and continued learning.

Mentoring

Identify and work with a mentor. Leadership is a performing art; becoming proficient at it requires continual and intensive coaching from an experienced practitioner who is invested in the student's development. There is a growing body of evidence to suggest that establishing an effective mentoring relationship is one of the most important factors separating successful from unsuccessful leaders.[54] To learn more about how to work with a mentor, read *Mentoring at Work: Developmental Relationships in Organizational Life.*[55]

Reflecting

Become a reflective leadership practitioner. Reflection is the key to learning from experience. Just as a winning sports team reviews its game films, so should the manager get in the habit of replaying and analyzing the leadership situations in which he or she has been involved. Schedule some time for reflection before each day ends. Reflect on both your successes and your failures. Ask yourself questions such as:

- Did you get the result anticipated? If so, why? If no, why not?
- What could or should you have done differently?
- What lesson have you learned from this experience?

Such reflection requires considerable discipline, but the effort pays off in more effective leadership.

Understanding Self

Continually seek to understand yourself better. All accomplished artists have an intimate knowledge of their tools. The primary tool of the leader is himself or herself. One particularly efficient way to gain enhanced self-understanding is through the feedback provided by self-administered leadership question-naires, instruments, and inventories. Many are available, and much can be gained by getting feedback on leadership behaviors and style.

Understanding Followers

It is virtually impossible to lead if you don't have an in-depth understanding of your followers. Invest the time and energy in getting to know each follower upon whom your effectiveness and success depends. Find out their aspirations, their wants and needs. Ask what they view as their most important competencies (that is, knowledge, skills, and experiences) and how the organization could make better use of them. Find out what motivates them most.

Constantly seek feedback from followers. Perceptions of ourselves are always somewhat at odds with how others perceive us. To be an effective and successful leader you must understand the impact you are having on others. The best way to gain such understanding is to ask questions. How am I coming across? What am I doing that helps you to be as effective, creative, or satisfied as you can be?

Continued Learning

Keep reading and studying. Experience is the single best teacher of leadership, but there are not enough hours in the day to acquire all the needed experience. Some has to be gained vicariously through reading.

Reading provides the essential models, concepts, and ideas that promote much more effective and efficient learning. There are thousands of books on leadership, and hundreds of new ones are published every year.

Each puts forth its own recipe for success. No one has the time, energy, patience, or money to consume even a small proportion of what is being written. The following books are recommended without reservation:

- Bennis W, Nanus B. *Leaders.* New York, NY: Harper & Row; 1985.
- Covey SR. *Principle Centered Leadership.* New York, NY: Simon & Schuster; 1990.
- DePree M. *Leadership Is an Art.* New York, NY: Doubleday; 1989.
- Gardner J. *On Leadership.* New York, NY: The Free Press; 1990.
- Kelley R. *The Power of Followership: How to Create Leaders People Want to Follow, and Followers Who Lead Themselves.* New York, NY: Doubleday/Currency; 1991.
- Kouzes JM, Posner BZ. *The Leadership Challenge: How to Get Extraordinary Things Done in Organizations.* San Francisco, Calif: Jossey-Bass; 1990.
- Senge P. *The Fifth Discipline: The Art and Practice of the Learning Organization.* New York, NY: Doubleday/Currency; 1990.
- Vail PB. *Managing as a Performing Art: New Ideas for a World of Chaotic Change.* San Francisco, Calif: Jossey-Bass; 1989.

CONCLUSION

A vital tool for the success of a public health agency is leadership. Without leadership the agency will not accomplish its mission or achieve its potential. This review illustrates some features of leadership and provides some suggestions for improving the leadership (or followership) you will provide. The key to success continues to be your commitment to being the best possible leader you can.

References

1. Katz D, Kahn RL. The taking of organizational roles. In: *The Social Psychology of Organizations.* New York, NY: John Wiley & Sons; 1966.
2. Jago AG. Leadership: perspectives in theory and research. *Manage Sci.* 1982;28:315-336.
3. Jennings WO. A review of leadership studies with a particular reference to military problems. *Psychol Bull.* 1947;44:540-579.
4. Stodgill RM. Personal factors associated with leadership: a survey of the literature. *J Appl Psychol.* 1948;32:35-71.

5. Stodgill RM. *Handbook of Leadership.* New York, NY: The Free Press; 1974.
6. Sartle CL. *Executive Performance and Leadership.* Englewood Cliffs, NJ: Prentice-Hall; 1956.
7. Lord AG, et al. A meta analysis of the relation between personality traits and leadership: an application of validity generalization procedures. *J Appl Psychol.* 1986;7:402-410.
8. Coska LS. A relationship between leader intelligence and leader rated effectiveness. *J Appl Psychol.* 1984;14:22-34.
9. Lewin K, et al. Patterns of aggressive behavior in experimentally created social climates. *J Soc Psychol.* 1939;10:271-276.
10. Stodgill R, Coon A, eds. *Leader Behavior: Its Description and Measurement.* Columbus: Bureau of Business Research, the Ohio State University; 1957.
11. Fleishman EA. Twenty years of consideration and structure. In: Fleishman EA, Hunt JG, eds. *Current Developments in the Study of Leadership.* Carbondale: Southern Illinois University; 1973:1-37.
12. Halpin AW. The leadership behavior and combat performance of airplane commanders. *J Abnorm Soc Psychol.* 1954;39:82-84.
13. Likert R. *New Patterns of Management.* New York, NY: McGraw-Hill; 1961.
14. Katz D, et al. *Productivity, Supervision and Morale in an Office Situation.* Ann Arbor: Institute for Social Research, University of Michigan; 1950.
15. Katz D, et al. *Productivity, Supervision and Morale among Railroad Workers.* Ann Arbor: Institute for Social Research, University of Michigan; 1951.
16. Blake J, Mouton R. *The New Managerial Grid.* Houston, Tex: Gulf Publishing; 1978.
17. Blake RR, Mouton JS. Theory and research for developing a science of leadership. *J Appl Behav Sci.* 1982;18:275-291.
18. Tannebaum R, Schmidt W. How to choose a leadership pattern. *Harvard Bus Rev.* 1973;51(3):162-180.
19. Fiedler FE. *A Theory of Leadership Effectiveness.* New York, NY: McGraw-Hill; 1967.
20. Fiedler FE, Chemers MM. *Leadership and Effective Management.* Glenview, Ill: Scott, Foresman; 1974.
21. Fiedler FE, et al. *Improving Leadership Effectiveness.* New York, NY: John Wiley; 1976.
22. Hall DD, Norgaim KE. The leadership match game: matching the man to the situation. *Organ Dynamics.* 1976;4: 6-16.
23. Stinson JE, Tracy L. Some disturbing characteristics of LPC scores. *Personnel Psychol.* 1974;27:477-485.
24. Nebeker DM. Situation favorability and perceived environmental uncertainty: an integrative approach. *Adm Sci Q.* 1975;20:281-294.
25. Vroom VH. *Work and Motivation.* New York, NY: John Wiley; 1964.
26. Porter LW, Lawler EE. *Managerial Attitudes and Performance.* Homewood, Ill: Richard D Irwin; 1968.
27. Evans MG. Leadership and motivation: a core concept. *Acad Manage J.* 1970;13:91-102.
28. Evans MG. The effects of supervisory behavior on the path-goal relationship. *Org Behav in Human Perf.* 1970;5:277-298.
29. House RJ. A path-goal theory of leader effectiveness. *Adm Sci Q.* 1971;16:321-323.
30. House RJ, Mitchell TR. Path-goal theory of leadership. *J Contem Bus.* 1974;3/4:81-98.
31. House RJ, Baetz ML. Leadership: some empirical generalizations and new directions. *Res Org Behav.* 1979;1:385-386.
32. Hershey P, Blanchard KH. *Management of Organizational Behaviors: Utilizing Human Resources.* Englewood Cliffs, NJ: Prentice-Hall; 1977.
33. Shaver KG. *An Introduction to Attribution Processes.* Hillsdale, NY: Eribaum Books; 1983.
34. Mitchell TR, et al. An attributional model of leadership and the poor performing subordinate: development and validation. *Res Org Behav.* 1981;3:197-234.
35. Lord RG, et al. A test of leadership categorization theory: internal structure, information processing and leadership perception. *Org Behav Human Perf.* 1984;34:343-378.
36. Mitchell TR. Attributions and actions: a note of caution. *J Manage.* 1982;8(1):65-74.
37. Burns JM. *Leadership.* New York, NY: Harper & Row; 1978.
38. Tishy NM, Devanna MA. *The Transformational Leader.* New York, NY: John Wiley; 1986.
39. Kuhnert KW, Lewis P. Transactional and transformational leadership: a constructive/developmental analysis. *Acad Manage Rev.* October 1987;12:649.
40. Liden RC, Dienesch RM. Leader-member exchange model of leadership: a critique and further development. *Acad Manage Rev.* 1986;11:618-634.
41. Bass BM. *Leadership Beyond Expectations.* New York, NY: The Free Press; 1985.
42. Eisenstadt SN. *Max Weber: On Charisma and Institution Building.* Chicago, Ill: University of Chicago Press; 1968:46.
43. House RJ. A 1976 theory of charismatic leadership. In: Hunt JG, Larson LL, eds. *Leadership: The Cutting Edge.*

Carbondale: Southern Illinois University Press; 1977:189-207.

44. Dow TE. The theory of charisma. *Sociol Q.* 1969;10:315.

45. Conger JA, Kanungo RN. Toward a behavior theory of charismatic leadership in organizational settings. *Acad Manage Rev.* 1987;12:637-647.

46. Management's new gurus. *Bus Week.* August 31, 1992: 44-52.

47. Bennis WG, Nanus BI. *Leaders.* New York, NY: Harper & Row; 1985.

48. Kouzes JM, Posner BZ. *The Leadership Challenge: How to Get Extraordinary Things Done in Organizations.* San Francisco, Calif: Jossey-Bass; 1988.

49. Morgan G. *Riding the Waves of Change: Developing Managerial Competencies for a Turbulent World.* San Francisco, Calif: Jossey-Bass; 1988.

50. Peters T. *Thriving on Chaos: Handbook for a Management Revolution.* New York, NY: Alfred A Knopf; 1987.

51. Senge PM. *The Fifth Discipline.* New York, NY: Doubleday/Currency; 1991.

52. Vail PB. *Managing as a Performing Art: New Ideas for a World of Chaotic Change.* San Francisco, Calif: Jossey-Bass; 1989.

53. Kelley RE. *The Power of Followership: How to Create Leaders People Want to Follow and Followers Who Lead Themselves.* New York, NY: Doubleday/Currency; 1991.

54. Dreher GF, Ash RA. A comparative study of mentoring among men and women in managerial professional and technical positions. *J Appl Psychol.* 1990;75:539-546.

55. Kram KE. *Mentoring to Work: Developmental Relationships on Organizational Life.* Glenview, Ill: Scott, Foresman; 1985.

CHAPTER
10

Healthy People:
Defining Mission, Goals, and Objectives

Emmeline Ochiai, J.D., M.P.H.
Carter Blakey, B.S.
Randolph F. Wykoff, M.D., M.P.H., and T.M.

HEALTHY PEOPLE 2010 OVERVIEW

Healthy People 2010 is a comprehensive set of health objectives with targets for the United States to achieve by the year 2010.[1] Released in January 2000, it has two overarching goals: first, to increase the quality and years of healthy life and, second, to eliminate disparities in health. To achieve these goals, Healthy People 2010 identifies 467 specific science-based health promotion and disease prevention objectives in 28 focus areas. Each focus area is the product of an extensive, multiyear consensus-building process that involved hundreds of scientists, practitioners, and other interested parties in both the public and the private sectors. Built on the most current scientific knowledge, with over 7,000 data elements drawn from almost 200 different sources, and with extensive documentation of racial and ethnic disparities in health, Healthy People 2010 is designed to provide a comprehensive picture of the nation's health at the beginning of the decade, set forth national goals and targets to be achieved by the year 2010, and monitor progress over time.

HISTORY

Healthy People 2010 is the most ambitious set of health promotion and disease prevention objectives yet developed in the United States. As the third iteration of the initiative, Healthy People 2010 builds on initiatives pursued over the past two decades, beginning with *Healthy People: The Surgeon General's Report on Health Promotion and Disease Prevention*, released in 1979.[2] In 1980, *Promoting Health/Preventing Disease: Objectives for the Nation* presented the first set of 10-year health objectives.[3] *Healthy People 2000: National Health Promotion and Disease Prevention Objectives*, released in 1990, identified national health objectives for the nation to achieve by the end of the twentieth century.[4] The development and oversight of all of these Healthy People documents was coordinated by the Office of Disease Prevention and Health Promotion (ODPHP) of the U.S. Department of Health and Human Services (DHHS). Like its predecessors, Healthy People 2010 establishes national health objectives and serves as the framework for developing state and community health promotion and disease prevention plans.

Healthy People: The First Two Decades

The 1979 document provided national goals for reducing premature deaths and preserving independence for older adults. Supporting those two overarching goals, the 1980 report spelled out 226 health objectives to be achieved by 1990.

The second set of national health objectives, Healthy People 2000, identified three broad goals: (1) increase the span of healthy life, (2) reduce health disparities, and (3) achieve access to preventive services. Healthy People 2000 set forth 319 specific objectives organized into 22 priority areas.

Realizing that progress toward a healthier America would depend substantially on improvements for certain populations at especially high risk, Healthy People 2000 set targets to narrow the gap between the total population and those population groups experiencing above-average incidences of disease, disability, and death. It also set targets for specific age groups.

Throughout the 1990s, the National Center for Health Statistics of the Centers for Disease Control and Prevention, working with ODPHP, produced a series of reviews tracking the nation's progress in achieving the Healthy People 2000 objectives.[5–10] Halfway through the decade, a midcourse review allowed for revisions and corrections to the objectives.[11]

A final review provided the final data for tracking the objectives in all priority areas and reported on two other elements of Healthy People 2000—the Health Status Indicators and Priority Data Needs.[12] (Table 10.1 provides examples of the final status of Healthy People 2000 objectives.)

Virtually all states embraced Healthy People 2000, and most developed more focused plans to reflect their unique priorities.[12] Close to 70 percent of local health departments used the strategies and guidelines of Healthy People 2000.[12]

DEVELOPMENT, PROCESS, AND MANAGEMENT

Healthy People 2010, the most comprehensive and most current national set of science-based health promotion and disease prevention objectives ever issued, was developed by a collaborative process that included substantial input from scientists, from government, academia, and the private sector.

Federal Leadership

Whereas Healthy People 2010 is a national prevention initiative, the federal government provided leadership in guiding its development. With the coordination of ODPHP, DHHS solicited input from private and voluntary organizations; local and state public health, mental health, substance abuse, and environmental agencies; federal government agencies; and individuals interested in improving health.

Focus Area Selection

Healthy People 2010's 28 focus areas are analogous to the 22 priority areas in Healthy People 2000. The term *focus area* was used to move away from an implied prioritization. New areas were added to reflect changes in health care and public health over the preceding decade and as a result of the comments received on a draft *Healthy People 2010* document (see Table 10.2).

Lead Agency Selection

The DHHS assistant secretary for health designated lead agencies with expertise in and responsibility for their respective focus areas. Each Healthy People 2010 focus area is led by one or more agencies of the federal government, including 10 agencies from DHHS, one from the U.S. Department of Agriculture, and one from the U.S. Department of Education (see Table 10.3).

Table 10.1. Healthy People 2000 Objectives: Progress during the 1990s

Over the course of the decade, progress was reported on over 60 percent of Healthy People 2000 objectives, of which approximately 20 percent were fully achieved and 40 percent showed substantial progress. About 15 percent showed that the nation moved in the wrong direction. Progress for the remaining objectives either could not be assessed or was mixed in some cases where multiple elements were used to measure a single objective. For example, the 2000 targets for reducing severe complications due to pregnancy and cancer deaths were achieved, and even surpassed, by the end of the decade, while the proportion of people with activity limitations due to asthma moved away from the target.

	Baseline	Final Data	2000 Target
Achieved Target			
14.7 Severe complications due to pregnancy	22 per 100 deliveries (1987)	13 per 100 deliveries (1999)	15 per 100 deliveries
16.1 Cancer deaths	134 deaths per 100,000 people (1987)	124 deaths per 100,000 people (1999)	130 deaths per 100,000 people
Moved in Right Direction			
13.4 Regular dental visits	54% (1986)	65% (1998)	70%
Moved in Wrong Direction			
17.4 People with activity limitation due to asthma	19.4% (1986–1988)	19.6% (1994–1996)	10%
Showed Mixed Progress			
9.14a States with safety belt use laws	33 (1989)	49 (1998)	50
9.14b States with helmet use laws	22 (1989)	21 (1999)	50

SOURCE: National Center for Health Statistics. *Healthy People 2000 Final Review.* Hyattsville, Md: US Government Printing Office. In press.

Table 10.2. Healthy People 2010 Focus Areas

1. Access to Quality Health Services
2. Arthritis, Osteoporosis, and Chronic Back Conditions
3. Cancer
4. Chronic Kidney Disease
5. Diabetes
6. Disability and Secondary Conditions
7. Educational and Community-Based Programs
8. Environmental Health
9. Family Planning
10. Food Safety
11. Health Communication
12. Heart Disease and Stroke
13. HIV
14. Immunization and Infectious Diseases
15. Injury and Violence Prevention
16. Maternal, Infant, and Child Health
17. Medical Product Safety
18. Mental Health and Mental Disorders
19. Nutrition and Overweight
20. Occupational Safety and Health
21. Oral Health
22. Physical Activity and Fitness
23. Public Health Infrastructure
24. Respiratory Diseases
25. Sexually Transmitted Diseases
26. Substance Abuse
27. Tobacco Use
28. Vision and Hearing

Table 10.3. Lead Federal Agencies and Focus Area Responsibilities

U.S. Department of Health and Human Services
Agency for Healthcare Research and Quality
- Access to Quality Health Care (Co-lead)
  Agency for Toxic Substances and Disease Registry
- Environmental Health (Co-lead)
  Centers for Disease Control and Prevention
- Arthritis, Osteoporosis, and Chronic Back Conditions (Co-lead)
- Cancer (Co-lead)
- Diabetes (Co-lead)
- Disability and Secondary Conditions (Co-lead)
- Educational and Community-Based Programs (Co-lead)
- Environmental Health (Co-lead)
- Heart Disease and Stroke (Co-lead)
- HIV (Co-lead)
- Immunization and Infectious Diseases (Lead)
- Injury and Violence Prevention (Lead)
- Maternal, Infant, and Child Health (Co-lead)
- Occupational Safety and Health (Lead)
- Oral Health (Co-lead)
- Physical Activity and Fitness (Co-lead)
- Public Health Infrastructure (Co-lead)
- Respiratory Diseases (Co-lead)
- Sexually Transmitted Diseases (Lead)
- Tobacco Use (Lead)
Food and Drug Administration
- Food Safety (Co-lead)
- Medical Product Safety (Lead)
- Nutrition and Overweight (Co-lead)
Health Resources and Services Administration
- Access to Quality Health Care (Co-lead)
- Educational and Community-Based Programs (Co-lead)
- HIV (Co-lead)
- Maternal, Infant, and Child Health (Co-lead)

- Oral Health (Co-lead)
- Public Health Infrastructure (Co-lead)
Indian Health Service
- Oral Health (Co-lead)
National Institutes of Health
- Arthritis, Osteoporosis, and Chronic Back Conditions (Co-lead)
- Cancer (Co-lead)
- Chronic Kidney Disease (Lead)
- Diabetes (Co-lead)
- Environmental Health (Co-lead)
- Heart Disease and Stroke (Co-lead)
- Mental Health and Mental Disorders (Co-lead)
- Nutrition and Overweight (Co-lead)
- Oral Health (Co-lead)
- Respiratory Diseases (Co-lead)
- Substance Abuse (Co-lead)
- Vision and Hearing (Lead)
Office of Disease Prevention and Health Promotion
- Health Communication (Lead)
Office of Population Affairs
- Family Planning (Lead)
President's Council on Physical Fitness and Sports
- Physical Activity and Fitness (Co-lead)
Substance Abuse and Mental Health Services Administration
- Mental Health and Mental Disorders (Co-lead)
- Substance Abuse (Co-lead)

U.S. Department of Agriculture
Food Safety and Inspection Service
- Food Safety (Co-lead)

U.S. Department of Education
National Institute on Disability and Rehabilitation Research
- Disability and Secondary Conditions (Co-lead)

SOURCE: *Healthy People 2010.*

Work Group Establishment

Lead agency duties include convening work groups of experts for each of the 28 focus areas. In addition to focus area work groups, work groups were established for specific population groups, such as adolescents, minority health, and women's health. To establish the work groups, HHS invited interested individuals and organizations to join the groups, which examined data, prevention science, and other information to draft objectives for inclusion in *Healthy People 2010.*

Chapter Development

The Healthy People 2010 focus area chapters were developed by the work groups with extensive public input. Draft chapters were circulated for public comment, and following the public comment period, two additional chapters were added, bringing the total to 28 chapters.

Healthy People Consortium

The Healthy People Consortium (the Consortium), an alliance of national membership organizations and state agencies committed to supporting the goals and objectives of Healthy People 2010, contributed to the development process by convening three national meetings in 1998. Consortium membership includes more than 600 state and territorial public health, mental health, substance abuse, and environmental agencies, and national membership organizations representing professional, voluntary, and business sectors, all working to advance health.

The Consortium was convened in 1988 when, at the request of the U.S. Public Health Service, the Institute of Medicine of the National Academy of Sciences invited national membership organizations representing professional, voluntary, and corporate sectors, as well as state and territorial public health agencies, to join the Healthy People 2000 Consortium. The members assisted in developing the Healthy People 2000 objectives and have played an important role in implementing, monitoring, and reporting on the nation's successes and challenges in health.

The Consortium grew in size during the 1990s, with the number of national membership organizations more than doubling since 1988. In 1995, state mental health, substance abuse, and environmental agencies joined the effort.

Secretary's Council on National Health Promotion and Disease Prevention Objectives for 2010

The Secretary's Council on National Health Promotion and Disease Prevention Objectives for 2010 (Secretary's Council) was established to guide and advise the development and implementation of Healthy People 2010. The secretary of health and human services chairs this council, with the assistant secretary for health sitting as vice chair. Members of the Secretary's Council include all former assistant DHHS secretaries for health and current heads of DHHS agencies, including the Administration on Aging, Administration for Children and Families, Agency for Healthcare Research and Quality, Centers for Disease Control and Prevention, Centers for Medicare and Medicaid Services, Food and Drug Administration, Health Research and Services Administration, Indian Health Service, National Institutes of Health, and Substance Abuse and Mental Health Services Administration. The Secretary's Council meets annually to address issues pertinent to the policy and implementation of Healthy People 2010.

Healthy People Steering Committee

The Healthy People Steering Committee (Steering Committee) is a standing committee of DHHS officials that monitors progress, steers the initiative, and contributes to the ongoing endeavors to implement Healthy People 2010 and improve the health of the nation. The Steering Committee is chaired by the deputy assistant secretary for health (disease prevention and health promotion). Composed of representatives from each of the DHHS agencies that serve on the Secretaries Council as well as representatives from the Office of Public Health and Science, the Steering Committee meets quarterly and provides significant ongoing direction to the Healthy People initiative.

Public Comment

In addition to the three national meetings conducted by the Healthy People Consortium, comments from the public were received during a series of five regional meetings during which individuals and organizations provided testimony on health priorities. More than 11,000 public comments on the draft objectives also were received during two public comment periods by mail or via the Internet from people in every state, the District of Columbia, and Puerto Rico.

HEALTHY PEOPLE GOALS FOR 2010

There are two overarching goals of Healthy People 2010:

- Goal 1: Increase quality and years of healthy life.
- Goal 2: Eliminate health disparities, including differences that occur by gender, race and ethnicity, education or income, disability, geographic location, or sexual orientation.

FOCUS AREAS

There are 28 focus areas in Healthy People 2010. Originally 26 focus areas were considered, but based on public comment, two additional focus areas (chronic kidney disease, and vision and hearing) were added.

Each focus area is managed by a designated lead agency or co-lead agency of the federal government. The lead agencies have expertise in and responsibility for their respective focus area. They are responsible for undertaking activities to move the nation toward achieving the year 2010 goals and for reporting progress on the focus area objectives over the decade. The focus area chapters were developed by work groups composed of experts in the subject area and through extensive public comment.

Each focus area chapter in the *Healthy People 2010* report presents background information about the topic, an overview about disparities and opportunities for future action, an interim report on progress of the relevant Healthy People 2000 objectives, a listing of related objectives from other Healthy People 2010 focus areas, definitions of chapter-specific terminology, and references. Each chapter also includes between 6 and 39 specific objectives that detail the current state of health within each focus area and identify a 10-year target for the nation.

OBJECTIVES FOR 2010

Healthy People 2010's 28 focus areas include 467 objectives. The objectives have data-based baselines and targets that will allow the measurement of progress over time. Approximately 75 percent of the objectives in *Healthy People 2010* were measurable with existing data sets at the time the report was published.

Approximately 25 percent of the objectives were not measurable at the time of publication of *Healthy People 2010*. These are referred to as developmental objectives. Developmental objectives provide a vision for a desired outcome or health status. Current national surveillance systems do not provide data on these subjects. The purpose of developmental objectives is to identify areas of emerging importance and to drive the development of data systems to measure them. Most developmental objectives have a potential data source with reasonable expectation of data points by the year 2004 to facilitate setting year 2010 targets in the mid-decade review. Developmental objectives with no baseline at the midcourse will be dropped.

Criteria for Developing Objectives

The criteria first published in *Developing Objectives for Healthy People 2010*[13] in September 1997 called for objectives to be useful to national, state, and local agencies as well as to the private sector and the public. The objectives must have certain attributes, including the following:

> The result to be achieved should be important and understandable to a broad audience and relate to the two overarching *Healthy People 2010* goals.
>
> Objectives should be prevention oriented and should address health improvements that can be achieved through population-based and health-service interventions.
>
> Objectives should drive action and suggest a set of interim steps that will achieve the proposed targets within the specified timeframe.
>
> Objectives should be useful and relevant. States, localities, and the private sector should be able to use the objectives to target efforts in schools, communities, worksites, health practices, and other settings.
>
> Objectives should be measurable and include a range of measures—health outcomes, behavioral and health-service interventions, and community capacity—directed toward improving health outcomes and quality of life.
>
> Continuity and comparability are important. Whenever possible, objectives should build on *Healthy People 2000* and those goals and performance measures already established.

Objectives must be supported by sound scientific evidence.

Population Group Data Table

Despite the United States' wealth, advances in technology, and new biomedical products, there are significant disparities in health from one population group to the next. Cognizant of the health disparities between racial and ethnic populations, genders, socioeconomic populations, and age groups, the second overarching goal of Healthy People 2010 is the elimination of health disparities. The elimination of health disparities is predicated on an understanding of health disparities, the ability to measure these health disparities, and the delivery of interventions to at-risk populations for which these disparities exist.

To facilitate consistency in tracking population groups, a standard data table is used to display the baseline information for each population group for which data are available, analyzed, and statistically reliable (see Table 10.4). The standard data table is used for those objectives that are population based (i.e., objectives that count people as opposed to schools, worksites, or states, etc.).

The data table (also referred to as a template) shown in Table 10.5 represents the minimum set of population variables for data collection for a population-based objective, including race and ethnicity, gender, and measures of socioeconomic status. Within each category in the table, groups are alphabetized or shown by some gradient or level (such as educational or income levels). Depending on the parameters of the objective, some tables show more detailed or additional breakouts of population groups. In addition, some tables include population groups for which data are provided for informational purposes; in such cases, these population groups will not be tracked over the decade.

Race and Ethnicity

Following guidance issued by the Office of Management and Budget (OMB), *Healthy People 2010* sets forth the current categories for reporting race and ethnicity. By act of Congress, federal data systems have until January 2003 to comply with the standards promulgated by OMB. According to OMB policy, "more than one race" will be displayed as a category when data are available.[14]

Gender

In many instances, data highlight the unique problem and disparities by gender. When this is the case, data for all population groups in the table are presented for both genders.

Socioeconomic Status (SES)

SES is shown as income or education level breakouts, or both. If income breakouts are used, data are presented in the following three groups: poor (below federal poverty level); near poor (100 or 199 percent of poverty level); and middle/high income (at least 200 percent of poverty level). In some objectives, programmatic data considerations may result in different income categories being displayed. For instance, for objectives related to the women, infants, and children (WIC) programs, income groups are displayed as lower income level (at or below 130 percent of federal poverty level) and upper income level (above 130 percent of federal level). If education was selected, data are presented in three groups: less than high school, high school graduate, and at least some college.

Age

Age is not included in the minimum table because showing inclusive age categories would add considerable complexity to the minimum set. Furthermore, age often is restricted as part of the objective definition (for example, Focus area 28: Vision and Hearing, objective 28-4. Reduce blindness and visual impairment in children and adolescents aged 17 years and under), and many objectives are relevant only for a subset of age groups. Age breakouts have been added to objectives where relevant and may not be inclusive of the total population. For example, data lines for elderly persons or children could be added to selected objectives without adding other groups.

Other Variables

Other population groups are shown in various objectives when scientific evidence and current knowledge

Table 10.4. Population Data Table from *Healthy People 2010*

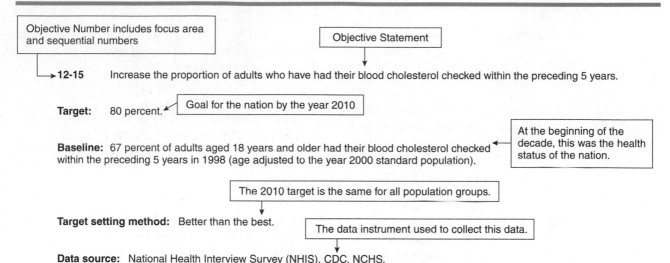

Objective Number includes focus area and sequential numbers

Objective Statement

12-15 Increase the proportion of adults who have had their blood cholesterol checked within the preceding 5 years.

Target: 80 percent. ← Goal for the nation by the year 2010

Baseline: 67 percent of adults aged 18 years and older had their blood cholesterol checked within the preceding 5 years in 1998 (age adjusted to the year 2000 standard population).

At the beginning of the decade, this was the health status of the nation.

The 2010 target is the same for all population groups.

Target setting method: Better than the best.

The data instrument used to collect this data.

Data source: National Health Interview Survey (NHIS), CDC, NCHS.

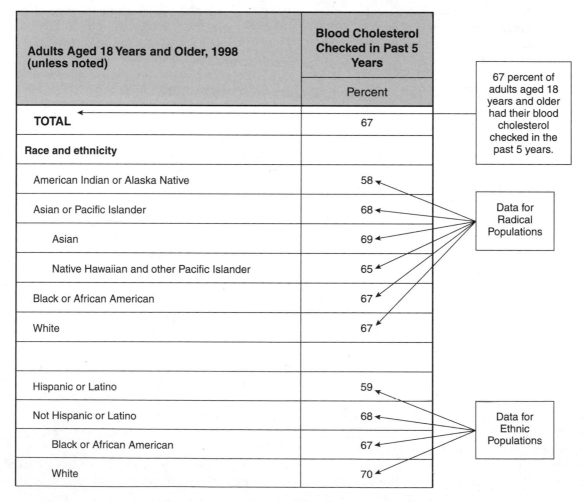

Adults Aged 18 Years and Older, 1998 (unless noted)	Blood Cholesterol Checked in Past 5 Years
	Percent
TOTAL	67
Race and ethnicity	
American Indian or Alaska Native	58
Asian or Pacific Islander	68
Asian	69
Native Hawaiian and other Pacific Islander	65
Black or African American	67
White	67
Hispanic or Latino	59
Not Hispanic or Latino	68
Black or African American	67
White	70

67 percent of adults aged 18 years and older had their blood cholesterol checked in the past 5 years.

Data for Radical Populations

Data for Ethnic Populations

Table 10.4. *(continued)*

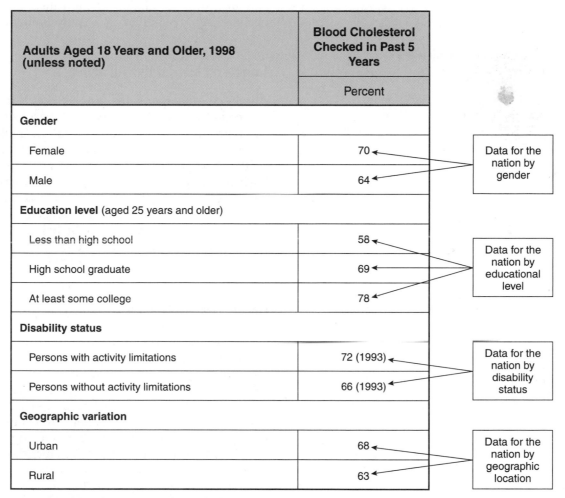

Adults Aged 18 Years and Older, 1998 (unless noted)	Blood Cholesterol Checked in Past 5 Years
	Percent
Gender	
Female	70
Male	64
Education level (aged 25 years and older)	
Less than high school	58
High school graduate	69
At least some college	78
Disability status	
Persons with activity limitations	72 (1993)
Persons without activity limitations	66 (1993)
Geographic variation	
Urban	68
Rural	63

Data for the nation by gender

Data for the nation by educational level

Data for the nation by disability status

Data for the nation by geographic location

DNA = Data have not been analyzed. DNC = Data are not collected. DSU = Data are statistically unreliable.
Note: Age adjusted to the year 2000 standard population

SOURCE: *Healthy People 2010.*

Table 10.5. Standard Table for Population Data

Population Group, Year	Condition Measure
TOTAL	
Race	
American Indian or Alaska Native	
Asian or Pacific Islander	
Asian	
Native Hawaiian and other Pacific Islander	
Black or African American	
White	
Ethnicity	
Hispanic or Latino	
Not Hispanic or Latino	
Black or African American	
White	
Gender	
Female	
Male	
Socioeconomic status	
Family income level	
Poor	
Near poor	
Middle/high income	
Education level	
Less than high school	
High school graduate	
At least some college	

The following are additional categories included where appropriate.

Geographic location
　Urban
　Rural
Health insurance status
　Private health insurance
　Public health insurance
　Medicare
　Medicaid
　No health insurance
Disability status
　Persons with disabilities or activity limitations
　Persons without disabilities or activity limitations
Sexual orientation
Select populations
　Age groups
　School grade levels
　Persons with select medical conditions

show that the group(s) may be at risk. Other population groups or breakouts that may be included are urban and rural populations, health insurance status, persons with disabilities or activity limitations, and sexual orientation.

Targets for Measurable Objectives

An objective's target is the number that is presented for achievement by 2010. Targets are based on the national baseline data. As a general rule, a single target is set for all population groups to reach by the year 2010. This supports the overarching goal of eliminating health disparities. Often this number was derived by using a "better than the best" approach, suggesting that the minimally acceptable target for all groups should be better than a rate that has already been achieved by one of the racial or ethnic groups.

DATA 2010

Data for Healthy People 2010 measures are updated on a quarterly basis at the Web site for Healthy People 2010 data known as DATA 2010 (http://www.cdc.gov/nchs/about/otheract/hpdata2010/aboutdata2010.htm). This Web site is maintained by the National Center for Health Statistics of the Centers for Disease Control and Prevention. DATA 2010 is an interactive database system that contains the most recent monitoring data for tracking Healthy People 2010 objectives. Data are included for all the measurable objectives and subgroups identified in *Healthy People 2010*. DATA 2010 contains primarily national data; however, state-based data are provided as available.

LEADING HEALTH INDICATORS

Whereas Healthy People 2010 continues an important public health tradition, it also introduces significant and useful innovations, including 10 leading health indicators (LHIs) (see Table 10.6 and Figures 10.1 and 10.2). Measured by a subset of objectives from *Healthy People 2010*, the LHIs highlight major risk factors Americans face and draw attention to the most signifi-

Table 10.6. The 10 Leading Health Indicators

Physical activity
Overweight and obesity
Tobacco use
Substance abuse
Responsible sexual behavior
Mental health
Injury and violence
Environmental quality
Immunization
Access to health care

cant areas where individual and community action regarding health improvements need to be made. Five of the factors relate primarily to individual behaviors, including physical activity, overweight and obesity, tobacco use, substance abuse, and responsible sexual behavior. The other five address mental health, injury and violence, environmental quality, immunization, and access to health care. The LHIs will be used to measure important determinants of the nation's health during the first decade of the twenty-first century.

The process for selecting the LHIs mirrored the extensive collaborative efforts undertaken to develop *Healthy People 2010*. The process was led by an interagency work group within HHS. Individuals and organizations provided comments at national or regional

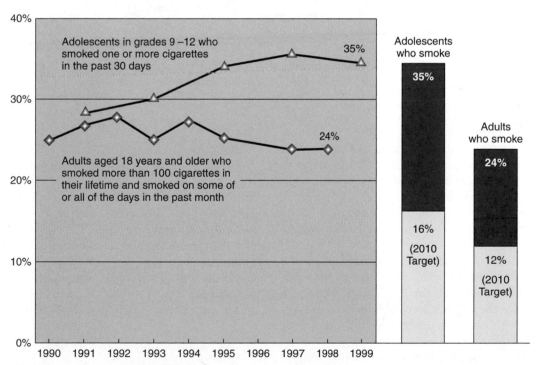

Figure 10.1. Tobacco Use: Leading Health Indicator. Cigarette smoking, United States, 1990–99.

SOURCES: Centers for Disease Control and Prevention. Youth Risk Behavior Survey; 1991–1999. Centers for Disease Control and Prevention, National Center for Health Statistics. National Health Interview Survey; 1990–1998.

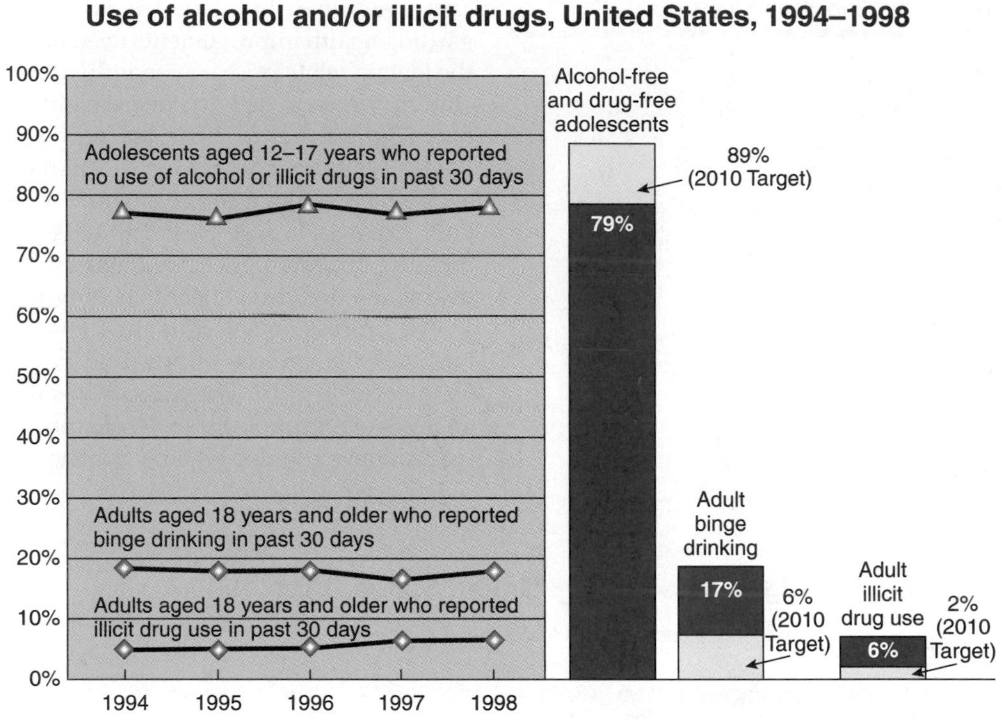

Use of alcohol and/or illicit drugs, United States, 1994–1998

Figure 10.2. Substance Abuse: Leading Health Indicator. Use of alcohol and/or illicit drugs, United States, 1994–98.

SOURCE: Substance Abuse and Mental Health Services Administration, Office of the Assistant Secretary. National Household Survey on Drug Abuse; 1994–1998.

meetings or via mail and the Internet. A report by the IOM provided several scientific models on which to support a set of indicators.[15] Focus groups were used to ensure that the indicators are meaningful and motivating to the public.

For program and policy planning and management purposes, the LHIs may serve as a valuable compass and resource. Similar to the index of leading economic indicators reported on by the New York-based Conference Board, the LHIs can provide a snapshot of the current health of the nation and forecast where the health of the nation may be in six months to a year.

By focusing public attention on the Healthy People message, it is hoped that the LHIs will serve as significant mechanisms to communicate important public health information to the media, to elected officials, and to the general public.

Leading Health Indicators Communications Strategy

Efforts are under way to develop additional strategies, based on a multiyear communication plan, to effectively communicate the LHIs to decision makers and the general public. The plan will include an approach to make key audiences aware of, and attuned to, the concept of the LHIs, and will dovetail with an LHI annual report on the health of the nation to increase awareness of public health issues.

THE CHALLENGE: IMPLEMENTATION

Healthy People 2010 is a tremendous resource for the nation. It is the basis for coordinated public health action on the national, state, and local levels and has been used as a teaching tool for the next generation of public health leaders. The challenge facing Healthy People 2010 is how to translate its exceptional potential energy into the kind of kinetic energy that will make a difference in the lives of the American people; that is, how to translate vision into action.

Using Healthy People 2010

There is a tremendous amount of data presented in Healthy People 2010. It can, therefore, be used as a descriptive encyclopedia of public health in the United States and as a textbook that describes public health opportunities for the next decade. But there are other sources of public health statistics and other more comprehensive textbooks of public health. Clearly, to reach its maximum potential and to justify its remarkable intellectual investment, Healthy People 2010 objectives must be applied to public health scenarios on a variety of levels.

Building Partnerships

Healthy People 2010 provides an opportunity for nongovernmental groups, organizations, and associations to identify areas of mutual interest and to begin or continue collaborative efforts to address these areas.

Through ODPHP, DHHS has engaged in strategic partnerships with nongovernmental groups, organizations, and associations that express a commitment to Healthy People 2010. These partnerships endeavor to identify common areas for collaboration, leverage resources, maximize program outreach and communication, draw on the expertise of nongovernmental organizations to relate to their membership and constituency, resonate the value of public-private partnerships, and recognize the nongovernmental organizations' commitment to improving the health of the American people through Healthy People 2010.

Enabling State and Local Action

The underlying premise of Healthy People 2010 is that the health of the individual is almost inseparable from the health of the larger community and that the health of every community in every state and territory determines the overall health status of the nation.

Nearly all states, the District of Columbia, and Guam developed their own Healthy People 2000 plans. Most states have built on the national objectives and virtually all states have adapted the national objectives to address their specific needs. A 1993 National Association of County and City Health Officials survey showed that 70 percent of local health departments used at least some Healthy People 2000 objectives. Many states, working with community coalitions, are now developing their own versions. The *Healthy People 2010 Toolkit: A Field Guide to Health Planning*,[16] developed by the Public Health Foundation under contract with ODPHP, provides examples of state and national experiences in setting and using objectives and is available online (www.health. gov/ healthypeople/state/toolkit). A network of state Healthy People coordinators exists to provide liaisons between DHHS and the states to foster communication among states and to serve as the central point of contact for residents. In some states, the state health official serves as the contact point; in others this responsibility is held by staff in the health statistics or planning branch. The DHHS Healthy People Web site (http://www.health.gov/healthypeople) lists all the state contacts. Making objectives setting and monitoring processes accessible to the public helps to increase citizen participation.

Community partnerships, particularly those that involve nontraditional partners, can be among the most effective tools for improving health in communities. For the past two decades, Healthy People has served as a strategic management tool for the federal government, states, communities, and other public- and private-sector partners. To assist groups in utilizing Healthy People 2010 to drive local action, ODPHP published a companion document titled *Healthy People in Healthy Communities: A Community Planning Guide Using Healthy People 2010*.[17] This document is a guide for building community coalitions, creating a vision, measuring results, and creating partnerships dedicated to improving the health of a community.

There are several other federal resources that can assist individuals and communities working to implement Healthy People 2010. Two of the most important are the *Guide to Clinical Preventive Services*[18] and the *Guide to Community Preventive Services*.[19]

The U.S. Task Force on Preventive Services systematically reviews evidence on preventive services and produces the *Guide to Clinical Preventive Services* (http://www.ahcpr.gov/clinic), recognizing preventive services as a key feature in improving quality of life and reducing health care costs. This guide reviews evidence for over 100 interventions to prevent 60 different illnesses and conditions, in order that clinicians can provide patients with screening, immunizations, counseling or other preventive services in the course of routine clinical care.

The *Guide to Community Preventive Services* (http://www.thecommunityguide.org), under development by the U.S. Task Force on Community Preventive Services, provides public health practitioners with recommendations for population-based interventions to promote health, and to prevent injury and premature death. These recommendations are based on systemic review of research in changing risk behaviors, reducing the prevalence and incidence of diseases, injuries, and impairments, and addressing environmental and ecosystem challenges.

International Action

Many countries and nations have adopted the health planning and management model espoused by Healthy People 2010. Egypt and Uruguay have modeled their own national health plan around the *Healthy People* document. In fall of 2000, Egypt launched Healthy Egyptians 2010.[20] In fall of 2001, Uruguay launched Salud Uruguay 2010.[21] Healthy Border, a project of the United States–Mexico Border Health Commission, has adopted Healthy People 2010 objectives. In addition, Chile, Brazil, Indonesia, Japan, and Australia are exploring the Healthy People model and objectives.

Assessing Performance

Many federal government agencies use Healthy People 2010 objectives as the metric for measuring their performance. In 1993, Congress enacted the Government Performance and Results Act (GPRA, Public Law 103-62). The principal purpose of the act is "to provide for the establishment of strategic planning and performance measurement in the Federal Government." In accordance with GPRA, federal agencies are required to identify performance measures and perform strategic planning for the purpose of increased efficiency, reduced waste, and improved accountability. Many federal agencies use Healthy People 2010 objectives as the basis for measuring their performance and reporting to Congress.

Healthy People objectives also have been used in other performance measurement activities. One example is the National Committee on Quality Assurance, which incorporated many Healthy People targets into its Health Plan Employer Data and Information Set (HEDIS) 3.0. HEDIS is a set of standardized measures that health care purchasers and consumers use in assessing the performance of managed care organizations in the areas of immunizations, mammography screening, and other clinical preventive services.

Healthy People 2010 objectives have been specified by Congress as the measures to be used for assessing progress under the American Indian Health Care Improvement Act, the Maternal and Child Health Block Grant, and the Preventive Health and Health Services Block Grant.

FUTURE OF HEALTHY PEOPLE 2010

As the Healthy People process enters its third decade it is important to carefully analyze how the process has evolved since 1979 and how Healthy People 2010 is being utilized by the public. A formal evaluation of *Healthy People 2010* has begun to determine who uses it, how it is being used, and what parts of it are used. The answers to these questions will allow the initiative to effectively target federal technical assistance for implementation of Healthy People 2010, and to create a more valuable *Healthy People 2020* document, in the future.

References

1. US Department of Health and Human Services. *Healthy People 2010.* 2nd ed. Washington, DC: US Government Printing Office; November 2000.

2. *Healthy People, Surgeon General's Report on Health Promotion and Disease Prevention.* Washington, DC: US Depart of Health Education and Welfare; 1979. PHS Publication 79-55071.

3. *Promoting Health/Preventing Disease: Objectives for the Nation.* Washington, DC: US Depart of Health and Services; 1980.

4. *Healthy People 2000: National Health Promotion and Disease Prevention Objectives.* Washington, DC: US Depart of Health and Human Services; 1990. PHS publication 91-50212.

5. National Center for Health Statistics. *Healthy People 2000 Review, 1992.* Hyattsville, Md: Public Health Service; 1992.

6. National Center for Health Statistics. *Healthy People 2000 Review, 1993.* Hyattsville, Md: Public Health Service; 1993.

7. National Center for Health Statistics. *Healthy People 2000 Review, 1994.* Hyattsville, Md: Public Health Service; 1994.

8. National Center for Health Statistics. *Healthy People 2000 Review, 1995-96.* Hyattsville, Md: Public Health Service; 1996.

9. National Center for Health Statistics. *Healthy People 2000 Review, 1997.* Hyattsville, Md: Public Health Service; 1997.

10. National Center for Health Statistics. *Healthy People 2000 Review, 1998-99.* Hyattsville, Md: Public Health Service; 1999.

11. US Department of Health and Human Services, Public Health Service. *Healthy People 2000: Midcourse Review and 1995 Revisions.* Washington, DC: US Government Printing Office; 1995.

12. National Center for Health Statistics. *Healthy People 2000 Final Review.* Hyattsville, Md. In press.

13. US Department of Health and Human Services. *Developing Objectives for Healthy People 2010.* Washington, DC: US Government Printing Office; 1997.

14. Office of Management and Budget. Standards for maintaining, collecting and presenting federal data on race and ethnicity. *Federal Register,* 1997. 62 FR 58781-58790.

15. Institute of Medicine, National Academy of Sciences. *Leading Health Indicators.* Washington, DC: National Academy Press, 1999.

16. Public Health Foundation. *Healthy People 2010 Toolkit: A Field Guide to Health Planning.* Washington, DC: Public Health Foundation; 1999.

17. US Department of Health and Human Services. *Healthy People in Healthy Communities: A Community Guide Using Healthy People 2010.* Washington, DC: US Government Printing Office; 2001.

18. US Preventive Services Task Force. *Guide to Clinical Preventive Services.* 2nd ed. Washington, DC: US Government Printing Office; 1996.

19. *Guide to Community Preventive Services.* Available at http://www.thecommunityguide.org.

20. Ministry of Health and Population. *A New Egyptian Health Care Model for the 21st Century* Cairo, Egypt; September 2001.

21. *Salud Uruguay.* In press.

CHAPTER

11

Community Assessment and Change: A Framework, Principles, Models, Methods, and Skills

Elizabeth A. Baker, Ph.D., M.P.H.
Robert M. Goodman, Ph.D., M.P.H.*

INTRODUCTION

Over the past 20 years, public health approaches to community health have undergone significant shifts in philosophy and orientation. The traditional approach to community health mainly involved direct service provision. Thus, community programs often were based in public or nonprofit organizations, implemented and managed by agency staff, and evaluated primarily on staff effort.[1] Several large-scale community trials for chronic diseases have had enormous influence in shaping public health programming in community settings over the last two decades. Of particular note are the 10-year community trials in the late 1970s and early 1980s, funded by the National Heart,

*The authors would like to thank the members of the Protective Social Factors Projects funded by the Centers for Disease Control and Prevention for their contributions to the thinking included in this chapter.

Lung, and Blood Institute (NHLBI), and directed at cardiovascular risk reduction.[2–5] All implemented numerous community activities that included risk factor screening, general and specific media messages, worksite physical activity, menu labeling at restaurants, grocery labeling, school programs, work with health practitioners, community-wide contests, community task forces, speakers bureaus, and others.[4] Great expense and effort went into such initiatives, but they produced modest results that some have attributed to the inadequacies of community interventions.[6–8]

Other lessons taken directly from these community trials reveal the need to alter program implementation and assessment strategies in ways that reflect the unique challenges of executing programs outside of organizational settings and in community settings. In reflecting upon the community trials, Green and McAlister[9] assert that "community or large-scale programs, even within large institutions, require a shift in perspective and the employment of the distinct set of analytic and programmatic tools from those used with patients, clients, or customers" (pp. 323–324). This formidable shift suggests that a transformation in community health frameworks may be required in producing more effective public health strategies in community settings. The community assessment and change processes that result are often referred to as "community-based public health."

This chapter begins with a brief definition of community, then refers to social ecology as a relevant framework for contemporary community-based public health interventions (see chapter 14 for an in-depth discussion of social ecology). Several principals for community-based practice and research follow, along with a number of popular models for community practice in public health. The chapter ends with a discussion of assessment strategies and core principles for community involvement.

Definitions of Community

Many programs purport to be community based or to be working with "the community." However, programs vary widely as to who is included in the definition of "community." For some, a *community* may be defined as a geographic area or neighborhood. For others, to be considered a community, members of the community must have a sense of shared identity with other members of the community, a sense of belonging and emotional connection to the community, and a set of shared values and norms.[10] For purposes of this chapter, a community is defined as a collection of individuals who live within a geographic area that can be specified. These individuals may have varied values and norms, and may self-identify as belonging to several different communities.

The Social Ecology Framework

In the last decade, the social ecology perspective has gained currency as a comprehensive framework for community-based public health (see chapter 14). The social ecology framework holds that individual, interpersonal, community (including cultural, social, and economic factors), organizational, and govern-

mental factors influence health directly and through individual behavior.[10,11] That is, individual lifestyle choices and behaviors are more likely to be health promoting when social ecology factors are taken into account, because such factors have a direct influence on the lifestyle and behavior choices. As Stokols, Allen, and Bellingham[12] write, ecological-informed programs address the "interdependencies between socioeconomic, cultural, political, environmental, organizational, psychological, and biological determinants of health and illness" (p. 247). They envision the shift to comprehensive ecological formulations as a needed transformation for program implementation because pockets of prevalence for ill health remain fixed in communities when interventions are limited in scope. Stokols and colleagues hold that such limited programs are the cause of high relapse and attrition rates.[10,11,13–15] Similarly, the Ottawa Charter for Health Promotion asserts that

> to reach a state of complete physical, mental and social well-being, an individual or group must be able to identify and realize aspirations, to satisfy needs, and to change or cope with the environment. Health is a positive concept emphasizing social and personal resources, as well as physical capacities. . . . The fundamental conditions and resources for health are peace, shelter, education, food, income, a stable eco-system, sustainable resources, social justice and equity. Improvement in health requires a secure foundation in these basic prerequisites.[16]

It is important to note that such multifaceted approaches are applicable whether the program is categorical (e.g., focused on a particular disease process), or a more broadly defined community program (e.g., community development). For example, a program that focuses on a disease category (e.g., breast cancer), and receives categorical funding to change individual behavior (e.g., mammography), may enhance its ability to influence behavior if it considers the impact of other factors (e.g., interpersonal, economic) and intervenes accordingly. This may entail providing low or no-cost mammograms, changing the state policy so that more women are eligible for low- or no-cost mammograms, or developing a lay health advisor approach to enhance breast cancer screening. Alternately, programs and policies may focus on changing physical, social, or economic factors (not a specific disease) because of the direct effects of these factors on health outcomes. These different programmatic and policy activities may occur simultaneously or sequentially.[10,17,18] As the example illustrates, multiple levels of intervention are at the core of community-based public health and require input from a wide variety of individuals with different and complementary expertise.

Levels of Engagement in Community Health Practice and Research

A comprehensive framework for community engagement has evolved over time and continues to grow as researchers, practitioners, and community members gain experience in implementing it. A recent IOM report[19] characterizes this evolutionary process in research projects as including three levels:

> 1) current proactive practice of academically driven research initiatives, 2) a more reactive practice for designing research in response to the needs and input of community agencies, and 3) the development of interactive practices that involve both academic researchers and the community as equal partners in all phases of a research project (p. 30).

The first type of research, Type 1, typically involves the researcher as the sole inquirer. The academician determines the questions to ask and defines the range of acceptable answers. In the second type of research, Type 2, nonacademicians assist in defining the question, but academicians still define the methods of inquiry and the range of answers. Using the third type of research, Type 3 or community-based public health research, the community and academicians jointly define the questions to ask, determine how to gather the answers, and decide what to do with the information that is gathered (i.e., dissemination of information and/or action).

Community-based public health interventions have gone through similar evolutionary processes and have similar gradations. There have been (1) collaborative efforts directed by public health practitioners with minimal input from community organizations and/or community members; (2) collaborative models that encourage community interaction using predetermined processes; and (3) efforts that involve joint definitions of processes and outcomes. Researcher- and practitioner-directed, or Type 1, approaches often usurp active and meaningful community involvement that results in disempowering rather than enhancing the building of community capacities to affect the population's health.[20–22] Thus, health professionals may require a new orientation to enhance the quality of their relationships with communities so that a community's capacity and control builds rather than diminishes. For many researchers, practitioners, and communities, this requires the development or modification of new and existing skills and tools including the following: knowledge and skills that enhance capacity for joint, collaborative control in decision making and action, including program design, implementation, and evaluation; nontrivial use of community resources, skills, and relationships; and cultivation of new capacities and partnerships among organizations and individuals.[22,23]

A program using Type 2 levels of engagement might use predetermined models or processes for assessment and intervention, but these models provide opportunities for community input. Using this approach, a community-based intervention may focus on changing multiple levels of the social ecology framework, but does so in a way that is rigidly defined and fixed.

The Type 3 level of engagement is founded on exacting principles in conducting community assessment and change programs[22,24–27] including:

1. All individuals must be respectful of each other.
2. All individuals must act in ways that build trust among partners, which often means letting go of individual needs in favor of collective desires.
3. All information gathered must be shared in understandable ways.
4. Actions should focus on and build community strengths and assets in a way that promotes social justice.
5. Organizational structures must ensure equal participation and influence of all affected by community assessments and change including community members and practitioners from public and private organizations.

6. Community assessment must be viewed not as an end in itself but rather as building toward community change.
7. Coalitions must act to create changes in systems and environments, not just individuals.
8. All participants in coalitions must recognize and act to minimize the institutional barriers to partnership development and action.
9. Partnerships must recognize that long-term relationships require flexibility and allowance for transition and interorganizational change.

In short, the Type 3 approach best fits a comprehensive framework for community-based public health because of its emphasis on collaborative principles that involve the community in a fashion that is inclusive, democratic, equitable from the outset, and is flexible and dynamic in the levels of the ecological framework that is the focus of the intervention.

Whereas the Type 3 principles are congruent with the desirable community practices, alternately, some consider communities to be defined by formal and informal collective associations or organizations. Therefore, many practitioners consider themselves to be working with "the community" when they are working with representatives of community-based organizations or associations. Traditionally community organizations were naturally occurring associations that brought together individuals to identify needs, and resources to address those needs and carry out actions to implement solutions. Recently, health professionals have recognized the need for community involvement in preventing disease and promoting healthy lifestyles, and have attempted to capitalize on these naturally occurring strengths, capacities, and structures to create health changes. In doing so, some have created new organizations while others have attempted to work with existing organizations through collaborations or coalitions. A *coalition* is defined as a group of community members and/or organizations that join together for a common purpose.[28,29] Some coalitions are focused on categorical issues, such as breast cancer. Other coalitions form to address broader public health issues.

Coalitions may differ considerably in the roles and responsibilities of each coalition member and the types of activities in which they wish to engage. This can be thought of as a continuum of integration.[28-30] On one end of the continuum is the desire of agencies and individuals to work together to identify gaps in services, avoid duplication of services, and exchange information to allow for appropriate client referral. The next level of integration involves agencies maintaining their autonomy, agendas, and resources, but beginning to share these resources to work on an issue that is identified as common to all agencies. The next level involves each of the agencies lessening their level of autonomy and beginning to develop joint agendas, joint goals, and joint resources.

The level of integration that is appropriate depends on the desires of the agencies and the length of time that the coalition has worked together. Some coalitions may decide to start at a low level of integration and move to higher levels over time; others may start with attempts to engage in projects that require full integration. What is most crucial is that all agencies agree on the level of integration and jointly define their common goals as well as objectives to reach these goals. The following section describes popular community intervention models that use community coalitions primarily within Type 1 and 2 levels of engagement.

Popular Models for Community Health Programming

There are a number of established models for assessing community resources and needs, and for developing and utilizing community coalitions to address health-related changes. The models discussed here include: Healthy Communities 2000, APEXPH, PATCH, and Healthy Cities. While a complete review of each is not possible within this chapter, a brief overview of each is presented below. References are provided for those wishing additional information on the specific models.

Healthy Communities 2000

Model Standards are at the core of Healthy Communities 2000 and were developed to provide communities with specific health status and process objectives that can be readily translated for use at the community level. These standards were published as a result of a collaborative effort of the American Public Health Association (APHA), the Association of State and Territorial Health Officials, the National Association of County and City Health Officials (NACCHO), the United States Conference of Local Health Officers, the Association of Schools of Public Health and the Centers for Disease Control and Prevention (CDC).[31] While the standards are laid out, and suggestions made for how to translate these locally, no specific guidelines are provided for communities interested in creating a coalition or developing programs to enhance community health; rather, recommendations are made to seek out these skills through other resources.

APEX*PH*

As with Healthy Communities 2000, APEX*PH* (Assessment Protocol for Excellence in Public Health) was created as part of efforts to create performance indicators and measures, but was not initially intended as an intervention model.[23] APEX*PH* was developed through the collaborative efforts of NACCHO and the CDC.[32] The assessment protocol includes an organizational capacity assessment (for health departments' self-assessment), a community assessment utilizing the earlier mentioned Healthy Communities 2000: Model Standards, and recommendations for the development of a community advisory committee. The organizational capacity assessment required that the health department director generate a team to examine the health department's authority and capacity to conduct a community assessment, develop policy, and manage related administrative tasks (e.g., financial, personnel, program management). This assessment was intended to lead to an organizational action plan. The second part of the APEX*PH* process was the community assessment to assess health status, identify priority areas, and set goals and objectives based on these priorities, that is, develop a community plan. To be effective, the health officer reviewed the community plan and used the organizational assessment to assess the capacity of the health department to assist the community in carrying out its plan.

As with Healthy Communities 2000, APEX*PH* provided little guidance for communities interested in creating a coalition or developing programs to enhance community health; recommendations are made to seek out these skills through other resources. Based on the lessons learned from APEX*PH*, NACCHO and CDC developed a new program, Mobilizing for Action through Planning and Partnerships (MAPP). MAPP provides additional guidance and tools on how to develop plans for improving community health ((http//www.naccho.org/project77.cfm). Similarly, the Protocol for Assessing Community Excellence in Environmental Health (PACE*EH*) is another NACCHO program that assists communities in the planning and implementation of community-based environmental health assessment (http://www.naccho.org/project78.cfm).

PATCH

PATCH (Planned Approach to Community Health) was initially created by the CDC and goes beyond the above assessment tools by providing specific guidelines for state and local health agencies to use to assess the health needs of communities and develop, implement, and evaluate health promotion programs.[33] The CDC provides materials and technical assistance to states, and in turn states taking part in PATCH provide local communities with resources. Although the PATCH model establishes interaction with community constituents prior to developing priorities, until recently, little guidance was incorporated for developing the structures and capacities that are prerequisites for meaningful community involvement.

Healthy Cities/Healthy Communities

This model was derived as a response to the World Health Organization's *Global Strategies for Health for all by the Year 2000*. It was developed by the World Health Organization (WHO) with the intention of developing solutions to broadly defined health related concerns by bringing together individuals and organizations from private, public, and voluntary agencies.[34–37] Technical assistance and training are provided to communities through WHO, but each community collects community-specific data and identifies site-specific solutions. These initiatives are a good example of broadly defined community-based health promotion that addresses individual, community, social, and economic factors.

Toronto, Canada, serves as an illustration. The city has worked extensively on its Healthy Cities/Healthy Communities program with the goal of establishing partnerships between community members and governmental and community organizations to ensure that "everyone has access to the basics needed for health; the physical environment supports healthy living; and communities control, define and direct action for health."[35,p37] This approach has resulted in efforts to address jobs, housing, air quality, smoking, AIDS, hunger, transportation, safety, and physical activity (e.g., individual, social, community, and economic factors). The approach takes into account the development and nurturing of community coalitions and is more commensurate than are other models with an ecologically informed framework and with Type 3 principles of engagement with community representatives and coalitions.

In general, each of the models offers unique and complementary approaches and tools. The models are useful in that they can minimize the likelihood that each community will reinvent such well-established approaches. One concern, however, is that the models may be brought to communities and viewed as canned approaches to issues that have been defined as "problems" by "experts" who offer solutions that are not consonant with the core needs expressed by a community. Also, the processes used to engage with communities often are in conflict with well-established community norms (e.g., Type 1 and 2 approaches).

To minimize the inappropriate use of these models, it is worthwhile to consider the key competencies and skills that the models suggest and to employ them in such a way that they are consistent with multifaceted approaches and Type 3 principles. For instance, in looking at community coalitions from the Type 3 level of engagement, coalition members jointly agree on the processes used and have joint training and discussions regarding the competencies required to engage in these processes. This avoids defining processes without community involvement (or domination of a few over the many) as well as ensuring that all can participate equally because all parties have had the opportunity to build skills jointly. Some of the processes and the skills necessary for community assessment and change are presented below.

Processes for Effective Community Engagement

Preformation and Initial Mobilization

Like many public health researchers and practitioners, we would like to believe that we are engaging in community-based public health. Yet, how many of us can say that, before even beginning to engage with communities and nurture community coalitions, we have made a concerted effort to understand the history of community relations, previous experiences with health projects, intergroup relations, and interorganizational relationships (particularly the levels of trust and respect among these individuals and groups), as well as community resources and values?[38] This context influences attitudes, behaviors, and structures that, in turn, affect how groups will form and interact and how behavior is created, maintained, and changed, and has direct impact on health and well-being.[38]

An exploration of already existing networks and organizations is another aspect of the community context that should be done at the outset of community engagement. It is important to include such existing community structures in the design and implementation of new community-based efforts. In addition, it is also important to include community members themselves. They may offer different perspectives than agency members because of different life experiences, education, or other factors. Moreover, there are multiple voices within any community (or community organization) and efforts must be made to include individuals from a variety of subgroups within a community.

Establishing Organizational Structure

Once community members have agreed to participate, practitioners and other core members should ensure that all members have similar opportunities to influence the processes and outcomes of the group. To do this, the organizational structure is jointly defined and established by coalition members. As trust and sincerity are critical to the ongoing relationship and capacity of the coalition to function, it is important from the outset that promises made are followed through, and that all individuals are treated with courtesy and respect.[38] More specifically, this step entails developing roles, decision-making structures, and group processes. In considering this, it is strategic to remember that individuals from different agencies and different community members each have different ways of engaging in these processes. Therefore, any choices regarding policies and procedures must consider the range of possibilities and include training opportunities so that all members of the coalition have the skills necessary to participate in whatever processes are decided on. These skills include leadership (democratic and supportive of member ideas and participation), decision making (collective decision making with equal voice and influence), group facilitation (including establishing ground rules for participation, developing agendas, running meetings, minute taking, and agenda development), communication (development of a common language, multiple channels of communication), problem solving and conflict resolution, and fiscal management (agreement regarding how funds are collected and distributed).[8,25,28,39–42]

The development of the organizational structure also needs to acknowledge cultural differences. These cultural differences may present themselves as differences in the culture of the organizations included in the coalition and/or in differences among individuals and communities. These cultural differences are likely to influence the way individuals and organizations interact and respond to any organizational structure that is created. Although the coalition literature contains relatively little regarding cultural competencies, a great deal can be drawn from health education, medical and health professions, as well as social work practice literatures. These include:

1. Be aware of your own cultural biases and prejudices and how these are communicated to others. Recognize what you do and do not know.
2. Be aware of differences in interaction styles and how these influence communication between individuals and organizations.

3. Be aware that different cultures may focus on different determinants of health and wellness and that these differences should be taken into account in both assessment and program intervention decisions.
4. Recognize that previous interactions with organizations may have been negative and created mistrust and fear of future interactions. More generally, recognize that the social fabric of discrimination on the basis of class and race influences all individuals and their actions regardless of their class background, culture, race, or ethnicity.
5. Be aware that asking individuals and/or organizations to change is likely to disrupt current adaptive behaviors.
6. Acknowledge differences within as well as between different cultural groups.

Suggestions for coalition building (including how to enhance these skills) can be found in the University of Kansas Workgroup on Health Promotion and Community Development's Community Toolbox, which can be accessed at http://ctb.lsi.ukans.edu. Johnson, Grossman, and Cassidy, and Wolff and Kaye also provide helpful hints as well as worksheets to enhance community efforts at this stage.[40,42] Additional information on establishing structures and cultural competencies is available in the literature.[38,39,41,43–45]

Assessment of Community Needs

A community assessment is necessary for coalitions to determine what programs or policies should be developed. Historically, many assessments focus on individual health problems, but recent work encourages the assessment of health concerns, organizational structures, community infrastructures and resources, as well as assessment of the cultural, historical, economic, political, social, and physical/geographic context that goes beyond the preformation assessments described earlier.[26]

Much of the data required to assess needs are available through surveillance systems and national and local data sets such as those available through hospital and other service provider records, the CDC (www.cdc.gov), local state health departments (e.g., http://www.health.state.mo.us/), and the U.S. Census Bureau (http://wonder.cdc.gov/censJ.shtml).

Such information includes current health status, rates of various risk behaviors and disease, and morbidity and mortality due to various causes. Some data sets provide county-level data and comparisons to state and national rates, while others allow users to get Zip Code-level data. There are also data available that provide information regarding existing programs and the populations they serve (http://www.communityconnection.org/). Healthy Communities 2000: Model Standards and APEX*PH* can be helpful in determining indicators to assess.[31,32]

Others have noted that it is also important to document the current knowledge and attitudes of potential program participants and/or those who will be affected by a policy with regard to various behaviors as well as to perspectives on current programs and reasons why these programs are or are not effective in meeting the defined needs.[46–48] These data can be collected through quantitative (questionnaires) or qualitative methods (individual or group interviews).

Tools for assessing organizational structures, community infrastructures, and resources as well as the cultural, historical, economic, political, social, and physical/geographic context are not as widely available.[46,48–50] Some data regarding resources and infrastructures are available through census data. Some of these data may be important in understanding community factors that influence health directly (e.g., housing density and crime rates) or that influence health behaviors (e.g., the number of grocery stores that sell fruit and vegetables and land-use patterns may influence dietary patterns and physical activity, respectively). Recent advances in geographic information systems (GIS) technology allows for increased availability and interpretation of these types of geographic or location-based information.[51] Others have developed community audits to assess these factors.[52]

Other advances in assessment are occurring as researchers have begun to explore some factors that could broadly be considered protective social factors. Recently, these factors have been combined to form multidimensional constructs such as collective efficacy, social capital, and community capacity.[21,53–56] Some of the dimensions included are psychosocial (such as social support), while others could arguably be considered more structural (job availability, civic engagement). Most of these constructs build upon the basic dimensions of social networks and social support and individual and community control.[10,57–61] As a result they have several common dimensions including aspects of social networks, civic engagement (voting, involvement in community-based activities and organizations), sense of belonging to one's community, and social (mis)trust. However, the conceptualization of these constructs varies in the extent to which they refer to individual resources versus community resources, how they operationalize key dimensions (e.g., some look at social networks or the structure of social ties, while others look at social support or the function of social ties) and the availability of valid and reliable measurement tools to assess the impact of the construct on health.[62] Some have suggested that these factors influence health directly (i.e., less access to health care, education, housing, etc.), while others suggest that perceptions of inequity affect health through psychological (stress, frustration, anger) and behavioral (eating, drinking, smoking) factors.[21,63,64] Still others have noted that it is important to understand the influence of the physical environment and resources or assets (e.g., recreation facilities, parks, libraries)[1] as well as historical and cultural factors and relationships (including classism and racism) that have not been explicitly included in many of the existing community constructs. Information on these factors can be collected via quantitative instruments (e.g., surveys), qualitative interviews, observational data (e.g., community audits), and census data.

Planning and Implementation

Once these assessment data are collected and analyzed, the community coalition as a whole decides the appropriate next step(s). As stated earlier, the desired level of integration may suggest a new referral network or more integrated services. However, should the coalition decide to work toward a common action or program, the assessments can be used to develop a program plan. A key component of the program plan is the development of a logic model or a program theory.[46–48,50,65,66] A logic model identifies specific activities and how they will lead to the accomplishment of objectives, and how these objectives will enhance the likelihood of accomplishing program goals. For exam ple, a logic model lays out what the program participants will do (e.g., attend an educational session on breast cancer screening at their church), what their activities will lead to (increased knowledge regarding risk factors for breast cancer and specific methods of breast cancer screening), what the short-range impact will be (increase breast cancer screening rates), and what long term outcome can be expected (decreased morbidity due to breast cancer). Depending on the focus of the coalition, Model Standards, APEX*PH*, or MAPP may be helpful in developing appropriate objectives.

Several authors have conceptualized this process somewhat differently,[47,50,65–67] yet the overall intent is that the program or policy be laid out with specific program objectives and activities that are expected to have an impact on clearly delineated outcomes in both the short and long term. While there are many unintended consequences of programs and policies, many argue that it is not possible to effectively evaluate a program until a logic model is specified. As stated by Rossi, Freeman, and Lipsey,[47] "evaluation in the absence of this results in a 'black box' effect in that the evaluation may provide information with regard to the effects but not the processes that produced or failed to produce these effects." Moreover, because so many of the long-term outcomes in health education and promotion are not evident until some time after a program is implemented (e.g., decreases in morbidity due to lung cancer), it is essential to ascertain if more short-term outcomes (e.g., decreases in current smoking rates) are being achieved.

The specific program or policy activities that will be developed should be determined by their ability to meet the objectives outlined in the logic model and should be based on sound theories or models of behavior and community change including social cognitive theory,[68,69] theory of reasoned action and theory of planned behavior,[70] and community development.[70–73] Program strategies should also be determined based on an assessment of the resources available (e.g., availability of recreation facilities, access to various types of foods) and the extent to which proposed programs complement rather than compete with existing programs. In addition, consideration

should be given to the extent to which the program strategies are appropriate for the intended program users, with particular attention paid to cultural appropriateness of strategies and materials and consistency with community norms.[38,74] Last, interventions are most likely to be effective when they target the root causes of the issues and intervene at multiple levels of the ecological framework.[1,75–79]

The PATCH and Healthy Cities/Healthy Communities materials are helpful for coalitions at this stage.[33–37] Other references also have worksheets and information that can be helpful.[40,52,80]

Evaluation

Evaluation of community-based public health initiatives is essential to understand the extent to which programs are meeting the intended objectives. Evaluation is typically broken down into three phases: process, impact, and outcome evaluation.

Process Evaluation

This type of evaluation addresses the questions of program implementation, for example, "To what extent is the program being implemented as planned?" "Are program materials and content appropriate for the population being served?" "Who is attending educational sessions?" "Are all potential participants participating equally?" "Does the program have sufficient resources?" "What percent of the program are most participants receiving (100%, 75%, 50%, 25%)?" These data are important to document changes that have been, and need to be, made to enhance program success and to enable the program to be implemented at other sites. Information for process evaluation can be collected through quantitative and qualitative methods including: observations, field notes, interviews, questionnaires, program records, and local newspapers and publications. Published examples of process evaluation exist in the literature.[81,82]

Impact Evaluation

Impact assesses the extent to which program objectives are being met.[46–48,83] Some also refer to this as an assessment of intermediate or proximal outcomes, both to acknowledge the importance of short-term outcomes and to acknowledge that impact evaluation can assess intended as well as unintended consequences.[48,84–88] Data collected for impact evaluation may be qualitative or quantitative.

Outcome Evaluation

This type of evaluation provides feedback on changes in health status, morbidity, mortality, and quality of life that can be attributed to the program. These more distal outcomes are difficult to attribute to a particular program because it takes so long for these effects to be seen and because changes in these outcomes are influenced by factors outside the confines of the program itself. Assessment of a program's influence on these outcomes, therefore, is often thought to require certain types of evaluation designs (experimental and quasi-experimental designs rather than observational) and long-term follow-up.

Because no evaluation can evaluate all program components, members of the community coalition should, prior to collecting data, agree on which objectives will be measured. This can be specified as part of the development of the logic model discussed above. It may be appropriate to alternate the types of data collected over months or years of a program to meet multiple programmatic and coalition member needs.

SUMMARY AND CONCLUSIONS

Community assessment and change processes are increasingly important given the essential public health roles of assessment, assurance, and policy development. However, while standardized models exist to assist practitioners who are interested in utilizing these approaches, it is essential that these be seen as providing guidelines and tools rather than as directives for proper action. It is advisable for health practitioners, community-based organizations, and community members to recognize that the lens through which they see the world is often limited. It is only by acting collaboratively that coalitions and other community groups can integrate each other's perspectives and obtain a more complete view of the world. Previous experiences within a community and experiences from other communities can help inform strategies, but each coalition will need to develop its own plan for action. There are no maps available for these endeavors; rather, coalitions engaging in community assessment and change will need to chart their course by walking together.

References

1. Altman DG, Goodman R, Community intervention. In: Baum A, Revenson T, Singer JE, eds. *Handbook of Health Psychology*. Mahwah, NJ: Lawrence Erlbaum Associates Publishers; 2001:591-612.
2. Elder J, et al. Organizational and community approaches to community-wide prevention of heart disease: The first two years of the Pawtucket Heart Health Program. *Prev Med.*, 1986;15:107-117.
3. Farquhar J, et al. The Stanford Five-City Project: Design and methods. *Am J Epidemiol.*, 1985;122:323-334.
4. Jacobs D, et al. Community-wide prevention strategies: Evaluation design of the Minnesota Heart Health Program. *J Chronic Dis.*, 1986;39:775-788.
5. Mittelmark MB, et al. Realistic outcomes: Lessons from community-based research and demonstration programs for the prevention of cardiovascular diseases. *J Public Health Policy.* 1993;14:437-462.
6. Krueter MW, Lezin N, Young L. Evaluating community-based collaborative mechanisms: Implications for practitioners. *Health Promotion Pract.* 2000;1:49-63.
7. Fisher EB. Editorial: The results of the COMMIT trial. *Amer J Public Health.* 1995;85:159-160.
8. Butterfoss F, Goodman R, Wandersman A. Community coalitions for prevention and health promotion: Factors predicting satisfaction, participation and planning. *Health Educ Q.* 1996;23(1):65-79.
9. Green L, McAlister A. Macro-intervention to support health behavior: Some theoretical perspectives and practical reflections. *Health Educ Q.* 1984;11:322-339.
10. Israel B, et al. Health education and community empowerment: Conceptualizing and measuring perceptions of

individual, organizational and community control. *Health Educ Q* 1994;21(2):149-170.

11. McLeroy K, et al. An ecological perspective on health promotion programs. *Health Educ Q.* 1988;15(4):351-377.

12. Stokols D, Allen J, Bellingham RL. The social ecology of health promotion: Implications for research and practice. *Am J Health Promotion.* 1996;10:247-251.

13. Green L, Kreuter M. *Health Promotion Planning: An Educational and Ecological Approach.* 3rd ed. Mountain View, Calif: Mayfield Publishing Co; 1999.

14. Green L, Kreuter M. CDC's planned approach to community health as an application of PRECEED and an inspiration for PROCEED. *J Health Educ.* 1992;23:140-147.

15. Shinn M. Special issue: Ecological assessment. *A Journal Community Psychol.* 1996;24(1).

16. World Health Organization, Health and Welfare Canada, and C.P.H. Association. Ottawa charter for health promotion. In: *International Conference on Health Promotion.* Ottawa, Ontario, Canada; 1986.

17. McGinnis J, Foege W. Actual causes of death in the United States. *JAMA.* 1993;270(18):2207-2212.

18. Patrick D, Wickizer T. Community and health. In: Amick B, et al., eds. *Society and Health.* New York, NY: Oxford University Press; 1995.

19. Institute of Medicine. *Linking Research and Public Health Practice: A Review of CDC's Program of Centers for Research and Demonstration of Health Promotion and Disease Prevention.* Washington, DC: National Academy Press; 1997.

20. Gottlieb B. Using social support to promote and protect health. *J Primary Prev.* 1987;8:49-70.

21. Hawe P, Shiell A. Social capital and health promotion: a review. *Soc Sci & Med.* 2000;51:871-885.

22. McKnight J. Rationale for a community approach to health improvement. In: Bruce T, Uranga McKane S, eds. *Community-Based Public Health: A Partnership Model.* Washington, DC: American Public Health Association; 2000.

23. Paxman D, Lee P, Satcher D. Public health status at the beginning of the twenty-first century. In: Bruce T, Uranga McKane S, eds. *Community-Based Public Health: A Partnership Approach.* Washington, DC: American Public Health Association; 2000.

24. Baker E, Brownson R. Community-based prevention: Blending community and scientific expertise. In: Novick L, Mays G, eds. *Public Health Administration: Principles of Population-Based Management.* Gaithersburg, Md: Aspen Publishers; 2001.

25. Bruce T, Uranga McKane S. *Community-Based Public Health. A Partnership Approach.* Washington, DC: American Public Health Association; 2000.

26. O'Fallon L, Tyson F, Dearry A. Successful models of community-based participatory research. In: *National Institute of Environmental Health Sciences.* Washington, DC: National Institutes of Health; 2000.

27. Israel B, et al. Review of community-based research: Assessing partnership approaches to improve public health. *Annu Rev Public Health.* 1998;19:173-202.

28. Butterfoss F, Goodman R, Wandersman A. Community coalitions for prevention and health promotion. *Health Educ Res.* 1993;8(3):315-330.

29. Parker E, et al. Coalition building for prevention. *J Public Health Manage and Pract.* 1998;4(2):25-36.

30. Alter C, Hage J. *Organizations Working Together: Coordination in Interorganizational Networks.* Newbury Park, Calif: Sage Publications; 1992.

31. US Department of Health and Human Services. *Healthy Communities 2000: Model Standards, Guidelines for Community Attainment of the Year 2000 National Health Objectives.* Washington, DC: US Department of Health and Human Services; 1991.

32. *APEX/PH, Assessment Protocol for Excellence in Public Health.* Washington, DC: National Association of County and City Health Officials; 1991.

33. Kreuter M. Health Promotion: The role of public health in the community of free exchange. In: *Health Promotion Monographs.* New York, NY: Center for Health Promotion, Columbia University; 1984.

34. World Health Organization. *Promoting Health in the Urban Context: Five-Year Planning Framework: A Guide to Assessing Health Cities.* Copenhagen, Denmark: World Health Organization regional office for Europe; 1988.

35. Toronto, CA. *Toronto's First State of the City Report. Produced for Healthy City Toronto.* Toronto, Canada: City Clerk, Communication Services Division; 1993.

36. World Health Organization. *Five-Year Planning Project: Healthy Cities Project.* Copenhagen, Denmark: World Health Organization; 1988.

37. World Health Organization. *Global Strategy of Health for All by the Year 2000.* Geneva, Switzerland: World Health Organization; 1981.

38. Gonzalez V, et al. *Health Promotion in Diverse Cultural Communities.* Palo Alto, Calif: Health Promotion Resource Center; 1991.

39. Braithwaite R, et al. Community organization and development for health promotion within an urban Black community: A conceptual model. *Health Educ.* 1989;20(5):56-60.

40. Johnson K, Grossman W, Cassidy A. *Collaborating to Improve Community Health: Workbook and Guide to Best Practices in Creating Healthier Communities and Populations.* San Francisco, Calif: Jossey-Bass; 1996.

41. Rowel R, Terry R. Establishing interorganizational arrangements between volunteer community-based groups. *Health Educ.* 1989;20(5):52-55.

42. Wolff T, Kaye G. *From the Ground Up! A Workbook on Coalition Building and Community Development.* Amherst, Mass: AHEC/Community Partners; 1991.

43. Diller J. *Cultural Diversity: A Primer for the Human Services.* Belmont, Calif: Wadsworth Publishing; 1999.

44. Lecca P, et al. *Cultural Competency in Health, Social and Human Services: Directions for the Twenty-first Century.* New York, NY: Garland Publishing Inc; 1998.

45. Holmes L, et al. *Enhancing Cultural Awareness and Communication Skills: A Training Program for HealthStart Providers.* Trenton, NJ: HealthStart Provider Education and Outreach Services; 1989.

46. Milstein R, Wetterhall S. *Framework for Program Evaluation in Public Health.* Atlanta, Ga: Centers for Disease Control and Prevention; 1999.

47. Rossi P, Freeman H, Lipsey M. *Evaluation: A Systematic Approach.* 6th ed. Thousand Oaks, Calif: Sage Publications; 1999.

48. Israel B, et al. Evaluation of health education programs: Current assessment and future directions. *Health Educ Q.* 1995;22(3):364-389.

49. Baker Q. et al. *An Evaluation Framework for Community Health Programs.* Durham, NC: The Center for the Advancement of Community Based Public Health; 2000.

50. Goodman R. Principles and tools for evaluating community-based prevention and health promotion programs. *J Public Health Manage and Pract.* 1998;4(2):37-47.

51. Richards T, et al. Geographic information systems and public health: mapping the future. *Public Health Rep.* 1999(114):359-373.

52. Kretzmann J, McKnight J. *Building Communities from the Inside Out: A Path toward Finding and Mobilizing a Community's Assets.* Chicago, Ill: ACTA Publications; 1993.

53. Goodman R, et al. Identifying and defining the dimensions of community capacity to provide a basis for measurement. *Health Educ and Behav.* 1998;25(3):258-278.

54. Coleman J. *The Foundations of Social Theory.* Cambridge, Mass: Harvard University Press; 1990.

55. Kawachi I, et al. Social capital, income inequality, and mortality. *Am J Public Health.* 1997;87(9):1491-1498.

56. Sampson R, Raudenbush S, Earls F. Neighborhoods and violent crime: A multilevel study of collective efficacy. *Science.* 1997;277:913-924.

57. Berkman L, Syme S. Social networks, host resistance and mortality: A nine-year follow-up study of Alameda county residents. *Am J Epidemiol.* 1979;109(2):186-204.

58. Cassel J. The contribution of the social environment to host resistance. *Am J Epidemiol.* 1976;104:108-123.

59. Cwikel J, et al. Mechanisms of pyschosocial effects on health: The role of social integration, coping style and health behavior. *Health Educ Q.* 1988;15(2):151-173.

60. House J, Umberson D, Landis K. Social relationships and health. *Science.* 1988;241:540-545.

61. Israel B, Rounds K. Social networks and social support: A synthesis for health educators. In: *Advances in Health Education and Promotion;* 1987:311-351.

62. Lochner K, Kawachi I, Kennedy B. Social capital: A guide to its measurement. *Health and Place.* 1999;5:259-270.

63. Lynch J, Kaplan G. Understanding how inequality in the distribution of income affects health. *J Health Psychol.* 1997;2(3):297-314.

64. Lynch J, et al. Income inequality and mortality: Importance to health or individual income, psychosocial environment, or material conditions. *British Med J.* 2000;320:1200-1204.

65. Goodman R, Wandersman A. FORECAST: A formative approach to evaluating the CSAP community partnerships. *J Community Psychol.* 1994; special issue: 6-25.

66. Patton M. *Qualitative Evaluation and Research Methods.* Newbury Park, Calif: Sage Publications; 1990.

67. Bartholomew L, Parcel G, Kok G. Intervention Mapping: A process for developing theory and evidence-based health education programs. *Health Educ & Behav.* 1998;25(5):545-563.

68. Bandura A. *Social Foundations of Thought and Action: A Social Cognitive Theory.* Englewood Cliffs, NJ: Prentice-Hall; 1986.

69. Bandura A. *Self-efficacy: The Exercise of Control.* New York, NY: Freeman; 1997.

70. Montano D, Kasprzyk D, Talin S. The theory of reasoned action and the theory of planned behavior. In: Glanz K, Lewis F, Rimer B, eds. *Health Behavior and Health Education.* 2nd ed. Jossey-Bass: San Francisco, Calif: 1997.

71. Lefebvre R, et al. Theory and delivery of health programming in the community: The Pawtucket Heart Health Program. *Prev Med.* 1987;16:80-95.

72. Bracht N, Kingsbury L. Community organization principles in health promotion: A five-stage model. In: Bracht N, ed. *Health Promotion at the Community Level,* Newbury Park, Calif: Sage Publications; 1990:66-88.

73. Bracht N, Tsouros A. Principles and strategies of effective community participation. *Health Promotion Int.* 1990:5(3):199-208.

74. Altman D, et al. Psychosocial factors associated with youth involvement in community activities promoting heart health. *Health Educ and Behav.* 1998;25(4):489-500.

75. Baker E, Brownson C. Defining characteristics of community-based health promotion programs. *J Public Health Manage and Pract.* 1998:4(2):1-9.

76. Cheadle A, et al. An empirical exploration of a conceptual model for community-based health promotion. *Int Q Community Health Educ.* 1993;13(4):329-363.

77. Elder J, et al. Community heart health programs: components, rationale and strategies for effective interventions. *J Public Health Policy.* 1993;4:463-479.

78. Mittelmark M, et al. Realistic outcomes: Lessons from community-based research and demonstration programs for the prevention of cardiovascular disease. *J Public Health Policy.* 1993;4:437-462.

79. Stokols D. Establishing and maintaining healthy environments: Toward a social ecology of health promotion. *Am Psychol.* 1992;47(1):6-22.

80. DiLima S. *Community Health Education and Promotion: A Guide to Program Design and Evaluation.* Gaithersburg, Md: Aspen Publishers; 1997.

81. Stone E, et al. Process evaluation in the multicenter Child and Adolescent Trial for Cardiovascular Health (CATCH). *Health Educ Q.* 1994;special issue(2):S1-S148.

82. Williams J, et al. Process evaluation methods of a peer-delivered health promotion program for African American women. *Health Promotion Pract.* 2001;2(2):135-142.

83. Herman J, Morris L, Fitz-Gibbon C. *Evaluator's Handbook.* Newbury Park, Calif: Sage Publications; 1987.

84. Resnicow K, et al. GO GIRLS! Results from a nutrition and physical activity program for low-income, overweight African American adolescent females. *Health Educ & Behav.* 2000;27(5):616-632.

85. COMMIT Research Group. Community Intervention Trial for Smoking Cessation: Summary of design and intervention. *J Nat Cancer Inst.* 1991;83:1620-1628.

86. COMMIT Research Group. Community Intervention Trial for Smoking Cessation: Cohort results from a four-year community intervention. *Am J Public Health.* 1995;85(2):183-192.

87. COMMIT Research Group. Community Intervention Trial for Smoking Cessation: Changes in adult cigarette smoking prevalence. *Am J Public Health.* 1995;85(2):193-200.

88. Clark N, et al. Impact of self-management education on the functional health status of older adults with heart disease. *Gerontologist.* 1986;32:438-443.

CHAPTER
12

Performance Measurement and Management in Public Health

Paul K. Halverson, M.H.S.A., Dr.P.H.
Glen P. Mays, M.P.H., Ph.D.

Public health organizations engage in a broad and expanding array of activities to protect and improve health at the population level. Tracking the work performed and results achieved in such complex institutional settings requires formal processes to measure public health outputs and outcomes, and valid methods to compare this production with established goals and expectations. The process of obtaining such measures and using them to evaluate the operation of an organization or program has become known as *performance measurement*. Similarly, the process of using such measures to enhance the production of desired outputs and the achievement of desired outcomes has become known as *performance management*.

These terms have achieved widespread use only recently in the field of public health, but the concepts they reflect have been familiar to public health professionals in the United States for most of the twentieth century. Contemporary methods of performance measurement and management derive from industrial quality improvement concepts that became popular in American business administration during the 1980s,[1] and later in public administration and health administration during the 1990s.[2–5] More recently, public health organizations at local, state, and national levels have begun to use these concepts together with basic principles of epidemiological investigation to monitor and improve the population-based activities carried out in public health.[6–9]

This chapter examines historical and contemporary trends in applying performance measurement concepts and methods to public health organizations in the United States. This exploration reveals that public health performance measurement initiatives, though still in their adolescence, are poised to have profound effects on the future structure and operation of public health organizations.

RATIONALE: WHY PERFORMANCE MEASUREMENT IN PUBLIC HEALTH?

Supporting Management

Performance measurement methods can be used in public health settings for a variety of purposes. Perhaps the most compelling rationale for using these methods stems from their utility as managerial tools for improving the quality, effectiveness, and efficiency of the programs and services produced in these settings.[7,9,10] Equipped with reliable information about how well various activities are performed within an organization or multiorganizational system, public health managers can reallocate resources and redesign work processes to address identified performance gaps. In this way, performance measurement activities can function as powerful tools for identifying problems and targeting solutions. Such tools are increasingly important to organizations operating in contemporary public health environments in which health risks and core institutional and financial structures are continually in flux. Public health organizations must adapt their operations on an ongoing basis in response to fluctuations in governmental spending for public health programs, realignments in the constellation of organizations that contribute to public health activities, and shifts in population demographics and disease patterns. In this context, managerial decision making can be substantially compromised without reliable and timely information about public health outputs and outcomes.

Ensuring Accountability

Performance measurement also holds the potential to generate external pressure for improvements in public health effectiveness and efficiency. Organizations that provide financial support or other resources to public health organizations can use performance measurement activities to ensure accountability for these resources and for the expectations and objectives that accompany them. For this reason, a growing number of state health agencies maintain performance measurement processes for the local public health agencies with which they work.[8] Performance measurement processes can also serve as the basis for performance-based contracting policies and performance-based payment systems that are designed to create incentives for efficiency and effectiveness in service delivery.[11,12]

Provisions of the federal Government Performance and Results Act of 1993 require federal agencies to develop these types of measurement and accountability systems as part of their contracting and grant-in-aid programs.[4] By the same token, public health organizations that depend on external sources of funding can use performance measurement activities to demonstrate their capacities and competencies to governmental policy makers, foundations, health plans, private purchasers, and other entities that control the allocation of resources in public health. Public health organizations then can enhance their ability to secure contracts, grants, governmental appropriations, and other vital public health resources. For this reason, performance measurement activities can serve as the basis for professional accreditation programs that provide organizations with a credential signaling their capacities and competencies. If broadly disseminated, these activities can also help raise public awareness of and support for public health capacities and needs, and address taxpayer concerns about the efficiency of government-funded services.[2]

Informing Policy

A third rationale for using performance measurement activities in public health stems from their ability to support rational policy development and resource allocation decisions. Public health organizations can use performance measurement activities to identify unmet resource needs and to target public health resources to meet these needs. The resource allocation decisions informed by such measurement activities may involve funding, deployment of personnel and technology, placement of programs and clinics, and dissemination of information and expertise. Public health policy makers may also use performance measurement activities to identify new ways of configuring public health delivery systems to ensure maximum coverage and to achieve operational efficiencies. For example, decision makers may use these measures to identify ways of consolidating public health delivery systems in order to pool their collective capacities and realize economies of scale. Moreover, performance measurement activities can be used to track and evaluate the effects of resource allocation and policy decisions on public health outputs and outcomes, thereby creating a feedback mechanism to inform subsequent policy and administrative decisions. In these ways, information produced by performance measurement activities potentially allows for a more efficient and equitable allocation of limited public health resources to populations in need.

Building a Research Base for Practice

A final rationale for using performance measurement activities in public health involves the opportunities for practice-based research and scientific discovery. When broadly and carefully implemented, performance measurement activities can support scientific investigations of the effects of specific public health resources, programs, and policies on public health outcomes.[7,13] Such practice-based observational studies have become the hallmark of the health outcomes research efforts carried out in medical care settings, and they have therefore fueled the development of clinical practice guidelines and the practice of evidence-based medicine in these settings.[14] The field of public health has lagged behind in comparable initiatives to develop evidence-based practice standards and guidelines, largely because the science base for public health practice has been slower to develop. Performance measurement activities can produce the information needed to fuel additional practice-based research initiatives in public health. A variety of methodological challenges must be overcome in using these observational data bases for scientific investigation.[13] Nonetheless, performance measurement activities potentially create exciting opportunities for investigating the effectiveness of public health programs and policies in actual practice settings.

HISTORY OF PUBLIC HEALTH PERFORMANCE MEASUREMENT

Early Foundations

Efforts to measure the outputs and outcomes of public health programs have occurred throughout the twentieth century (for a complete review, see the excellent analysis by Turnock and Handler).[15] The American Public Health Association (APHA) created the foundation for modern public health performance measurement through a series of studies targeted at local public health agencies during the 1920s through the 1940s (Figure 12.1).[16–22] The objectives of these efforts were twofold: to develop practice standards for local public health agencies to build public health capacity across the nation; and to generate comparative information on public health practice to encourage agencies to improve their performance and to mobilize public and political support for public health practice.[9,15] These objectives have remained paramount for virtually all of the public health performance measurement activities that followed these early efforts.[7,23]

The APHA's initiatives relied on voluntary participation by public health agencies, and most were based wholly on quantitative measures of the outputs produced by these agencies, such as the number of immunizations administered or the number of prenatal home visits delivered. In the initial efforts, measures were collected through site visits made to participating agencies by appraisers. Later, when broad participation became the focus, measures were collected using a self-assessment appraisal form completed by agency administrators. A numerical scoring process was devised to create an aggregate rating of each agency's performance, and ratings were made available to agencies, government officials, and the public to support comparisons across agencies. The APHA's performance measurement instrument was eventually expanded to include some measures of public health outcomes, such as statistics on infant mortality and motor vehicle deaths.[19,21] In the expanded instrument, performance scores were summarized by size and type of agency to facilitate comparisons among agencies of similar structure. On the

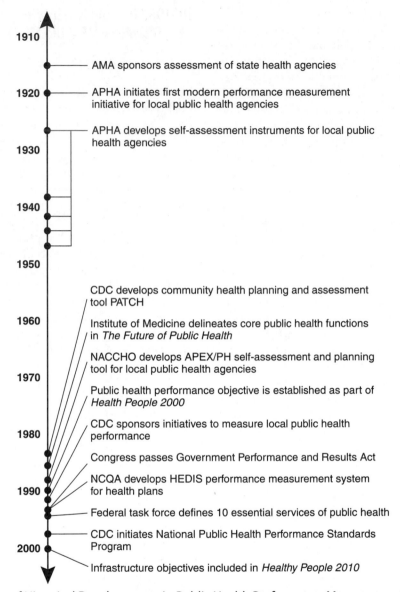

Figure 12.1. Time Line of Historical Developments in Public Health Performance Measurement
Source: Authors.

whole, public health administrators found these early performance measurement activities to be helpful in managing their programs and organizations.[15] Nonetheless, most of these activities were discontinued in the 1950s as the APHA's interests turned to other issues.[9]

Efforts to measure the performance of state public health agencies have occurred less frequently than those focusing on the local level. The earliest state-level initiative, sponsored by the American Medical Association in 1914, relied on a quantitative scoring system that reflected the scope of services provided by state health agencies and the extent of their efforts to develop local public health units.[15,24] Much later, the Association of State and Territorial Health Officials developed a national reporting system that tracked annual trends in state health agency expenditures and services throughout much of the 1970s and 1980s.[9] These efforts supported basic comparisons of state public health infrastructure, but they lacked the detailed and quantitative measures of outputs and outcomes that would be necessary for a more complete analysis of public health capacity and performance.

A Second Generation of Measurement

The Institute of Medicine's (IOM) 1988 study of the nation's public health system sparked a revival of interest in and support for performance measurement in public health.[25] This renewed interest was fueled not only by the alarming gaps in public health performance and capacity profiled in the report, but also by the report's delineation of the concept of "core public health functions."[26] These concepts provided public health scholars and practitioners with a simple and intuitive framework for describing the scope of public health activity, and a framework from which performance measures and performance standards could be derived. The Institute's report also raised awareness about the fundamental activities that support and inform the delivery of specific programs and services, such as needs assessment, coalition-building, advocacy, education, policy development, and planning. As a consequence, the performance measurement activities that developed subsequent to the IOM's report were more reflective of these basic public health activities than previous efforts.[9]

Soon after publication of the report, the U.S. Public Health Service established Objective 8.14 as one of its national Healthy People 2000 objectives for the year 2000, which called for 90 percent of the U.S. population to be served by a local health department that effectively carries out the core functions of public health.[27] In response to this objective, the U.S. Centers for Disease Control and Prevention (CDC) sponsored an array of research and development efforts during the 1990s designed to identify the specific

practice elements that comprise core public health functions, and to develop ways of measuring the extent to which these elements are performed by public health agencies.

A variety of self-assessment tools and planning protocols were developed during this period to assist public health agencies in improving their performance, many of which used measures of public health processes, outputs, and outcomes to evaluate performance. One of the most prominent of these tools, the Planned Approach to Community Health (PATCH), was originally developed by the (CDC) in 1985.[28] Expanding on this effort, the APHA developed an assessment protocol in 1991, *Healthy Communities 2000: Model Standards,* based on measures that linked directly with the national health objectives identified in the U.S. Public Health Service's *Healthy People 2000* planning document.[29]

Another assessment and planning tool, the Assessment Protocol for Excellence in Public Health (APEX*PH*), was developed by the National Association of County and City Health Officials (NACCHO) with sponsorship from CDC in 1991 to serve as a self-assessment workbook for public health officials.[30] The workbook included measures for assessing the internal capacity of public health organizations as well as the external capacity of other organizations serving the community. The workbook used an array of indicators measuring public health structures and outputs (processes), including those addressing public health authority, community relations, community health assessment, policy development, financial management, personnel management, program management, and governing board procedures. Subsequent refinements and expansions of this protocol, including the Assessment and Planning Excellence through Community Partners for Health (APEX-*CPH*) and the Mobilizing for Action through Planning and Partnerships (MAPP), have developed new measures of community capacity to reflect the contributions of a broader array of community organizations and activities.[31,32]

The public health assessment and planning tools developed during this period were designed to stimulate improvements in performance within individual public health organizations. Building on these efforts, the CDC sponsored a series of research initiatives during the 1990s to measure and compare performance of core public health functions across the nation's local public health system, in order to track progress toward Objective 8.14 of *Healthy People 2000*. Several of these efforts were designed around a set of 10 public health practices, each of which were derived from one of the IOM's three public health functions by a workgroup convened by the CDC.[33] All of these initiatives relied on measures of public health outputs or processes, such as whether the local population is surveyed routinely for behavioral risk factors, or whether adverse health events are investigated on a routine basis.

One group of studies focused specifically on activities performed by local governmental public health agencies.[34–38] A second group of studies used measures that reflected the activities performed by not only local public health agencies, but also the range of other organizations that potentially contribute to public health activities at the local level.[39–41] Ultimately, indicators from the two groups of studies were combined into a merged set of performance measures and used in several national surveys of local public health performance.[42] Interestingly, all of the CDC-sponsored performance measurement activities undertaken during the 1990s produced similar results indicating that, on average, about half of the activities regarded as important elements of public health practice are performed at the local level (Table 12.1).[15]

Individual states also became active in implementing performance measurement activities for local public health agencies during the decade of the 1990s. In some cases, these activities were developed in response to the demands of state legislatures and taxpayers for greater accountability in the use of public funds. In other cases, these efforts were undertaken as strategies to enhance the capacity of state and local public health delivery systems in the wake of the 1988 IOM report.

A 1998 survey of the nation's state health agencies revealed that 22 agencies currently had a local public health performance measurement process in place, and another 13 agencies were in the process of developing such a process.[8] Only 4 agencies indicated that they did not currently face a substantial need for a performance measurement process. Among the agencies with a measurement process in place or under development, 73 percent indicated that the process was designed to operate statewide, whereas 27 percent indicated that the process covered only a subset of local public health jurisdictions. Nearly two-thirds of these agencies used externally developed performance measures as part of their process, while the remaining one-third developed all of their measures internally. The most commonly reported use of performance measures was state-level planning and policy development (39 percent), followed by information provision to local agencies (20 percent), state resource allo-

Table 12.1. Estimates of Local Public Health Performance Produced by Recent Studies

Study	Year	Population/Sample size	Estimate
NACCHO	1990	All U.S. agencies/$N=1{,}967$	50%
NACCHO	1992–1993	All U.S. agencies/$N=2{,}191$	46%
Miller et al.	1992	Nonrandom selection of local jurisdictions/$N=14$	57%
Turnock et al.	1993	All U.S. agencies/$N=208$	50%
Richards et al.	1993	All local jurisdictions in 6 states/$N=370$	56%
Halverson et al.	1992–1993	Nonrandom selection of local jurisdictions/$N=64$	51%
Rohrer et al.	1995	All Iowa county agencies/$N=96$	61%
Turnock et al.	1994	All U.S. agencies/$N=298$	56%
Mays et al.	1998	All U.S. jurisdictions with at least 100,000 residents/$N=356$	65%

Source: Turnock BJ, Handler AS. From measuring to improving public health practice. *Annu Rev Public Health.* 1997;18:261-282.

cation decision making (16 percent), state legislature budgetary negotiations (7 percent), and public health program evaluation (5 percent). Several states developed formal accreditation and certification programs for local public health agencies based on their performance measurement systems.

Public and Private Sector Stimuli

The movement toward performance measurement in public health was fueled during the 1990s by federal efforts to address concerns about governmental inefficiency and accountability by developing new systems to monitor the activities and results of federal programs. In 1993 Congress passed the Government Performance and Results Act, which required federal agencies to develop systems for measuring the performance of all federally funded programs. In response to this legislation, the U.S. Department of Health and Human Services proposed the creation of Performance Partnership Grants that would require the use of performance measurement methods in federal block grant programs that support state activities in public health, substance abuse, and mental health services. A performance measurement process based on the essential public health services has already been developed and implemented for state programs funded under the Maternal and Child Health Services Block Grant,[43] and similar processes are under development for other federal grant programs. The National Research Council identified an extensive set of performance measures and data systems that could be used for these purposes.[44]

Public health performance measurement activities were also stimulated and informed during the 1990s by a variety of private-sector initiatives to measure and improve the performance among health care institutions. The most visible of these initiatives has been the Health Plan Employer Data and Information Set (HEDIS), a voluntary performance measurement system developed for health plans in 1991 by a coalition of large health care purchasers that eventually formed the National Committee for Quality Assurance (NCQA). Designed to inform purchasing decisions, the NCQA collects and compares annual measures of health plan performance

in areas such as health care effectiveness, accessibility, utilization, cost, and patient satisfaction. The HEDIS system includes detailed standards for data collection, measurement, and auditing that participating plans were required to meet.[45] The HEDIS system has been administered by the NCQA since 1992, and is used as part of the NCQA's accreditation program for health plans. Another major performance measurement initiative was launched by the Joint Commission on Accreditation of Healthcare Organizations (JCAHO) in 1996 to enhance its accreditation process for hospitals and other health care facilities. Known as Project ORYX, the JCAHO's initiative allows participating organizations some flexibility in the types of measures that are used to track their performance.

Several other large-scale performance measurement initiatives were launched during the 1990s for health care institutions, including a system for medical groups developed by the Medical Group Management Association, and a system for physician practices developed by the American Medical Association (the American Medical Accreditation Program). In response to the proliferation of performance measurement processes, several initiatives formed to develop consensus around core sets of health care performance measures, and to facilitate the dissemination and use of these measures by health care providers, consumers, and purchasers. One of these initiatives, the Foundation for Accountability (FACCT), was formed in 1995 to facilitate the use of performance measures by health care consumers. The National Forum for Health Care Quality Measurement and Reporting was launched in 1999 to develop a coordinated national strategy for performance measurement among health care institutions in the public and private sectors.[46]

Most recently, the CDC has begun to develop and implement a national performance measurement initiative for public health organizations that builds upon many of the measurement activities that have been undertaken to date.[7] As part of the National Public Health Performance Standards Program, the CDC convened a broad group of public health scientists and practitioners to develop standards of practice in various public health settings, along with measures and surveillance instruments that track progress toward these standards. The program, which is based on the voluntary participation of public health organizations, pursues three interrelated goals: improved quality, enhanced public accountability, and expanded scientific investigation in public health practice.

At present, separate but related sets of performance standards and measurement instruments have been developed for local public health systems, state public health systems, and public health governing boards. Performance standards and measures have been specified at the level of the public health system—which comprises the full range of public and private organizations that contribute to public health—rather than at the level of the individual public health agency. Each performance standard is linked directly to 1 of the 10 essential public health services identified by a workgroup of major public health stakeholders in 1994.[47] Once fully operational, the National Public Health Performance Standards Program promises to be an unparalleled resource for informing administrative, policy, and clinical decision making in public health.

Anticipating the capabilities of this program, a series of national health objectives related to public health infrastructure have been included in the *Healthy People 2010* planning document developed by the U.S. Department of Health and Human Services.[48] A total of 17 infrastructure objectives were developed, including those related to public health data and information systems, the public health workforce, public health organizations, public health resources, and prevention research. Progress toward each of these objectives will be monitored and encouraged through the CDC's National Public Health Performance Standards Program (Table 12.2). Objective 23-11 directly addresses the ability of the program to engage the nation's public health organizations performance measurement and improvement initiatives, by calling for an increase in "the proportion of state and local public health agencies that meet national performance standards for essential public health services."[48]

CRITICAL ISSUES IN PERFORMANCE MEASUREMENT

A variety of measurement issues have come to light during the nation's 80-year experiment with performance measurement activities in public health. These issues include both conceptual problems and methodological challenges that must be considered implicitly or explicitly when designing, managing, or participating in a performance measurement process. Key among these issues are:

- the unit of analysis (whose performance is measured, and who is accountable for this performance);
- the scope of activity (which domains of performance are examined);
- the indicators of performance (what information is used to provide evidence of performance in each domain);
- the methods for measuring indicators of performance (how the information is obtained); and
- the methods for comparing and evaluating performance (what standards are used and how they are applied).[13,49]

Each of these issues is explored in detail below.

Unit of Analysis

Public health activities are carried out through an array of important actors and instruments, all of which can be examined through the lens of performance measurement. It is possible to measure and evaluate performance at the level of the individual, the team, the program or division, the organization, and various multi-institutional settings. The appropriate unit of analysis is contingent on the objectives of the performance measurement activity. If the primary goal is to improve performance within a specific program or organization, then measurement should focus on the intraorganizational elements that determine this performance.

A variety of management tools and processes now exist for assessing the function and performance of individuals and teams within an organization, and for creating feedback mechanisms and incentive systems

Table 12.2.   Public Health Infrastructure Objectives Included in Healthy People 2010

Coal:	Ensure that Federal, Tribal, State, and local health agencies have the infrastructure to provide essential public health services effectively.

Objective

Date and Information Systems

23-1   Increase the proportion of Tribal, State, and local public health agencies that provide Internet and e-mail access for at least 75 percent of their employees and that teach employees to use the Internet and other electronic information systems to apply data and information to public health practice

23-2   Increase the proportion of Federal, Tribal, State, and local health agencies that have made information available to the public in the past year on the Leading Health Indicators, Health Status Indicators, and Priority Data Needs

23-3   Increase the proportion of all major National, State, and local health data systems that use geocoding to promote nationwide use of geographic information systems (GIS) at all levels

23-4   Increase the proportion of population-based Healthy People 2010 objectives for which national data are available for all population groups identified for the objective

23-5   Increase the proportion of Leading Health Indicators, Health Status Indicators, and Priority Data Needs for which data—especially for select populations—are available at the Tribal, State, and local levels

23-6   Increase the proportion of Healthy People 2010 objectives that are tracked regularly at the national level

23-7   Increase the proportion of Healthy People 2010 objectives for which national data are released within 1 year of the end of data collection

Workforce

23-8   Increase the proportion of Federal, Tribal, State, and local agencies that incorporate specific competencies in the essential public health services into personnel systems

23-9   Increase the proportion of schools for public health workers that integrate into their curricula specific content to develop competency in the essential public health services

23-10   Increase the proportion of Federal, Tribal, State, and local public health agencies that provide continuing education to develop competency in essential public health services for their employees

Public Health Organizations

23-11   Increase the proportion of State and local public health agencies that meet national performance standards for essential public health services

23-12   Increase the proportion of Tribes, States, and the District of Columbia that have a health improvement plan and increase the proportion of local jurisdictions that have a health improvement plan linked with their State plan

23-13   Increase the proportion of Tribal, State, and local health agencies that provide or assure comprehensive laboratory services to support essential public health services

23-14   Increase the proportion of Tribal, State, and local public health agencies that provide or assure comprehensive epidemiology services to support essential public health services

23-15   Increase the proportion of Federal, Tribal, State, and local jurisdictions that review and evaluate the extent to which their statutes, ordinances, and bylaws assure the delivery of essential public health services

23-16   Increase the proportion of Federal, Tribal, State, and local public health agencies that gather accurate data on public health expenditures, categorized by essential public health service

23-17   Increase the proportion of Federal, Tribal, State, and local public health agencies that conduct or collaborate on population-based prevention research

Source: U.S. Department of Health and Human Services. *Healthy People 2010: Conference Edition*. Washington, DC: U.S. Dept of Health and Human Services; 2000.

to improve performance.[50] The application of such tools is usually context-specific—highly contingent on the structure and size of the institution, the scope and scale of its production processes, and the composition of its workforce. Alternatively, if the overarching goal of the performance measurement activity is to improve performance on a large (e.g., state or national) scale, it is often desirable to focus measurement activities at the organizational and/or multiorganizational levels. The rationale for this choice is that performance measurement at these higher levels motivates organizations to undertake interorganizational improvement efforts in ways that are appropriate to their specific institutional contexts.[4,51]

Public health activities are performed by a variety of organizations operating in different institutional, governmental, and geographic settings. Most of the large-scale public health performance measurement activities carried out to date have focused on the activities performed by governmental public health agencies at the local and/or state levels. In most U.S. settings, these agencies assume primary responsibility for managing the programs and resources that are dedicated to improving population health. Many important public health activities, however, are carried out by other public and private organizations—either alone or in partnership with governmental public health agencies.[8,41] Performance measures that do not account for these outside contributions may provide an incomplete or biased representation of public health capacity in some settings. Consequently, recent initiatives have focused on measuring performance at the level of the public health system, which is specified as the collection of public and private institutions that contribute to public health for a defined population.[7,39,41] The appropriate choice between agency-level and systems-level measures ultimately depends on the overall purpose of the performance measurement activity. Agency-level measures may be appropriate for activities that are concerned exclusively with the structure and operation of governmental public health agencies, independent of other actors within the public health system.

To measure performance at the system level, it is first necessary to identify the common population that this system serves. For purposes of epidemiological investigation, populations can be defined in myriad ways, such as by geographic area of residence, sociodemographic characteristics, health status, or characteristics associated with disease risk. For purposes of public health performance measurement, however, the population of interest is typically defined by the geopolitical jurisdiction to which and for which governmental public health agencies are accountable.[39] Although these agencies do not directly perform all of the public health activities that occur within their jurisdictions, they are ultimately accountable for these activities (or lack of activities) and their effects on population health. Consequently, public health performance measurement activities typically focus on the jurisdictions served by local and/or state public health agencies.

Choosing the unit of analysis for a performance measurement process has important implications for the downstream activities of developing specific measures of performance and collecting data for these measures. Measuring the activities undertaken by governmental public health agencies is often straightforward compared to the task of measuring activities undertaken by a loose collection of public and private institutions that comprise a public health system. No single entity within the system is likely to have full and unbiased knowledge about the public health activities performed by all contributing institutions. At the same time, it may not be feasible to collect information from all of the institutions that potentially contribute to public health activities for a given population. For these reasons, each unit of analysis may entail unique sources of bias and measurement error. The choice of unit of analysis must be made with regard to not only the purposes of the performance measurement activity, but also to the inherent tradeoffs among feasibility, cost, bias, and precision.[13] These issues are revisited in the discussion on measuring indicators of performance.

Scope of Activity

Public health performance is inherently a multidimensional construct, because public health organizations and systems do not produce a single product or service.[13] An essential early step in the performance measurement process is to identify the scope of activities that should be performed by the organizations or systems under study. These activities represent general domains of performance for which specific measures and indicators will be developed. These domains should clearly reflect the overall mission, goals, and objectives of the public health programs, organizations, or systems to be covered by the performance measurement system.[4] If the performance measurement process is designed to enhance accountability and outcomes for a specific public health program or funding stream, as is the case for the U.S. Department of Health and Human Services' Performance Partnership Grants, these goals and objectives may be relatively narrow and well defined in scope. If, however, the measurement process is designed to improve accountability and outcomes among public health organizations and systems more generally, as is the case for the CDC's National Public Health Performance Standards Program and many state-level measurement activities, then a broader range of goals and objectives may be required.

In most cases, performance domains are defined to reflect the ideal or expected scope of performance rather than the actual scope of performance, so that measurement initiatives can be used to track progress toward expectations and goals.[51] It is also desirable for performance measurement systems to use a relatively limited number of performance domains, so that the information produced by these systems can be readily understood by public health practitioners, and so that this information creates clear and unambiguous incentives for performance improvement.[4] Nevertheless, performance measurement systems should cover the full scope of activities needed to achieve the overall mission and goals of public health programs, organizations, and/or systems under study.

The appropriate domains of performance in the field of public health are those activities that are regarded as core elements of practice because of their utility in protecting and improving population health. Perceptions about these core elements may vary over time and across different practice settings; however, several large-scale efforts have been undertaken in recent years to define the ideal scope of activity for public health practice. These efforts have proven very useful in identifying the domains of performance for many current performance measurement activities in public health.

Perhaps the best-known conceptual model of public health practice is the one developed in the Institute of Medicine's 1988 report on public health.[25] This model consists of three core functions of public health—assessment, policy development, and assurance—to be carried out by public health organizations at every level of practice. The primary limitation of this model for performance measurement activities is its lack of specificity. Each of the core functions potentially encompasses a broad scope of activities and services. To address this limitation, the CDC convened a panel of experts in 1992 to identify a set of specific public health activities that were viewed as components of the core functions defined by the IOM. The result of this effort was a set of 10 public health practices, each of which was linked with one of the core functions (Table 12.3).[33] These practices were used as the domains of performance in several large-scale public health performance measurement initiatives conducted at the local level during the 1990s.[37–41]

Table 12.3. Ten Core Practices of Public Health

Assessment

1. Assess the health need of the community
2. Investigate the occurrence of health effects and health hazards of the community
3. Analyze the determinants of identified health needs

Policy Development

4. Advocate for public health, build constituencies and identify resources in the community
5. Set priorities among health needs
6. Develop plans and policies to address priority health needs

Assurance

7. Manage resources and develop organizational structure
8. Implement programs
9. Evaluate programs and provide quality assurance
10. Inform and educate the public

Source: Dyal WW. Ten organizational practices of public health: a historical perspective. *Am J Preven Med.* 1995;11 (6 suppl):6-8.

A more recent model of public health practice was developed by a workgroup convened by the U.S. Department of Health and Human Services as part of the national health care reform debates in 1994. This panel of experts identified 10 essential public health services that were considered core components of practice (Table 12.4).[47] The elements of this model were conceptually similar to the CDC's 10 public health practices and the IOM's core functions, although these elements did not correspond exactly with components of the earlier models. The essential services framework has been used to track public health expenditures in states and localities, and to monitor state expenditures under the federal Maternal and Child Health Services Block Grant.[52] More recently, this framework was used to define domains of performance for the CDC's National Public Health Performance Standards Program currently under development.

Another effort to define the scope of public health practice was initiated by the World Health Organization (WHO) in 1997, drawing on the knowledge and experiences of an international collection of public health experts.[53] Using a Delphi process with 145 public health administrators, educators, researchers, and practitioners, the WHO study identified and prioritized a list of 37 essential public health functions that fell within nine general categories:

- Prevention, surveillance, and control of communicable and noncommunicable diseases
- Monitoring the health situation (health status, determinants, risks, and interventions)
- Health promotion
- Occupational health
- Protecting the environment
- Public health legislation and regulations
- Public health management
- Specific public health services (school health, emergency services, and laboratory services)
- Personal health care for vulnerable and high-risk populations

With straightforward modifications, the conceptual models developed by IOM, CDC, DHHS, and

Table 12.4. Essential Services of Public Health

1. Monitor health status to identify and solve community health problems
2. Diagnose and investigate health problems and health hazards in the community
3. Inform, educate, and empower people about health issues
4. Mobilize community partnerships and action to solve health problems
5. Develop policies and plans that support individual and community health efforts
6. Enforce laws and regulations that protect health and assure safety
7. Link people to needed personal health services and assure the provision of health care when otherwise unavailable
8. Assure a competent work force—public health and personal health care
9. Evaluate effectiveness, accessibility, and quality of personal and population-base health services
10. Research for new insights and innovative solutions to health problems

Source: Public Health Functions Steering Committee. *Public Health in America.* July 1995.

WHO approximate each other, but it is unlikely that any one of them represents the last word for defining the complex role of public health in modern society.[26] A 1998 survey of state public health agencies revealed that many of them are using the above models in their efforts to measure and improve public health performance, but that few of them use any single approach in an unaltered form.[8] Many use locally developed concepts of public health practice to supplement existing conceptual frameworks. What matters most for the purposes of performance measurement is not the specific framework used to develop a measurement strategy, but rather the ability to define the overarching mission, objectives, and activities of public health in clear and measurable terms. Various conceptual models can be helpful in accomplishing this task.

Performance Indicators

Another important issue for performance measurement activities involves the specific indicators that are used to measure performance in each domain of activity. Performance indicators can generally be classified into one of three basic types: indicators of structure or capacity; indicators of process or outputs; and indicators of outcomes.[54] First, *structural indicators* reflect the basic resources and institutional capacities that are available in a given performance domain. Examples of structural indicators in the field of public health practice include: the amount and type of human resources available for public health activities; the amount and sources of funding available; the number and type of institutions involved in the public health system; the data, information, and communication systems available to the public health system; and the governmental authority and powers granted to the public health system.

Second, *process indicators* reflect the specific activities performed and outputs produced in a given performance domain. Examples in public health may include: the scope, volume, and coverage of clinical and population-based services produced by public health agencies and systems (e.g., age-appropriate immunizations, prenatal care and counseling, age-appropriate screening services); the processes used for community health needs assessment and priority setting (e.g., frequency, scope of issues examined, stakeholders involved); the processes used for disease surveillance (e.g., frequency, coverage, data collection methods, and scope of diseases included); and the processes used for health education and information dissemination (e.g., frequency, coverage, and scope of information).

Finally, *outcome indicators* capture the effects of specific activities and outputs on the population(s) of interest and outcomes. Examples include disease-specific mortality rates; incidence rates for preventable diseases; incidence rates of adolescent pregnancy; and measures of the prevalence of behavioral risk factors such as smoking, unsafe sexual activity, obesity, and alcohol and other drug abuse. Outcome indicators can also be specified in terms of financial outcomes (e.g., the economic burden of preventable disease) and measures of public satisfaction or dissatisfaction with public health activities and services.

Good performance indicators in public health share a number of important attributes. First, indicators should be closely linked to a specific performance domain and a specific program or policy objective.[4] Indicators having a weak or ambiguous association with performance domains and program objectives may provide very little insight about how well an organization or system carries out its public health responsibilities. In many cases, public health program and policy objectives are defined in terms of population health status goals such as those established in *Healthy People 2010* (e.g., improvements in infant mortality, reductions in the incidence of infectious diseases). For this reason, outcome indicators of performance often have the strongest empirical association with program and policy objectives. Unfortunately, the scientific evidence concerning the association between structural or process indicators of performance and population health status is often quite limited. In these cases, good performance indicators should at least be consistent with expert opinions about the activities and elements that constitute effective public health practice. The indicators and domains used for performance measurement purposes should therefore evolve as standards of public health practice change over time, and as new evidence about public health impact becomes available.[13]

Good indicators should also reflect a process or condition that is substantially within the control or influence of the public health organizations under study. This trait helps ensure that indicators are sensitive to changes in public health performance over time and across different organizations or systems (*measurement sensitivity*). This trait also helps ensure that indicators can be used to identify public health performance exclusive of other phenomena outside the domain of public health practice (*measurement specificity*). For these reasons, structure and process indicators are used more frequently than outcome indicators in public health performance measurement activities. Population-based health outcome indicators (e.g., statistics on mortality and disease incidence) are influenced by many factors outside the immediate control of the public health system, such as population demographics and mobility patterns, and socioeconomic conditions. Consequently, in some cases these measures may not be sufficiently sensitive nor specific to public health interventions to merit using them for performance measurement purposes. In other cases, it may be possible to adjust these measures using statistical methods to make them suitable indicators of public health performance. Some outcome indicators may also pose problems for performance measurement applications because of the long time lag that may be required for public health activities to exert a measurable impact on the indicator. Mortality statistics, for example, often present this problem. In these cases, process indicators or intermediate outcome measures may be preferred to outcome measures.

Finally, good performance indicators show substantial variation across organizations or jurisdictions and across time. Variation helps ensure that indicators can be used to detect meaningful differences in performance among the organizations and populations under study. Indicators that are likely to show little variation in the population of interest (e.g., the proportion of public health agencies with at least one full-time employee) may not be helpful in distinguishing high-performing and low-performing organizations or systems. Nonetheless, for some applications it may be useful to include indicators of rare but important events that provide strong evidence of high or low performance. Such sentinel events may include specific preventable diseases, causes of hospitalization, or causes of death.

Public health performance indicators can be developed at various levels of detail to measure progress toward program goals and objectives, to achieve the desired attributes of measurement sensitivity and specificity, and to address the constraints of feasibility and cost in data collection. In some cases, indicators are defined around specific health risks and populations at risk, such as the proportion of children age two and younger who are up-to-date on immunizations for vaccine-preventable diseases. Such detailed indicators are often used to track progress toward

specific program or policy objectives, such as those specified in the *Healthy People 2010* set of national health objectives.[27] The National Research Council recently identified a series of such population-specific and disease-specific indicators suitable for use in public health performance monitoring activities (Table 12.5).[4]

In other cases it may be sufficient to use indicators that capture only general categories of activity, such as whether or not the local public health system surveys the population for behavioral risk factors at least every three years. These types of indicators were used in several performance measurement systems developed during the 1990s to measure progress toward the more generic Healthy People 2000 objective of increasing the proportion of the population served by a local health department that effectively carries out core public health functions (Table 12.6).[37–42] Generic indicators may be easier to derive from broad program and policy objectives, but they may also be more difficult to measure reliably due to heterogeneity in how such indicators are interpreted by respondents.

Methods for Measuring Performance

The utility of any performance measurement system hinges on its ability to obtain valid and reliable measures of performance indicators. Valid measures capture the information that is expected and intended for the purposes of evaluation and comparison.[55] Reliable measures reflect performance consistently across observations and over time. Some level of measurement error is unavoidable in most empirical applications, but systematic gaps in measurement reliability undermine the utility of the measures that are produced. A number of alternative measurement strategies are possible for collecting useful information about public health performance. Each of these strategies requires a different amount of time and resources to implement, and each entails a different mix of advantages and disadvantages for obtaining valid and reliable measures of performance.[49] Issues of feasibility, validity, and reliability must be balanced carefully when selecting and using public health performance measures.

Table 12.5. Health Performance Indicators Identified by the National Research Council

Tobacco

Percentage of (a) persons age 18-24 and (b) persons age 25 and older currently smoking tobacco

Percentage of persons age 14-17 (grades 9-12) currently smoking tobacco

Percentage of women who gave birth in the past year and reported smoking tobacco during pregnancy

Percentage of employed adults whose workplace has an official policy that bans smoking

Nutrition

Percentage of persons age 18 and older who eat five or more servings of fruit and vegetables per day

Percentage of persons age 14-17 (grades 9-12) who eat five or more servings of fruit and vegetables per day

Percentage of persons age 18 and older who are 20 percent or more above optimal body mass index

Exercise

Percentage of persons age 18 and older who do not engage in physical activity or exercise

Percentage of persons age 14-17 (grades 9-12) who do not engage in physical activity or exercise

Preventive Screenings and Tests

Percentage of persons age 18 and older who had their blood pressure checked within the past 2 years

Percentage of women age 45 and older and men age 35 and older who had their cholesterol checked within the past 5 years

Percentage of women age 50 and older who received a mammogram within the past 2 years

Percentage of adults age 50 and older who had a fecal occult blood test within the past 12 months or a flexible sigmoidoscopy within the past 5 years

Percentage of women age 18 and older who received a Pap smear within the past 3 years

Percentage of persons with diabetes who had HbA1C checked within the past 12 months

Percentage of persons with diabetes who had a health professional examine their feet at least once within the past 12 months

Percentage of persons with diabetes who received a dilated eye exam within the past 12 months

Infectious Diseases

Incidence rates of selected STDs

Incidence rates of HIV infection

Prevalence rates of selected STDs

Prevalence rates of HIV infection

Consumer satisfaction with STD, HIV, and tuberculosis treatment programs

Rates of sexual activity among adolescents age 14-17

Rates of sexual activity with multiple sex partners among people age 18 and older

Rates of condom use during last episode of sexual intercourse among sexually active adolescents age 14-17

Rates of condom use during last episode of sexual intercourse among sexually active adolescents age 18 and older with multiple sex partners

Rates of condom use during last episode of sexual intercourse among men having sex with men

Rates of injection drug use among adolescents and adults

Completion rates of treatment for STDs, HIV infection, and tuberculosis

Immunization

Reported incidence rate of representative vaccine-preventable diseases

Age-appropriate vaccination rates for target age groups (children age 2 years; children entering school at approximately 5 years of age; and adults age 65 years and older) for each major vaccine group

Source: Perrin EB, Koshel JJ. *Assessment of Performance Measures for Public Health, Substance Abuse, and Mental Health*. Washington, DC: National Academy Press; 1997.

Table 12.6. Twenty Indicators of Local Public Health Performance

Assessment

1. In your jurisdiction, is there a community needs assessment process that systematically describes the prevailing health status in the community?

2. In the past three years in your jurisdiction, has the local public health agency surveyed the population for behavioral risk factors?

3. In your jurisdiction, are timely investigations of adverse health events conducted on an ongoing basis—including communicable disease outbreaks and environmental health hazards?

4. Are the necessary laboratory services available to the local public health agency to support investigations of adverse health events and meet routine diagnostic and surveillance needs?

5. In your jurisdiction, has an analysis been completed of the determinants of and contributing factors to priority health needs, the adequacy of existing health resources, and the population groups most effected?

6. In the past three years in your jurisdiction, has the local public health agency conducted an analysis of age-specific participation in preventive and screening services?

Policy Development

7. In your jurisdiction, is there a network of support and communication relationships that includes health-related organizations, the media, and the general public?

8. In the past year in your jurisdiction, has there been a formal attempt by the local public health agency to inform elected officials about the potential public health impact of decisions under their consideration?

9. In your local public health agency, has there been a prioritization of the community health needs that have been identified from a community needs assessment?

10. In the past three years in your jurisdiction, has the local public health agency implemented community health initiatives consistent with established priorities?

11. In your jurisdiction, has a community health action plan been developed with community participation to address priority community health needs?

12. In the past three years in your jurisdiction, has the local public health agency developed plans to allocate resources in a manner consistent with community health action plans?

Assurance

13. In your jurisdiction, have resources been deployed as necessary to address priority health needs identified in a community health needs assessment?

14. In the past three years in your jurisdiction, has the local public health agency conducted an organizational self-assessment?

15. In your jurisdiction, are age-specific priority health needs effectively addressed through the provision of or linkage to appropriate services?

16. In your jurisdiction, have there been regular evaluations of the effects of public health services on community health status?

17. In the past three years in your jurisdiction, has the local public health agency used professionally recognized process and outcome measures to monitor programs and to redirect resources as appropriate?

18. In your jurisdiction, is the public regularly provided with information about current health status, health care needs, positive health behaviors, and health care policy issues?

19. In the past year in your jurisdiction, has the local public health agency provided reported to the media on a regular basis?

20. In the past three years in your jurisdiction, has there been an instance in which the local public health agency has failed to implement a mandated program or service?

Source: Turnock BJ. *Public Health: What It Is and How It Works.* Gaithersburg, Md: Aspen Publishers; 1997.

Self-Reported Assessment Instruments

Most of the performance measurement initiatives that have occurred to date in public health have relied on measures that are self-reported by public health organizations. A compelling advantage of these types of measures is their ability to be collected relatively quickly and cost effectively, thereby providing timely data with limited respondent burden. Several self-reported performance assessment instruments have been developed for use with the administrators of public health organizations, including an 84-indicator instrument and a 26-indicator screening survey developed by Miller and colleagues to measure performance within local public health systems,[39,40] several instruments developed by Turnock and colleagues to measure the performance of local public health agencies,[37,38,56] and an instrument developed by Halverson and colleagues to measure the local public health contributions made by organizations other than the local public health agency.[41] More recently, a 20-indicator screening instrument was developed from elements contained in both the Miller and Turnock survey protocols (Table 12.6).[42] This instrument has been used in several national surveys of local public health systems and is currently used as part of the CDC's National Public Health Performance Standards Program.

Several reliability issues emerge from performance measures that are constructed from self-reported data. The reliability of these data is conditional on whether the appropriate people in the appropriate organizations are consistently recruited to report performance data. To report performance data accurately and consistently, respondents must have sufficient knowledge, expertise, and access rights to the necessary information. Respondent selection is therefore a critically important element of research design and management. Unreliable performance measures can result from a variety of data collection situations, including:

- Systematic differences in respondent knowledge and information across organizations or over time (e.g., due to staff turnover within the organizations under study)

- Systematic differences in how respondents interpret performance measures across organizations or over time (e.g., due to incomplete or ambiguous case definitions for measures)
- Systematic differences in the content and quality of information systems used by organizations in reporting performance measures

Efforts to ensure the comparability of respondents and information systems across organizations and over time can help reduce these potential threats. First, clear and specific case definitions should be provided for each measure to reduce differences in how measures are interpreted. Second, performance measurement systems may require respondents to meet detailed reporting standards regarding what information should be used to respond to each measure, and how this information should be collected, maintained, and documented by the responding organization. These standards can be periodically verified by audit, as is done in the HEDIS system that monitors health plan performance. Finally, where possible, performance measures should be based on objective, observable criteria rather than on criteria that are subject to the perceptions of the respondents. In the absence of objective information, however, perception-based measures may still offer some insight about practice-patterns and performance among public health organizations and systems.

Performance measures designed to assess the public health contributions of multiple organizations serving a common population are subject to additional reliability issues. One measurement approach is to rely on the governmental public health agency as the key informant about public health contributions made by other organizations.[39–41,57] It is important to recognize that the reliability of such measures is contingent on the agency's access to information about the activities of other organizations. In most cases the governmental agency may be the best single source for this information. Nevertheless, where information gaps or differences in perception exist, systematic reporting biases may arise. Another strategy for obtaining these measures is to survey directly the range of other organizations that contribute to public health performance, requiring these organizations to report information about their own activities. This strategy is likely to be considerably more time- and resource-intensive than strategies that target the public health agency only. Additionally, this strategy may encounter problems of measurement reliability due to systematic differences across organizations in how performance measures are interpreted.

Reliability tests can be used to detect inconsistencies in performance measure reporting.[58] Interrater reliability tests use reports of performance from multiple independent raters. If these reports are highly correlated, then measurement reliability is confirmed. Reliability can also be confirmed through internal consistency tests. These tests are carried out by collecting multiple measures of the same performance dimension from each organization or jurisdiction under study. A high correlation among the multiple measures suggests sufficient reliability. Reliability can also be evaluated by collecting repeated observations of the same measure over time, and testing for longitudinal consistency. Finally, external audits and direct-observation site visits can be used to confirm the reliability of self-reported performance measures. These types of reliability tests may be particularly important for performance measures designed to assess the public health contributions of multiple organizations serving a common population.

To guard against potential reliability problems, care must be taken in how performance measurement data are used. Self-reported performance measures are particularly vulnerable to problems of gaming, wherein respondents inflate their reported measures to create the impression of high performance or significant performance improvement over time. The incentives for systematic reporting bias may be particularly powerful if performance data are publicly disseminated or used for purposes other than to support internal quality improvement and practice-based research. For example, if performance measures are used to allocate resources or enforce contracts, then respondents face clear incentives to up-code their reports. Consequently, the implicit incentives for reporting bias should be considered carefully when developing and using performance measures in public health.

As mentioned above, one strategy for enhancing measurement reliability is to require respondent compliance with rigorous data collection and reporting standards. This strategy allows researchers to ensure that the organizations participating in measurement activities have sufficient capacities for the collection, documentation, verification, and validation of performance data. Performance measurement systems in other fields of practice require such standards (e.g., the HEDIS system for health plans and the ORYX system for hospitals and health systems). The disadvantage of rigorous reporting standards is that they necessarily limit the range of organizations that are eligible to participate in performance measurement systems, thereby diminishing the degree to which measures are representative of the larger population of organizations. The trade-off between reliability and representativeness in performance measurement is an issue that researchers must consider carefully.

Other Measurement Approaches

Public health performance measures can be constructed using a number of other data sources. Secondary data from state vital and health statistics systems, disease registries, immunization registries, and notifiable disease reporting systems can be used to construct a variety of disease-specific and population-specific process and outcome measures that may function as valuable components of performance measurement systems.[4] Other potential data sources include the administrative data systems maintained by federal and state agencies for specific public health programs (e.g., Medicaid, WIC), and the hospital discharge data systems maintained by many state health data organizations. These data elements often do not entail the same measurement reliability problems that are commonly encountered in self-reported measures. Across-state variation in data system structure and content, however, may introduce new reliability challenges for performance measurement activities that span multiple states.[59,60] Problems with measurement sensitivity and specificity are also more likely to arise with the use of measures constructed from secondary data, because these measures are likely to be influenced by many factors outside the control of the public health systems being studied.

State-level measures relevant to public health performance can also be constructed from the large national health surveys conducted periodically by federal agencies. Among the most widely used surveys for public health applications are the National Health and Nutrition Examination Survey and the National Health Interview Survey conducted by the National Center for Health Statistics, as well as the Medical Expenditure Panel Survey conducted by the Agency for Healthcare Research and Quality. State-level measures of behavioral risk factors can also be obtained from the CDC's Behavioral Risk Factor Surveillance System. Although useful for national and state-level measurement activities, these national data sources use sampling methods that prevent them from being able to produce measures of performance at substate and local levels.[61] For some state and local performance measurement initiatives, it may also be desirable and feasible to establish new primary data collection systems, such as population-based surveys of public health risks and outcomes, or to modify existing surveillance systems to address the need for reliable performance measures. As with any public health surveillance activity, the expected utility of the information obtained from such systems must be weighed against the expected cost of acquiring the information.

Each of the available methods for public health performance measurement offers a different mix of costs, risks, and benefits, whether based on self-reported assessment instruments, population-based surveys, or secondary data sources. The ideal measurement strategy for a specific application necessarily depends upon the scope of activities to be measured, the availability of secondary data sources, and the resources available to support primary data collection and measurement. Where possible, it may be advantageous to use a combination of self-reported measures and measures obtained from more objective and verifiable secondary data sources and surveillance systems. By avoiding reliance on any single type of measurement strategy, this strategy may be better able to detect and address common problems with measurement validity and reliability.

Performance Comparison and Evaluation

Performance measurement processes are powerful tools for quality improvement because of their ability to support comparisons of performance across organizations and systems as well as over time. Such comparisons allow organizations to chart progress toward established goals and objectives, to benchmark themselves against similar organizations, and to monitor the effects of administrative and policy changes on performance. Once valid and reliable measures of public health performance have been developed and collected, a remaining methodological issue concerns how measures are evaluated and compared cross-sectionally as well as longitudinally.[62] A number of methodological issues may complicate the task of evaluating and comparing performance measures, including the following:

- *Measurement signal:* For some dimensions of performance it remains an open question as to whether meaningful differences in performance exist across organizations and systems, and as to how such meaningful differences should be defined empirically. A key conceptual and methodological challenge therefore lies in determining whether empirical performance measures signal meaningful differences in practice and outcomes.
- *Measurement noise:* Some differences in performance measures may result from random variation that is unrelated to true performance levels or quality of practice. An important methodological challenge therefore lies in distinguishing this noise from true differences in performance across organizations and systems and over time.
- *Measurement bias:* Observed differences in performance measures across organizations and systems may result from true differences in the effectiveness and efficiency of public health practice, or from underlying, systematic differences in factors outside the control of public health organizations—such as the sociodemographic characteristics, economic conditions, and intractable health risks (i.e., genetic profiles) of the populations served by these organizations. Failure to account for systematic differences

in these underlying characteristics can lead to biased performance measures and performance comparisons. A third methodological challenge therefore lies in correcting for these potential sources of measurement bias.

Several basic approaches can be used alone or in combination for evaluating and comparing performance measures: using performance standards as a basis for comparison; using "benchmark" comparisons among similar organizations and systems; and using statistical "risk-adjustment" methods to make cross-sectional and longitudinal comparisons. Each of these approaches is examined below.

Performance Standards

One common strategy for evaluating performance involves the use of established performance standards. Using this strategy, performance measures are simply compared with a priori standards to determine the extent to which these standards are met (the measurement signal). Standards are most often established using either a dichotomous "pass/fail" metric or a graduated continuum of performance levels that range from low to high. Dichotomous standards are often criticized for creating a ceiling effect such that organizations are not encouraged to pursue additional improvements in performance after achieving the specified threshold.[51] For this reason, graduated performance standards are preferred as a means for motivating continual improvement. Regardless of the type of standard used, simple bivariate statistical tests can be used to determine whether specific groups of observations exceed a performance standard after accounting for measurement noise. The power of these tests to detect differences in performance depend upon the number of observations that are included in the performance measurement process.

Ideally, performance standards are established based on empirical studies that indicate the performance levels needed to achieve desired outcomes, such as the vaccination coverage rates that are required to bring infectious disease risks within certain acceptable ranges, or the purification standards for public water sources that are required to bring waterborne disease risks within acceptable ranges. In the absence of strong scientific evidence, performance standards are often based on the practical experiences of public health professionals. Standards can be developed, therefore, by convening panels of experienced public health professionals, and identifying consensus opinions about appropriate public health practices and expected public health outcomes. A variety of structured group process methods can be used to identify such consensus opinions, with the most widely used methods being the Nominal Group Technique and the Delphi Method—both of which rely on an iterative, anonymous process of generating opinions, rating opinions, and reflecting on the ratings given by other panel members.[63] Less structured consensus development processes, such as brainstorming and facilitated discussion, are also commonly used in specifying performance standards. A variety of electronic technologies are now available to facilitate both structured and unstructured consensus development processes, ranging from anonymous computerized polling devices to Internet-based discussion forums (for an example of the former see the recent study by Mays and Halverson).[64]

The CDC's National Public Health Performance Standards Program uses a multiphased process for standards development that relies initially on consensus conferences and expert panels to define the standards for local and state public health systems.[7] During the first phase, the CDC convened a broad range of public health stakeholders to reach consensus about these standards, including representatives from the National Association of County and City Health Officials, the Association of State and Territorial Health Officials, the Public Health Foundation, the American Public Health Association, and numerous representatives from state and local public health agencies as well as academic schools of public health. These consensus panels identified a set of performance standards for each of the 10 essential public health services, with separate standards for local systems and state systems. A graduated continuum of performance levels was identified for each performance standard (for an example standard see Table 12.7).

Table 12.7. Example Performance Standard Used in the National Public Health Performance Standards Program

Essential Service 1: Monitor Health Status to Identify Community Health Problems

Indicator 1.3:   Maintenance of Population Health Registries

Performance Standard: The Local Public Health System (LPHS) develops, maintains, and regularly contributes to health-related registries. Data is collected for registries in accordance with standards that assure comparability of data from public/private and local/state/regional/national sources. The LPHS utilizes established criteria for reporting identified health events to the appropriate registry and creates and supports systems to assure accurate, timely, and unduplicated reporting by data providers. Collaboration among multiple partners facilitates the aggregation of individual data to compile a population registry used to inform policy decisions, program implementation, and population research. Registries track health-related events such as disease patterns and preventive health services delivery (i.e., cancer registries facilitate the tracking over time of cancer incidence, cancer stage at diagnosis, treatment patterns, and survival probability; vaccine registries provide the real time status of vaccine coverage for specified age groups in the community).

Performance Measures:

1. Does the LPHS contribute information to one or more health registries [Y/N]?

    If Yes:

    1.1 Are there established criteria and processes for reporting health events to the registry [Y/N]?

    1.2 Are there established partnerships to facilitate the collection and aggregation of data [Y/N]?

2. Does the LPHS use information from one or more registries [Y/N]?

    If Yes:

    2.1 Is the information used to inform policy decisions [Y/N]?

    2.2 Is the information used to design and implement programs [Y/N]?

    2.3 Is the information used to conduct population research [Y/N]?

3. In the past year, has the LPHS accessed information from one or more health registries [Y/N]?

    If Yes, which type(s) of registries were accessed:

    3.1 Immunization status of children [Y/N]?

    3.2 Immunization status of adults [Y/N]?

    3.3 Cancer [Y/N]?

    3.4 Syphilis serology [Y/N]?

    3.5 Newborn screening [Y/N]?

    3.6 Birth defects and developmental disabilities [Y/N]?

    3.7 Trauma [Y/N]?

    3.8 Occupational injury [Y/N]?

    3.9 Environmental exposures [Y/N]?

4. Does the LPHS operate one or more health registries [Y/N]?

    If Yes:

    4.1 Are there standards for data collection [Y/N]?

5. To what extent does the local public health agency achieve the model standard

    [Not at all or minimally/Partially/Substantially/Fully or almost fully]?

6. To what extent does the LPHS (including the local public health agency) achieve the model standard

    [Not at all or minimally/Partially/Substantially/Fully or almost fully]?

Source: Centers for Disease Control and Prevention. *National Public Health Performance Standards Program: Local Public Health System Performance Assessment Instrument, Version Field Test 5b.* Atlanta, Ga: Centers for Disease Control and Prevention; 2000.

During subsequent phases of the standards development process, the CDC plans to use the results from its performance measurement activities to update and revise established performance standards. Extensive analytical work will be completed to examine the relationships among measures of public health processes and measures of public health outcomes, to examine variations in performance measures across systems, and to examine rates of change in public health performance over time. New evidence-based standards will then be developed based on the results of these studies. After several successive iterations of performance measurement activities, analytical forecasting techniques may be used to identify performance improvement expectations and improvement trajectories, and then to establish future standards based on these results.

Benchmarking

Another approach for evaluating performance measures involves conducting comparisons among groups of organizations or systems that are closely related in structure and operation. These benchmarking comparisons are frequently used as part of continuous quality improvement initiatives because they create a "moving target" for organizations to work toward, rather than an absolute standard.[5] Under this approach, organizations are stratified into comparison groups of similar organizations based on observable structural and operational characteristics such as the size and demographic composition of the jurisdiction, and the scope of services offered. Statistical clustering procedures may be used to group organizations based on similarities across multiple characteristics. Performance measures for individual organizations are then compared with norms from the peer group of similar organizations. Bivariate statistical tests can be used to determine whether an individual organization is significantly above or below the average performance level of its group after accounting for measurement noise. By making comparisons only among similar organizations and systems, this approach reduces, but not eliminates, the risk of measurement bias resulting from unobserved differences across organizations and systems. Consequently, the benchmarking approach offers a potentially powerful strategy for motivating improvements in public health performance based on empirical observation and comparison.

Researchers at the University of South Florida have developed a community health tracking system for Florida counties that uses this benchmarking strategy for making comparisons among county-level measures of community health resources, processes, and outcomes.[65] This system integrates secondary data from a variety of sources to create measures that can inform local public health decision making. A similar method was used by investigators at the University of North Carolina at Chapel Hill to profile measures of public health performance and community health outcomes on a national scale across local public health jurisdictions.[66] For this study, investigators collected measures from all U.S. local public health departments serving populations of at least 100,000 residents (response rate = 71 percent) using a self-reported assessment instrument. After analyzing measures for validity and reliability, a customized report was developed that compared each jurisdiction's measures with U.S. and "peer group" averages (for an example see Figure 12.2). Peer groups were defined using a statistical clustering algorithm based on jurisdictional population size, ethnic composition, and the scope of services offered by the local health department. Reports were sent back to each responding jurisdiction, and follow-up telephone interviews were conducted with a subset of respondents to assess the perceived utility of this benchmarking method. Follow-up interviews indicated that local public health administrators found the comparative results to be useful in developing improvement goals and strategies for their organizations.

If performance measures are collected longitudinally, then another form of benchmarking can be carried out using multiple observations from the same organizations or systems. Simple trend analysis can be used to examine the direction and magnitude of change in performance measures over time, thereby benchmarking an organization or system against itself. Additionally, measures of the magnitude and rate of performance improvement can be computed for each organization and then benchmarked with measures from similar organizations using the meth-

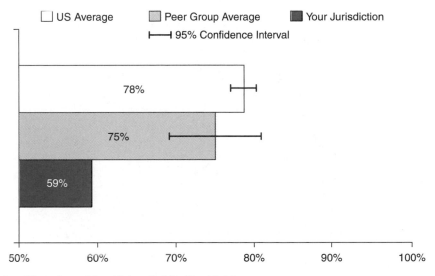

Figure 12.2. Example of Benchmarking Using Public Health Measures

Source: Mays GP, Miller CA, Halverson PK, et al. *Assessing Organizational Performance in the Nation's Largest Public Health Jurisdictions.* American Public Health Association 126th Annual Meeting. Washington, DC: American Public Health Association; 1999.

ods described above. For these improvement comparisons, organizations may be grouped based on their baseline performance measures and/or based on other characteristics. Similar benchmarking methods can be used when multiple cross-sectional measures of performance are collected within the same organizations or systems. In these cases, performance is compared across different domains of activity rather than across different time periods. It is also possible to use longitudinal and cross-sectional benchmarking methods simultaneously, as was done in a recent case study analysis of eight local public health jurisdictions using the performance measurement instrument developed by Miller and colleagues.[67] For this study, performance measures were compared across 10 domains of public health practice as defined in Dyal[33] and across two time periods (1993 and 1996; see Figure 12.3).

Risk Adjustment

Another set of strategies for evaluating and comparing performance measures involve the use of statisti-

cal methods to control for potential sources of measurement bias. In one approach, performance measures are adjusted only for factors that influence performance but are fully beyond the control of the public health organizations under study. These factors may include sociodemographic and health status characteristics of the populations served by public health organizations, as well as market and policy characteristics that are determined outside the public health organizations' spheres of influence. These types of controlled comparisons or risk-adjustment methods are especially useful for studies that evaluate the effects of policies and programs that are externally imposed on public health systems.[68] As in most types of observational research, the need to control for a large number of characteristics dictates the use of multivariate statistical methods rather than simple stratified comparisons. These methods can be used to compute adjusted performance scores that then can be compared among organizations or over time using benchmarking techniques. Adjusted performance scores can also be compared with a priori performance standards.

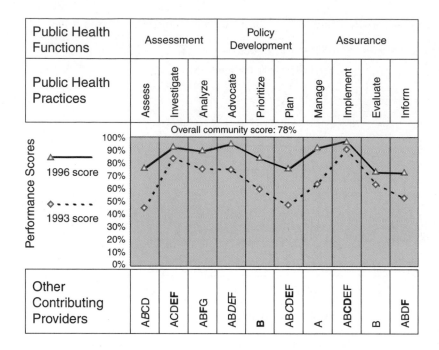

Figure 12.3. Public Health Performance Profile for a Sample Jurisdiction

Source: Miller CA, Moore KS, Richards TB, Monk JD. A proposed method for assessing the performance of local public health functions and practices. *Am J Public Health.* 1994;84(11)1743–1749.

A second method for risk adjustment must be used when analysts wish to examine performance variation due to factors that are within the control of the organizations or systems under study. For example, a researcher may want to examine how performance varies with the number of full-time-equivalent staff available in each organization under study. In these cases, standard statistical modeling techniques often produce estimates that are biased, because they do not account for the fact that both public health outputs/outcomes (e.g., vaccination coverage rates) and public health inputs/structures (e.g., staffing levels) are simultaneously determined by the organization under study. In this example, public health agency staffing decisions may be based in part on local economic conditions that also influence health insurance coverage and the demand for health services such as vaccinations. Failure to control for this simultaneous relationship may lead to incorrect inferences regarding the effect of staffing on vaccination coverage. Advanced statistical methods such as structural equation modeling and instrumental-variables analysis can be used to test and control for possible sources of bias due to simultaneous relationships.[69] Specifica-

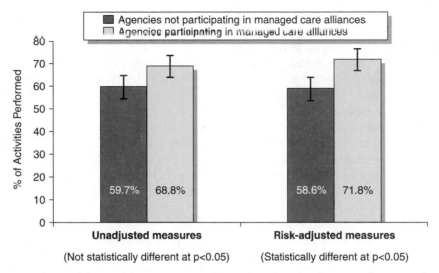

Figure 12.4. Proportion of 20 Public Health Activities Performed in the Jurisdictions of U.S. Local Public Health Agencies Serving at Least 100,000 Residents, 1998

Source: Mays GP, Halverson PK, Stevens R. The contributions of managed care plans to public health practice: Evidence from the nation's largest local health departments. *Public Health Rep.* In press.

tion tests can be applied to help researchers decide whether problems of simultaneity exist in their data and what can be done to address these problems.

This approach was used in one recent study to compare performance measures for local public health agencies that did and did not participate in partnerships with managed care plans.[57] Because such partnerships are at least partly under the control of the public health agencies, a simple comparison of measures between participating and nonparticipating agencies may lead to incorrect inferences about the effects of partnerships on performance. The main performance measure used for this study was the proportion of 20 public health activities that were performed in the jurisdiction served by each agency, and the study population included all local public health agencies in the United States serving a population of at least 100,000 residents ($N=397$, response rate=71%). Using instrumental-variables estimation, researchers were able to adjust performance measures for the effects of other confounding variables—including the effects of public health agency decisions to form partnerships with managed care plans. Results indicated that performance measures were

higher among agencies that formed partnerships with managed care plans, and that this difference was statistically significant only when risk-adjusted measures were used (Figure 12.4). Although these risk-adjustment methods have been developed in the fields of econometrics and health services research, they are nonetheless readily applicable to performance measurement applications in public health.

A third method of multivariate risk adjustment may be used for applications that collect multiple measures of performance for each organization or system. Rather than analyzing each measure separately, multivariate statistical models can be used to examine the relationships among multiple performance dimensions while simultaneously adjusting for confounding variables that are beyond the control of the public health system. By analyzing multiple performance measures using this pooled method known as multivariate signal extraction, additional statistical power is gained (due to the larger effective sample size) for use in untangling measurement noise from measurement signals.[70] Additionally, by examining the relationships among multiple measures of performance, analysts can identify and compare patterns of performance across organizations and systems, rather than comparing single performance measures. This type of practice pattern analysis (which is similar in methodology to factor analysis and principal components analysis) can also be useful in identifying how specific combinations of public health structures and processes affect public health outcomes. For example, one recent study examined 20 different performance measures collected from all U.S. local public health agencies that serve populations of at least 100,000 residents ($N=397$, response rate=71%). Multivariate factor analysis methods were used to identify groups of measures that were strongly correlated after controlling for a variety of confounding variables.[71] This study identified three dominant practice patterns from the measures: one that emphasized ensuring the delivery of health services to populations in need; one that emphasized assessing and prioritizing community health needs; and one that emphasized planning for public health interventions and resource allocation decisions (Table 12.8). Based on these results, additional studies can examine the relative effects of these three practice patterns on specific public health outcomes of interest. It is important to

Table 12.8. Practice Pattern Analysis Based on 20 Public Health Performance Measures: Results From a Factor Analysis of Risk-Adjusted Measures

	Factor Loadings (Correlations)		
1. Community health needs assessment	0.21	**0.57****	0.28
2. Behavioral risk factor survey	0.18	0.50**	0.21
3. Adverse health events investigation	0.25	0.16	0.03
4. Laboratory services	0.19	0.10	−0.03
5. Analysis of health determinants	0.23	**0.69****	0.11
6. Analysis of preventive services	0.14	**0.41****	0.04
7. Support and communication networks	0.39	0.16	0.11
8. Information for elected officials	**0.41****	0.13	0.29
9. Prioritization of health needs	0.25	**0.55****	0.38
10. Implementation of initiatives	0.51**	0.21	0.24
11. Community action plans	0.12	0.23	**0.74****
12. Plans for resource allocation	0.10	0.13	**0.78****
13. Resources for priority needs	0.43**	0.36	0.35
14. Self-assessment	0.32	0.06	0.27
15. Provision/linkage of services	0.37	0.21	0.03
16. Evaluation of services	**0.43****	0.28	0.22
17. Process/outcome measures	**0.41****	0.20	0.13
18. Public information	**0.61****	0.21	0.11
19. Media information	**0.52****	0.01	0.10
20. Performance of mandated programs	0.13	0.12	0.00
**Statistically significant at $p<0.05$			
Practice Pattern Grouping:	Assurance-intensive	Assessment-intensive	Planning-intensive

Source: Mays GP, Miller CA, Halverson PK, et al. *Assessing Organizational Performance in the Nation's Largest Public Health Jurisdictions.* American Public Health Association 126th Annual Meeting. Washington, DC: American Public Health Association; 1999.

note that all of the multivariate risk-adjustment methods described here can be implemented using longitudinal data (through time-series and panel-data models) as well as cross-sectional data.

All of the methods available for evaluating and comparing performance measures require good information about the structural and operational characteristics of public health organizations and systems. This information is needed to group organizations and systems for the purposes of benchmarking, and to construct statistical controls for confounding sources of variation in risk adjustment models. The information required for such tasks may include data on the geographic extent of public health jurisdictions; the sociodemographic and health status characteristics of populations residing within these jurisdictions; the workforce characteristics of the professionals that staff public health organizations; information on public health funding sources and expenditures; information on the administrative and legal authority of public health organizations, including any governance structures; and information on the array of official and nonofficial organizations that potentially contribute to public health activities. One excellent source of such information is the *National Profile of Local Health Departments* collected periodically by the National Association of County and City Health Officials.[31] Similarly, basic sociodemographic and health resources information can be obtained from the *Area Resource File* maintained by the U.S. Health Resources and Services Administration.[72] Other data elements necessary for these analytic activities may need to be obtained from administrative data systems maintained by individual federal and state agencies. These existing data sources provide a useful starting point for implementing performance measurement activities; however, it is clear that more detailed, comprehensive, and longitudinal data about the nation's public health infrastructure will be needed to support advanced applications in public health performance measurement and evidence-based decision making.

THE FUTURE OF PUBLIC HEALTH PERFORMANCE MEASUREMENT

The movement toward performance measurement activities in public health has been under way for most of the twentieth century. This movement has accelerated dramatically during the 1990s as public health decision makers have faced new pressures to improve the effectiveness, efficiency, and accountability of their organizations. The pressures for performance measurement appear likely to grow in intensity as new and emerging threats to population health continue to develop, and as citizens and policy makers continue to demand evidence that public resources are being used optimally. Contemporary performance measurement applications have been limited, however, by the types of information that are readily available and easily collected concerning public health structures, processes, and outcomes. New investments in public health information and surveillance systems—which are being made at local, state, and national levels—are steadily overcoming these limitations and expanding the opportunities for performance measurement. Key among these new developments is the CDC's National Public Health Performance Standards Program, which promises to provide a rich longitudinal data source for public health organizations to use in monitoring their own performance over time, comparing performance with peer institutions, and identifying performance gaps in need of improvement. Other important developments include: the CDC's Bioterrorism Preparedness and Response Initiative, which endeavors to expand the surveillance and information technology capacities of public health organizations across the United States; the U.S. Department of Health and Human Services' Performance Partnership Grants, which propose to link federal public health funding with measurable performance objectives; and numerous state-level initiatives to expand the surveillance and performance measurement capacities of state and local public health organizations.

These developments uniformly suggest that public health organizations will require the ability to produce reliable and timely measures of performance for their organizations and jurisdictions, and to use these measures appropriately for administrative and policy decision making. To operate successfully in this new environment of performance measurement, public health organizations are likely to need a variety of new skills and strategies:

- *Technical resources.* Public health organizations will require the information and communication systems necessary to collect and report verifiable, timely data on resources consumed, outputs produced, and outcomes achieved. The additional costs of such systems may be substantial in some cases, but the benefits of more informed administrative and policy decision making will justify the investment—particularly if these systems are integrated with the organization's other information management and surveillance systems.

- *Interorganizational relationships.* Public health organizations will require the ability to measure and monitor the performance of the public health *system* in which it participates, which necessarily entails sharing data and information with the other public and private institutions that contribute to this system. Consequently, the ability to develop and manage effective interorganizational relationships for the purposes of performance measurement becomes essential. Public health administrators must be able to mobilize shared interest in and support for performance measurement among all major stakeholders within the system. Correspondingly, administrators must play key roles in helping these stakeholders understand and use performance measures to achieve their own institutional objectives.

- *Analytical expertise.* To take full advantage of the information generated by performance measurement activities, public health organizations will require strong expertise in evaluating and comparing performance measures, and in deriving implications for organizational strategy and public health policy. Ideally this expertise should extend to the technical details of the benchmarking and risk-adjustment methods described earlier in this chapter. Of course, all public health organizations need not maintain this level of analytical expertise in-house, as long as effective mechanisms are in place to obtain this expertise from external sources such as academic institutions and state and federal agencies.

- *Improvement processes.* Public health organizations will require effective institutional and interorganizational processes for using the information generated through performance measurement to improve public health operations and outcomes.

Successful processes are likely to follow the basic principles of continuous quality improvement, which emphasize active participation by the broad array of stakeholders that influence specific process or outcome under study.[5] Most often, these processes include iterative cycles of identifying a problem, developing a potential solution, testing and evaluating the solution, and modifying the solution to achieve further improvements in performance. For public health organizations, the problems to be addressed often involve multiple organizations, which add additional complexity to the improvement process.[12,73,74]

- *Dissemination, outreach, and marketing strategies.* Finally, public health organizations will require the ability to disseminate information on performance measurement activities to the broad range of institutions and individuals that can use this information to improve health-related decision making. These stakeholders may include policy makers involved in resource allocation decisions in public health; health plans, hospitals, employers, and other institutions that currently or potentially engage in partnerships with public health organizations; clients that use specific services provided by public health organizations; and other members of the public that have a general interest in population health and the use of public resources. One important challenge lies in making this information understandable and usable by such a diverse audience, through targeted dissemination and outreach strategies. Another challenge lies in using performance measurement information to encourage personal decision making and policy decision making that improves population health. This task, which is fundamentally a marketing problem, may include efforts to encourage greater public participation in the health education and prevention services offered by public health organizations (i.e., personal decision making), as well as efforts to encourage additional governmental support for public health programs and services (i.e., policy decision making).[75]

Performance measurement applications in public health will continue to evolve in form and function as new data, analytical methods, and information technologies become available. Developing and using these applications are certain to remain key priorities for public health organizations for the foreseeable future. Performance measurement will remain a priority in part because of formal efforts to institutionalize these activities within mainstream public health practice. Such institutionalization efforts include the development of public health infrastructure goals as part of the Healthy People 2010 national health objectives, and the implementation of a National Public Health Performance Standards Program. More important, however, performance measurement will remain a priority because of the growing imperatives to improve the nation's defenses against existing and emerging public health threats. Public health organizations form the core of the nation's response to problems as varied as new and resurgent infectious diseases, persistent disparities in population health, and the looming threat of bioterrorism. It becomes possible to improve this response only when a true understanding is obtained about the work produced and outcomes achieved by the nation's public health organizations. Performance measurement provides the mechanism to achieve this understanding and to prepare for the public health challenges of the future.

References

1. Walton M, Deming WE. *Deming Management Method.* New York, NY: Perigee; 1988.
2. Lynch TD, Day SE. Public sector performance measurement. *Public Adm Q.* 1996;19(4):404-419.
3. Tankersley WB. Performance measurement. *J Public Adm Res Theory.* 1997;7(1):163-171.
4. Perrin E, Durch J, Skillman SM. *Health Performance Measurement in the Public Sector: Principles and Policies for Implementing an Information Network.* Washington, DC: National Academy Press; 1999.
5. McLaughlin CP, Kaluzny AD. *Continuous Quality Improvement in Health Care: Theory, Implementation, and Applications.* Gaithersburg, Md: Aspen Publishers; 1999.
6. Scutchfield FD, Zuniga de Nuncio ML, Bush RA, Fainstein SH, LaRocco MA, Anvar N. The presence of total quality management and continuous quality improvement processes in California public health clinics. *J Public Health Manage Pract.* 1997;3(3):57–60.
7. Halverson PK; Nicola RM; Baker EL. Performance measurement and accreditation of public health organizations: a call to action. *J Public Health Manage Pract.* 1998;4(4):5-7.
8. Mays GP, Halverson PK, Miller CA. Assessing the performance of local public health systems: a survey of state health agency efforts. *J Public Health Manage Pract.* 1998;4(4):63-78.
9. Turnock BJ. Performance measurement and improvement in public health. In: Novick L, Mays GP, eds. *Public Health Administration: Principles for Population-based Management.* Gaithersburg, Md: Aspen Publishers; 2000:431-456.
10. Kearney RC, Berman EM. *Public Sector Performance: Management, Motivation and Measurement.* Columbia: Institute of Public Affairs, University of South Carolina; 2000.
11. Byrnes P. Performance measurement and financial incentives for community behavioral health services provision. *Int J Public Adm.* 1997;20(8):1555-1579.
12. Mays GP, Hatzell T, Kaluzny AD, Halverson PK. Continuous quality improvement in public health organizations. In: McLaughlin CP, Kaluzny AD, eds. *Continuous Quality Improvement in Health Care: Theory, Implementation, and Evaluation.* Gaithersburg, Md: Aspen Publishers. 1999:360-403.
13. Roper WL, Mays GP. Performance measurement in public health: conceptual and methodological issues in building the science base. *J Public Health Manage Pract.* 2000;(5):66-77.
14. Clancy CM, Eisenberg JM. Outcomes research: measuring the end results of health care. *Science.* 1998;282(5387):245-246.
15. Turnock BJ, Handler AS. From measuring to improving public health practice. *Annu Rev Public Health.* 1997;18:261-282.
16. American Public Health Association, Committee on Municipal Health Department Practice. First report, part 1. *Am J Public Health.* 1922;12(2):7-15.
17. American Public Health Association, Committee on Municipal Health Department Practice. First report, part 2. *Am J Public Health.* 1922;12(2):138-347.
18. American Public Health Association, Committee on Administrative Practice. Appraisal form for city health work. *Am J Public Health.* 1926;16(1 suppl):1-65.

19. Walker WW. The new appraisal form for local health work. *Am J Public Health.* 1939;29(5):490-500.

20. Krantz FW. The present status of full-time local health organizations. *Public Health Rep.* 1942;57:194-196.

21. Halverson WL. A twenty-five year review of the work of the committee on administrative practice. *Am J Public Health.* 1945;35(12):1253-1259.

22. American Public Health Association, Committee on Administrative Practice. *Evaluation Schedule for Use in the Study and Appraisal of Community Health Programs.* New York, NY: American Public Health Association; 1947.

23. Halverson PK. Performance measurement and performance standards: old wine in new bottles. *J Public Health Manage Pract.* 2000;6(5):vi-x.

24. Vaughan HF. Local health services in the United States: The story of CAP. *Am J Public Health.* 1972;62:95-108.

25. Institute of Medicine, National Academy of Sciences. *The Future of Public Health.* Washington, DC: National Academy Press; 1988.

26. Miller CA, Halverson PK, Mays GP. Flexibility in measurement of public health performance. *J Public Health Manage Pract.* 1997;3(5):1-2.

27. US Department of Health and Human Services. *Healthy People 2010: Conference Edition.* Washington, DC: US Government Printing Office; 2000.

28. Greene LW. PATCH: CDC's Planned Approach to Community Health, an application of PRECEED and an inspiration for PROCEED. *J Health Educ.* 1992;23(3):140-147.

29. American Public Health Association. *The Guide to Implementing Model Standards. Eleven Steps Toward a Healthy Community.* Washington, DC: American Public Health Association; 1993.

30. National Association of County and City Health Officials. *Assessment Protocol for Excellence in Public Health (APEXPH).* Washington, DC: National Association of County and City Health Officials; 1991.

31. National Association of County and City Health Officials. *Assessment Planning Excellence through Community Partners for Health* (APEXCPH). Washington, DC: National Association of County and City Health Officials; 1999.

32. National Association of County and City Health Officials. *Mobilizing for Action through Planning and Partnerships (MAPP).* Washington, DC: National Association of County and City Health Officials; 2000.

33. Dyal WW. Ten organizational practices of public health: a historical perspective. *Am J Prev Med.* 1995;11(6 suppl):6-8.

34. National Association of County and City Health Officials. *1989-90 National Profile of Local Health Departments.* Washington, DC: National Association of County and City Health Officials; 1992.

35. National Association of County and City Health Officials. *1992-93 National Profile of Local Health Departments.* Washington, DC: National Association of County and City Health Officials; 1995.

36. National Association of County and City Health Officials. *1996-97 National Profile of Local Health Departments.* Washington, DC: National Association of County and City Health Officials; 1997.

37. Turnock BJ, Handler A, Dyal WW, et al. Implementing and assessing organizational practices in local health departments. *Public Health Rep.* 1994;109(4):478-484.

38. Turnock BJ, Handler AS, Hall W, Potsic S, Nalluri R, Vaughn EH. Local health department effectiveness in addressing the core functions of public health. *Public Health Rep.* 1994;109:653-658.

39. Miller CA, Moore KS, Richards TB, McKaig CA. A proposed method for assessing public health functions and practices. *Am J Public Health.* 1994;84(1):1743-1749.

40. Richards TB, Rogers JJ, Christenson GM, Miller CA, Taylor MS, Cooper AD. Evaluating local public health performance at a community level on a statewide basis. *J Public Health Manage Pract.* 1995;1(4):70-83.

41. Halverson PK, Miller CA, Kaluzny AD, et al. Performing public health functions: the perceived contribution of public health and other community agencies. *J Health Hum Serv Adm.* 1996;18(3):288-303.

42. Turnock BJ, Handler AS, Miller CA. Core function-related local public health practice effectiveness. *J Public Health Manage Pract.* 1998;4(5):26-32.

43. Maternal and Child Health Bureau, Health Resources and Services Administration (US). *Guidance and Forms for the Title V Application/Annual Report.* Rockville, Md: Health Resources and Services Administration; 1997.

44. Perrin EB, Koshel JJ. *Assessment of Performance Measures for Public Health, Substance Abuse, and Mental Health.* Washington, DC: National Academy Press; 1997.

45. National Committee for Quality Assurance. *HEDIS 3.0.* Washington, DC: National Committee for Quality Assurance; 1997.

46. Miller T, Leatherman S. The National Quality Forum: a "me-too" or a breakthrough in quality measurement and reporting? *Health Aff.* 1999;18(6):233-237.

47. Baker EL, Melton RJ, Stange PV, et al. Health reform and the health of the public. Forging community health partnerships. *JAMA.* 1994;272(16):1276-1282.

48. US Department of Health and Human Services. *Healthy People 2010: Conference Edition.* Washington, DC: U.S. Dept of Health and Human Services; 2000.

49. Eddy DM. Performance measurement: problems and solutions. *Health Aff.* 1998;17(4):7-25.

50. Brannick MT, Salas E. *Team Performance Assessment and Measurement: Theory, Methods, and Applications.* New York, NY: Lawrence Erlbaum; 1997.

51. Kazandjian VA, Lied TR. *Healthcare Performance Measurement: Systems Designs and Evaluation.* Chicago, Ill: American Society for Quality; 1999.

52. Barry MA, Centra L, Pratt E, Brown CK, Giordano L. *Where Do the Dollars Go? Measuring Local Public Health Expenditures.* Washington, DC: Public Health Foundation; 1998.

53. Bettcher DW, Sapirie S, Goon EHT. Essential public health functions: results of the international Delphi study. *World Health Stat Q.* 1998;51(1):44-54.

54. Donabedian A. *The Definition of Quality and Approaches to Its Assessment.* Ann Arbor, Mich: Health Administration Press; 1980.

55. Shadish WR, Cook TD, Leviton LC. *Foundations of Program Evaluation: Theories of Practice.* Newbury Park, Calif: Sage Publications; 1991.

56. Handler AS, Turnock BJ, Hall W, et al. A strategy for measuring local public health practice. *Am J Prev Med.* 1995;11(supp 2):29-35.

57. Mays GP, Halverson PK, Stevens R. The contributions of managed care plans to public health practice: evidence from the nation's largest local health departments. *Public Health Rep.* In press.

58. Silva F. *Psychometric Foundations and Behavioral Assessment.* Newbury Park, Calif: Sage Publications; 1993.

59. Mendelson DN, Salinsky EM. Health information systems and the role of state government. *Health Aff.* 1997; 16(3):106-119.

60. Starr P. Smart technology, stunted policy: developing health information networks. *Health Aff.* 1997;16(3):91-105.

61. Lee CV. Public health data acquisition. In: Novick L, Mays GP, eds. *Public Health Administration: Principles for Population-based Management.* Gaithersburg, Md: Aspen Publishers; 2000:171-201.

62. Gerzoff RB. Comparisons: the basis for measuring public health performance. *J Public Health Manage Pract.* 1997;3(5):11-21.

63. Patton, MQ. *Qualitative Research and Evaluation Methods.* Third edition. Newbury Park, Calif.: Sage Publications; 2001.

64. Mays GP, Halverson PK. Conceptual and methodological issues in public health performance measurement: results from a computer-assisted expert panel process. *J Public Health Manage Pract.* 2000;6(5):59-65.

65. Studnicki J, Steverson B, Myers B, Hevner AR, Berndt DJ. A community health report card: comprehensive assessment for tracking community health (CATCH). *Best Practices & Benchmarking in Healthcare.* 1997;2(5):196-207.

66. Mays GP, Miller CA, Stevens R, et al. Developing a model report card of community health. 2001. (Manuscript under review)

67. Mays GP, Miller CA, Halverson PK. *Local Public Health Practice: Trends and Models.* Washington, DC: American Public Health Association; 2000.

68. Iezzoni LI. *Risk Adjustment for Measuring Health Care Outcomes.* Chicago, Ill: Health Administration Press; 1997.

69. Newhouse JP, McClellan M. Econometrics in outcomes research: the use of instrumental variables. *Annu Rev Public Health.* 1998;19:17-34.

70. Koopman SJ, Shephard N, Doornik JA. Statistical algorithms for models in state space using SPack 2.2. *The Econometrics J.* 1999;2(1):107-161.

71. Mays GP, Miller CA, Halverson PK, et al. *Assessing Organizational Performance in the Nation's Largest Public Health Jurisdictions.* American Public Health Association 126th Annual Meeting. Washington, DC: American Public Health Association; 1999.

72. US Health Resources and Services Administration. *Area Resource File 1998.* Fairfax, Va: Quality Resource Systems; 1999.

73. Institute of Medicine, National Academy of Sciences. *Improving Health in the Community: A Role for Performance Monitoring.* Washington, DC: National Academy Press; 1997.

74. Stoto MA. Evaluation of public health interventions. In: Novick L, Mays GP, eds. *Public Health Administration: Principles for Population-based Management.* Gaithersburg, Md: Aspen Publishers: 2000:324-358.

75. Doner L, Siegel M. Public health marketing. In: Novick L, Mays GP, eds. *Public Health Administration: Principles for Population-based Management.* Gaithersburg, Md: Aspen Publishers; 2000:474-510.

Health Data Management for Public Health

Stephen B. Thacker, M.D., M.Sc.
Donna F. Stroup, Ph.D., M.Sc.
Richard C. Dicker, M.D., M.Sc.

PRINCIPLES AND PRACTICE OF EPIDEMIOLOGY

To understand the uses of data in public health, we first define and discuss epidemiology as the basic science of public health. Next, we describe the basic principles of public health surveillance and review selected sources of health data and the usefulness of each. We then discuss the use of descriptive and comparative/analytic studies in epidemiology. Finally, we close with a discussion of selected special issues for data management in public health, including data sources for the public health response to bioterrorism and the increasingly important area of public health informatics.

Defining Epidemiology

The definition of epidemiology has two dimensions—one related to science, the other to public health practice. *The Dictionary of Epidemiology* reflects both dimensions in its definition of epidemiology as the study of the distribution and determinants of health-related states or events in specified populations, and the application of this study to the control of health problems.[1]

The phrase *health problem* is used in this definition in place of the word *disease* because epidemiologists and public health agencies now find themselves responsible for a range of health problems. In addition to infectious diseases (e.g., tuberculosis), noninfectious health problems (e.g., automobile crash injuries in adolescents, exposure of miners to coal dust in mines, and unintended pregnancies to teenagers) are also high-priority public health problems in many countries.

The term *distribution* in the definition addresses the relationship of health events to person, places, and time; in other words, the relationship between the health problem and the population in which it exists. The characteristics of the population are usually given in terms of age, sex, and the places where people live and where the health event occurs.

The word *determinants* refers to both the direct causes of the health problem and the factors that determine the risk for the problem. These factors are often classified into three groups: (1) host factors, (2) agent factors, and (3) environmental factors. **Host factors** are those that characterize persons afflicted with the health problem and their susceptibility to it. **Agent factors** are those that characterize the mechanisms that lead to disease or injury. **Environmental factors** are those that determine the exposure of the host group to the agent.

In an epidemic of food poisoning, for example, the host group includes the persons who ate the food and became ill. The agent factors are those related to the cause of the problem (e.g., the *salmonella bacillus*) that may contaminate turkey or egg dishes. The environmental factors are those that provide suitable circumstances for the agent to survive (e.g., improper handling of food) and those that determine the exposure of the host group.

The Tasks of Epidemiologic Practice

Even though epidemiology is regarded as the basic science of public health, a science is often best defined by what the scientist does. Alexander Langmuir was the first chief epidemiologist of the Communicable Disease Center (now the Centers for Disease Control and Prevention, or CDC). He is credited with conceptualizing modern disease surveillance. Langmuir articulated in simple words what the epidemiologist does: "The basic operation of the epidemiologist is to count cases and measure the population in which they arise," so that rates can be calculated and the occurrence of a health problem can be compared in different groups of people.[2] The contemporary epidemiologist has unique responsibilities that can be stated in more detail. These basic responsibilities are surveillance, investigation, analysis, and evaluation. In addition, the epidemiologist has responsibilities, such as clear communication, effective management, consultation, group or public presentation, and human relations skills.

Public Health Surveillance

Public health surveillance is the ongoing systematic collection, analysis, and dissemination of health data to those who need to know. The final link in the surveillance chain is the application of these data to disease prevention and injury control. Surveillance in public health is information in action.

Investigation

The epidemiologic investigation includes field work and office (or computer) work—follow-up of individual case reports of adverse health events, assessment of risk in a community, and conduct of epidemiologic studies to identify causal relationships. An epidemiologic investigation may focus on an epidemic (e.g., an outbreak of infection), a cluster of events (e.g., injuries or leukemia), or the presence of risk factors for disease (e.g., tobacco use or an occupational exposure).

Analysis

The analysis of epidemiologic data includes not only manipulation of numbers, but also transforming numbers into information that can lead to the control or prevention of a health problem. Such data analysis must be interpreted in the context of social, cultural, and environmental factors that might affect public health decisions.

Evaluation

Evaluation has been defined as systematic investigation of the merit, worth, or significance of an object.[3,4] During the past three decades, the practice of evaluation has evolved as a discipline with new definitions, methods, approaches, and applications to diverse subjects and settings.[4-7] Evaluation of an operating surveillance system aims at increasing the system's utility and efficiency.

Additional Essential Tasks

Dealing with health data and management requires a public health practitioner to do more than those tasks that are uniquely epidemiologic. Clearly communicating the findings from epidemiologic studies to the public and to health professionals is needed if community cooperation with control and prevention measures is to be effective.

Management of the persons who are needed to conduct epidemiologic studies and carry out control and prevention programs makes it essential for public health practitioners to be skilled in this area. Because practitioners skilled in working with health data and management problems are often called on for advice, competence in consultation is also important. Finally, proficiency in human relations is required of every public health practitioner who deals with colleagues in carrying out tasks related to health data and the management of community health problems.

Relationships with Other Health Practitioners

Health data and its management are important for many public health practitioners with a range of special competencies. Statisticians play a special role in accessing and managing data sources and evaluating and interpreting results. Laboratory staff have an important part to play in carrying out tests that identify the exact cause of a health problem and confirm the presence of the problem in those persons who show symptoms and signs of the condition.

Health policy makers need to understand health data if effective strategies are to be designed to control and prevent a community health problem. Health service and program managers need to understand the findings of studies and policy analyses if they are to be persuaded to provide services and conduct effective programs.

SURVEILLANCE SYSTEMS: THEIR ESTABLISHMENT AND USE

In the late 1940s, Langmuir broadened the concept of surveillance beyond watching individuals at risk for specific disease at quarantine stations and changed the focus of attention to diseases such as malaria and smallpox. He emphasized rapid collection and analysis of data on a particular disease with quick dissemination of the findings to those who needed to know.[8]

Now this credo of rapid reporting, analysis, and action applies to nearly 100 infectious diseases and adverse health events of noninfectious etiology at the local, state, and national levels. Many ongoing systems of reporting have resulted from local or national

emergencies such as contaminated lots of polio vaccine (the so-called Cutter Incident of 1955), pandemic Asian influenza in 1957, shellfish-associated hepatitis A in 1961, toxic shock syndrome in 1980, Hanta pulmonary syndrome in the Four Corners area in 1994, widespread outbreaks of *Escherichia coli* 0157:H7 in 1994–1999, and an outbreak of West Nile encephalitis in the northeast in 1999. Within days following the investigation of L-tryptophan-induced eosinophilia-myalgia syndrome (EMS) in 1990, a national reporting system was put into place for a previously rare and nonreportable condition.

Public health surveillance is essential to making competent, well-informed public health policy decisions that are based on quantitative data. As a public health activity, surveillance is conceptualized by practicing epidemiologists as follows:

> Public health surveillance is the ongoing systematic collection, analysis, and interpretation of health data essential to the planning, implementation, and evaluation of public health practice, closely integrated with the timely dissemination of these data to those who need to know. The final link in the surveillance chain is the application of these data to prevention and control.[9]

Surveillance versus Research

Surveillance must be defined in terms of what it is *not* as well as what it is. Public health surveillance is not research in the sense of data collection for generalizable knowledge subject to rigorous and lengthy human subjects review. The need for timeliness and for rapid dissemination is essential for effective public health surveillance. This attribute is not as important for research, whose finding must be subject to careful and deliberate contemplation by scientists rather than by public health decision makers.[10]

Surveillance data must be disseminated quickly to public health practitioners, including those who originally gathered the data, as well as to decision makers throughout the public health organization and, depending on the character of the information, to other public service agencies and the community. Surveillance data are more often related to identifying a public health problem than to problem solving. The dissemination of surveillance data frequently stimulates the search for additional data that may come from other sources.

Using Health Information Systems for Surveillance

Surveillance systems are also different from health information systems. Health information systems span a broad range of health data, which may include interviews, abstracted hospital records, birth certificates, death certificates, physician office visit abstracts, and medical prescriptions. Data from a health information system may be used for surveillance, just as death certificates may be an indispensable component of a cancer surveillance system, but surveillance systems differ from health information systems in at least three ways:

- Surveillance systems must be ongoing; health information systems may not be.
- Surveillance systems must be integrated with timely dissemination.
- Surveillance systems must be applicable to public health actions, such as control and prevention.

The Purpose of Public Health Surveillance

Public health surveillance has specific purposes that are fundamental to decision making, policy development, program implementation, and sometimes crisis management. The following are the key purposes of a surveillance system:

- Describing trends and the natural history of health problems
- Detecting epidemics
- Providing details about patterns of disease
- Monitoring changes in disease agents through laboratory testing
- Planning and setting health program priorities
- Evaluating the effects of control and prevention measures
- Detecting critical changes in health practice
- Evaluating hypotheses about the cause of health problems

- Detecting rare but important cases of disease, such as botulism
- Generating hypotheses for research

To be certain that a surveillance system meets the needs of public health decision makers and their communities, the objectives of the system must be specified in detail. Everyone who might make decisions based on the surveillance data needs to be involved in the process.

The Surveillance Cycle

Public health surveillance is conducted in a systematic cycle that has four major steps. These steps and their most important characteristics include:

- Collection of data: pertinent, regular, frequent, prompt, timely
- Consolidation and interpretation of data: orderly, descriptive, evaluative, prompt, timely
- Dissemination of information: prompt, timely; disseminated to all who need to know, such as data providers (for confirmation and support), policy makers, and action takers
- Action: to control and prevent problems

The surveillance cycle is a concept that may be used for the entire spectrum of public health problems. Originally applied to infectious diseases, the surveillance cycle is now used in prevention and control programs for injury, cancer, certain cardiovascular diseases, and high-risk and unintended pregnancies. Understanding this cycle, especially the need for promptness in data collection and timely, accurate reporting, is essential for public health policy makers and action-oriented health program managers.

Specifically, the surveillance cycle highlights three important points for policy makers and program managers:

- Promptness is important at every step of the cycle and is given priority over meticulousness. As a result, changes may occur in surveillance data that do not occur in vital statistics or in most health survey data.

- Reports based on surveillance data are highly descriptive; that is, for the most part surveillance data provide the numerator numbers for estimated rates of disease occurrence. Surveillance reports generate hypotheses and suggest causes of health problems rather than confirm or establish them.
- Under rare circumstances surveillance systems may be brought to an end. When smallpox was eradicated, for example, surveillance was terminated because the smallpox virus was no longer a public health threat.

Establishing a Surveillance System

At the beginning, one needs to understand clearly the purpose of the surveillance program—what data are necessary, and how and when they are to be used. A particular surveillance system may have more than one goal (e.g., including monitoring the occurrence of both fatal and nonfatal disease or injury, evaluating the impact of a public health intervention, or detecting epidemics for control and prevention). A single health event (e.g., influenza or cervical cancer) may require multiple surveillance systems to track morbidity, mortality, laboratory tests, exposures, and risk factors. The key question to be answered is, "What action will be taken?" There must be a specific, action-oriented commitment to use the data effectively for public health action.

Attributes of a Surveillance System

A public health surveillance system has the following eight attributes:[11]

1. Simplicity: elegance of design and limitation of size, as well as ease of operation.
2. Flexibility: the ability of the system to adapt to changing needs such as the addition of new conditions or data-collection elements.
3. Acceptability: the willingness of individuals and organizations to participate in the surveillance system, including persons outside the sponsoring agency who are asked to report.
4. Sensitivity: the completeness of case reporting—the proportion of cases of a disease or health event

that are detected by the surveillance system. Also used to denote the ability of the surveillance system to detect epidemics.
5. Positive predictive value: the proportion of persons identified as case-patients who actually have the condition being monitored.
6. Representativeness: the extent to which the data collected in the system accurately describe the occurrence of a health event over time and its distribution in the population by place and person. Includes concepts of case ascertainment bias (discussed below), as well as bias in descriptive information about a reported case (e.g., diagnostic misclassification).
7. Timeliness: the delay between any two (or more) steps in a surveillance system, best assessed by the ability of the system to take appropriate public health action.
8. Cost: the resources used to operate the surveillance system, including costs of data collection and analysis as well as costs of disseminating information resulting from the system.

In many ways, these attributes are interdependent. Simplicity is essential if data quality is to be maintained and if consolidation, interpretation, and dissemination are to be carried out promptly. Acceptability is required because voluntary cooperation from both patients and busy public health practitioners is the cornerstone of data collection. Sensitivity and a high positive predictive value are important because surveillance is one approach to screening for the health problems of a community, especially for epidemic diseases and a clusters of health events, such as injuries.

Flexibility is critical because surveillance systems often prove to be the only mechanism for detecting new and emerging public health problems. This was the case in detecting West Nile encephalitis and in finding penicillinase-producing *Neisseria gonorrhoeae*. Representativeness is necessary if the system is to reflect accurately the occurrence of health problems in all sectors of a geographic area. Finally, timeliness must be an integral part of any surveillance system that is expected to detect health problems and to lead to the institution of effective control and prevention measures.

Analysis and Dissemination of Surveillance Data

Surveillance practitioners should ensure that surveillance data from surveillance systems they manage are analyzed appropriately and disseminated in a timely manner. Programmed data-analysis packages are a first step to data analysis, but results of these analyses should be reviewed and customized analysis done as needed. Surveillance information must be analyzed in terms of time, place, and person. More sophisticated methods such as cluster and time-series analyses and computer-mapping techniques may be appropriate subsequently.

Critical to the usefulness of surveillance systems is the timely dissemination of surveillance data to those who need to know. Publication of analyses together with interpretation of surveillance data should be done on a regular basis. Whatever format is chosen, it must be appropriate for the intended audience; the audience will affect data collection and interpretation as well as the dissemination process. Regular and timely data dissemination allows effective control and prevention. Because "those who need to know" include persons with little epidemiologic knowledge or background (i.e., policy makers and administrators), the reports should be simple and easy to understand.

Evaluation of a Surveillance System

Evaluation of surveillance systems should address three questions: (1) Is the health event under surveillance of continuing public health importance? (2) Is the surveillance system useful and cost effective? (3) Are the attributes of the quality of the surveillance system (i.e., sensitivity, specificity, representativeness, timeliness, simplicity, flexibility, and acceptability) addressed adequately? In addition, with the continuing advancement of technology and importance of informatics, you may wish to recommend that certain informatics criteria also be reviewed (e.g., hardware/software, interface, data format/coding, and quality checks). The decision to establish, maintain, or deemphasize a surveillance system should be guided by assessments based on these questions. Ultimately, that decision rests on whether a health event under surveillance is a public health priority and whether the surveillance system is useful and cost effective.

SOURCES OF DATA FOR MONITORING HEALTH

The idea of collecting data, analyzing them, and considering a reasonable public health response stems from Hippocrates.[12] Perhaps the first public health action that can be attributed to the use of surveillance data occurred in the 1300s when public health authorities in a port near the Republic of Venice prevented passengers from coming ashore during the time of epidemic bubonic plague in Europe. Since that time, a diversity of sources of health data have been used by countries and smaller areas for monitoring health. These sources include vital statistics, morbidity reporting systems, laboratory systems, surveys, registries, and other administrative systems. Table 13.1 describes selected examples of these systems.

Vital Statistics

The documentation of vital events (births and deaths) is one of the oldest and most complete public sources of health information. The first Bill of Mortality was issued in London in 1532 as a consequence of fear of a plague epidemic. John Graunt's treatise *Natural and Political Observations on the Bills of Mortality* (1662) is generally recognized as one of the first documents to describe use of numerical methods for monitoring public health.[9] In 1776 Johann Peter Frank advocated a more extensive monitoring of health in Germany that would support public health efforts related to the health of schoolchildren, prevention of injuries, maternal and child health, and public water and sewage disposal. As superintendent of the Statistical Department of the General Registrar's Office in Great Britain from 1839 to 1879, William Farr collected, analyzed, and interpreted vital statistics and disseminated the information in weekly, quarterly, and annual reports.[13] To standardize the data on vital statistics, the first international list of causes of death was developed in 1893.[12]

Today, each birth or death certificate contains an individual identifier, geographic location, date, and personal characteristics (e.g., sex, race, and marital status

Table 13.1.   Selected Data Sources and Web Sites

Data Source	Web Site
AIDS Public Use Data	http://wonder.cdc.gov/aids00
Behavioral Risk Factor Surveillance System	http://www.cdc.gov/nccdphp/brfss
Cancer: Surveillance, Epidemiology and End Results (SEER) Data	http://wonder.cdc.gov/seerj
Consumer Product Safety Commission (CPSC) Data	http://www.cpsc.gov
Council of State and Territorial Epidemiologists (CSTE)	http://www.cste.org
Department of the Interior Water Quality Data	http://www.doi.gov
Department of Transportation: Fatality Analysis Reporting System (FARS)	http://www-fars.nhtsa.dot.gov
Food and Drug Administration (FDA) Data	http://www.fda.gov
Hazardous Substance Release/Health Effects Database	http://www.atsdr.cdc.gov/hazdat
Healthy People 2010 Data	http://wonder.cdc.gov/data2010
International Classification of Disease (ICD) Codes	http://www.cdc.gov/nchs/about/major/dvs
International Vital Statistics (WHO)	http://www.who.int/dsa/cat98
National Health and Nutrition Examination Survey	http://www.cdc.gov/nchs/nhanes
National Health Care Survey	http://www.cdc.gov/nchs/nhcs
National Health Interview Survey	http://www.cdc.gov/nchs/nhis
National Immunization Survey	http://www.cdc.gov/nchs/nis
National Institute on Drug Abuse (NIDA) Data	http://www.nih.nida.gov
National Maternal and Infant Health Survey	http://www.cdc.gov/nchs/nmihs
National Mortality Follow-back Survey	http://www.cdc.gov/nchs/nmfs
National Notifiable Diseases Surveillance System	http://www.cdc.gov
National Survey of Family Growth	http://www.cdc.gov/nchs.nsfg
National Vital Statistics System	http://www.cdc.gov/nchs/nvss
PulseNet	http://www.cdc.gov/ncidod/dbmd/pulsenet
State and Local Area Integrated Telephone Survey	http://www.cdc.gov/nchs/slaits
Youth Risk Behavior Surveillance System	http://www.cdc.gov/nccdphp/dash/yrbs

[http://www.cdc.gov/nchs/data]). Data from birth certificates are generally more complete than those of deaths and include length of pregnancy, birthweight, time and place of birth, and some information on maternal characteristics (e.g., smoking during pregnancy).[14] Linked birth-death files can be used for maternal and infant mortality studies (http://www.cdc.gov/nchs/about/major/lbid/linked.htm). At the local level, data from vital statistics systems are timely and have been used for surveillance of mortality associated with acute events (e.g., heat waves and influenza).

Despite these uses, data from vital statistics systems pose several problems for public health decision makers. They might not be edited, aggregated, or made accessible in a timely manner. For example, na-

tional mortality data are not available for up to three years, although a 10 percent sample is available within 12 months of the close of the calendar year,[15] and lack of data on external cause (E-code) limits usefulness for injury prevention and control. Weekly reporting of deaths from 122 American cities to CDC has been integral to the surveillance of influenza epidemics in the United States.[16] In addition, automated systems for coding mortality information are both expanding and improving internationally.[17]

For a more detailed description of circumstances surrounding deaths (including autopsy reports, toxicology studies, and police reports), medical examiner and coroner records may be useful. In the United States, however, these reports are most representative of deaths caused by intentional and unintentional injuries and other unnatural causes.[18–20]

Unfortunately, not all characteristics are reported with full accuracy. Reporting of race is particularly problematic for certain population subgroups.[21] Furthermore, information on geographic location should be interpreted with care because the data may indicate the location where the certificate was completed (e.g., hospital) rather than the place where the vital event occurred (e.g., home or workplace). Finally, use of coding schemes organized according to organ system, rather than prevention activity, may hinder utility of these data for public health activities.[22]

The most basic health statistics are limited in many developing countries, with death registration inadequate or nonexistent. Use of the verbal autopsy, which uses a caretaker interview to determine the cause of death, may assist in following mortality patterns in places without routine death registration.[23–25] Sensitivity in establishing an accurate cause of death may be lower for some acute febrile conditions such as malaria than for conditions such as maternal causes, injuries, tuberculosis, and AIDS,[26] and different techniques in conducting verbal autopsies may result in different sensitivities for specific conditions.[27]

In all countries, the accuracy and specificity of many diagnoses is limited, and changes in the use of diagnostic categories and codes over time, together with variation in the quality of information, are limiting factors. For example, a 1978 study revealed that seven countries in Europe and North America coded the underlying cause of death the same for only 53 percent of a sample of 1,246 death certificates sent to these countries.[28]

Despite these limitations, vital statistics, particularly mortality statistics, are used to support many surveillance activities. For example, death certificates have been used in maternal mortality surveillance as a source of data to demonstrate progress toward reduction in maternal mortality in association with increased use of prenatal care and other factors. Analyses of death certificates in the United States have highlighted racial differences in mortality rates over time, differences in maternal mortality rates for women age 35 or older, and premature mortality specific to different populations. Because maternal mortality rates are often based on number of live births, this surveillance system also depends on birth certificate information.[29]

Morbidity Reporting

In 1899 the United Kingdom began compulsory notification of selected infectious diseases. In 1907 the *Office International d'Hygiene Publique*, predominantly composed of European member states, was created to collect morbidity data.[30] In the United States, national morbidity data collection on plague, smallpox, and yellow fever was initiated in 1878, and by 1925 all states were reporting weekly to the United States Public Health Service on the occurrence of selected diseases.

In the United States, traditional morbidity surveillance is illustrated by the National Notifiable Disease Surveillance System.[31] Physicians, laboratorians, and other health care providers are required by state law to report all cases of health conditions that are notifiable, most of which are infectious diseases (Table 13.1; http://www.cste.org). Authority to modify the list of notifiable diseases is often granted to the state health officer; in some states, each change must be newly legislated. Completeness and timeliness of reporting is influenced by the disease severity, availability of public health measures, public concern, ease of reporting, and physician appreciation of public health practice in the community.[32]

Reporting is generally incomplete for most notifiable diseases.[33,34] If persons are asymptomatic or have only mild symptoms, they may not seek health care. Patients and physicians may conceal diseases that carry a social stigma, such as sexually transmitted diseases. Health care providers also may fail to report because they might be unaware of regulations or because they may treat the symptoms without a complete laboratory investigation. Completeness of reporting may also be significantly influenced by factors such as medical community interest and publicity;[35] the most important is probably the intensity of surveillance efforts, which is linked to availability of resources.[36] For example, a study of underreporting of acute viral hepatitis in the United States demonstrated that homosexual men with hepatitis B and blood transfusion recipients with non-A non-B hepatitis were less likely to be reported than members of other risk groups.[37]

Many incomplete data may serve their purpose, however. Epidemics, as well as general temporal and geographic trends, can be determined as long as the proportion of cases detected remains consistent over time and across geographic areas. A comparison between cases of viral hepatitis reported by practitioners in private practice and cases reported in a population covered by an insurance plan in Israel demonstrated that, although completeness of reporting by the physicians was only 37 percent, the distribution of reported cases by season and age was similar to that recorded in the insured population.[38]

Sentinel Providers

Networks of health care providers have been organized as sentinel systems to gather information on selected health events. Most have been organized by practicing physicians on a voluntary basis; in many European countries, these networks have formed firm relationships with both public health authorities and academic centers, and often form the basis for morbidity surveillance.[39]

The strengths of sentinel provider systems include the commitment of the participants, the possibility of collecting longitudinal data, the flexibility of the system to address a changing set of conditions, and the ability to gain information on all patient-provider encounters, regardless of severity of illness. The most severe limitation of this type of system is that the population served by these physicians may not be representative of the general population. In addition, the illness must be fairly common to provide representative incidence data from a small sample of physician contacts.

For example, a voluntary network of general practitioners in Belgium was initiated in 1978.[40] Practitioners were selected who were representative of Belgian general practitioners according to age and sex and who were geographically distributed to ensure coverage of the country. Participants were to report weekly and results were to be sent to the participants on a quarterly basis. The list of health problems has included selected vaccine-preventable diseases, res-

piratory conditions, and suicide attempts, with some health problems such as mumps and measles reported continuously and others on a less frequent basis. A high level of participation has been documented, with the degree of form completion and continuity of reporting as criteria for assessment. The network has been evaluated in terms of its possible biases, such as nonparticipation of practitioners and difficulties in estimating the population at risk for the health problems under study; methods have been developed to reduce these biases.[41]

Risk Factors

For many chronic conditions, morbidity data typically comes from population surveys, registries, and health services sources (to come later in this section) to assess the magnitude and changes in known risk factors, daily living habits, health care, major social and economic features, and morbidity and mortality.[42] The surveillance of risk factors for a condition is a particularly useful approach for chronic diseases both because of long latency between exposure and disease and the multifactorial etiology of many chronic conditions.

Morbidity surveillance in environmental public health involves hazards and exposures as well as outcomes.[43] An example of a hazard surveillance source is the environmental air monitoring data from 4,000 state and local monitoring sites in the United States, which are mandated by the Clean Air Act. Data are collected and published routinely for six air pollutants covered by the national air quality standards (e.g., carbon monoxide, lead, nitrogen dioxide, ozone, particulate matter, and sulfur dioxide). An example of exposure surveillance is the use of the results of blood lead testing among children. Such surveillance is used to assess the effectiveness of programs designed to reduce environmental lead hazards.

Sentinel Health Events

CDC's National Institute of Occupational Safety and Health has maintained a sentinel health event verification system for occupational risk, which is a state-based network of health care providers that focuses on reporting specific occupational conditions.[44] Insurance records and workers' compensation claims have been useful sources of morbidity data for injuries and illnesses in specific geographic locales. Because regulations governing completion and submission of forms differ both among and within jurisdictions, data derived from these systems cannot easily be compared. In addition, the use of medical claims data for surveillance may be limited by lack of comparability among data from different jurisdictions (because of varying regulations governing completion of forms) or the accuracy of diagnostic recording.[45] For example, in an evaluation of claims for workers' compensation as an adjunct to an occupational lead surveillance system, the usefulness of claims was demonstrated: the likelihood that a company had a case of lead poisoning strongly correlated with the number of claims against the company.[46]

Laboratory Sources

Surveillance of routinely collected laboratory reports has been particularly useful for certain infectious conditions. For instance, in the United States, reporting from many public health laboratories is automated.[47] In England, nearly all microbiology laboratories report specified infections each week to the Communicable Disease Surveillance Centre. The advantages of a laboratory-reporting system are its specificity, its flexibility in adding new diseases, its rapidity, and the amount of detail about the infectious agent that can be provided. Reports can indicate trends or the appearance of rare infections originating from a common source that could not be identified by a single laboratory. One disadvantage is that the number of persons from whom specimens are collected and tested is usually not reported. In addition, the persons tested may not be representative of the population at risk. Also, whereas laboratory reporting provides details about the microorganism, it often lacks important information about the patient (e.g., risk factors or exposures). For some infections, such as toxic shock syndrome, there is no laboratory test, and for many common illnesses a specimen may not be taken (e.g., influenza).

Nosocomial Infections

Nosocomial infection surveillance is often based on review of laboratory records by an infection-control nurse or other designated staff.[48] In 1970, the National Nosocomial Infection Study was initiated to monitor the frequency and trends of nosocomial infection in U.S. hospitals. Approximately 160 hospitals participate in what is now a voluntary national surveillance system, with microbiology studies reported on 90 percent of infected patients.[49] A network of laboratories of different medical centers around the world has been established to conduct surveillance of antibiotic resistance for various pathogens.[50]

Laboratory Data

In addition, the use of molecular tools to enhance surveillance of pathogens is growing in many countries. PulseNet enables comparison of state-specific data by linking U.S. public health laboratories that perform DNA "fingerprinting" on bacteria that may be foodborne. The network permits rapid comparison of these patterns through an electronic database at the CDC. Similar pulsed field gel electrophoresis patterns of *E. coli* 0157:H7 bacteria isolated from ill persons suggest that the bacteria come from a common source, for example, a widely distributed contaminated food product.[51]

Surveys

Household surveys of the general population, such as the National Health Interview Survey conducted in the United States (http://www.cdc.gov/nchs) or the General Household Survey in England and Wales,[52,53] have provided information at the national level on personal health practices such as alcohol use and smoking, on disabilities, and on physician encounters. In the People's Republic of China, in addition to mandated information on acute infectious conditions, sentinel sites, known as disease surveillance points, are chosen through a statistical sample of provincial areas. These sites collect data on health events and medical encounters for the entire population within their jurisdiction.[54,55]

Although national estimates may be gained more efficiently from such surveys, local programs may benefit from involvement in data collection and the flexibility to adapt data collection to their particular needs. Interview surveys such as the Behavioral Risk Factor Surveillance System conducted by telephone and in person can obtain personal health-related information with only minor differences in the reported prevalence of various health conditions between the two techniques. In developed countries where most residences have telephones, telephone interviews have the advantages of lower cost and ease of supervising interviewers.[56] To obtain information concerning sexual activity, many states have begun periodic administration of the school-based Youth Risk Behavior Survey, a multistage sampling survey of high school students.[57]

Surveys using hospital records and other medical care records may be useful for information on diagnoses, surgical procedures, and patient demographic characteristics. Although computerization of parts of these records has allowed their use for routine surveillance, a major limitation has often resulted when identifiers are not recorded because repeat admissions and discharges by individual patients usually cannot be identified.

Hospital discharge surveys have been useful for surveillance of many medical care technologies, such as trends in the use of hysterectomies in the United States (particularly by geographical region), in the rate of coronary artery bypass graft procedures by sex and race, and in the assessment of outcome with carotid endarterectomies.[58–60]

Other sources of morbidity health information from surveys may include United Nations International Children's Emergency Fund (UNICEF), the World Health Organization (WHO), international conferences, nongovernmental organizations, and population laboratories (e.g., International Center for Diarrheal Disease Research, Bangladesh). Although health problems are similar in many low-resource settings, relying on data from other countries can create major problems when geographic differences are present in the incidence of the condition. In addition, the health impact associated with certain conditions such as hepatitis B, rotavirus, or malaria may be different in different regions and countries.

Registries

Registries are comprehensive longitudinal listings of persons with particular conditions, which may include detailed information about diagnostic classification, treatment, and outcome.[61] Registries have also been used to ensure the provision of appropriate care and to evaluate changing patterns of medical care; unlike other disease information systems, they cut across the different levels of severity of illness and may provide information over time about individual persons.

Population-based cancer registries generally have relied on multiple sources of data, including most importantly clinical pathology laboratories and hospital diagnoses. Death certification is also important, and other records such as those from oncology or radiotherapy units are also useful where available. Adherence to internationally recognized data collection and reporting standards has been increasing and the resulting data are used to compare the incidence of cancer in different geographic locations and distinct ethnic groups.[62] In the United States, several population-based registries based on the Surveillance of Epidemiology and End Results (SEER) model have been developed that conduct surveillance for cancer, and the national Coordinating Council for Cancer Surveillance was organized in 1995 to facilitate a collaborative approach among the involved organizations and to ensure maximal efficiency.[63] In many developing areas of the world, population-based surveillance systems may not be feasible,[64] but surveillance in selected institutions or laboratories may still be useful.

Surveillance for birth defects was first initiated in many parts of the world in response to the thalidomide tragedy; registries were established to provide reliable baseline rates for specific birth defects and to detect increases in the prevalence of birth defects as a means of rapidly identifying human teratogens.[65] CDC has conducted birth defects surveillance in metropolitan Atlanta since 1967 by using multiple sources of ascertainment of all serious birth defects observed in stillborn and liveborn infants or recognized by signs and symptoms apparent in the first year of life.[66] This birth defects registry system has been a valuable resource for monitoring rates of change of specific defects[67] and for conducting numerous genetic and epidemiologic investigations of risk factors for birth defects.[68] In addition to monitoring birth defect rates and serving as the basis for epidemiologic studies, the data from these state registries are used to evaluate the effectiveness of prevention activities and to refer children for health services and early intervention programs.[69]

Other Administrative Systems

Other federal agencies are involved in the collection of data that may be useful for public health. For example, the Food and Drug Administration (FDA) conducts postmarketing surveillance of adverse reaction to drugs,[70] and the Consumer Product Safety Commission (CPSC) conducts surveillance on product-related injuries.[71] The Hazardous Materials Information System of the Department of Transportation, established in 1971, provides reporting of spills associated with interstate commerce on a voluntary basis.[72] Such data, although incomplete, often are the only available source of information of particular issues of public health importance. These systems, however, frequently are not integrated at the state and national levels of public health surveillance and prevention activities.

Medical records are gaining increasing recognition for potential use in the field of public health. At the national level, Medicare data have been adapted for research purposes; locally and regionally, managed care organizations have established research activities based on their patient populations.[73]

EPIDEMIOLOGIC STUDIES

As noted earlier in the chapter, the practice of epidemiology includes the study of the distribution and determinants of health-related states or events. In practical terms, the distribution—the relationship of health events to person, place, and time—is called descriptive epidemiology. The study of determinants—causes and risk factors—is the domain of analytic epidemiology. Both aspects are necessary to provide a complete picture of the health event in the population. Just as a newspaper reporter must describe the what, who, when, where,

and why of a story, the epidemiologist must address the health event itself, as well as its person, time, and place characteristics, and finally its causes.

Case Definition

A case definition is a set of standard criteria for determining whether a person should be categorized as having a particular disease or health-related condition. A case definition consists of clinical criteria and, sometimes, limitations on time, place, and person. The clinical criteria usually include confirmatory laboratory tests, if available, or combinations of symptoms, signs, and other findings. For example, the case definition for human rabies requires laboratory confirmation (Table 13.2). In contrast, the case definition for Kawasaki syndrome, a febrile rash illness of children with no known cause and no pathognomonic laboratory findings, is based on the presence of fever, at least four of five specified clinical findings, and no other explanation for the findings.

Use of a standard case definition ensures that a diagnosis is consistent over time, locale, and clinical practice. Thus, the current number of cases of hepatitis A in one area can be compared with the numbers in the same area over time, and to the numbers in surrounding areas. When standard case definitions are used, an excess number of observed cases is likely to represent a true outbreak rather than variation in diagnostic criteria.

Case definitions may vary with varying purposes and in different settings. In conducting surveillance for a rare but serious communicable disease, a sensitive case definition is appropriate. The local health officials would want to hear about a patient with clinical findings consistent with plague or food-borne botulism, even if confirmatory laboratory results are still pending, so they could begin planning the appropriate public health measures that might be needed. Similarly, in areas of the world where malaria is endemic but diagnostic tools are rare, the case definition for malaria may be as simple as "fever." On the other hand, when conducting epidemiologic research into the cause of disease, it is important that the cases have the disease under study. Therefore, the investigator is likely to prefer a specific or "strict" case definition.

Table 13.2.   Selected Case Definitions

Rabies, Human

Clinical Description

Rabies is an acute encephalomyelitis that almost always progresses to coma or death within 10 days after the first symptom.

Laboratory Criteria for Diagnosis

- Detection by direct fluorescent antibody of viral antigens in a clinical specimen (preferably the brain or the nerves surrounding hair follicles in the nape of the neck); or
- Isolation (in cell culture or in a laboratory animal) of rabies virus from saliva, cerebrospinal fluid (CSF), or central nervous system tissue; or
- Identification of a rabies-neutralizing antibody titer greater than or equal to 5 (complete neutralization) in the serum or CSF of an unvaccinated person.

Case Classification

Confirmed: a clinically compatible case that is laboratory confirmed.

Comment

Laboratory confirmation by all of the above methods is strongly recommended.

SOURCE: CDC. Case definitions for infectious conditions under public health surveillance. *MMWR*. 1997;46:RR10.

Kawasaki Syndrome

Clinical Case Definition

A febrile illness of greater than or equal to 5 days' duration, with at least four of the five following physical findings and no other more reasonable explanation for the observed clinical findings:

- Bilateral conjunctival injection; or
- Oral changes (erythema of lips or oropharynx, strawberry tongue, or fissuring of the lips); or
- Peripheral extremity changes (edema, erythema, or generalized or periungual desquamation); or
- Rash; or
- Cervical lymphadenopathy (at least one lymph node greater than or equal to 1.5 cm in diameter).

Laboratory Criteria for Diagnosis

None.

Case Classification

Confirmed: a case that meets the clinical case definition.

Comment

If fever disappears after intravenous gamma globulin therapy is started, fever may be of less than five days' duration, and the clinical case definition may still be met.

SOURCE: CDC. Case definitions for infectious conditions under public health surveillance. *MMWR*. 1990;39:RR13.

Descriptive Epidemiology

In descriptive epidemiology, data on the health problem in the population are organized and summarized by time, place, and person. Decades ago, these aspects were usually addressed simply, but sometimes quite thoroughly. Now, advanced laboratory, statistical, and graphical methods allow much more sophisticated and complex assessments.

The approach of carefully compiling and systematically analyzing epidemiologic data by time, place, and person serves several purposes. First, this approach allows the public health worker conducting the analysis to become familiar with the data and with the dimensions of the public health problem. Second, the approach provides a thorough characterization of the public health problem that can be communicated easily to others. Third, the approach provides an indication of which populations or persons with particular characteristics are at greatest risk for acquiring a particular disease. This, in turn, provides important clues regarding etiology of disease. These clues can be turned into hypotheses that can be tested using analytic epidemiology.

Numbers and Rates

Counting the number of events—the number of new cases of hepatitis A reported this week, the number of infants who died this year, the number of doses of influenza vaccine administered this month—is a common and essential activity of a health department. The numbers can be added or grouped by time, place, and person to provide an informative description of the magnitude and pattern of a health problem or service. The numbers may indicate clusters or outbreaks of disease in the community. The numbers can also be used to guide health policy and resource allocation—the number of hospital beds needed, the best location of a satellite clinic, or the dollar amount to request for HIV counseling in next year's budget.

The use of counts alone has limitations, however. Because counts do not take into account population size or dynamics, they are insufficient for assessing an individual's or a population's risk of some adverse health event. To characterize risk, rates rather than counts must be used. Calculating rates for different subgroups by age, sex, geographic location, exposure history, or other characteristics can identify groups at increased risk for disease. Identification of these high-risk groups is vital to the development and targeting of effective control and prevention strategies. Rates are also preferred over counts for comparing health conditions in a population over time or among different populations, because rates take into account the size of the population and the specific period.

To calculate a rate, the count must be divided by an appropriate denominator. The denominator is usually an estimate of the population that gave rise to the counts in the numerator. For example, if the numerator is the number of women diagnosed with breast cancer as identified by a statewide cancer registry during the past year, an appropriate denominator might be the estimated midyear female population of the state based on census figures. If the numerator is restricted to women above a certain age, the denominator should be similarly restricted. These rates provide an estimate of the one-year risk of breast cancer among women in that population. In practice, such rates are usually expressed per 1,000 population or per 100,000 population. Use of these standard population units facilitate comparisons of disease or death rates among different groups.

As illustrated by this example, denominators for public health data are often population estimates from the United States Bureau of the Census. Based on the census conducted every 10 years, the bureau provides detailed breakdowns of the population by age, race or ethnic group, sex, and census track. Between census years, the bureau provides less-detailed estimates. Many states develop more-detailed estimates for use in their own jurisdictions for the years between the national censuses.

Common Measures

The most common health outcomes measured by health agencies are those related to morbidity (illness, injury, disability), mortality (death), and natality (birth). Morbidity measures include disease incidence and prevalence. Mortality measures include crude, specific, and standardized mortality rates as well as years of potential life lost. Some of the most commonly used measures are described in the following material (Table 13.3).

Morbidity Measures

Morbidity measures quantify a population's likelihood of developing or having an illness, injury, disability, or other adverse health condition.

An incidence rate, sometimes referred to simply as incidence, is the rate at which new events, such as new cases of disease, occur in a population in a stated

Table 13.3. Commonly Used Epidemiologic Measures

Natality Measure	Numerator	Denominator	Expressed per Number At Risk
Crude Birth Rate	live births reported during a given time interval	estimated total population at midinterval	1,000
Crude Fertility Rate	live births reported during a given time interval	estimated number of women age 15–44 years at midinterval	1,000
Morbidity Measure			
Incidence Rate	new cases of a specified disease reported during a given time interval	average or midpoint population during time interval	variable: 10^x where $x = 2,3,4,5,6$
Attack Rate	new cases of a specified disease reported during an epidemic period of time	population at start of the epidemic period	variable: 10^x where $x = 2,3,4,5,6$
Point Prevalence	current cases, new and old, of a specified disease at a given point in time	estimated population at the same point in time	variable: 10^x where $x = 2,3,4,5,6$
Period Prevalence	current cases, new and old, of a specified disease identified over a given time interval	estimated population at midinterval	variable: 10^x where $x = 2,3,4,5,6$
Mortality Measure			
Crude Death Rate	total number of deaths reported during a given time interval	estimated midinterval population	1,000 or 100,000
Cause-Specific Death Rate	deaths assigned to a specific cause during a given time interval	estimated midinterval population	100,000
Death-to-Case Ratio (case-fatality rate, case-fatality ratio)	deaths assigned to a specific disease during a given time interval	new cases of that disease reported during the same time interval	100
Neonatal Mortality Rate	deaths under 28 days of age during a given time interval	live births during the same time interval	1,000
Infant Mortality Rate	deaths under one year of age during a given time interval	live births reported during the same time interval	1,000

SOURCE: *Self-Study Course 3030-G: Principles of Epidemiology.* 2nd ed. Atlanta, Ga: Centers for Disease Control; 1992.

period of time. The numerator is the number of persons who develop new cases of illness during a specified period of time. The denominator is either a sum of the time during which all persons were observed (person-time rate) or the average or midperiod size of the population.

An attack rate or cumulative incidence is a measure of incidence calculated most commonly in the investigation of an acute outbreak of disease. It is simply the proportion of the population that developed illness during a specified period of time. The numerator is the number of new cases. The denominator, however, is the size of the population at the beginning of the observation period. The attack rate is a measure of the probability or risk of developing illness.

The prevalence rate, often referred to simply as prevalence, is the proportion of persons in a population who have a particular disease or attribute at a specific point in time or during a specified period. Prevalence differs from incidence in that prevalence includes all cases, both old and new, in the population during the specified time, whereas incidence is limited to new cases only. Prevalence is most often measured from cross-sectional surveys of a population.

Point prevalence refers to prevalence measured at a particular point in time; that is, the proportion of persons with a particular disease or attribute on a particular date. Period prevalence refers to prevalence measured over an interval of time; that is, the proportion of persons who had a particular disease or attribute at any time during the interval.

Mortality Measures

The mortality rate or death rate quantifies the frequency of occurrence of death in a defined population during a specified period.

The crude death rate (or crude mortality rate) is the number of deaths from all causes for the entire population, divided by the population. In the United States in 1998, a record high total of 2,337,256 deaths were recorded. The 1998 estimated midyear population was 270,298,524. The crude mortality rate was, therefore, 864.7 deaths per 100,000 population, similar to death rates since the mid-1970s.[74]

To assess or compare the mortality experience of different subpopulations, death rates may be calculated specifically for those subpopulations. An age-specific death rate is a death rate limited to a particular age group. Similarly, a sex-specific or race-specific death rate is limited to one sex or one racial group, respectively.

The infant mortality rate, a type of age-specific death rate, is used by all nations as an important public health indicator. The numerator is the number of deaths among children under one year of age reported during a given period, usually a calendar year. The denominator is the number of live births reported during the same period. The infant mortality rate is usually expressed per 1,000 live births. In 1998, the U.S. infant mortality rate was 7.2 infant deaths per 1,000 live births.[74]

A cause-specific death rate is the mortality rate from a specified cause for a population. The numerator is the number of deaths attributed to a specific cause. The denominator is the same as the crude death rate, that is, an estimate of the entire population. Cause-specific death rates are usually expressed per 100,000 population. In the United States, diseases of the heart and malignant neoplasms have had the two highest cause-specific death rates since at least 1950, but the gap between the two has narrowed considerably.[74]

Often, one wishes to compare the mortality experience of different populations, or of the same population over time. However, because death rates increase with age, a higher crude death rate in one population than another may simply reflect that the first population is older, on average, than the second. When the underlying age distribution of two (or more) populations varies, one could either compare age-specific death rates or compute age-standardized (or age-adjusted) death (or mortality) rates.

Age-standardized death rates are based on statistical techniques that eliminate the effects of different age distributions in different populations. In effect, an age-standardized rate is a "what if" rate—what would the overall death rate be if the age distributions of the two (or more) populations were the same. This is accomplished by applying the observed age-specific rates from each population to some standard population. For many years the standard population recommended by the National Center for Health Statistics (NCHS) was the 1940 U.S. population. However, in the new millennium, the 2000 U.S. population will be the standard.[74]

Years of potential life lost (YPLL) is a measure of the impact of premature mortality on a population.[75] For a person who dies "prematurely" (usually defined as either before age 65 or before the average life expectancy is reached), YPLL is calculated as the difference between that defined end point and the actual age at death. For an entire population, the YPLL is the sum of the individual YPLLs. Cause-specific YPLL can be calculated for specific causes of death.

The YPLL rate represents years of potential life lost per 1,000 population who are below the specified end point in age. YPLL rates are used to compare premature mortality in different populations, because YPLL alone does not take into account differences in population size. Furthermore, YPLL rates may be standardized by age to adjust for differences in the underlying age distribution of populations.

Quality-adjusted life years (QALYs) is the standard unit of measure in a cost-utility analysis that reflects the quality of life, or desirability of living, as well as the duration of survival. Quality of life is integrated with length of life using a multiplicative formula and discounting length of life by quality of life expected.[76] The measures are based on surveys of individuals, where individuals are asked to weigh a particular health state against perfect health and against death using methods such as person trade-off, time trade-off, and standard gamble.[77]

Disability-adjusted life years (DALYs) is a variant of QALYs used by the World Health Organization that measures the burden of disease, not only from premature mortality, but also from disability.[78] It is a composite measure (sum) of time lost due to premature mortality (YPLL, with life expectancy currently of 82.5 years for females and 80 years for males), and time lived with a disability, adjusted for the severity of the disability. An expert panel weighs the severity of disability using methods similar to those used for QALYs. Also included in the calculation of DALYs are age weights (different values of life for each age) and discounted future years of life.[79]

Time, Place, Person

Time

Characterizing a health event in a population by time is critical in determining historical trends, baseline levels and epidemics, and projections for the future. The time pattern of interest varies with the health condition of interest. For most chronic diseases, the time pattern of interest is the secular trend, the annual number or rate of disease over many years (Figure 13.1). For many injuries, the most revealing time pattern may be by day of the week and time of day (Figure 13.2). For acute infectious diseases, the choice may be seasonal patterns or an epidemic period during which the reported number of cases exceeds the usual number of cases (Figure 13.3).

Place

Characterizing a health event in a population by place provides insight into the geographic extent of the problem. Characterization by place includes assessment of occurrence according to place or residence (country, state, county, census tract, street address, map coordinates), birthplace, employment, and school district. Place also considers disease occurrence by categories such as urban or rural, domestic or foreign, institutional or noninstitutional, and so forth.

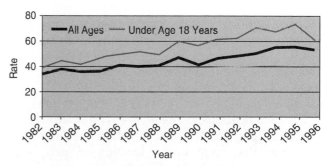

Figure 13.1. Rate* of Asthma by Age and Year— United States, 1982–1996

*Per 100,000 population.

Source: Centers for Disease Control and Prevention. *CDC Fact Book, 2000/2001.* Atlanta, GA: Centers for Disease Control and Prevention; 2000.

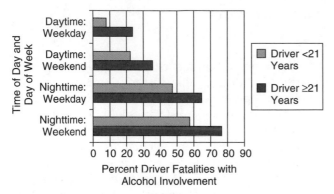

Figure 13.2. Percentage of Driver Fatalities in Which Blood Alcohol Concentration Exceeded 0.1% and a Single Vehicle Was Involved, by Driver Age, Time of Day, and Day of Week—United States, 1998

Source: *1998 Motor Vehicle Crash Data, Traffic Safety Facts 1998.* National Traffic Safety Administration.

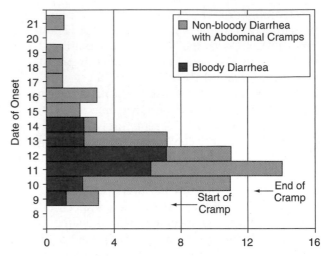

Figure 13.3. Number of *E. coli* 0111:H8-Associated Illnesses, by Symptoms and Date of Onset—Texas, June 1999

Source: Centers for Disease and Control Prevention. E. coli 011:H8 outbreak among teen campers—Texas 1999. *MMWR*. 2000;49:321–324.

Analysis of data by place can suggest hypotheses regarding reservoirs, vehicles, manner of spread, and causes. The association of disease occurrence with place implies that risk factors are present either in the persons living there (host factors) or in the environment or both. For example, communicable diseases are spread from person to person more rapidly in urban areas than in rural areas, primarily because the greater population density of the urban area provides more opportunities for susceptible persons to come in contact with a source of infection. On the other hand, diseases that are transmitted from animals to humans often have a greater incidence in the rural and suburban areas as a result of greater opportunity for humans to come into contact with disease-carrying animals, ticks, and the like. For example, lyme disease has become more common as humans have moved to wooded areas where they come into contact with infected ticks.

Characterization of a health event by place may be simple or complex. The simplest characterization is a spot map that displays the location of each case-patient's home on a map. On the other hand, geographic information systems (GIS) are data management systems that organize and display map data from several sources and facilitate the analysis of re-

lationships between the mapped features. GIS technology has been used to create a variety of atlases of disease and has been used in a number of field investigations.[80,81]

Person

Persons can be described in terms of their inherent characteristics (age, sex, race), acquired characteristics (marital status, vaccination status), behaviors and activities (occupation, leisure activities, use of medications, tobacco, seat belts), and the circumstances under which they live (socioeconomic status, access to health care). These characteristics, activities, and conditions determine to a large degree which persons will be at increased or decreased risk for various diseases and other adverse health events. As with time and place, characterization by person provides the investigator with insights into the distribution of the health condition in the population and may provide hypotheses about disease etiology.

Analytic Epidemiology

Analytic epidemiology is concerned with the search for causes and effects, or the *why* or *how*. The key feature is the presence of a comparison group. With a case report or case series, apparently unusual features may be described for one or more persons with disease, but no information is provided to tell how unusual those features really are. In an analytic epidemiologic study, the comparison group explicitly provides that information. If persons with a particular characteristic are more likely than those without the characteristic to develop a certain disease, then the characteristic is said to be *associated* with the disease. The characteristic may be a demographic factor such as age or sex; a constitutional factor such as blood group or immune status; a behavior such as smoking or having eaten the potato salad; or a circumstance such as living near a toxic waste site. These factors help identify populations at increased risk for disease, which may lead to appropriate targeting of public health prevention and control activities as well as ideas for future etiologic research.

For example, in an outbreak of hepatitis A, almost all of the case-patients ate pastries from a particular bakery and drank city water. An epidemiologic study was conducted in which consumption by cases was compared with consumption by a comparable group without hepatitis A. Almost all members of the comparison group drank city water, but few had eaten pastries. The study therefore implicated the bakery rather than the city water as the source of the outbreak, which would have remained unknown without the comparison group.[82]

Types of Studies

Epidemiologic studies fall into two broad categories: experimental and observational. In an experimental study, the investigator determines the exposure category for each individual (clinical trial) or community (community trial), then follows the individuals or communities to identify effects. More commonly, epidemiologists conduct observational studies, in which the investigator simply observes the exposure and outcome status of each study participant.

The two most common types of observational studies are the cohort study and the case-control study. A cohort or prospective study is similar conceptually to the experimental study—subjects are categorized on the basis of their exposure and followed for the subsequent development of the health events under study. The difference is that, in a cohort study, the epidemiologist observes rather than dictates the exposure status of the participants. After a sufficient period of follow-up, the rate of disease occurrence among the exposed group is compared with the rate of disease development among the unexposed group. The length of follow-up varies for different diseases, ranging from a few days for acute diseases to several decades for cancer, cardiovascular disease, and other chronic diseases. The Framingham study is a well-known cohort study in which over 5,000 residents of Framingham, Massachusetts, have been followed since the early 1950s to determine the rate of and risk factors for cardiovascular disease.[83]

The second and more common type of observational epidemiologic study is the case-control or retrospective study. In a case-control study, a group of persons with disease ("cases" or "case-patients") and a comparable group of persons without disease ("controls") are enrolled. The exposure or risk factor status of each enrollee is ascertained, and the exposure pattern of cases is compared with the exposure pattern of controls. The purpose of the control group is to provide an estimate of the expected or baseline exposure level or pattern in the population from which the cases arose. An exposure that is more common among cases than among controls is said to be associated with the disease, as in the study of hepatitis A cited previously. The key to well-designed case-control studies is to select an appropriate control group that provides a valid estimate of the baseline exposure.

The Two-by-Two Table

A two-by-two table is a cross-tabulation of the exposure and disease data from a cohort or case-control study. The traditional data layout for a two-by-two table is shown in Table 13.4. Each cell contains the

Table 13.4. Data Layout and Notation for a Standard Two-by-Two Table

	Ill/Cases	Well/Controls	Total	Attack Rate
Exposed	a	b	a + b	a/(a + b)
Unexposed	c	d	c + d	c/(c + d)
Total	a + c	b + d	a + b + c + d	(a + c)/(a + b + c + d)

Table 13.5. Consumption of Ham and Risk of Gastroenteritis Following an Easter Sunday Dinner, State A, April 2000

	Ill	Well	Total	Attack Rate
Ate ham	16	11	27	59.3%
Did not eat ham	1	6	7	14.3%
Total	17	17	34	50.0%

number of study subjects with the exposure status as indicated in the row heading to the left and with the disease status indicated in the column heading above. For example, *c* represents the number of persons in the study who were not exposed, but who became ill or case subjects nonetheless.

Data from the investigation of an outbreak of gastroenteritis following an Easter Sunday dinner are presented in Table 13.5 (Cassius Lockett, personal communication, 2000). The table provides a cross-tabulation of ham consumption (exposure) by presence or absence of gastroenteritis (outcome). Attack rates (59.3 percent for those who ate ham; 14.3 percent for those who did not) are given to the right of the table.

Measures of Association

A measure of association quantifies the strength or magnitude of the association between the exposure and the health outcome of interest. Measures of association are sometimes called measures of effect because, if the exposure is causally related to the disease, the measures quantify the effect of being exposed on the risk of disease. In cohort studies, the measure of association of choice is the risk ratio or rate ratio. In case-control studies, the measure of choice is the odds ratio.

A risk ratio or relative risk compares the risk of disease or other health outcome between two groups, such as an exposed and unexposed group. It is calculated as the ratio of two risks (attack rates, cumulative incidences):

$$\text{Risk Ratio} = \frac{\text{risk}_{\text{exposed}}}{\text{risk}_{\text{unexposed}}} = \frac{a/a + b}{c/c + d}$$

The risk ratio based on the data presented in Table 13.4 is 59.3/14.3 = 4.1. That is, persons who ate ham were 4.1 times more likely to develop gastroenteritis than those who did not eat ham. Note that the risk ratio will be greater than 1.0 when the risk in the exposed group is greater than the risk in the unexposed group. The risk will be equal to 1.0 if both groups have the same risk of disease, that is, if exposure is unrelated to risk of disease. The risk will be less than 1.0 if the risk of disease in the exposed group is less than the risk in the unexposed group, as would be expected when the exposure is a protective one such as vaccination or prophylactic antibiotic use.

In most case-control studies, the size of the exposed and unexposed groups are unknown, and the number of controls is decided by the investigator. Without true denominators, attack rates (risks) cannot be calculated, so risk ratios cannot be calculated either. However, the odds ratio can be calculated as its

Table 13.6. Legionnaires' Disease and Exposure to Hospital A, State B, 1998

	Cases	Controls	Total
Visited hospital	12	4	16
Did not visit hospital	1	18	19
Total	13	22	35

own measure of association, and when the disease is relatively rare, the odds ratio approximates the risk ratio. The odds ratio is calculated as:

$$\text{Odds Ratio} = \frac{ad}{bc}$$

In an outbreak of Legionnaires' disease, 13 cases occurred among residents of a small community. Controls were selected from local physician logs. Ironically, visiting the local hospital appeared to be associated with illness, as shown in Table 13.6 (Joel Ackelsberg, personal communication, 2000). The odds ratio, calculated as $12 \times 18/(4 \times 1)$, was 54.0. This odds ratio indicates a very strong association. Subsequent cultures of the cooling tower atop the hospital grew *Legionella pneumophila* with patterns indistinguishable from clinical samples from the patients.

Incidence rates and prevalence rates in different populations can also be compared. A rate ratio and a prevalence ratio compare two incidence rates or prevalence rates, respectively, by dividing one by the other. A prevalence odds ratio is calculated as the odds ratio described below, but uses prevalent cases rather than incident cases.

Finally, the standardized mortality ratio and the standardized morbidity ratio (both abbreviated as *SMR*) are measures of association commonly used in occupational epidemiology, wherein the number of observed deaths (or new cases) is divided by the expected number, taking into account the age distribution of the population.[84]

Measures of Public Health Impact

A measure of public health impact puts the association between exposure and disease into a public health context. It quantifies how much of the disease occurrence in a population may be attributed to the exposure being studied. For example, for an exposure that apparently increases one's risk of disease, such as smoking and lung cancer or undercooked hamburgers from Restaurant A and diarrhea, the attributable risk percent quantifies the amount of disease allegedly caused by the exposure. This measure can also be interpreted as the amount of disease that could be (or could have been) avoided if the exposure could be removed (or had never existed). For an exposure such as vaccination that reduces one's risk of disease, the prevented fraction quantifies the reduction in disease burden attributable to the exposure.[84] For example, in one of their classic papers on smoking, Doll and Hill reported that the lung cancer mortality rates for smokers and nonsmokers were 1.30 and 0.07 per 1,000 persons per year, respectively.[85] Because only 0.07 deaths per 1,000 would be expected in the absence of smoking, the proportion of deaths among smokers attributable to their smoking (attributable risk percentage) was $100\% \times (1.30 - 0.07)/1.30 = 95\%$. Although smoking also contributed to an increase in cardiovascular disease deaths, the attributable risk percent was much smaller, only 23 percent.

Tests of Statistical Significance

Not every elevated risk ratio or odds ratio indicates a causal relationship between exposure and disease. Particularly when the risk ratio or odds ratio is only slightly deviant from 1.0, or when a study has only a few subjects, the apparent association could simply be a chance finding. Tests of statistical significance are tools to evaluate the role of chance in explaining the finding.

The test of an association for statistical significance begins with the assumption that the exposure is *not* related to disease. This assumption is known as the null hypothesis. (The alternative hypothesis, which may be adopted if the null hypothesis proves to be implausible, is that exposure *is* associated with disease.) A statistical test appropriate for the data is then selected and applied—for the data in a two-by-two table, either a Fisher Exact Test (which is best for studies with relatively few subjects) or a chi-square test. The test of significance provides the probability of finding an association as strong as, or stronger than, the one observed if the null hypothesis were really true. This probability is called the P value. A very small P value indicates that one is very unlikely to observe such an association if the null hypothesis were true. When the P value is smaller than some cutoff specified in advance, such as 0.05, the null hypothesis is discarded as implausible, in favor of the alternative hypothesis. Note that, in practice, most tests have more than one formulation, which occasionally lead to different conclusions.

The statistical test for the data in Table 13.4 yielded a P value of 0.046. Because this P value is smaller than the specified cutoff of 0.05, we would reject the null hypothesis and adopt the alternative hypothesis that eating ham was indeed associated with an increased risk of becoming ill. Note that a P value of approximately 0.05 indicates 5 percent of the time we may observe data that supports an association, even if there is none—not likely, but certainly within the realm of possibility. If the ham had come directly from a commercial processor, the investigator might prefer a greater level of statistical assurance, that is, a smaller P value of less than 0.01 or 1 out of 100, before claiming that a company's hams are associated with illness and should be recalled from supermarket shelves.

The P value for the data in Table 13.6 is 0.00004. Therefore, the likelihood that the association of visiting the hospital and developing legionellosis can be attributed to chance is extremely small, and the null hypothesis would be rejected.

Confidence Intervals

Another technique for quantifying the statistical likelihood of an observed measure of association is the confidence interval. A confidence interval surrounds the observed value, and provides an indication of its statistical precision. The confidence interval is a range of values that has a given probability (often 95 percent) of containing the true value of the association. A narrow confidence interval reflects high precision in the observed value, whereas a wide confidence interval reflects more variability and less precision. Investigators often infer that the confidence interval is the range of values consistent with the data in the study. As a result, a confidence interval can also be used as a test of statistical significance—a 95 percent confidence interval that includes the null hypothesis value of 1.0 cannot reject the null hypothesis, while a 95 percent confidence interval that does not include 1.0 can reject the null hypothesis. Note that different formulas for the 95 percent confidence limits can occasionally give quite different results.

For example, the 95 percent confidence interval for the data in Table 13.5 (odds ratio = 54.0) is from 5.4 to 544.0. This interval does not include 1.0, so, as with the chi-square test, the null hypothesis would be rejected. The interval is quite wide, indicating that the actual observed value of 54.0 is not very precise. Nonetheless, all of the values in the interval, even those at the lower end, indicate a very strong association between visiting the hospital and developing legionellosis.

Interpretation and Inference

An elevated risk ratio or odds ratio does not necessarily indicate a causal relationship between the exposure and the health outcome. In fact, other explanations of the apparent association should be assessed first. These possible explanations are chance, selection bias, information bias, confounding and investigator error.

Chance is one possible explanation for an observed association. The role of chance is assessed through the use of tests of statistical significance. A very small P value indicates that it is unlikely for us to observe these data if the null hypothesis is true, and that chance is an improbable explanation for the observed association. Note that statistical tests and P values only address the role of chance—they do not address problems in how the study may have been designed, conducted, and analyzed; thus, these measures will not address any bias that may exist.

A second explanation for an observed association is selection bias. Selection bias is a systematic flaw in how participants were selected, enrolled, or categorized that results in an erroneous estimate of the association between exposure and disease. Consider a hypothetical case-control study of toxic shock syndrome at the time when its association with tampon use was suspected but not confirmed. The diagnosis was not well known at the time, but physicians may have been reminded of the diagnosis if they knew the patient had been using a tampon. If diagnosis-based-on-exposure had been common, the effect on the two-by-two table would have been to load up the *a* cell, resulting in an artificially elevated odds ratio. Bias can also result from other selection, enrollment, and categorization problems such as differences between persons who agree versus those who decline (or are too sick) to participate, from the use of volunteer controls who have their own reasons for participating, and by enrolling persons with asymptomatic disease as controls.

A third explanation for an observed association is information bias. Information bias is a systematic flaw in the information collected from or about the participants in the study that results in an erroneous estimate of the association between exposure and disease. If cases are more likely to recall an exposure than controls, then that exposure will appear to be associated with illness. If interviewers probe more thoroughly when interviewing cases than controls, or data abstractors review hospital charts of cases more vigorously than charts of controls, then again the exposure will appear to be associated with illness.

A fourth explanation for an observed association is confounding. Confounding is a mixing of two effects, specifically when an unstudied risk factor is associated with both the exposure and outcome under study. Consider a hypothetical, poorly randomized clinical trial in which more cancer patients with early-stage disease receive investigational drug A than tried-and-true drug B, and more cancer patients with late-stage disease receive tried-and-true drug B than investigational drug A. Assume that persons with early-stage disease survive longer than persons with late-stage disease. Even if investigational drug A is no

better than tried-and-true drug B, drug A will appear to be associated with improved survival in comparison with drug B, because drug A was preferentially administered to persons with early-stage disease. In this example the unstudied risk factor is stage of disease, resulting in an apparent association between drug A and improved survival when no such effect truly exists.

A fifth explanation for an observed association is investigator error. Investigator error may result from erroneous data entry or manipulation, inappropriate analysis, or misinterpretation. It may be unintentional or intentional.

Assuming that an observed association does not appear to be attributable to chance, selection bias, information bias, confounding, or investigator error, a causal relationship might well be the explanation. Several criteria have been proposed for helping an investigator decide whether an association might be considered causal. These criteria include the magnitude of association (the larger the risk ratio or odds ratio, the more plausible), biologic plausibility, consistency with other studies, dose-response effect (increasing exposure associated with increased risk of disease), and exposure preceding disease. These criteria involve judgment, and reasonable people can disagree about whether the available evidence is sufficient to demonstrate causality.

SPECIAL ISSUES IN DATA MANAGEMENT FOR PUBLIC HEALTH

System Integration

Historically, data systems, as discussed in this chapter, have been developed around the study of specific diseases or health events (e.g., tuberculosis, sexually transmitted diseases, birth defects). Subsequently, independently developed disease-specific computer applications for use at the state and local level for the collection, entry, analysis, and transmission of data have arisen. These categorical systems result from distinct funding streams, mechanisms for delivering clinical care and health services, and organizational systems. Although these systems have played an important role in standardizing data collection and reporting across the nation for their respective systems, lack of integration among specific diseases or health events hinders usefulness. Variables common to multiple systems, classification and coding schemes, user interfaces, database formats, and methods for data transmission and analysis have not been standardized and/or reused. Thus, personnel at local and state health departments must use multiple systems that are not linked or merged.[86] This disease-based approach has resulted in lack of utility of data collected,[87] incomplete reporting,[88] and delays and burdens in reporting.[89]

A more integrated approach to data collection is motivated by an interest in data from new sources (e.g., pharmacy data or school absenteeism), access in electronic format, and concerns about security and confidentiality. In 1996, the U.S. Congress passed the Health Insurance and Portability Act (HIPAA; P.L. 104-191) which mandated the development and implementation of standards for exchanging financial and administrative data related to health care and concurrent changes in technology to allow timely and secure data reporting and access to data across governmental and geographic boundaries.[90]

The HIPAA, drafted at the request of the industry that finances health care, mandates the development, implementation, and use of standards for exchanging financial and administrative data related to health care.[91] Since 1999, this has resulted in standards for electronic transactions related to health (e.g., insurance claims, eligibility, encounters, and identifiers).[92] These mandated standards have brought together groups previously not working together; for example, the National Library of Medicines' Unified Medical Language System and the U.S. College of American Pathologists' Systematized Nomenclature of Medicine (SNOMED). Having similar standards and coding for data will enable data sharing between agencies interested in population health, privacy protections for medical information, and security of data transmission and storage.[93] As an example, CDC has developed agencywide Internet security standards for transmission of public health surveillance data consistent with these guidelines (http://www.cdc.gov/cic). One of the standards mandated by HIPAA is the creation of a unique health identifier for individuals; such an identifier would allow longitudinal and geographic linkages among health care records, facilitating information available for public health surveillance and control activities. To be most effective, public health must take advantage of other information development activities to be able to use data from any different sources, with rapid and secure dissemination of data to those who need to act to improve communities' health.

Computers and Informatics

The increase in availability of computers to analyze and transmit data and the decrease in the cost of such technology offers increased opportunity for surveillance. *Epi Info* is a public health computer program designed to assist data management and analysis that is available over the Internet;[94] the tool has been used successfully in both developed and developing countries in seven languages (English, French, Spanish, Arabic, Russian, Chinese, and Serbo-Croatian). The manual or portions of it have been translated into these languages as well as into Italian, Portuguese, German, Norwegian, Hungarian, Czech, Polish, Romanian, Indonesian, and Farsi.

The explosive development of technology includes the development of high-capacity storage devices, expansion of the capabilities of the Internet, use of local- and wide-area networks for entry of surveillance data at multiple computers simultaneously, and development of new programming tools, video and computer integration, and voice and pen input. Integration of systems, including data standards, is needed to allow maximal use of these advancements.[86]

In addition to the widespread use of computers in surveillance,[31] standards for exchanging information are critical to the future utility of all public health surveillance and information systems. HIPAA also encourages the development of standards for data related to health care.[95] The passage of this legislation has increased the level of activity related to integration of clinical information in the United States.[96]

Computerization has also been helpful in transmitting molecular data on isolates of certain pathogens, such as the previously discussed pulsed field gel electrophoresis patterns of *Escherichia coli*

0157:H7 through PulseNet (http://www.cdc.gov/ ncidod/dbmd/pulsenet/pulsenet.htm). In addition, computerization may facilitate and enhance regular and personal contact among public health officials, health care providers, and others who participate in such activities as a closed electronic mail system. The Emerging Infections Network, in which hundreds of infectious diseases practitioners participate in the United States, uses an electronic mail conference for online discussion when new insights into disease occurrence are needed and allows for close communication between public health officials and health care providers.[97]

Updating Records

Surveillance data often need to be updated. Information that was initially unattainable may become available, follow-up investigations yield supplemental information, persons initially classified as meeting or not meeting a case definition may be reclassified, errors in reporting may be identified and corrected, and duplicate case reports may be recognized and culled. One approach to handling these and other changes is to maintain both provisional and final records, including separate publications for provisional and final data. When analyzing trends, it is often useful to compare provisional data in one period with provisional data from another period because bias in preliminary data may change when data are updated. Provisional reports may satisfy immediate information needs, whereas final and more delayed reports can accommodate corrections and updates to a reasonable limit and can serve an archival function. Computerization facilitates record updates.

Privacy and Confidentiality

Preventing inappropriate disclosure of surveillance data is essential both to the privacy of persons with reported cases of disease and to the trust of participants in the surveillance system. The protection of confidentiality begins with limiting data collection and transmission to a minimum and includes ensuring the physical security of surveillance records, the discretion of surveillance staff, and legal safe-

guards.[98] To elicit public health surveillance information from the public and from health care providers, strong laws that ensure a careful procedure for maintaining and reporting data are frequently necessary to ensure the privacy of personal information[99] (see also Chapter 5). As applied to personally identifiable information (as opposed to aggregate data or data about institutions), *confidentiality* refers to a status accorded to information that indicates it is sensitive for stated reasons, must be protected, and access to it controlled. Privacy refers to the claim of individuals, and the societal value representing that claim, to control the use and disclosure of personal data. *Security* includes the safeguards (administrative, technical, physical) in an information system that protect it and its information against unauthorized disclosure and limit access to authorized users in accordance with an established policy.[100]

Privacy regulations in the United States are currently based on a patchwork of state and local legislation and may not adequately protect electronic health information. Recent bills introduced in the U.S. Congress include definitions of protected information and descriptions of disclosures that may occur with or without consent. Sometimes forgotten in the discussion of health information privacy is the concept that use of electronic information systems can often improve the security of data.

Physical protection of records is accomplished by rules of conduct for persons involved in the design, development, operation, or maintenance of any surveillance system. For example, confidential records should be kept locked up at all times when not in use. When confidential records are in use, they must be kept out of the sight of persons not authorized to work with the records. Except as needed for operational purposes, copies of confidential records should not be made. When confidential surveillance records are in the possession of other agencies, provision should be made for their protection.

Provision of data-containing identifiers of individuals or establishments should be held to the minimum number deemed essential to perform public health functions. Categories should be sufficiently broad to avoid inadvertent identification of a person or institution. In particular, release of information for small geographic areas must be carefully considered to protect confidentiality. Other methods of data security involve statistical disclosure techniques such as addition of "noise" (random data) while preserving aggregate statistics.[101]

Bioterrorism

The need for a strong infrastructure for data and information systems is being reemphasized today not only as countries face the emergence and reemergence of infectious diseases,[102] but also as a result of the increasing threat of biological and chemical terrorism.[103] Plans for detecting terrorist events include strengthening current surveillance systems as well as establishing new ones, such as surveillance of emergency calls for medical assistance and admissions of patients to intensive care units for respiratory conditions.[104] The purposeful dispersion of anthrax spores in the fall of 2001 demonstrated the need for concern

and preparedness (see chapters 3, 22, and 29). Bioterrorism is the subject of best-selling novels and nonfiction books.[105] Such awareness can fuel the enhancement of disease surveillance systems to ensure an effective response to acts of bioterrorism, especially at the local level.[106]

CONCLUSION

Public health decisions are best driven by data that are collected carefully and analyzed rigorously. Such data must be communicated clearly to policy makers so that public health practice is conducted effectively. Public health surveillance is the cornerstone of public health practice, and epidemiologic research is the basic science of public health. Both require high-quality data appropriate to the needs of the population at risk for diseases, injury, and disability. Only then can we ensure the public's health is served.

References

1. Last JM. *A Dictionary of Epidemiology.* 3rd ed. New York, NY: Oxford University Press; 1995.
2. Langmuir AD, Andrews JM. Biological warfare defense. 2. The Epidemic Intelligence Service of the Communicable Disease Center. *Am J Public Health.* 1952;42:235-238.
3. Scriven M. Minimalist theory of evaluation: the least theory that practice requires. *Am J Eval.* 1998;19:57-70.
4. Shadish WR, Cook TD, Leviton LC. Foundations of program evaluation: theories of practice. Newbury Park, Calif: Sage Publications; 1991.
5. Weiss CH. Evaluation: methods for studying programs and policies. 2nd ed. Upper Saddle River, NJ: Prentice Hall; 1998.
6. Worthen BR, Sanders JR, Fitzpatrick, JL. Program evaluation: alternative approaches and practical guidelines. 2nd ed. New York, NY: Longman; 1996.
7. Patton MQ. Utilization-focused evaluation: the new century text. 3rd ed. Thousand Oaks, Calif: Sage Publications; 1997.
8. Langmuir AD. The surveillance of communicable diseases of national importance. *N Engl J Med.* 1963;268:182-192.
9. Thacker SB. Historical development. In: Teustch SM, Churchill RE, eds. *Principles and Practice of Public Health Surveillance.* New York, NY: Oxford University Press; 2000:1-16.
10. Snider DE, Stroup DF. Ethical issues. In: Teustch SM, Churchill RE, eds. *Principles and Practice of Public Health Surveillance.* New York, NY: Oxford University Press; 2000:194-214.
11. Romaguera RA, German RR, Klaucke DN. Evaluating public health surveillance. In: Teutsch SM, Churchill RE, eds. *Principles and Practice of Public Health Surveillance.* Vol 2. New York, NY: Oxford University Press; 2000:176-193.
12. Eylenbosch WJ, Noah ND, eds. *Surveillance in Health and Disease.* London, England: Oxford University Press; 1988.
13. Langmuir AD. William Farr: founder of modern concepts of surveillance. *Int J Epidemiol.* 1976;5: 13-18.
14. McKay AP, Rochat R, Smith JC, Berg CH. The check box: determining pregnancy status to improve maternal mortality surveillance. *Am J Prev Med.* 2000;29:35-39.

15. Kovar MG. Data systems of the National Center for Health Statistics. Hyattsville, Md: National Center for Health Statistics, Centers for Disease Control; 1989. *Vital and Health Statistics,* Series 1. DHHS Publication (PHS)89-1325.

16. Choi K, Thacker SB. An evaluation of influenza mortality surveillance, 1962-1979. I. Time series forecasts of expected pneumonia and influenza deaths. *Am J Epidemiol.* 1981;113:215-226.

17. Freedman MA, Weed JA. The national vital statistics system. In: Martin E, ed. *Public Health Informatics and Information Systems.* New York, NY: Aspen Publishers; in press.

18. Jones TS, Liang AP, Kilbourne EM, et al. Morbidity and mortality associated with the July 1980 heat wave in St. Louis and Kansas City, Missouri. *JAMA.* 1982;247:3327-3331.

19. Parrish RG, Tucker M, Ing R, Encarnacion C. Sudden unexplained death syndrome in southeast Asian refugees: a review of CDC surveillance. In: *CDC Surveillance Summaries. MMWR.* 1987;36(SS):43-53.

20. Koo D, Birkhead GS. Prospects and challenges in implementing firearm-related injury surveillance in the United States. Not a flash in the pan. *Am J Prev Med.* 1998;15(suppl 3)120-124.

21. Hahn RA, Stroup DF. Race and ethnicity in public health surveillance: criteria for the scientific use of social categories. *Public Health Rep.* 1994;109:7-15.

22. Pinner RW, Teutsch SM, Simonsen L, Klug LA, Graber JM, Clarke MJ, et al. Trends in infectious diseases mortality in the United States. *JAMA.* 1996;275:189-193.

23. Kaufman JS, Asuzu MC, Rotimi CN, Johnson OO, Owoaje EE, Cooper RS. The absence of adult mortality data for sub-Saharan Africa: a practical solution. *Bull World Health Organ.* 1997;75:389-395.

24. Tollman SM, Kahn K, Garenne M, Gear JS. Reversal in mortality trends: evidence from the Agincourt field site, South Africa, 1992-1995. *AIDS.* 1999;13:1091-1097.

25. Fantahun M. Patterns of childhood mortality in three districts of north Gondar administrative zone. A community-based study using the verbal autopsy method. *Ethiopian Med J.* 1998;36:71-81.

26. Chandramohan D, Maude GH, Rodrigues LD, Hayes RJ. Verbal autopsies for adult deaths: their development and validation in a multi-centre study. *Trop Med Int Health.* 1998;3:436-446.

27. Quigley MA, Armstrong SJR, Schellenberg JR, Snow RW. Algorithms for verbal autopsies: a validation study in Kenyan children. *Bull World Health Organ.* 1996;74:147-154.

28. Percy C, Dolman A. Comparison of the coding of death certificates related to cancer in seven countries. *Public Health Rep.* 1978;93:335-350.

29. Kaunitz A, Rochat RW, Hughes JM, Smith JC, Grimes DA. Maternal mortality surveillance, 1974-1978. In: *CDC Surveillance Summaries. MMWR.* 1984;33(SS-1):5-8.

30. World Health Organization. The first ten years of the World Health Organization. *1958.* Geneva, Switzerland: World Health Organization.

31. Koo D, Wetterhall SF. History and current status of the National Notifiable Diseases Surveillance System. *J Public Health Manage Pract.* 1996;2:4-10.

32. Thacker SB, Stroup DF. Future directions for comprehensive public health surveillance and health information systems in the United States. *Am J Epidemiol.* 1994;140:383-397.

33. Hinman AR. Analysis, interpretation, use and dissemination of surveillance information. *PAHO Bull.* 1977;11:338-343.

34. Vogt RL, LaRue D, Klaucke DN, Jillson DA. Comparison of active and passive surveillance systems of primary care providers for hepatitis, measles, rubella and salmonellosis in Vermont. *Am J Public Health.* 1983;73:795-797.

35. Davis JP, Vergeront JM. The effect of publicity on the reporting of toxic-shock syndrome in Wisconsin. *J Infect Dis.* 1982;145:449-457.

36. Buehler JW, Berkelman RL, Stehr-Green JK. The completeness of AIDS surveillance. *J Acquir Immune Defic Syndr.* 1992;5:257-264.

37. Alter MJ, Mares A, Hadler SC, Maynard, JE. The effect of underreporting on the apparent incidence and epidemiology of acute viral hepatitis. *Am J Epidemiol.* 1987;125(1):133-139.

38. Brachott D, Mosley JW. Viral hepatitis in Israel: the effect of canvassing physicians on notifications and the apparent epidemiological pattern. *Bull World Health Organ.* 1972;46:457-464.

39. Valleron AJ, Bouvet E, Garnerin P, et al. A computer network for the surveillance of communicable diseases: the French experiment. *Am J Public Health.* 1986;76:1289-1292.

40. Stroobant AW, Van Casteren V, Thiers G. Surveillance systems from primary care data: surveillance through a network of sentinel general practitioners. In: Eylenbosch WJ, Noah ND, eds. *Surveillance in Health and Disease.* London, England: Oxford University Press; 1988:62-74.

41. Lobet MP, Stroobant A, Mertens R, et al. Tool for validation of the network of sentinel general practitioners in the Belgian health care system. *Int J Epidemiol.* 1987;16:612-618.

42. Thacker SB, Stroup DF, Rothenberg RB, Brownson RC. Public health surveillance for chronic conditions: a scientific basis for decisions. *Stat Med.* 1995;14:629-641.

43. Thacker SB, Stroup DF, Parrish RG, Anderson HA. Surveillance in environmental public health: issues, systems, and sources. *Am J Public Health.* 1996;86:633-638.

44. Baker EL. Sentinel event notification system for occupational risks (SENSOR): the concept. *Am J Public Health.* 1989;79(suppl):18-20.

45. Pollack ES, Ringen K. Risk of hospitalization for specific nonwork-related conditions among laborers and their families. *Am J Indus Med.* 1992;23:417-425.

46. Seligman PJ, Halperin WE, Mullan RJ, Frazier TM. Occupational lead poisoning in Ohio: surveillance using worker's compensation data. *Am J Public Health.* 1986;76:1299-1302.

47. Bean NH, Martin SM, Bradford H Jr. PHLIS: an electronic system for reporting public health data from remote sites. *Am J Public Health.* 1992;82:1273-1276.

48. Brachman PS. Surveillance. In: Evans AS, Feldman HH, eds. *Bacterial Infections of Humans.* New York, NY: Plenum Medical; 1982:49-61.

49. Gaynes RP, Culver DH, Emori, TG, et al. The national nosocomial infections surveillance system: plans for the 1990s and beyond. *Am J Prev Med.* 1991;91(3B):116S-120S.

50. Stelling JM, O'Brien TF. Surveillance of antimicrobial resistance: The WHONET program. *Clin Infect Dis.* 1997;24 (suppl 1):S157-S168.

51. Centers for Disease Control and Prevention. Outbreak of *salmonella* serotype *muenchen* infections associated with unpasteurized orange juice—United States and Canada. *MMWR.* 1999;48:582-585.

52. Fraser P, Beral V, Chilvers C. Monitoring disease in England and Wales: methods applicable to routine data-collecting systems. *J Epidemiol Community Health.* 1978;32:294-302.

53. Twigg L. Choosing a national survey to investigate smoking behavior: making comparisons between the General Household Survey, the British Household Panel Survey and the Health Survey for England. *J Public Health Med.* 1999;21:14-21.

54. Cheng C. Disease surveillance in China. In: Wetterhall SE, ed. Proceedings of the 1992 International Symposium on Public Health Surveillance. *MMWR.* 1992;41(supp):111-122.

55. Yang G. Selection of DSP points in second stage and their representation. *Chinese J Epidemiol.* 1992;13:197-201.

56. Siegel PZ, Brackbill RM, Frazier, EL, et al. Behavioral risk factor surveillance, 1986-1990. In: *CDC Surveillance Summaries. MMWR.* 1991;40(SS-4):1-23.

57. Kann L, Warren CW, Harns WA, Collins JL, Williams BI, Ross JG. Youth risk behavior surveillance—United States, 1995. In: *CDC Surveillance Summaries. MMWR.* 1996;45(SS-4):1-83.

58. Sattin RW, Rubin GL, Hughes JM. Hysterectomy among women of reproductive age, United States, update for 1979-1980. In: *CDC Surveillance Summaries. MMWR.* 1983;32(SS):1-7.

59. Thacker SB, Berkelman RL. Surveillance of medical technologies. *J Public Health Pol.* 1986;7:363-377.

60. McBean AM, Gornick M. Differences by race in the rates of procedures performed in hospitals for Medicare beneficiaries. *Health Care Financing Rev.* 1994;15:77-90.

61. Weddell JM. Registers and registries: a review. *Int J Epidemiol.* 1973;2:221-228.

62. Raymond L. Techniques of registration. In: Parkin DM, Whelan SL, Ferlay J, Raymond L, Young J, eds. *Cancer Incidence in Five Continents.* Vol VII. Lyon, France: IARC Scientific Publications, 1997.

63. Swan J, Wingo P, Clive R, et al. Cancer surveillance in the U.S.: can we have a national system? *Cancer.* 1998;83:9.

64. Parkin DM, ed. Cancer occurrence in developing countries. Lyon, France: International Agency for Research on Cancer; 1986.

65. Holtzman NA, Khoury MJ. Monitoring for congenital malformations. *Annu Rev Public Health.* 1986;7:237-266.

66. Edmonds LD, Layde PM, James LM, Flynt JW Jr, Erickson JD, Oakley GP Jr. Congenital malformations surveillance: two American systems. *Int J Epidemiol.* 1981;10:247-252.

67. Yen H, Khoury MJ, Erickson JD, James LM, Waters GD, Berry RJ. The changing epidemiology of neural tube defects in the United States. *Am J Dis Child.* 1992;146:857-861.

68. Erickson JD. Introduction: birth defects surveillance in the United States. *Teratology.* 1997;56:1-4.

69. Edmonds LD. Birth defects surveillance at the state and local level. *Teratology.* 1997;56:5-7.

70. Faich GA, Knapp D, Dreis M, Turner W. National adverse drug reaction surveillance—1985. *JAMA.* 1987;257:2068-2070.

71. Rivara FP, Bergman AB, Lo Gerfo JP, Weiss NS. Epidemiology of childhood injuries. *Am J Dis Child.* 1982;136:502-506.

72. US Congress, Office of Technology Assessment. *Transportation of Hazardous Materials.* Washington, DC: US Government Printing Office; 1986. OTA Publication SET-304.

73. Health Care Financing Administration. Medicare enrollment, 1986-87. Baltimore, Md: US Depart of Health and Human Services, Health Care Financing Administration, 1989; HCFA Publication 03282.

74. Murphy SL. Deaths: Final data for 1998. *National Vital Statistics Reports.* Vol 48, No. 11. Hyattsville, Md; National Center for Health Statistics, Centers for Disease Control and Prevention; 2000. PHS Publication 2000-1120.

75. Wise RP, Livengood JR, Berkelman RL, Goodman RA. Methodologic alternatives for measuring premature mortality. *Am J Prev Med.* 1988;4:268-273.

76. Farnham PG, Ackerman SP, Haddix AC. Study design. In: Haddix AC, Teutsch SM, Shaffer PA, Duñet DO, eds. *Prevention Effectiveness: A Guide to Decision Analysis and Economic Evaluation.* New York, NY: Oxford University Press; 1996:12-26.

77. Dasbach E, Teutsch SM. Cost-utility analysis. In: Haddix AC, Teutsch SM, Shaffer PA, Duñet DO, eds. *Prevention Effectiveness: A Guide to Decision Analysis and Economic Evaluation.* New York, NY: Oxford University Press; 1996:130-137.

78. The GBD's Approach to Measuring Health Status. In: Murray CJL, Lopez AD, eds. *Summary: The Global Burden of Disease.* Cambridge, Mass: Harvard University Press; 1996:6-7.

79. Hennekens CH, Buring JE. *Epidemiology in Medicine.* Boston, Mass: Little Brown; 1987.

80. Casper ML, Barnett E, Halverson JA, et al. Women and heart disease: An atlas of racial and ethnic disparities in mortality. 2nd ed. Atlanta, Ga: Centers for Disease Control and Prevention; 2000.

81. Bales NE, Dannenberg AL. Use of geographic information systems in epidemiologic field investigations [abstract]. *Am J Epidemiol.* 2001;153:s262.

82. Schoenbaum SC, Baker O, Jezek Z. Common-source epidemic of hepatitis due to glazed and iced pastries. *Am J Epidemiol.* 1976;104:74-80.

83. Dawber TR, Kannell WB, Lyell LP. An approach to longitudinal studies in a community: the Framingham Study. *Ann NY Acad Sci.* 1963;107:539-556.

84. Kahn HA, Sempos CT. *Statistical Methods in Epidemiology.* New York, NY: Oxford University Press; 1989.

85. Doll R, Hill AB. Mortality in relation to smoking: Ten years' observation of British doctors. *Br Med J.* 1964;1:1399-1410, 1460-1467.

86. Morris G, Snider D, Katz M. Integrating public health informatics and surveillance systems in the United States. *Am J Epidemiol.* 1996;2:24-27.

87. Brackbull RM, Sternberg MR, Fishbein M. Where do people go for treatment of sexually transmitted diseases? *Fam Plan Perspect.* 1999;31:10-15.

88. Marier R. The reporting of communicable diseases. *Am J Epidemiol.* 1977;105:587-590.

89. Birkhead G, Chorba TL, Root S, Klaucke DN, Gibbs NJ. Timeliness of national reporting of communicable diseases; the experience of the National Electronic Telecommunications Systems for Surveillance. *Am J Public Health.* 1991;81:313-315.

90. National Research Council. For the record: protecting electronic health information, computer science and telecommunications board, commission of physical sciences, mathematics and applications. Washington, DC: National Academy Press; 1997.

91. Curtin L, Simpson R. HIPAA: what's hot. . . . *Health Manage Technol.* 2000;21:42-44.

92. Tribble DA. The Health Insurance Portability and Accountability Act: security and privacy requirements. *Am J Health Syst Pharm.* 2001;58:763-770.

93. Lanser EG. Capitalizing on HIPAA compliance. *Healthc Exec.* 2001;16:6-11.

94. Dean AG. Epi Info and Epi Map: Current status and plans for Epi Info 2000. *J Public Health Manage Pract.* 1999;5:54-57.

95. Chute CG, Cohn SP, Campbell JR. A framework for comprehensive health terminology systems in the United States: development guidelines, criteria for selection and public policy implications. *J Am Med Informatics Assoc.* 1998;5:503-510.

96. College of American Pathologists. SNOMED RT and READ Codes to be combined in an international terminology of health. Joint development agreement by the College of American Pathologists and United Kingdom's Secretary of State for Health [press release]. March 1999. Available at: http://www.cap.org/ html/public/snomed_intl.html

97. Executive Committee of the Infectious Diseases Society of America Emerging Infections Network. Emerging Infections Network: A new venture for the Infectious Diseases Society of America. *Clin Infect Dis.* 1997;25:34-36.

98. Federal Committee on Statistics. *Private Lives and Public Policies.* Washington, DC: Federal Committee on

Statistics, US Dept of Health and Human Services; 1994.

99. Gostin LO, Burris S, Lazzarini Z. The law and the public's health: A study of infectious disease law in the United States. *Columbia Law Rev.* 1999;99:59-128.

100. O'Brien DG, Yasnoff WA. Privacy, confidentiality, and security in information systems of state health agencies. *Am J Prev Med.* 1999;16:351-358.

101. Jabine TB. Procedures for restricted data access. *J Off Stat.* 1993;9:537-589.

102. Heymann DL, Rodier GR. Global surveillance of communicable diseases. *Emerg Infect Dis.* 1998;4: 362-365.

103. Henderson DA. The looming threat of bioterrorism. *Science.* 1999;283:1279-1282.

104. Rotz LD, Koo D, O'Carroll PW, Kellogg RB, Lillibridge SR. Bioterrorism preparedness: Planning for the future. *J Public Health Manage Pract.* 2000;6:45-49.

105. Alibeck K, Handelman S. *Biohazard. The Chilling True Story of the Largest Covert Biological Weapons Program in the World—Told from Inside by the Man Who Ran It.* New York, NY: Random House; 1999.

106. Hamburg MA. Bioterrorism: a challenge to public health and medicine. *J Public Health Manage Pract.* 2000;6:38-44.

CHAPTER
14

Theories and Structures
of Public Health Behavior

John P. Elder, Ph.D., M.P.H.
Gregory A. Talavera, M.D., M.P.H.
Pamina M. Gorbach, M.H.S., Dr. P.H.
Guadalupe X. Ayala, Ph.D. (ABD), M.P.H.

INTRODUCTION

Health promotion is the branch of the public health sciences that emphasizes health-related behavior change. Whether it is for the teen at risk of smoking, the automobile passenger who forgets to wear a seat belt, or the mother deciding whether to breastfeed, human behavior represents a key element of a person's and population's health. This chapter examines several theories of health behavior current in the field, most of which derive from psychology, health education, and other health-related areas. Second, a "structural model" of ecological health behavior is presented, integrating these previous formulations while emphasizing the predominant note of the physical and social environment. Finally, we describe applications of this structural model to tobacco use prevention, nutritional health promotion, mammography screen utilization, and the prevention of sexually transmitted infections in the developing world.

Popular current psychosocial theories are based on Western notions of individual autonomy and purpose.[1] The Health Belief Model,[2] the Social Cognitive Theory,[3] the Theory of Reasoned Action,[4] Self Regulation and Self Control,[5] and other psychological theory formulations emphasize individual perceptions and attitude formation as they relate to health behavior. In other words, the emphasis of these theories is on how a person thinks rather than on what he or she does.

However, concepts such as "reasoned action" and "behavioral intentions"—as applied to individuals—

The authors are deeply indebted to Lisa Kondrat-Dauphin for her competent coordination of the writing efforts and processing of this manuscript.

are less relevant to many communities and cultures where individual self-identity is still grounded in familial and community roles.[6] Second, if we want to know what people are thinking, we have to ask them. Many cognitive theories imply or require detailed, thorough individual measurement, making them less practical for people not accustomed to questionnaires or with limited literacy, or for programs with no resources for such measurement. Third, scientific support for cognitive mechanisms driving health behavior is largely correlational, not causal. Few studies have shown that large-scale behavior change can be achieved by first changing thought patterns. Psychologically based theories are often more connected to the understanding of individual cognitive processes than to intervention design per se. As applied to health, they are more suited to focused interventions for high-risk groups than for entire populations.[7,8]

Ecological and Structural Models

Ecological models acknowledge the role of cognitive variables but place emphasis on the pervasive influences of social-environmental and physical-environmental factors. For example, McLeroy et al[9] and Stokols[10] have described the social ecological model for health promotion as representing five major sources of influence on behavior, four of which (interpersonal, organizational, community, and policy factors) comprise forces external to the individual.

Other health behavior models have increasingly emphasized environmental settings and structures for planning health promotion interventions. Green and Kreuter's[11] widely used Precede ("predisposing, reinforcing and enabling constructs in educational and ecological diagnosis and evaluation") and Proceed ("policy, regulatory and organizational constructs in educational and environmental development") Model has been a mainstay in health education for two decades. It acknowledges the preeminence of policy and environmental changes in promoting healthy behavior. However, in spite of consistent findings in the epidemiological and health education literature demonstrating the central role of environmental factors in various health behaviors,

and the long-standing documentation of the effectiveness of behavior modification through altering the social and environmental consequences of behavior, there has been a surprisingly limited amount of emphasis on the environment in health behavior change programs. Instead, many programs continue to focus on knowledge and attitude changes as an indirect path to improving health behavior.

In contrast, ecological theories highlight the direct interaction between human behavior and the environment in which it occurs. Cast in the context of ecological theory,[12,13] Cohen et al.[7] propose a structural model of health behavior change. Four specific factors delineated within this model are availability, physical structures, social structures, and cultural and media messages. Availability refers to the accessibility of health-related consumer products (e.g., fiber or fat-rich foods, guns and ammunition, over-the-counter medications, condoms, and cigarettes). Physical structures are those aspects of products or environments that make health-related behavior more or less likely to occur (e.g., single-use needles for IV drug users, bike lanes and well-marked pedestrian crossings, and child safety bars over windows). Social structures refer to laws and policies that require or restrict health behaviors, and to their enforcement (e.g., restrictions on alcohol sales and where it can be consumed, immunization requirement for enrolling in public schools). Informal social control mechanisms (e.g., friends taking away car keys from inebriated drivers) are central to this category as well. Finally, cultural and media messages are those which individuals are exposed to every day (e.g., health messages and alcohol beverage ads), which inform them about specific health behaviors and denote social norms underpinning these behaviors.

An example of a structural change with both direct and indirect effects on health behavior is represented by alcohol taxation on alcohol consumption and reducing sexually transmitted infection (STI) rates among youth.[14] Between 1982 and 1994 there were 34 instances of a state beer tax increase in the United States. Evaluators compared the changes in STI rates in states with and without a tax increase over the same period and evaluated the effect of the level of beer taxation on the changes in STI rates, controlling for legal minimum drinking age, per capita income, and state and year differences. The results showed that in 26 (77 percent) of the states with an increase in beer tax, there was a greater decrease in gonorrhea rates among males in both the 15–19 and 20–24 age groups as compared to the change among the states without a tax increase. Similar patterns were observed for females. It was estimated that a $0.15 tax increase on a six-pack of beer would reduce gonorrhea incidence rates by roughly 10 percent among the 15–19 age group.

In application, substantial overlap exists among these four structures. Availability can be influenced by the physical nature of an environment or entities therein. For example, mass transportation accessible within a 20-minute walk would make physical activity more "available" and at the same time reduce automobile pollution. Policies and other changes in social structures can mandate reductions in environmental tobacco smoke and air pollution in general. Health communication typically emphasizes individual behavior change. However, through its incarnation as "media advocacy,"[15] communication has increasingly mobilized public support for policy change, again showing how changes in one structure can result in changes in another. Structural and ecological analyses offer a blueprint for most or all of effective public health behavior change interventions. Of special interest is that only the final of the four factors (cultural/media) implies knowledge and attitude change before behavior change can occur. Although not presented as a psychosocial theory itself, this structural model brings into question the validity of emphasizing personality and cognitions in efforts to study and change public health behavior.

Less dependent on notions of individual personality constructs or hypothesized cognitive processes, health communication models and learning theory reflect through their key tenets these four structures of public health behavior. These two conceptual foundations yield specific guidelines not only for measuring health behavior, but also for behavior change interventions.

HEALTH COMMUNICATION: BEHAVIORAL AND STRUCTURAL CHANGES VIA THE MEDIA

Communication "Inputs"

Central to the field of health communication is McGuire's[16] Communication-Persuasion Model, which presents an input-output matrix to describe stages (outputs) leading to behavior change, and how progress through these stages is aided by communication in its various forms (inputs). The *inputs* represent qualities of the communicated message that can be manipulated and controlled by campaign designers, whereas outputs represent the information-processing steps that must be stimulated in those receiving the message. Specifically, the inputs include the "source" (who), "message" (saying what), "channel" (by what medium), "receiver" (to whom), and "destination" (for what purpose). Source characteristics refer to the communicator of the message. Persuasive impact may be influenced by such source factors as age, gender, ethnicity, credibility, and socioeconomic status. Message refers to the information that is communicated, and important factors include delivery style, content organization, length, and repetition. Channel comprises the mode of communication, including face-to-face, print (newspaper, brochures, etc.), and broadcast. Receiver characteristics include age, education, intelligence, and demographic variables considered when creating a public health campaign. Finally, the destination describes the targeted behaviors and issues to be considered, including long-term versus short-term change and specific versus general behaviors (see Figure 14.1).

Communication "Outputs"

Outputs reflect the temporal process and stages of change from initial exposure to communication to long-term maintenance of change within the intended receiver. The eleven output steps are:

1. exposure;
2. attention;
3. attraction to the message;

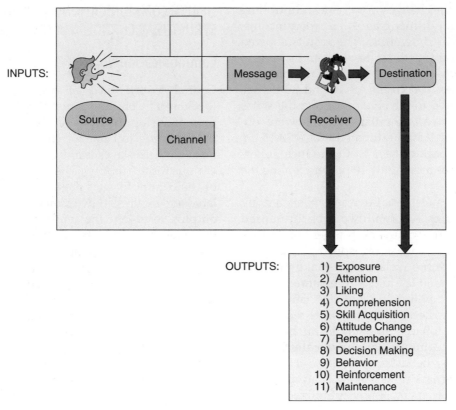

Figure 14.1. The Communication-Persuasion Model

4. comprehension;
5. skill acquisition;
6. attitude change;
7. remembering;
8. making a decision;
9. behaving in accordance with the decision;
10. reinforcement; and
11. maintenance of the behavior change.

The theory assumes that these output processing steps are contingent upon each other and, therefore, must occur more or less in the specified sequence. A strength of McGuire's theory is that it lends itself both to program design and to evaluating specific changes related to a communication effort. There have been several variations on this theory that incorporate different output processing routes, that account for behavior change leading to attitude change instead of

vice versa, or that focus on activating information that is already possessed by the individual and increasing the salience of message components that support current beliefs.

Outputs and Stages of Change

In important ways, the Communication-Persuasion Model (especially its output dimension) parallels the widely used "Stages of Change" or Transtheoretical Model (TTM).[17,18] In the TTM, stages represent the periods of time in which particular changes occur[18] as well as a continuum of readiness to take and sustain action.[19] The TTM characterizes individuals as moving from precontemplation (not intending to change) to contemplation (intending to change in the near future), to preparation (actively planning immediate change), to action (overtly making changes), and finally to maintenance (taking steps to sustain the change). To be considered in "action," individuals are required to meet some behavioral criterion at least for some minimal period of time (e.g., six months), after which the individual enters the maintenance stage. The TTM conceptualizes change as a dynamic, non-linear process, with many individuals relapsing and returning to earlier stages of change before successfully reaching maintenance.[20] More than the TTM, however, McGuire's[21] conceptualization has guided the field of public health communication, especially in the use of mass media.

Increasing the Effectiveness of Health Communication

Public health communication includes a variety of techniques, but specifically emphasizes a few practical and simple messages through as many channels as possible. The success of a communication program is determined by a variety of factors including: (1) how much access the target audience has to the information (e.g., does a large percentage of the target audience own televisions or have Internet access?); (2) whether people were actually exposed to the media advertisement (e.g., did the freeway billboard ad stay up long enough for people to see it?); (3) whether the target audience acquired sufficient knowledge and skills to perform the target behavior (especially relevant to complex behaviors such as the safe operation of an automobile, or glucose self-monitoring); (4) whether the target audience actually has the opportunity to perform the behavior (e.g., new physical activity skills should be taught with reference to the appropriate season); and (5) whether this trial and subsequent short-term adoption can be reinforced naturally through subsequent communication approaches.

Health communication typically attempts to persuade a target audience to engage in a certain behavior through informing them about the benefits of the behavior. When such benefits are attractive or compelling, and barriers are minimal (e.g., preventing infant car accident deaths by putting their safety seat in the back of the vehicle), communication may be effective.[22] Inattention to consequences, however, may render the communication effort ineffective.

Social Marketing

Largely a hybrid of the fields of communication and marketing, *social marketing*[23–25] has recently been defined as a mutual fulfillment of self-interest in which marketers promote a product (or behavior), service, or idea by delivering benefits and reducing barriers associated with their adoption.[22] This can be accomplished only if the marketer understands the needs of the target audience, and if the audience sees clear advantages over alternative behaviors. This emphasis on behavior-consequence relationships reflects social marketing's partial grounding in learning theory.

LEARNING THEORY

While the Communication-Persuasion and Transtheoretical Models provide the context for "communication and media messages" structure,[7] learning theory may better explain the other principal aspects of structural models (availability, social structures, physical structures) and general social ecological theory. The term *learning theory* is most closely connected with Skinner[26] and his work in operant psychology (which he referred to as the "experimental analysis of behavior"). Bandura,[27] the person most closely identified with Social Learning Theory, demonstrated how individuals need not personally experience reinforcement, punishment, or other consequences to learn from them. In this chapter, "learning theory" is used broadly to refer to research and applications that emphasize direct or vicarious learning through the interaction between behaviors and consequences. This behavior-consequence emphasis distinguishes learning theory from most health communication models, which primarily focus on modifying behaviors through changing antecedents.

Health communication and social marketing techniques are considered valuable and effective procedures for altering protective or risk-related behavior. Indeed, marketing strategies may be particularly useful in prompting an initial behavioral change. However, communication should not be expected to sustain behavioral change except where the new behavior is reinforced by the environment.

Social marketing and applied learning theory differ in a variety of other important ways. Most health communication campaigns attempt to change cognitive factors such as the consumer's attention, attitude, knowledge, or beliefs. The theoretical assumption underlying these campaigns is that new cognitive processes will lead to informed decisions to change behavior since they have changed their beliefs with respect to the behavior. From a learning theory perspective, the tactics used to change knowledge, attitudes, and beliefs are largely "antecedent-oriented" educational procedures. In other words, they represent stimuli that set the stage for the occurrence of the behavior through forging antecedent-behavior or A-B links. Learning theory-based procedures, in contrast, emphasize behavior-consequence (B-C) associations, or "contingencies."

Behavior Modification

Behavior modification, or more specifically "contingency management," has been defined as the systematic application of principles derived from learning theory to altering environment-behavior relationships in order to strengthen adaptive and weaken maladaptive behaviors.[28] These environment-behavior relationships that cause and maintain behavior are referred to by Skinner[26] as contingencies of reinforcement. Hence, contingency management is the application, removal, or discontinuation of consequences that results in a strengthening or weakening of a behavior. Applying pleasant consequences or removing or discontinuing unpleasant ones will strengthen behaviors through the processes of positive reinforcement, negative reinforcement, or response facilitation, respectively. Removing a pleasant consequence, applying an aversive consequence, or discontinuing a pleasant consequence will weaken behaviors. The first two of these latter contingencies are technically referred to as "punishment," (e.g., stiff fines for drunk drivers, increased prices for tobacco, and the enforcement of indoor smoking bans) whereas the latter is referred to as "extinction."[28,29] Understanding the processes of how behaviors are formed or eliminated is critical to developing campaigns, policies, and other behavior change interventions.

The HealthCom project[30] identified various criteria for selecting target behaviors, including: (1) the health impact of the behavior; (2) its perceptible positive reinforcers and any punishers or barriers to its performance; (3) whether the behavior is compatible with and similar to existing practices; and (4) the ease or complexity of engaging in the behavior in general and specifically at the rate and duration required to alleviate a health problem. Program planners can weigh these criteria differentially in the design of campaigns, environmental interventions, or policies that promote adaptive and/or weaken unhealthy behavioral alternatives.

Skill versus Performance Deficits

Less-than-optimal levels of behavior may result from either a "performance" or "skill" deficit. In the former case, contingency management procedures are in order, whereas when skill deficits are present, additional training with appropriate skill-building supervision would be indicated.[31] Alternatively, application of Social Learning Theory concepts of modeling (vicarious learning through the observation of others), self-efficacy (confidence in a skill or being able to handle a specific situation), and outcome expectations (subjective estimation of the probability that a reinforcer or punisher will follow the performance of a behavior) afford the opportunity for the learning to occur without personal experience of consequences. The individual would need to see other people performing the behavior, develop the necessary confidence around the particular act, and believe that reinforcement will be optimal and/or punishment minimal. According to Bandura,[27] meeting these criteria should be sufficient to promote behavior change.

Health communication and learning theory-based models provide divergent perspectives on planning and implementing public health behavior change interventions. One additional model, media advocacy, complements and integrates these primary intervention approaches.

MEDIA ADVOCACY: LINKING HEALTH COMMUNICATIONS WITH LEARNING THEORY APPLICATIONS

Wallack[32] advocates the use of media to advance social change. He points out that although mass media can be an important source of health information, it is a primary source of health misinformation as well, and even promotes unhealthy lifestyles. Moreover, Wallack asserts that the media usually represent health as an individual responsibility rather than the product of societal forces. Counter to a public health understanding of the problem, for example, news media often depict the youth violence problem as the product of "bad kids" who need to be punished and removed from society.[33] Media role models and advertising add to the promotion of instant gratification and the minimization of risks associated with this gratification. Noting that mass media generally reinforce existing arrangements without stimulating social change, he calls for more creative and aggressive approaches in health promotion's use of the media.

Wallack and Dorfman[15] suggested reorientation away from traditional health communication approaches toward a methodology that sets the public agenda away from individual and toward societal responsibility for health. "Media advocacy" maintains a behavior change focus-only in this case, on the behavior of corporate executives, policy makers, and other power brokers rather than that of individual citizens. Members of the legislative and executive branches of government at all levels are responsible for structuring the physical and social environments that reinforce healthy behaviors and make unhealthy ones less appealing. Policy makers are unlikely to fund universal child health care, raise taxes on tobacco and alcohol, pass clean indoor air acts, control gun sales, or promote conservation without pressure from the public to do so. Executives responsible for the manufacturing of dangerous products (e.g. alcohol, weapons, and cigarettes) are unlikely to rein in their advertising unless forced to do so.

Wallack[32] noted that appeals to change health behavior in exchange for gratification that is delayed until the distant future will have little success in maintaining behavior change. Media advocacy integrates the knowledge and attitude change approaches of social marketing and health communication with policy changes and other interventions that alter availability and social and physical structures. Media advocacy provides both carrots and sticks to back up the promise of health communication. It shifts the burden of behavior change to the powerful.

This chapter examines structural change approaches to diverse public health problems including smoking prevention, nutritional behavior change, sexually transmitted infection (STI) control, and mammography promotion. Ways in which learning theory and health communication alter availability, social and physical structures, and media messages are examined as individual or integrated programs.

PREVENTING TOBACCO USE

Tobacco use is responsible for more than one of five deaths in the United States and remains the single most preventable cause of death and disease in our society. The age at which smokers initiate tobacco use has steadily declined over the years. Approximately 90 percent of those who take up smoking currently do so prior to the age of 18.[34] Once teenagers experiment with smoking, their chances of becoming regular smokers and developing a physiological addiction are increased significantly.[35] According to de Moor et al,[36] those youth who were exposed to adult tobacco use in the home had a significantly higher probability of regular tobacco use than those who reported no exposure. Sociodemographic variables related to ever-smoking groups were similar to those reported in the literature for this age group (i.e., older, male, lower income students living with a single parent and exposed to both parents' and friends' smoking were at highest risk of smoking).

Reduction of tobacco use has been identified in *Healthy People 2010* as the most important of the priority areas for the prevention of cancer. In the 1990s, smoking prevention programs emphasized information about the effects of tobacco use (e.g., social and physiological), information about social influences on tobacco use (e.g., media, peers, and parents), and training (e.g., modeling and practice) in refusal skills. However, experience since then has indicated that more aggressive structural approaches to preventing smoking may be needed. Objectives from *Healthy People 2010* focus on the need to establish tobacco-free environments and include tobacco use prevention in the curricula for all elementary, middle, and secondary schools as part of a comprehensive school health education program.[37] This section reviews recent environmental change experiences in protecting youth from acquiring the smoking habit.

Recognizing the limits of victim-focused cessation and clinical interventions, more aggressive tobacco control measures, such as closing down retailers who sell cigarettes to minors without checking IDs and eliminating advertisement directed at youth, gained preeminence in the 1990s. This has been achieved in spite of the tobacco industry's extraordinary financial and political power. On August 10, 1995, President Clinton approved Food and Drug Administration (FDA) proposals that would: (1) prohibit the sale of cigarettes to minors; (2) severely limit advertising; (3) ban cigarette vending machines; (4) eliminate mail-order sales and free sample promotions; and (5) require the tobacco industry to fund a $150 million per year antismoking education campaign. This action set the stage for a variety of new battles against youth smoking, to be played out in the arenas of availability, physical and social structures, and media messages. The coming years promise decisive battles for community tobacco control.

Media and Cultural Messages

Recognizing the futility of trying to get people to withdraw from an established addiction, especially among "hard-core" smokers, programs shifted their attention to the prevention of first-time or regular smoking. These programs specifically addressed peer pressure to begin smoking and interpersonal skills designed to counteract this pressure. Again, the bulkiness (e.g., requiring 10 to 20 classroom hours over two or more school years) and limited effectiveness of many prevention programs limited their widespread adoption. Attention turned naturally to mass media.

Mass media-based messages and programs are included among the earliest smoking prevention efforts of federal agencies and voluntary health organizations. Much of this early programming was in response to the first Surgeon General's Report on Smoking and Health in 1964, the Fairness Doctrine Act (1967–1970), and the ban on broadcast advertising of cigarettes. For the purpose of this discussion, "mass media" is any form of communication that uses print, electronic, interpersonal, or display media. Messages range from antismoking exhortations delivered through the newspapers, television, and radio, to educational brochures and more comprehensive educational curricula that make use of the media.

The mass media have tremendous capacity for modeling desired behaviors and can contribute to the redefining of social norms in support of prevention (e.g., making it "cool" not to smoke). Radio and television are the optimal channels, since electronic media reach the largest number of people in our society and are heavily used by all socioeconomic groups, all educational levels, and all racial/ethnic minorities. A mediating factor is that media can be played at optimal viewing or listening times by target audience members. However, media programs alone are typically not effective[38,39] in preventing tobacco use.

Over time, tobacco control experts sought more aggressive and accessible structural changes to promote tobacco control. Mass media spots to counter the tobacco industry image, taken off the airways as part of an American congressional compromise with the industry thirty years ago, once again came into vogue. Not only did these spots aim to encourage prevention and cessation, but they were also used to question the very legitimacy of the tobacco industry and its marketing. Mass media interventions have helped lower smoking initiation in the United States.[40,41] Provocative themes and messages may be especially attractive to adolescents and may boost the preventive power of such spots.[42]

Perhaps educational and media approaches to smoking prevention are guilty of a common fault: they place the onus of responsibility for resisting tobacco on the young nonsmoker. Mass media can perhaps be used most effectively by promoting the acceptance of and participation in changes in social and physical structures and availability. Innovative media spots and Web sites (such as thetruth.com) encourage youth to become social activists by ripping tobacco ads out of magazines and destroying them, as well as by communicating directly with politicians and the tobacco industry about the exploitation of youth that occurs through the promotion of tobacco use.

Availability

Several approaches for reducing tobacco availability to minors have been described in the literature, including: (1) restricting distribution; (2) regulating how cigarettes are sold; (3) enforcing minimum age laws (18 or 19 in all states); (4) easing the burden of enforcement by allowing civil rather than criminal penalties for illegal sales; and (5) providing merchant training regarding the laws and how to comply with them. Recent years have witnessed substantial progress in reducing availability of tobacco products. Free samples are no longer distributed to adolescents nor in general to the public. The ban of sales of single cigarettes is enforced, and proposals for mandatory larger minimal packages have been circulated. Vending machines, for more than a generation the source of choice among adolescent smokers, have been restricted to adult-only establishments or banned altogether.

Physical Structures

Three decades ago, adults and even youth were allowed to smoke cigarettes in numerous and varied public places, including on school grounds. Today, proscriptions on indoor environmental tobacco smoke (ETS) inhibit not only youth but also adult smoking, thereby reducing physical harm to the non-smoker while communicating to the adolescent the social undesirability of the habit. Other physical structural interventions include the design of vending machines so that they may be electronically locked or require special tokens purchased from the merchant. The elimination of self-service tobacco displays also may reduce sales to minors.[43]

Social Structures

Recent research[44] has shown that adolescents are less likely to smoke in societies where tobacco prices are higher, where tobacco tax revenues must be spent on antitobacco activities, where there are statutes that strictly limit public smoking, and where bans on retailing to youth are strictly enforced. Tax increases may be especially effective at dissuading low-income youth from smoking.[45] At a community level, Forster and colleagues[46] showed that localities that developed new ordinances and policies and ways of enforcing these policies, especially regarding sales to minors, experienced lower rates of adolescent tobacco use as a result.

By involving adolescents themselves in enforcement, the impact of social structural changes may be enhanced. In numerous states and communities, adolescent "sting" operations are coordinated by local police, whereby underage youth enter a store, attempt a purchase, and then record the vendor's response (e.g., asked for identification and refused the sale or proceeded with the illegal sale). The vendor or owner may then be cited for an illegal sale or reinforced for obeying the law.

NUTRITION

Second to tobacco use, the leading causes of death in the United States are attributable to dietary factors and physical activity.[47] Dietary factors include the underconsumption of the recommended number of fruits and vegetables and the overconsumption of added fats.[48,49] The prevalence of healthy eating varies by region. For example, 68 percent of the population in Minnesota and 91 percent in Arizona eat less than five servings of fruits and vegetables per day.[49] Related to both poor nutrition and physical inactivity, the median prevalence of overweight among adults in the United States is 54.5 percent.[50] This trend toward unhealthy eating and overweight appears to be getting worse.[48,50]

In a series of articles on social ecology, Stokols[51] suggested a positive movement toward strengthening community support for healthier lifestyles. Although this may be true in general, the nutrition field in particular is guilty of placing responsibility for healthy eating on the individual. For example, there are numerous interventions targeting individual-level behavior and a dearth of research promoting structural change.[52] This is not to suggest that individuals may not benefit from empirically supported, individually based interventions for improving food choices and food quantities; rather, concurrent changes in the environment need to occur for lasting change. Similar arguments are made by Jeffrey[53] regarding the causes of risk behavior and by Leviton,[54] who addresses the growing convergence of psychology and public health. Jeffrey noted that if the purpose of research is to study individual differences, then it is appropriate to study individual-level characteristics. However, if the goal is to examine differences in the prevalence of a condition across populations, then it becomes necessary to examine factors that discriminate between these populations. Structural factors such as availability and the physical and social structures of the environment are some examples of population-based variables. The goal in this section is to acquaint the reader with current nutrition research and areas of future research that target structural factors in nutrition.

Mass Media

Mass media interventions in the nutrition field have been designed primarily to increase awareness, provide models of healthy behavior, and promote skill development. Although some work has been done attempting to change community norms through the use of mass media, efforts paralleling those in tobacco control (e.g., challenging the industries responsible for promoting unhealthy dietary behaviors) have not been forthcoming. Positive models of mass media use include the "5-a-Day" program for promoting greater consumption of fruits and vegetables using multiple communication channels.[55] Research on the use of the Nutrition Food Facts Label suggests that usage does impact food evaluation and purchase intentions.[56] Future research efforts should use accessible sources of media (e.g., television) to covertly introduce positive role models and promote healthier lifestyles via vicarious learning.[57]

Availability

There is no argument that availability is a key determinant of nutrition behavior. If a product is not readily available, it is unlikely to be purchased and consumed. Conversely, if a product is easily accessible, it is more likely to be consumed. Availability has been suggested as one reason for the disparity in nutrition among poorer families. For example, grocery stores in some inner-city communities are less likely to have fresh fruits and vegetables, lean meats, and low-fat dairy products.[58] Similarly, products may be available but they are priced out of the reach for low-income families.[59] Availability in general, and with respect to food portion sizes, has been suggested as one determinant in the increasing prevalence of overweight and obesity.[60] Our society's obsession with getting the most for our money may be responsible for the trend in "super-sizing" menu items. It is difficult to implement strategies for behavioral control in the face of increasing food portion sizes that are deemed normative because of their availability. Attempts at increasing the accessibility of healthy food options (e.g., vending machines, healthy menu items, school cafeterias) are beginning to take hold.[61,62] Nevertheless, targeting availability by increasing shelf space for healthier foods, offering smaller portions of food at a reduced price, stocking vending machines with healthier options, and limiting the availability of unhealthy foods in schools will go a long way toward improving nutritional habits.

Physical Structures

One area of research that has been woefully neglected in the nutrition field is the impact of physical structures on food choices and consumption behavior. Physical structures can include such things as the location of products in a grocery store or the location of restaurants in a community. To date, researchers have studied and intervened at the physical structure level by installing kiosks and introducing shelf labeling to increase awareness of healthy options.[63] However, little to no work has been done in the public health field on the impact of playgrounds in fast-food restaurants or the proximity of fast-food restaurants to freeways and commuter traffic. Current efforts to map communities and assess community factors (e.g., proximity of farmer's markets, fast-food restaurants) affecting dietary behaviors are promising.[64]

Social Structures

Unlike tobacco, few laws and policies have been developed targeting improvements in nutrition. Efforts to change community norms by regulating the environment are only beginning to emerge in the nutrition field.[65] The proposed "snack tax" is one of the few examples of a barrier to purchasing and consuming high-fat, low-fiber foods. Informal social structures, including family connectedness and integration around eating, send messages to children about the importance of meal setting and the type and quantity of foods consumed. Research efforts utilizing community health workers are an important avenue for promoting healthier lifestyles around dietary behaviors.[66]

The integration of these four structural factors for change provide multiple approaches for improving dietary behaviors. For example, Hill and Peters[60] suggest "regulating the food and restaurant industry . . . to take responsible action by reducing portion sizes . . ." (p. 1373). Similarly, the Nutrition Food Facts Label implemented in the 1980s is an example of a policy and mass media approach for increasing awareness and educating the public. Structural approaches, in combination with well-validated behavioral approaches, engage both the community and the individual in a process of change that is likely to lead to maintenance of the behavior. Finally, concurrent efforts promoting increases in energy expenditure are necessary to halt the increasing prevalence of overweight and obesity.

BREAST CANCER SCREENING AMONG WOMEN

Clinical preventive services for the early detection of diseases are one method of reducing morbidity and mortality among women.[67] Mammography screening, although increasing, is still underutilized as an early detection procedure. Timely mammography screening among women older than age 40 could pre-

vent 15–30 percent of all deaths from breast cancer. Nevertheless, among women in the United States only 65.6 percent have had a mammogram in the last year.[68] Furthermore, there is evidence that differential use of mammography among racial/ethnic groups may explain some of the variation reported for breast cancer incidence.[69] Breast cancer screening rates among older women are also low.[70]

The four structural factors described above affect mammography utilization in a complex way. As applied to mammography, these categories include: (1) availability of mammograms in the community; (2) discomfort and/or embarrassment related to the procedure; (3) the policy of requiring a clinician visit before the procedure is obtained; and (4) the strong cultural messages that create misconceptions about the utility of mammograms.

Media and Cultural Messages

There are three important channels of health communication for women to receive information and motivation for mammography: mass media, physicians/clinicians, and social networks. In contrast to the first two, social messages such as those from family members, friends, and neighbors are more powerful influences on adherence to mammography screening.[71] Within their social networks, women communicate fear, anxiety, embarrassment, and other emotional responses when considering or undergoing screening. This can lead to inadequate, misleading, or inaccurate information about breast cancer screening. Embarrassment associated with clinical breast exam and mammography, for example, has been identified as a barrier among older women of all cultures.[72] Inaccurate risk perceptions and elevated levels of psychological distress among relatives of breast cancer patients may serve as barriers to mammography use in this population[73] who have surprisingly low rates of mammography, despite their increased risk.[74] These sociocultural messages are powerful because they come from trusted sources.

The success of community health advisor (CHA) programs[75–77] in promoting mammography exemplifies the importance of social networks as a source of cultural messages.[78] Typically coming from the immigrant or disadvantaged communities that they serve, the CHAs are volunteer outreach workers trained with knowledge and skills to promote mammography. They then use existing social networks to provide the public health message within the target population. The strategy is useful because the channel of communication is through informal mechanisms such as church groups, neighbors, and apartment complexes. Through these channels of communication, the CHAs can address the fears, anxiety, embarrassment, and other emotional issues surrounding mammogram screening.

Resource Availability

Unlike many other behaviors promoted in public health programs, getting a mammogram requires the "permission" of a medical clinician. In general, an asymptomatic woman who desires a screening mammogram must first make an appointment with a clinician, have a past medical and family history reviewed by the clinician, and usually go through a clinical breast exam before a referral can be obtained for routine screening mammography. It is currently not possible for a woman to order her own mammogram or go to a "mammogram screening clinic," as is the case for diabetes or cholesterol screening. This medical circumstance significantly reduces availability in the environment.[70,79,80]

Mobile mammography has been one method to increase service availability.[81,82] Mobile mammography usually involves special equipment and a certified mammographer to provide this service under the legal authority of a certified radiologist. Although the idea seems practical, it is costly and requires significant planning to achieve the volume of activity for the method to achieve cost-effectiveness.[83] Other limitations of the mobile units are the clinical case management required to return results and to follow up for abnormalities and additional imaging.[84]

For women with limited or no health insurance, availability becomes more challenging. Cost factors pertain to more than just the cost of a mammogram, and include the costs of lost wages, child care, and transportation. The medical community and public desire for high-quality mammography has also created decreased availability. With the passage of the 1992 Mammography Quality Standards Act (MQSA), mammography is now confined to dedicated mammography centers that follow the FDA guidelines. The push for reliable mammography centers has also been fueled by the medical-legal liability of mammography interpretation over recent years. The consequence of this movement is the decreased availability of mammography in small rural and urban ambulatory clinics.

Physical Structures

Mammography utilizes ionizing radiation to create images of the breast tissue. The examination is performed by compressing the breast firmly between a plastic plate and an x-ray cassette, which contains special x-ray film. For routine screening, examination films are taken in two views. Recent improvements in the quality of design and its physical characteristics are evident in federal manufacturing and safety laws. Under the MQSA enacted by Congress in 1992, all facilities that perform mammography must be certified by the FDA. This mandate has resulted in improved mammography techniques, lower radiation dose, and better training of personnel. Image contrast has improved with the use of lower kilovoltage, specialized aluminum grids, and higher film optical density. The 1998 MQSA Reauthorization Act requires that patients receive a written lay-language summary of mammography results.[85]

Physical changes in the mammography "product" can improve outcomes without changing attitudes, beliefs, or behaviors. The first digital mammography system received U.S. Food and Drug Administration approval in 2000.[85] Only facilities that have been certified to practice conventional mammography and have FDA approval for digital mammography may offer the digital system. Currently, women considering digital mammography need to speak with their doctor or contact a local FDA-certified mammography center to find out if this technique is available in their location. However, when digital mammography becomes a standard of care, there may be advantages that improve health outcomes. The images can be stored and retrieved electronically, which could make long-distance consultation with another physician possible. The improved accuracy of digital mammography could reduce the number of follow-up procedures. These physical changes in the product could be more effective in finding cancer than conventional mammography.[85]

Social Structures

Now that mammography availability and screening guidelines are well established in the medical community, the greatest increases in adherence to recommended mammography guidelines will be made by altering social structures affecting utilization. The laws and policies that affect mammography relate to the adoption of consensus panel screening guidelines for different age groups of women in the United States, insurance coverage, and federal programs supporting mammography.

Screening guidelines have changed significantly over the last decade. The most significant discussion has been the policy recommendations for women between the ages of 40 and 49. In 1997, a national consensus conference, sponsored by the National Cancer Institute (NCI), determined that there was no statistical increase in survival of breast cancer from mammography screening among women 40 to 49 years of age.[86,87] Two months after the consensus conference, the recommendation was made public. Under pressure from the medical profession and certain advocacy groups, however, the NCI issued a new recommendation that women in their forties have a screening mammogram every year or two.[88] The American Cancer Society went further and issued the recommendation that women in this age group be screened every year. These consensus guidelines are important examples of how policies can influence physicians and insurance companies in the delivery of clinical preventive services such as mammography. Once the mammography screening guidelines were changed, individual medical providers and health insurance companies were forced to act. As clinicians became aware of the new guidelines for women 40 to 49, they began to order more screening mammograms for women in this age group to be in compliance. As health insurance companies became aware of the

changes, they were obligated to include this service in the insurance plan possibly to avoid litigation.[87] Changes in both the medical and insurance companies were a result of policy-level changes.

Often, the federal government can affect adherence to clinical services by enacting entitlement laws. Recognizing the value of screening and early detection, Congress passed the Breast and Cervical Cancer Mortality Prevention Act of 1990, which established the CDC's National Breast and Cervical Cancer Early Detection Program (NBCCEDP).[89] The NBCCEDP provides screening services, including clinical breast examinations, mammograms, pelvic examinations, and Pap tests, to underserved women. The NBCCEDP also funds postscreening diagnostic services, such as surgical consultation and biopsy, to ensure that all women with abnormal results receive timely and adequate referrals. Providing federal funds to remove financial barriers to mammography is one way in which laws improve the social structures. Now in its 11th year, the NBCCEDP has provided more than 2.7 million screening examinations. The program has diagnosed more than 8,600 breast cancers, 39,400 precancerous cervical lesions, and 660 cervical cancers. The NBCCEDP operates in all 50 states, the District of Columbia, 6 U.S. territories, and 12 American Indian/ Alaska Native organizations. Fiscal year 2001 appropriations of about $174 million will enable CDC to increase education and outreach programs for women and health care providers, improve quality assurance measures for screening, and improve access to screening and follow-up services.[90]

CONTROL OF SEXUALLY TRANSMITTED INFECTIONS INCLUDING HIV

The control of sexually transmitted infections (STIs) including HIV is a challenge for behavior change programs for two reasons: (1) these are infectious diseases that require two people for transmission; and (2) the targets for change comprise the individual's most private and intimate behaviors. Although an individual certainly must adopt a behavior that exposes him or her to an STI (e.g., engage in sexual activity), the same behavior carries differential risks depending on the context in which it is carried out. For example, a woman living in Missoula, Montana, who engages in unprotected vaginal sex with a man she meets in a bar is much less likely to acquire an STI than a woman of the same age in New Orleans, Louisiana, who practices the same behavior, simply because there is a higher prevalence of STIs among young men living in New Orleans. In other words, the behavior (vaginal sex with a new partner) practiced in one community carries a different risk than the same behavior practiced in another community. Similarly, a man who has vaginal sex with a monogamous partner is engaging in the same behavior as a man who has vaginal sex with a commercial sex partner. But the latter man is much more likely to get an STI than the former, simply because there is a higher prevalence of STIs among commercial sex workers than among women with few sex partners. Therefore, messages for behavior change to reduce community prevalence of STIs vary by types of sexual partners, and within the geosocial context. The probability of exposure to STIs depends on the prevalence of disease in the partner's pool, the characteristics of the disease, and specific sexual behaviors.

Consistent with an ecological model, the classic transmission dynamics model for STIs reflects the fact that both environment and behavior make up one part of an individual's risk of being infected with an STI. This is represented by

$$R_0 = \beta * C * D$$

where R_0 = case reproduction rate; β = efficiency of transmission; C = mean rate of partner change; D = duration of infectiousness. The higher the value of R_0, the greater spread of an infection within a community. In this model, individual behavior may affect β if condoms are used, in that this reduces the efficiency of transmission. However, β is also strongly affected by the biology of the organism transmitted, as some are more efficiently transmitted than others. Individual behavior directly affects C, the mean rate of partner change, as individuals can choose how many partners they will engage in sexual activity with and how often. Finally, duration is affected by both the biology of the organism and individual health-seeking behavior. Individuals who rapidly acquire treatment for their infections, even if chronic and not curable such as with HIV and herpes simplex virus (HSV),

may greatly reduce the infectiousness of these STIs. Therefore, STI/HIV control programs focus on different components of the transmission dynamics model, thereby reducing efficiency of transmission through promoting condom use, decreasing partner change rates by encouraging monogamy, or decreasing duration of infections by promoting symptom recognition, screening, and health-seeking behavior of STIs.

Media and Cultural Messages

There has been little direct evidence that mass media campaigns have achieved reductions in sexual risk behavior. Mass media campaigns have been stymied by sociocultural, religious, and governmental restrictions on content. For example, it has been a challenge to develop messages about how to use condoms that are clear and precise without being too sexually explicit for mass media. A further challenge is that the messages to reduce community prevalence of these diseases are about harm reduction, not cessation of behaviors. It seems relatively straightforward to advise the public to quit smoking, not use crack cocaine, or get flu shots once a year. But it is neither possible nor rational to instruct individuals not to have sex, pronouncements from the current U.S. government notwithstanding. Behavior change messages and programs must, therefore, focus on selection of sexual partners, and the type of sexual activities to be avoided. This requires a level of detail about sexuality that the public is not accustomed to receiving on their televisions, through their radios, or on their buses as public service announcements. However, the HIV/AIDS epidemic has created an urgent health need to communicate about topics that have never before entered the public debate.

Structural Approaches to Reducing STI/HIV

Structural approaches to STI control have been proven effective by operating through the mechanisms identified in the Transmission Dynamics Model. Yet one important difference between STI control and other health problems discussed in this chapter is that given the infectious nature of these diseases, structural change and control programs are most effective when targeting segments of populations that are most likely to transmit and acquire STIs. These segments are known as *core groups*. In most countries, there is a disproportionately large number of STIs that result directly or indirectly from a small subgroup of the people experiencing infection, or the "STI core group."[91] The core group concept has gained credence among those involved in STI/HIV prevention and research and has been identified in various countries and populations. A "core group" is defined as a highly vulnerable group of individuals characterized by high rates of partner change (often with each other), longer duration of infection often related to poor access to acceptable health care, and highly efficient transmission of infection per exposure, all contributing to high rates of STIs.[92] Core group theory suggests that the prevention of STIs in these groups will lower a community's STI rate more than prevention among other groups or the general population.[93] Examples of core groups include female sex workers (FSWs), men who have sex with men (MSM), and intravenous drug users (IVDUs). These individuals often have higher rates of partner change than the rest of the population, an important component in STI transmission dynamics as described above. Therefore, structural change aimed at these groups may reduce the prevalence of STIs within the group, and as a result within the broader population.

STI prevention efforts with the greatest impact include structural interventions, often involving policy changes. Perhaps the best example of policy-level changes that impacted HIV as well as other STIs were those adopted by the Thai HIV/AIDS Control Program, which required 100 percent condom use by commercial sex workers. Evaluations of the effectiveness of this program were based on reductions in STI cases in government clinics, and declines in STI/HIV observed through surveys of men and commercial sex workers. Between 1989 and 1993, rates of condom use in commercial sex reported by female sex workers increased from 14 to 94 percent and the number of cases of five major STIs decreased by 79 percent in men.[94] Additionally, a comparison of two cohorts of military conscripts showed a decline in HIV incidence from 2.48 per 100 person-years of exposure between 1991 and 1993 to 0.55 per 100 person-years of expo-

sure between 1993 and 1995. STI incidence declined even more, with an overall tenfold decrease between 1991 and 1993, and 1993 and 1995.[95] The most recent analysis of trends in prevalence of HIV infection among young men conscripted into the military during May or November each year, show that the prevalence peaked in 1992 to 1993 and has been declining since, with possible leveling off in the most recent group of conscripts.[96] Thailand is now recognized as the developing country with one of the earliest and most successful STI/HIV control programs implemented early in its HIV epidemic and without a biomedical intervention. Thailand has become a model for national behavior change success and is credited with averting many new infections of HIV and saving the lives of millions of its inhabitants.

Governmental regulation and provision of services for female sex workers may result in a reduction in both incidence and prevalence of STIs. One example of a program addressing availability as well as physical and social structures affecting STIs, comes from a South African mining community. In this community, STI treatment services (including periodic presumptive treatment and prevention education) were provided to a core group of high-risk women living in areas around the mines from October 1996 to June 1997. A mobile clinic service was established near a commercial area surrounded by three mine hostels and provided examinations, counseling, and presumptive treatment for bacterial STIs for high-risk women. These women were asked to return monthly for further examination and treatment. Prevalence of *Neisseria gonorrhoeae* (GC) and/or *Chlamydia trachomatis* (CT) in women declined from 24.9 to 12.3 percent at the first monthly return visit; genital ulcers were found in 9.7 percent of these women at baseline and declined to 4.4 percent after one month. In the miner population, the prevalence of *N. gonorrhoeae* (GC) and/or *C. trachomatis* (CT) was 10.9 percent at baseline and 6.2 percent at the nine-month follow-up examination. The prevalence of genital ulcer disease (GUD) by clinical examination was 5.8 percent at baseline and 1.3 percent at follow-up examination. Rates of symptomatic STIs seen at mine health facilities decreased among miners in the intervention area compared with miners living farther from the site and with less exposure to the project. The study demonstrated that increasing the physical availability of STI treatment services to a core group of high-risk women significantly reduced their burden of disease, and may contribute to a reduction in community STI prevalence.[97]

The results of this study suggest that provision of effective curative and preventive services to high-risk women may have a significant impact on STD rates in these women and on community STD prevalence. The South African study suggests the utility of a core group approach to STD control. Periodic presumptive treatment, combined with preventive education and syndrome management of symptomatic women, is a viable option for STD service delivery in this population of high-risk women.

Another structural intervention that consisted of enhancing community STI services has become a landmark in HIV prevention. In Tanzania, communities were randomized to assess the effect of a community-level intervention that included establishment of an STI reference clinic, staff training in syndromic management,[98] regular supervisory visits to health facilities and provision of antimicrobials, and general population health education about STI and health care seeking for STI symptoms. A random cohort of 1,000 adults, 15 to 54 years of age, from each community was surveyed at baseline and at follow-up two years later. HIV incidence was compared in six intervention communities and six pair-matched comparison communities. Improved syndromic management of STI at the primary health care level reduced HIV incidence by about 40 percent[99] over the two years. This was the first randomized trial to demonstrate an impact of a preventive intervention on HIV incidence in a general population.

A subsequent HIV-prevention trial in Uganda tried to build on the concept that treating STIs at the community level would reduce incidence of HIV. Rather than restrict STI treatment to the clinic visits level, this second trial treated individuals at the household level in their homes, regardless of symptoms. Clusters of villages were randomized to mass treatment of STI every ten months versus antiparasitic treatment alone. Serologic screening and treatment for syphilis, and syndromic management for STI, were offered both to intervention and control villages. The study showed no effect on HIV incidence, but significant improvements in pregnancy outcomes.[100] The differences in outcome of the Tanzanian and Ugandan studies are intriguing. The Tanzanian project focused on treatment of symptomatic STI only, whereas the Ugandan program provided antimicrobials to the entire population, only some of whom had prevalent STI. It may have been differences in the relative prevalence of STI and HIV in the two study populations (higher prevalence of HIV infection in Uganda) and basic differences in study design and in the nature of the interventions that resulted in the differences in outcome.[101] Although many explanations have been posited as to the reason one community trial to control STIs succeeded while the other failed, one simple explanation may be that because the biomedical intervention (i.e., treatment of symptomatic STIs) in Tanzania was clinic based, counseling for condom use and risk reduction was included. In Uganda, however, the distribution of treatment for STIs was home based and not linked to symptoms, thus reducing an opportunity for counseling. Additionally, Tanzanians receiving treatment were symptomatic and the experience of having an STI symptom may well have served as a trigger for behavior change absent in Uganda, where many of the individuals treated did not have symptoms.

SUMMARY

Product availability, physical and social structures of products and environments, and media and cultural messages account for much of health-related behavior and provide a blueprint for public health promotion. The integration of these four structural factors for change provide multiple approaches for improving screening and dietary behaviors, and reducing smoking acquisition and sexually transmitted infections. Public health officials and program planners have begun to take notice of the potential inherent in structural changes. For example, Hill and Peters[50] suggest "regulating the food and restaurant industry . . . to take responsible action by reducing portion sizes. . . ." (p. 1373). New laws and lawsuits have increasingly made cigarette advertising, vending machines, and the extraordinary profitability of tobacco sales a thing of the past. Progress in mammography screening rates in the United States and STI control in developing countries have been made possible by improved use of media and reduced environmental and physical barriers to tar-

geted screening and preventive behaviors. Structural approaches, in combination with well-validated individual behavior change approaches, engage both the community and the individual in a process of change that is likely to lead to maintenance of the behavior.

References

1. Elder JP. *Behavior Change & Public Health in the Developing World.* Thousand Oaks, Calif: Sage Publications; 2001.
2. Janz NK, Becker MH. The health belief model: A decade later. *Health Educ Q.* 1984;11:1-47.
3. Bandura A. *Social Foundations of Thought and Action: A Social Cognitive Theory.* Englewood Cliffs, NJ: Prentice Hall; 1986.
4. Ajzen I, Fishbein M. *Understanding Attitudes and Predicting Social Behavior.* Englewood Cliffs, NJ: Prentice-Hall; 1980.
5. Kanfer FH. Self-management methods. In: Kanfer F, Goldstein A, eds. *Helping People Change.* New York, NY: Pergamon; 1975:309-356.
6. King R, Estey J, Allen S, Kegeles S, Wolf W, Valentine C, Serufilira A. A family planning intervention to reduce vertical transmission of HIV in Rwanda. *AIDS.* 1995;9(suppl 1):45-51.
7. Cohen D, Scribner R, Farley T. A structural model of health behavior: A pragmatic approach to explain and influence health behaviors at the population level. *Prev Med.* 2000;30:164-154.
8. McKinlay JB, Marceau LD. A tale of 3 tails. *Am J Public Health.* 1999;89(3):295-298.
9. McLeroy KR, Bibeau D, Steckler A, Glanz K. An ecological perspective on health promotion programs. *Health Educ Q.* 1988;15(4):351-377.
10. Stokols D. Establishing and maintaining healthy environments: Toward a social ecology of health promotion. *American Psychol.* 1992;47(1):6-22.
11. Green LW, Kreuter M. *Health Promotion Planning: An Educational and Ecological Approach.* 3rd ed. Mountain View, Calif: Mayfield; 1999.
12. Sallis J, Owen N. *Physical Activity and Behavioral Medicine.* Newbury Park, Calif: Sage Publications; 1999.
13. Baker EA, Goodman RM. *Community Assessment and Change: A Framework Principles, Models, Methods, and Skills.* Clifton Park, NY: Delmar Learning; 2002.

14. Chesson HW, Harrison P, Kassler WJ. Sex under the influence: The effect of alcohol policy on sexually transmitted disease rates in the US. *J Law and Econ.* 2000;XLIII: 215-238.
15. Wallack L, Dorfman L. Media advocacy: A strategy for advancing policy and promoting health. *Health Educ Q.* 1996;23:293-317.
16. McGuire WJ. Theoretical foundations of campaigns. In: Rice RE, Atkins CK, eds. *Public Communication Campaigns.* 2nd ed. Newbury Park, Calif: Sage Publications; 1989:43-65.
17. DiClemente CC, Prochaska JO. Self-exchange and therapy change of smoking behavior: A comparison of processes of change in cessation and maintenance. *Addict Behav.* 1982;7:133-142.
18. Prochaska JO, DiClemente CC. Stages and processes of self-change in smoking: Towards an integrative model of change. *J Consult Clin Psychol.* 1983;51:390-395.
19. Elder JP, Ayala GX, Zabinski M, Prochaska J, Gehrmann C. Theories, models, and methods of health promotion in rural settings. In: Quill BE, Loues, eds. *Handbook of Rural Health.* New York, NY: Plenum; 2001.
20. Prochaska JO, DiClemente CC. Towards a comprehensive, transtheoretical model of change: Stages of change and addictive behaviors. In: Miller WR, Heather N, eds. *Treating Addictive Behaviors.* 2nd ed. New York, NY: Plenum; 1998:3-24.
21. McGuire T. Theoretical foundations of public communication campaigns. In: Rice R, Paisley W, eds. *Public Communication Campaigns.* Beverly Hills, Calif: Sage Publications; 1981:41-70.
22. Maibach E, Rothschild M, Novelli W. Social marketing. In: Glanz K, Rimer B, Lewis F, eds. *Health Behavior and Health Education.* 3rd ed. San Francisco, Calif: Jossey-Bass; in press.
23. Andreasen AR. *Marketing Social Change: Changing Behavior to Promote Health, Social Development, and the Environment.* San Francisco, Calif: Jossey-Bass; 1995.

24. Kotler P, Roberto EL. *Social Marketing Strategies for Changing Public Behavior.* New York, NY: Free Press; 1989.

25. Lefebvre RC, Rochlin L. Social marketing. In: Glanz K, Lewis FM, Rimer BK, eds. *Health Behavior and Health Education: Theory, Research, and Practice.* 2nd ed. San Francisco, Calif: Jossey-Bass; 1997.

26. Skinner BF. *Science and Human Behavior.* New York, NY: Macmillan; 1953.

27. Bandura A. *Social Learning Theory.* Englewood Cliffs, NJ: Prentice Hall; 1977.

28. Elder JP, Geller ES, Hovell MF, Mayer JA. *Motivating Health Behavior.* Albany, NY: Delmar; 1994:128, 129-131.

29. Sulzer-Azaroff B, Mayer GR. *Behavior Analysis for Lasting Change.* Fort Worth, Tex: Harcourt Brace; 1991.

30. Academy for Educational Development. *A Tool Box for Building Health Communication Capacity.* Washington, DC: Author; 1995.

31. Graeff J, Elder JP, Booth E. *Communications for Health Behavior Change: A Developing Country Perspective.* San Francisco, Calif: Jossey-Bass; 1993.

32. Wallack L. Improving health promotion: Media advocacy and social marketing approaches. In: Atkin C, Wallack L, eds. *Mass Communication and Public Health.* Newbury Park, Calif: Sage Publications; 1990:147-163.

33. Wallack L, Dorfman L, Woodruff K. Communications and public health. In: Keck CW, Scutchfield FD, eds. *Principles of Public Health Practice.* Albany, NY: Delmar; 1997:183-194.

34. Wald N, Hackshaw AK. Cigarette smoking: An epidemiological overview. *Br Med Bull.* 1996;52(1):3-11.

35. Pierce JP, Choi WS, Gilpin EA, Farkas AJ, Berry C. Tobacco industry promotion of cigarettes and adolescent smoking. *JAMA.* 1998;279:511-515.

36. de Moor C, Elder JP, Young R, Wildey MB, Molgaard C. Generic tobacco use among four ethnic groups in a school-age population. *J Drug Educ.* 1989;19(3):257-270.

37. US Department of Health and Human Services. The Healthy People 2010 page. Available at: http://www.health.gov/healthypeople/. Accessed June 11, 2001.

38. Flay BR. Psychosocial approaches to smoking prevention: A review of findings. *Health Psychol.* 1985;4(5):449-88.

39. Flay BR, Brannon BR, Johnson CA, et al. The Television, School, and Family Smoking Prevention and Cessation Project. I. Theoretical basis and program development. *Prev Med.* 1998;17(5):585-607.

40. Biener L, Siegel M. Tobacco marketing and adolescent smoking: More support for a causal inference. *Am J Public Health.* 2000;90:407-411.

41. Worden JK, Flynn BS, Solomon LJ, Secker-Walker RH, Badger GJ, Carpenter JH. Using mass media to prevent cigarette smoking among adolescent girls. *Health Educ Q.* 1996;23:453-468.

42. Hafstad A, Aaro LE, Engeland A, Andersen A, Langmark F, Stray-Petersen B. Provocative appeals in anti-smoking mass media campaigns in adolescents—the accumulated effect of multiple exposures. *Health Educ Res.* 1977;12:227-236.

43. Biedell MP, Furlong MJ, Dunn DM, Koegler JE. Case study of attempts to enact self-service tobacco display ordinances: A tale of three communities. *Tob Control.* 2000;9:71-77.

44. Chaloupka FJ, Pacula RL. Limiting youth access to tobacco: The early impact of the Synar Amendment on youth smoking. Paper presented at the Third Biennial Pacific Rim Allied Economic Organizations Conference. Bangkok, Thailand; January 14, 1998.

45. Biener L, Aseltine RJ, Cohen B, Anderka M. Reactions of adult and teenaged smokers to the Massachusetts tobacco tax. *Am J Public Health.* 1998;88:1389-1391.

46. Forster JL, Murray DM, Wolfson M, Blaine TM, Wagenaar AC, Hennrikus DJ. The effects of community policies to reduce youth access to tobacco. *Am J Public Health.* 1998;88(8):1193-1198.

47. McGinnis JM, Foege WH. Actual cases of death in the United States. *JAMA.* 1993;270:2207-2212.

48. American Institute for Cancer Research (AICR). *Food, Nutrition, and the Prevention of Cancer: A Global Perspective.* Washington, DC: World Cancer Research Fund; 1999.

49. US Department of Health and Human Services, Centers for Disease Control and Prevention. *Chronic Diseases and Their Risk Factors: The Nation's Leading Causes of Death.* Atlanta, Ga: US Dept of Health and Human Services; 1999.

50. Flegal KM, Carroll MD, Kuczmarski RJ, Johnson CL. Overweight and obesity in the United States: Prevalence and trends, 1960-1994. *Int J Obesity & Related Metab Disord.* 1998;22(1):39-47.

51. Stokols D. Translating social ecological theory into guidelines for community health promotion. *Am J Health Promotion.* 1996;10(4):282-298.

52. Glanz K, Mullis RM. Environmental interventions to promote healthy eating: A review of models, programs, and evidence. *Health Educ Q.* 1988;15(4):395-415.

53. Jeffrey RW. Risk behaviors and health. *Am Psychol.* 1989;44(9):1194-1202.

54. Leviton LC. Integrating psychology and public health. *Am Psychol.* 1996;51(1):42-51.

55. National Institutes of Health. The Welcome to 5-a-day page. Available at: http://www.nci.nih.gov/5aday/ WLCOME.html. Accessed June 26, 2001.

56. Burton S, Garretson JA, Velliquette AM. Implications of accurate usage of nutrition facts panel information for food product evaluations and purchase intentions. *J Acad Marketing Sci.* 1999;27(4):470-480.

57. Larson MS. Health-related messages embedded in prime-time television entertainment. *Health Commun.* 1991;3(3):175-184.

58. Nader P, Sallis J, Patterson T, et al. A family approach to cardiovascular risk reduction: Results from the San Diego Family Health Project. *Health Educ Q.* 1989;16:229-244.

59. Turrell G. Structural, material, and economic influences on the food-purchasing choices of socioeconomic groups. *Australian and New Zealand J Public Health.* 1996;20(6):611-617.

60. Hill JO, Peters JC. Environmental contributions to the obesity epidemic. *Science.* 1998;280:1371-1374.

61. Glanz K. Progress in dietary behavior change. *Am J Health Promotion.* 1999;14(2):112-117.

62. Wechsler II, Devereaux RS, Davis M, Collins J. Using the school environment to promote physical activity and healthy eating. *Prev Med.* 2000;31(2,Pt.2). S121-S137.

63. Winett RA, Anderson ES, Bickley PG, et al. Nutrition for a Lifetime System: A multimedia system for altering food supermarket shoppers' purchases to meet nutritional guidelines. *Comput Hum Behav.* 1997;13(3):371-392.

64. Kirby RS, Foldy SL. *The Role of Geographic Information Systems in Population Health.* Proceedings from the Third National Conference: Geographic Information Systems in Public Health; 1998.

65. Curry SJ, Wagner EH, Cheadle A, et al. Assessment of community-level influences on individuals' attitude about cigarette smoking, alcohol use, and consumption of dietary fat. *Am J Prev Med.* 1993;9(2):78-84.

66. Ayala GX, Elder JP, Campbell NR, et al. Nutrition communication for a Latino community: Formative research foundations. *Fam Comm Health,* in press.

67. US Preventive Task Force (USPTF). *The Guide to Clinical Preventive Services.* 2nd ed. Available at: http://text.nlm.nih.gov/ftrs/dbaccess/cps. Accessed June 15, 2001.

68. US Department of Health and Human Services, Centers for Disease Control and Prevention. The Office of Women's Health: Breast and cervical cancer page. Available at: http://www.cdc.gov/od/owh/whbc.htm. Accessed June 5, 2001.

69. May DS, Lee NC, Richardson LC, Giustozzi AG, Bobo JK. Mammography and breast cancer detection by race and Hispanic ethnicity: Results from a national program (United States). *Cancer Causes and Control.* September 2000;11(8):697-705.

70. California Department of Health Services, Cancer Detection Section. *Healthcare Providers and Women: Partners in Communication: A Literature Review of Obstacles to Breast Cancer Screening.* Sacramento: University of California-Davis; 1996.

71. National Cancer Institute. *Knowledge, Attitudes and Behavior of Immigrant Asian American Women Ages 40 and Older Regarding Breast Cancer Screening.* NIH Publication No. 00-4809; 1999.

72. King ES, Resch N, Rimer B, Lerman C, Boyce A, McGovern-Gorchov P. Breast cancer screening practices among retirement community women. *Prev Med.* 1993;22:1-19.

73. Kash KM, Holland JC, Halper MS, Miller DG. Psychological distress and surveillance behavior of women with a family history of breast cancer. *J Natl Cancer Inst.* 84.24-30. In: Schwartz MD, Rimer BK, Daly M, et al. A randomized trial of breast cancer risk counseling: The impact on self reported mammography use. *Am J Public Health.* 1992;89:924-926.

74. Rutledge DN, Hartman WH, Kinman PO, Winfield AC. Exploration of factors affecting mammography behaviors. *Prev Med.* 1988;17:412-422.

75. Castro F, Elder J, Coe K, et al. Mobilizing churches for health promotion in Latino communities: Companeras en la Salud. *J Natl Cancer Inst Monogr.* 1995;18:127-135.

76. Navarro AM, Senn KL, Kaplan RM, McNichols L, Campo MC, Roppe B. Por La Vida intervention model for cancer prevention in Latinas. *J Natl Health Instit.* 1995;18:137.

77. Talavera GA. *Compañeros En Acción: Promoting breast cancer screening among indigent women.* Presented at the 128th Annual Meeting of the APHA in Boston, Mass; November 2000.

78. Tessaro I, Eng E, Smith J. Breast cancer screening in older African-American women: Qualitative research findings. *Am J Health Promotion.* March-April 1994; 8(4):286-292.

79. California Department of Health Services. The Breast and Cervical Cancer Master Plan Task Force. *California Plan to Prevent and Control Breast and Cervical Cancer: Strategies for Cancer Prevention and Control for Tears 2000-2005.* January 2000; 13-14.

80. Rimer BK, Keintz MK, Kessler HB, Engstrom PF, Rosan JR. Why women resist screening mammography; Patient-related barriers. *Radiology.* 1989;172(1):243-246.

81. Ruben E, Frank MS, Stanley RJ, Bernreuter WK, Han SY. Patient-initiated mobile mammography: Analysis of the patients and the problems. *Southern Med J.* 1990;83(2):178-184.

82. American Association of Retired Persons. *Educating Older Women About Mammography: A Guide for Program Planners and Volunteer Leaders.* Washington, DC: AARP; 1993.

83. Parker K. Owner/Director of Mobil Mammography of San Diego. Personal communication; 1999.

84. Dershaw DD, Liberman L, Lippin BS. Mobile mammographic screening of self-referred women: Results of 22,540 screenings. *Radiology.* August 1992;18(2):415-419.

85. National Cancer Institute. The Cancer Facts: Improving Methods for Breast Cancer Detection and Diagnosis; Fact Sheets page. Available at: http://cis.nci.nih.gov/fact/5_14.htm. Accessed June 15, 2001.

86. Freund K. Breast cancer screening for women ages 40-49. *Medscape Women's Health.* 1997;2(2).

87. Lawson HD, Henson R, Bobo JK, Kaeser MK. Implementing recommendations for the early detection of breast and cervical cancer among low-income women. Division of Cancer Prevention and Control, National Center for Chronic Disease Prevention and Health Promotion. *MMWR.* March 31, 2000;49(RR02):35-55.

88. Evans N, Martin AR. The Pathways to Prevention: Eight Practical Steps—From the Personal to the Political—Toward Reducing the Risk of Breast Cancer page. *The Breast Cancer Fund.* Available at: http://www.breastcancerfund.org. Accessed May 16, 2001.

89. Koplan JP. The National Breast and Cervical Cancer Early Detection Program: At a Glance page. Available at: http://www.cdc.gov/cancer/nbccedp/bccpdfs/bccaag01.pdf. Accessed April 17, 2001.

90. US Department of Health and Human Services, Centers for Disease Control and Prevention. The National Breast and Cervical Cancer Early Detection Program: At a Glance page. Available at: http://www.cdc.gov/cancer.htm. Accessed April 17, 2001.

91. Thomas JC, Tucker MJ. The development and use of the concept of a sexually transmitted disease core. *J Infect Dis.* 1996;174(suppl 2):S134-43.

92. Aral SO, Holmes KK, Padian NS, Cates W Jr. Overview: Individual and population approaches to the epidemiology and prevention of sexually transmitted diseases and human immunodeficiency virus infection. *J Infect Dis.* 1996;174(suppl 2):S127-33.

93. Brunham RC, Plummer FA. A general model of sexually transmitted disease epidemiology and its implications for control. *Med Clin North Am.* 1990;74:1339-1352.

94. Hanenberg RS, Rojanaithayakorn W, Kunasol P, Sokal DC. Impact of Thailand's HIV-control programme as indicated by the decline of sexually transmitted diseases. *Lancet.* 1994;344:243-245.

95. Nelson KE, Celentano DD, Eiumtrakul S, et al. Changes in sexual behavior and a decline in HIV infection among young men in Thailand. *N Engl J Med.* 1996;335:297-303.

96. Celentano DD, Nelson KE, Lyles CM, et al. Decreasing incidence of HIV and sexually transmitted diseases in young Thai men: Evidence for success of the HIV/AIDS control and prevention program. *AIDS.* 1998;12:F29-F36.

97. Steen R, Vuylsteke B, DeCoito T, et al. Evidence of declining STD prevalence in a South African mining community following a core-group intervention. *Sex Transm Dis.* January 2000;27(1):1-8.

98. Dallabetta GA, Laga M, Lamptey PL, eds. *Control of Sexually Transmitted Diseases: A Handbook for the Design and Management of Programs.* Arlington, Va: AIDSCAP/Family Health International, V-X11; 1996.

99. Grosskurth H, Mosha F, Todd J, et al. A community trial of the impact of improved sexually transmitted disease treatment on the HIV epidemic in rural Tanzania: 2 Baseline survey results. *AIDS.* 1995;9(8):927-934.

100. Wawer MJ, Sewankambo NK, Serwadda D, et al. Control of sexually transmitted diseases for AIDS prevention in Uganda: A randomized community trial. Rakai Project Study Group. *Lancet.* February 13, 1999;353(9152):525-535.

101. Aral SO, Holmes KK. Social and behavioral determinants of the epidemiology of STDs: Industrialized and developing countries. In: Holmes KK, Sparling PF, Mardh PA, et al, eds. *Sexually Transmitted Diseases.* 3rd ed. New York, NY: McGraw-Hill; 1999:39-76.

CHAPTER
15

The Management of Public Health Organizations

Joel M. Lee, Dr.P.H.

INTRODUCTION

Excellence in management is an essential activity to provide the highest quality public health services. Although many definitions of management in health care organizations exist, most share common characteristics related to the optimal coordination of human, capital, and material resources in achievement of the organization's goals. The responsibilities of public health practice are broad and complex, and require many staff members with different types of professional education, skills, and personalities. It is the role of the manager to organize staff and other resources to obtain optimal performance for the organization and its customers.

Managers in many sectors of the economy are formally educated to be managers, and management education may be a criterion for employment. In health care, and particularly in public health, most of the personnel with management responsibilities are edu-

cated and employed based upon their expertise in functional areas, such as nursing, medicine, health education, or environmental science, rather than as managers. As highly capable practitioners of a clinical or technical specialty, many of these professionals are promoted into positions with management responsibilities. With limited preparation beyond intuitive skills, many public health personnel are expected to be managers responsible for getting things done. New managers are expected to assume management responsibilities and address topics such as planning, human resources, and allocation of limited resources immediately upon assuming a supervisory position.

Many books and journals address the concept of management in for-profit and not-for-profit businesses, and specifically in health care organizations. Although less has been written about management of public health services than business or other health and medical settings, a body of literature on management of public health programs does exist. The breadth and depth of this content are complex and significant, and cannot be addressed in a single chapter of this book. Consequently, this chapter is designed as an introduction to the basic management functions using public health examples. More detailed general reference sources include Griffith,[1] Longest et al.[2] and Novick and Mays.[3]

It is important to note that management in public health is different from management in other sectors of the economy. Differences in public health setting management include divergent goals, organizations that focus on reducing future services through prevention, differences with traditional economic models, decision making by providers rather than consumers, and discretionary price setting by providers. Additionally, some argue that public health organizations as government bodies lack incentives to maximize productivity. Public health organizations also differ in focus from other types of health organizations exclusively providing direct medical care services, and therefore management of these organizations will be different.

Although there are differences in organizations providing public health services, medical services, and other products or services, there are common frameworks that may be applied. Management research suggests that whereas management style may vary with the external environment, strategy, and structure of the organization, the functional framework of management will be the same in all organizations. One of the most common frameworks is to organize around four functions of management: planning, organizing, directing, and controlling. These four functions address the responsibilities of managers in all types of organizations producing products or services in for-profit, not-for-profit, and government settings.

PLANNING

All organizations must make current decisions as a means to address the future. If appropriate action is not taken at the present time, a desired future state is not likely to occur. The planning function is intended to help an organization anticipate the future, and decide how the organization will achieve desired outcomes. Planning is a continuous process, and no plan is ever finished.

There is a long history of federal planning policy in health care. The initial planning focus was on resource-based activities such as hospital bed need under the 1946 Federal Hill Burton funding for hospitals. Federal and state planning continued with the Comprehensive Health Planning and Health Systems Agency planning programs of the 1960s through the 1980s, and to the present Healthy People 2000 and 2010 efforts as detailed in chapter 10. The most recent planning efforts have shifted from planning for resources to focus on the outcome of services provided. Managers of public health organizations must function in a continuously changing environment. To accomplish this task, health managers must use planning techniques to solve problems in a systematic way. Planning creates a framework of plans and procedures based upon institutional goals and objectives.

Planning activities in public health may be divided into two functions, tactical and strategic planning. *Tactical planning* (also known as operational planning), is short time range, narrow in focus, and addresses the achievement of specific organizational objectives. In contrast, *strategic planning* is long time range, broad in focus, and concentrates on formulation of organizational goals. The longer the effect of a plan and the more difficult it is to reverse once implemented, the more strategic the nature of the plan. In addition, the greater the emphasis upon policy, the more strategic the plan. Organizations conduct strategic and operational plans concurrently and these activities are complementary.

As an example of the relationship of the two types of plans, a public health organization may establish a strategic plan to reduce deaths in the general population associated with cigarette smoking, while setting operational goals for changes 10 years into the future. To achieve this strategy, the organization may establish a tactical plan to reduce smoking by middle school students over the next 2 years.

Health care organizations have not always viewed planning in a positive light. In public health care organizations, current planning efforts have followed historic efforts. When asked to plan, participants do what they know best, what they have done in the past, or what they are told to do. Consequently, a great deal of planning has been less than effective, and has diminished enthusiasm for future planning efforts. In contrast, effective planning contributes to success in the mission of the organization and can have the enthusiastic support of the organization's staff and governing body. There are many approaches to planning public health services, and there is not one model that is appropriate for all situations. Consequently, the selection of an appropriate planning model is contingent upon the task, organization, and external milieu.

Planning Theory

Planning theory is the basis for design of all planning activities. Planning may be categorized into four distinct planning approaches: the rational, incremental, mixed-scanning, and radical models. When selecting a model for planning decisions, each of the planning approaches has strengths and weaknesses, and selection of a model is linked to the specific situation under consideration. Normally one of the four approaches will be best for a specific public health planning purpose.

Rational Strategy

The first approach is the *rational* (also known as comprehensive) strategy of planning. Rational planning focuses on development of a comprehensive list of all possible opportunities for intervention by decision makers. The strategy identifies the consequence of each possible action, and selects the action that would result in the most desired set of outcomes. This is a relatively complex process, as it requires enumeration of all possible opportunities and consequences of actions. The rational strategy is most applicable to situations where there are technical decisions to be made, if values are implied, where the primary goal is efficiency, and/or if the future appears stable with clear trends.

Planning related to substance abuse is an example of a situation appropriate for rational planning. Such a plan would consider the costs and benefits of every potential activity in the areas of education and treatment of each abused substance, in all cohorts of the

population. Following this inventory of actions, the best strategies would be selected for implementation. Knowledgeable authorities and technical personnel capable of identifying all factors under consideration best conduct rational planning.

Incremental Strategy

The *incremental* strategy of planning emphasizes repeated comparisons of planning options. The approach assumes that change is gradual and focuses on a series of small incremental steps, each making a slight improvement in the outcome. Incremental strategy is most effective when addressing problems of scarce resources, where there is not agreement on policy, and compromise is important. Other factors that influence the selection of the incremental strategy include decisions that are not theoretical and situations where there is little detailed information on preference.

Incremental strategy may be best used for an activity such as the reduction of infant mortality. Although it would be desirable for no infants to die, it is unlikely this would be achieved in the short term, if at all. If the current infant mortality rate is 7.2 per 1,000 live births, an incremental reduction to 7.1 next year, 7.0 the following year, and 6.9 the following year may be achievable as well as desirable. In contrast, a decrease from 7.2 to 5.0 per 1,000 deaths in one year may be unachievable. Incremental planning is best conducted by the individuals most affected by the planning decisions. Incremental planning may also be useful when there is not agreement on policy or use of resources and when a small change will be acceptable to all parties involved.

Mixed-Scanning Strategy

The third model, the *mixed-scanning* approach to planning, is a blend of the first two strategies. All opportunities and consequences for intervention may be considered on a comprehensive basis, and then narrowed to a manageable set of options. Incremental decisions are then made for implementation. For example, in the case of bioterrorism, all factors might be considered and the most likely events selected as priorities. If a biological threat might be addressed through immunization with a vaccine in limited supply, immunization could be done incrementally, targeting groups at greatest risk first. Availability of resources (time, money, and data) defines the balance between the two strategies. The mixed-scanning planning method is most appropriate to a rapidly changing environment requiring a great deal of flexibility. Who conducts mixed-scanning planning is situational to the issues.

Radical Strategy

A final planning approach is the *radical* strategy or model. This method emphasizes innovation, spontaneity, and experimentation, and may address an innovative or extreme strategy contrasting with traditional approaches to a problem. A radical strategy might be national decriminalization of abused drugs, along with a needle exchange program. Due to their nature, radical strategies are the least common planning approach, and are most likely where there is a profound dissatisfaction with the status quo.

The rational planning approach is most appropriate to topics such as a long-range master plan, planning methods such Program Evaluation and Review Technique (PERT), and economic studies such as cost benefit analysis. The incremental strategy is most useful for gradual change, public budgeting, and policy. The mixed-scanning model would be very appropriate to clinical decision making, and the radical model would be appropriate for a major policy change such as a universal health insurance program. Each planning model is appropriate for specific planning issues in specific environments. In some cases, multiple methods may be appropriate for planning in a public health organization.

Strategic Planning Model

Following selection of a planning strategy, development of a strategic plan is a useful and necessary tool in management. The plan may then be used as a step toward the achievement of a desired future outcome. Planning activity should never be an objective; it is a management process to achieve objectives. Strategic planning seeks to define the organization and its future. Planning emphasizes designing and causing a desired future state, rather than designing and implementing programs to achieve specific written objectives.

Whereas a variety of approaches to strategic planning exist, these models offer a generalized concept for planning. This can be illustrated by a model based upon the work of Coopers and Lybrand (Figure 15.1).[4] This model divides the strategic planning process into four sets of activities, answering four specific questions:

1. Where are we now?
2. Where should we be going?
3. How should we get there?
4. Are we getting there?

These questions focus upon the activities of planning. To answer the question "Where are we now?" requires a situational analysis where participants must collect and assemble data addressing the organization's environment and operations. This leads to the use of an assessment tool such as a Strengths/Weaknesses/Opportunities/Threats (SWOT) analysis, and concludes with the establishment of a set of issues and challenges for the organization. The question "Where should we be going?" can be answered with goal formulation, including exploration of alternative strategies, and development of organizational direction in the form of statements of vision, mission, goals, and objectives. Strategy formulation answers the question "How should we get there?" Strategy includes development of actions to achieve goals, and assessment of resources to achieve each strategy, including budgets. Following implementation of operations, evaluation and control are addressed through the final question, "Are we getting there?" Monitoring requires collection and analysis of data, followed by using this performance feedback to adjust where the organization should be going. Operations are then managed to achieve these outcomes.

The planning process is continuous, and upon completion the model is repeated from the beginning, using the evaluation data as input for the next situational analysis, and further refinement of the strategic planning process. This model of strategic planning simplifies a complex process of decision making, but requires a great deal of time and effort. In developing

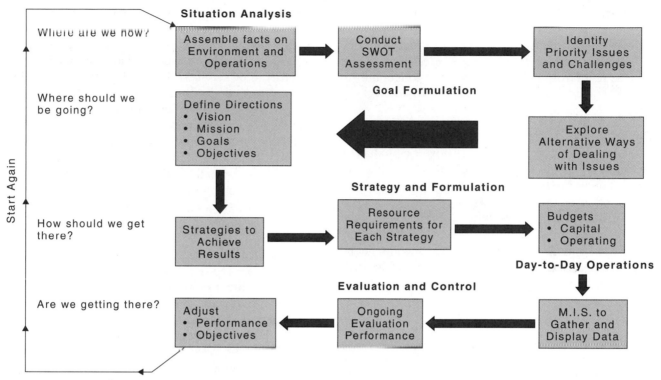

Figure 15.1. Strategic Planning Model

Source: Adapted from Keck RK Jr., 1986. Strategic planning in the health care industry: Concentrate on the basics. *Health Care Issues* (September). Reprinted in the *Handbook of Business Strategy 1985/1986 Yearbook*, Coopers & Lybrand.

such a plan it is important to remember that the objective is not to write a plan, but to get something accomplished, and to take action regarding the future direction and financial viability of the organization.

Marketing Model

In considering the planning function, managers may also consider a marketing model. Planning and marketing are very closely related functions, and planning components may be complemented using marketing concepts and definitions. Although planning and marketing are closely related both conceptually and operationally,[5] it is the former that has received more considerable attention in terms of governmental policy, whereas the latter has received greater attention in the private sector. Both planning and marketing have merit in the public health setting, and marketing in public health has received increased attention in recent years.[6]

The fundamental concept of marketing is that an organization's most precious asset is its relationship with customers, and this relationship is defined by quality, service, and price. Although many people think of marketing as advertising, marketing is a far more complex set of activities. At the most basic level, marketing can be defined as an exchange between two parties to satisfy their needs. In public health, this is an exchange of public health services for appropriate compensation. Marketing activity can be described in the context of the four "Ps" of marketing: product, place, price, and promotion.

Product

The first "P" represents the product or service that defines the activity of the organization. In the private sector, manufacturing activity results in a product to be exchanged. In public health we normally offer a service. The product or service can be described as the set of activities focused on a particular public health need such as acquired immunodeficiency syndrome, or food inspection. Alternatively, a product or service can be described as the benefit provided to the client, such as relief from pain and anxiety, or longer life.

Place

The second "P" stands for the place or location where the service is offered. Place defines how the product or service will be delivered to the client. This marketing concept refers not only to the location of the service, but also to other factors such as operating hours, referral mechanisms, and enablers or barriers to access for the service. These access factors may be based on the characteristics of the external marketplace such as public transportation, or internal organizational factors such as barriers to access for a wheelchair-bound client.

Price

The third "P" of marketing addresses the price or fees exchanged for a service. Price addresses not only the charge for a service (which in public health is usually not paid directly by the client), but also everything that the organization requires the client to go through to use the service including social costs such as the waiting time for care, missing work, or the stigma associated with obtaining the service. Price links the organization's revenue and the consumer's satisfaction. This presents a potential conflict of interest between providing the highest quality public health service and increasing an organization's revenue.

Promotion

Finally, the fourth "P," promotion, includes activities to acquaint the prospective client with the organization and the services offered. Promotion is a matter of communication of information between an organization and the external market. Promotion describes how the patient becomes aware of the services offered, and how the patient develops an interest in using one or more of these services. Promotion addresses the education of clients about public health services and the reasons to use these services or to support funding of public health.

Additional strategic concepts in marketing include product or service differentiation from alternative services, price competition with alternative providers, market segmentation for specific cohorts of the population by socioeconomic variables, product segmentation for special population groups, and mass marketing/advertising of services. A subcategory of marketing with a direct relationship to health care is social marketing, which focuses on behavior; for example, changing health behaviors such as smoking or diet. Social marketing is discussed in greater detail in chapter 14. Although these marketing concepts have been used historically in the private sector, they are equally valuable in designing future public health services to meet the needs of the population.

The Relationship of Planning and Marketing

Whereas planning and marketing are overlapping concepts, planning focuses more on change over time, while marketing addresses the design of relationships between providers and consumers of services. A critical stage of both marketing and planning is needs assessment. In needs assessment, the public health organization attempts to characterize the needs of the population served to define current and future activities to meet the needs of the population. In public health, this involves such items as morbidity profiles, described specifically in terms of the incidence and prevalence rates of acute and chronic disease. Marketing strategies can also incorporate epidemiologic measures. Product or service definition, for instance, depends on the description of public needs. The development of a women's health "product" can be defined based on the dimensions of need for this service, much of which is epidemiologically derived. For example, a women's health need that could result in a public health product is the prevalence of breast and cervical cancer. The price of the service may increase or decrease utilization. Strategies regarding place include an assessment of barriers to access to care. Promotional activities may include motivational messages, based in part on epidemiologic studies. Primary prevention, such as cancer screening, can be promoted by encouraging clients to consider the advantages of early- versus late-stage diagnosis in terms of survival studies. Marketing has clear epidemiologic roots, to the extent that behaviors such as smoking, diet, and sexual behaviors have been epidemiologically linked to morbidity.

ORGANIZING

The management function of organizing addresses successful completion of management tasks through structure, delegation, and communication. Organizing focuses on the relationships between tasks and activities to achieve organizational goals and explains lines of authority and supervision in the public health organization.

Organizational Design

Organizations may be structured in a variety of ways to improve the management function. Public health services may be organized by function, geography, client, and/or purpose. An organization built on function organizes its work activities into units based upon common management functions such as home health, human resources, and finance.

Geographic organization would focus on division of the service area into specific regions of the public health department's service area. A third method is organization by client, where functions serve specific populations such as children, teenagers, adults, and senior citizens. A final approach is organization by purpose, where all activities are structured by a common reason or objective for their existence. This approach is organized around the outcomes to be achieved. Examples might include the departmentalization around well-baby services, health promotion, or substance abuse. Simplified illustrations of each of the four models are presented in Figure 15.2.

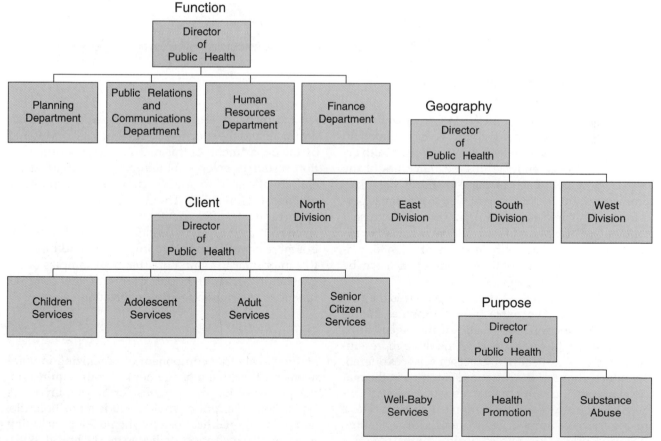

Figure 15.2. Four Models of Organization

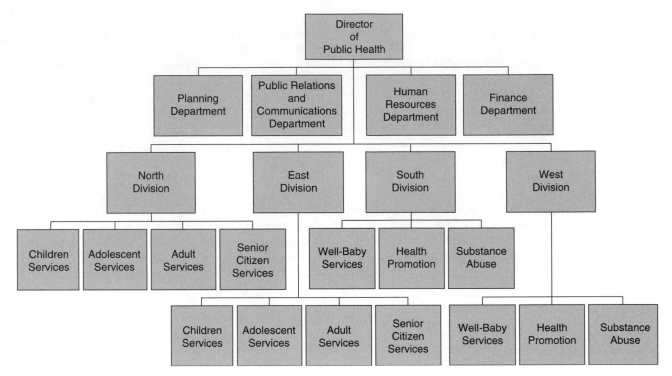

Figure 15.3. Mixed Organizational Structure

Selection of an optimal method of organization for a public health department should be based upon an assessment of the external environment, the health organization's goals, and the desired outcomes of the services provided. Each of these methods organizes common resources in a different way to maximize performance. In some cases, an organization may use a combination of the four organizational models. For example, a large public health department might organize using a combination of these models to achieve the greatest level of effectiveness (Figure 15.3).

An alternative method of management is the matrix organization. The matrix model combines and organizes the functional approach of management as columns of a table, with rows of the table representing specific public health products or services offered. The intersections of the rows and columns in the matrix represent tasks, or resources (such as staff) required to achieve the organization's objectives. There are a variety of approaches to matrix organization; one appropriate for public health might organize around managerial functions of a public health department and the specific products or services offered by the department. In this matrix model of organization, resources belong to the functional departments, and are allocated to specific projects or purposes as required (Figure 15.4). The matrix model creates an opportunity to offer greater flexibility and responsiveness than the four traditional models. However, it is a more complex model to implement and manage. It is important to again note that the examples of organization are oversimplifications of the complex functions of a public health organization.

Staffing

Staffing is another component of organizing in management. Effective management of staff requires development of job descriptions for all employees. A typical job description would include a position title, and detailed qualifications for the position including education, registration or licensure, technical skills,

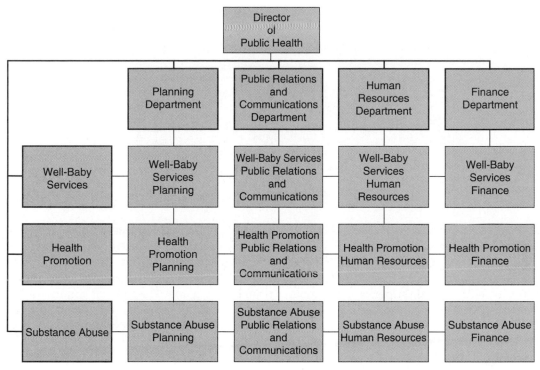

Figure 15.4. Matrix Organization

and prior experience. In addition, the position description would address specific responsibilities as general categories and performance standards, criteria for performance appraisal, and the salary range. Staffing will also address the management responsibilities of personnel, identifying front-line, mid-level, and senior managers who are directly responsible for the activities of the organization, and staff who support the work of managers. The basic management literature describes management theory and principles of supervision, including division of work among staff and specialization of work.

On an organizational chart, personnel are categorized by line or staff functions. *Line* is the term used to define supervisory authority within the organization, and roles such as director, associate director, and department head. The organizational chart demonstrates the hierarchy of managers and subordinates they supervise. *Staff* is the term used to identify personnel with specialized and technical skills who provide support to the supervisory line personnel, but

who do not have supervisory authority over others. In the example presented in Figure 15.5 the Director and Associate Directors are line positions with supervisory authority over other personnel, and a part-time Medical Director and Executive Assistant are staff positions providing technical support without supervisory responsibilities. These staff relationships help in defining the expectations of personnel and their interrelationships. In the purest form of organization, these roles are discrete; line personnel always supervise other personnel, and staff personnel do not. In most organizations and particularly smaller organizations, the distinction may be less clear.

Management Theory

Effective management is based upon a body of theory. A simplification of theory would present two principal approaches to management, the classical and behavioral models. The classical approach advocates that structure be kept simple with as few levels of line

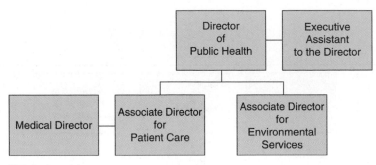

Figure 15.5. Line and Staff Relationships

and staff employees as possible, with clear-cut authority and responsibility for each position. Each employee is confined to a single specialized function. Supervision addresses unity of command and a clear chain of authority, with a single superior directing an employee and staff communication taking place exclusively through managers, each supervisor having a limited number of subordinates. Classical managers assume that their employees are solely motivated by financial reward and that they do not value their contribution to the organization's work. Consequently, classical theory managers believe subordinates must be constantly supervised and that they will not do their jobs well if they are not. Classical theory managers also believe this approach is the best and the only way to effectively manage an organization.

The behavioral approach assumes that people can enjoy work, and if conditions are favorable they can exercise control over their performance. The behavioral model of management explains that the classical theory makes demands on individuals that are incongruent with their needs, and questions the classical attitude toward workers and aggressive supervision as the only way to motivate staff. In place of the assumption that financial reward is the only source of motivation, behavioral managers believe that people are motivated by the desire to do a good job, and by the opportunity to interact with peers. This would result in decentralization of the organization, enlarged and unspecialized responsibilities for staff, employee participation in decision making, and upward and lateral communication between personnel. Although it oversimplifies the approach, behavioral managers

believe happy employees are good employees. Just as the advocates of classical management advocate one best way to manage, the advocates of human relations management would substitute an alternative universal best way to manage in all situations.

A third and more contemporary approach to management describes a contingency or situational approach to management. In the contingency model, planning, organizing, directing, and controlling are dependent upon the organizational environment and tasks. Contingency managers propose a situational approach, where managers may supervise some personnel and activity using the classical approach, and others using the behavioral approach. Contingency management shifts from universal principles or methods of management and recognizes that each organization and management problem will be unique. As a result, management strategies must be developed differently for each situation. In a public health organization, supervision of registered nurses conducting home visits may be managed differently than the supervision of a data entry clerk. Rather than selecting a single best way to manage, contingency managers evaluate a specific management situation and select an appropriate management strategy for that situation. All managers must consider these alternatives and select an appropriate management style in the context of their unique organization and its personnel.

Competencies for Public Health Professionals

An excellent example for organizing staff in public health is presented by the Council on Linkages Between

Academia and Public Health Practice's 2001 project to develop a list of core competencies for public health professionals. This model may also be applied to the discussion of controlling, later in this chapter. The Council states that the core competencies represent a set of skills, knowledge, and attitudes necessary for the broad practice of public health; that competencies transcend the boundaries of the specific disciplines within public health, and help to unify the profession. The Council on Linkages believes that these competencies can be used for several purposes including education, and as a framework for hiring and evaluating public health staff in practice settings. The Council has developed eight public health domains each with a set of skills and knowledge levels, followed by important attitudes about the practice of public health. These domains are:

1. Analytical Assessment Skills (11 Specific Competencies)
2. Policy Development/Program Planning Skills (11 Specific Competencies)
3. Communications Skills (6 Specific Competencies, 1 Attitude Competency)
4. Cultural Competency Skills (11 Specific Competencies, 2 Attitude Competencies)
5. Community Dimensions of Practice Skills (8 Specific Competencies)
6. Basic Public Health Sciences Skills (7 Specific Competencies, 1 Attitude Competency)
7. Financial Planning and Management Skills (10 Specific Competencies)
8. Leadership and Systems Thinking Skills (8 Specific Competencies)

The Council defines the specific core competencies as they apply to three levels of mastery of the competency: a basic level (aware), an intermediate level (knowledgeable), and an advanced level (proficient). Although the Council on Linkages notes limitations in the use of these broadly defined job categories (frontline staff, senior-level staff, and supervisory and management staff), this model offers potential benefits in staffing decisions. Table 15.1 presents a graphic representation of this framework and definitions of job categories and levels of mastery.[7] These competencies are also discussed in chapter 3 and appendix C.

Public Health as a Profession

Another important aspect of staffing in public health is the definition of the public health profession. Effective planning and decision making for public health requires an understanding of a variety of categories of public health personnel and their professional competencies. Although it is feasible to identify the number of personnel budgeted and employed in local, state, and federal public health agencies, the job descriptions, educational backgrounds, and professional skills of these personnel are not standardized. Complicating this further is the absence of information about personnel employed in public health functions in private industry, and personnel intersecting public health with another profession such as medicine, health administration, or education.

In contrast to professions such as medicine, dentistry, or law, public health professionals do not share a single standardized and accredited educational degree as a requisite for state licensure. Further, as public health professionals rather than as practitioners of a technical skill, personnel are not required to participate in ongoing public health continuing education.

Enumeration of the public health workforce is currently not possible. In *The Public Health Workforce: Enumeration 2000*, Gebbie discusses the educational and technical diversity of public health workers in the United States and notes the difficulties in estimating the public health workforce, as "there has been no systematic accumulation of the necessary information."[8] This lack of information complicates staffing decisions in public health organizations.

When formally establishing a profession, specific characteristics must be identified to define the nature of the profession. This applies to definition of the public health professional. First, the profession must require a body of scientific knowledge and technical skill that serves the needs of the public. Second, professionals have autonomy or independent control of their work. Third, there should be a clear differentiation between the public health professional and support staff. This means that public health professionals would be self-directing, and have a degree of autonomy and authority in work activities. As professionals, public health workers would have the expertise to

Table 15.1.   Council on Linkages, Framework of Individual Skills Desirable for the Delivery of Essential Public Health Services

Public Health Staff Category:	Front-Line Staff:	Senior-Level Staff:	Supervisory and Management Staff:
	Individuals who carry out the bulk of day-to-day tasks (e.g., sanitarians, counselors, nurses and other clinicians, investigators, lab technicians, health educators). Responsibilities may include basic data collection and analysis, fieldwork, program planning, outreach activities, programmatic support, and other organizational tasks.	Individuals with a specialized staff function but not serving as managers (e.g., epidemiologists, attorneys, biostatisticians, health planners, health policy analysts). They have increased technical knowledge of principles in areas such as epidemiology, program planning and evaluation, data collection, budget development, grant writing, etc. and may be responsible for coordination and/or oversight of pieces of projects or programs.	Individuals responsible for major programs or functions of an organization, with staff who report to them. Increased skills can be expected in program development, program implementation, program evaluation, community relations, writing, public speaking, managing timelines and work plans, presenting arguments and recommendations on policy issues.

Levels of Mastery:

Aware:

Basic level of mastery of the competency. Individuals may be able to identify the concept or skill but have limited ability to perform the skill.

Knowledgeable:

Intermediate level of mastery of the competency. Individuals are able to apply and describe the skill.

Proficient:

Advanced level of mastery of the competency. Individuals are able to synthesize, critique, or teach the skill.

make decisions in their area of competence; control the production of public health personnel; determine the application of knowledge and skills in the public health work they perform; and direct support staff in public health matters. Other characteristics defining a profession include formal certification or licensure as a requirement, regional or national professional associations, and a code of ethics.

To manage personnel in public health it would be valuable to define staff in professional and support roles. In evaluating whether public health is a profession, there is clearly a body of public health knowledge in the core areas of behavioral health, biostatis-tics, epidemiology, environmental health, and health administration. This knowledge is defined by the accrediting organization for academic programs in public health (the Council on Education in Public Health). Although accreditation is not mandatory for universities awarding degrees to public health professionals, the establishment of this entity contributes to control over professional education. Specific public health disciplines such as environmental health and health administration do offer specialized professional certification. However, disciplinary certification is not limited exclusively to graduates of public health programs or individuals in public health. In the United States, there is an absence of required licensure or certification for practicing public health professionals.

Complicating this further is the public health interest and specialization of other professions such as medicine, nursing, and education with overlapping roles. Autonomy and authority in public health work activities currently seem situational to specific work activity and organizations and complicates supervision.

Public health may be noteworthy as a profession for its historic lack of a professional code of ethics. In 2000, the Public Health Code of Ethics Work Group (consisting of public health professionals from local and state public health organizations, academia, the Centers for Disease Control and Prevention, and the American Public Health Association) initiated development of a code of ethics for public health. The Public Health Leadership Society that leads this effort states that the code will clarify the distinctive elements of public health and the ethical principles that follow from, or respond to those distinct aspects, and "serve as a goal to guide public health institutions and practitioners and as a standard to which they could be held accountable."[9] The Society reports that its code is intended principally for public and other institutions in the United States that have an explicit public health mission, and notes that the code will not specify the criteria for professional competence. This would have to be specified by individual professions, such as epidemiology and health education. As a result, a generic code with professional relevance will be established.

Status of public health as a profession has direct relevance to staffing decisions in public health and the relationship of public health personnel to other health professionals. Consequently, although issues related to academic accreditation, professional competencies, and professional ethics continue to evolve, debate continues regarding whether public health is, should be, or can become a distinct profession.

DIRECTING

The directing function of management focuses upon effective communication as a management tool. Effective communication enables employees to understand what their responsibilities are and how they relate to achieving the organization's goals. Communication will include the functions of motivating and leading staff. These attributes are addressed in chapter 9.

CONTROLLING

The controlling process of management addresses monitoring and adjusting management activities to achieve organizational goals. The process creates standards, monitors activities, compares results with external standards, and takes corrective actions or adjustments to realign management activities with organizational goals. The control function requires evaluation of organizational status. Traditional methods include budgeting as a decision-making process and using financial ratios to address cash flow and capital expenditures.

The National Public Health Performance Standards Program

More innovative methods of controlling in public health may also be considered as management tools. The National Public Health Performance Standards Program (NPHPSP) offers an example of an effort to improve the performance of public health organizations. In 2000, after two years of effort, the Centers for Disease Control and Prevention (CDC) and a coalition of national public health organizations developed and released a draft of public health performance standards. The participants are seeking to develop state and local governance performance standards and measurement tools related to essential public health services. The tools will enable public health systems, organizations, and governing bodies to assess their overall performance against optimum standards of practice. NPHPSP states that the practice standards are predicated on the axiom, "what gets measured gets done." The program proposes a vision, mission, and goals for public health performance:

> Vision: Excellence in public health practice defined by recognized performance standards

Mission: To improve the practice of public health by providing leadership in research, development, and implementation of science-based performance standards

Goals: Quality improvement, accountability, and enhanced science base for public health practice[10]

As an example of monitoring and adjusting management activities, the National Public Health Performance Standards Program seeks to explore how performance standards and measurement data can be molded into a national surveillance system for public health practice. The NPHPSP partnership reports that it is identifying and addressing issues related to the collection, analysis, and use of performance data for meeting the three goals of the program, (quality improvement, improving accountability, and further developing a science base for the practice of public health) delineating systemwide strengths and deficiencies and identifying best practices. The National Public Health Standards Program is discussed in greater detail in chapter 12.

Quality as a Tool for Control

The issue of quality of service has received growing attention, first as a management tool in private industry, then in medical care, and now in public health. Ideas such as total quality management and continuous quality improvement have received a great deal of interest in industry with varying outcomes, and have recently received increasing attention from health care organizations. Many managers have become advocates of these tools, whereas others view these same applications as "fads." Traditional industrial total quality improvement evaluation tools may be used to evaluate public health quality improvement,[11] financial ratio analysis,[12] and general health measurement.[13]

In considering the use of quality management tools in public health, the first question to ask is: "In a time of diminishing resources, why would an organization wish to invest resources in this type of time-consuming and expensive effort?" Quality in management allows an opportunity for an organization to improve

its service and be viewed as the best provider. This perception can redefine the community's image of a public health organization, change its public perception, and gain new clients'/patients' respect.

In addition, these efforts may reduce complaints from the clients/patients while improving employee job satisfaction. A second consideration is: "Who decides what quality is?" In medical or other scientific matters, it may be a scientific construct; however, in most things, the consumer decides on quality and will not use services viewed as being of poor quality. Consumer perceptions of poor quality may result in reduced use and consequently smaller budgets, based upon services provided and/or politically determined allocations.[14]

Examples of quality measurement tools in health care include accreditation models such as the Joint Commission on Accreditation of Health Care Organizations (JCAHO) and National Commission on Quality Assurance (NCQA) and its Health Plan Employer Data and Information Set (HEDIS). Details may be found at http://www.jcaho.org and http://www.ncqa.org. The Ernest A. Codman Award is presented to health care organizations for achievement in the use of process and outcome measures to improve organization performance and, ultimately, the quality of care provided to the public (http://www.jcaho.org/codman/codman.html). HealthGrades (http://www.healthgrades.com) helps to assess and improve the quality of health care in a variety of settings including hospitals, nursing homes, home health, hospices, and emergency services, as well as the quality of providers such as physicians, dentists, and acupuncturists. Each of these models offers valuable information for public health organizations seeking to improve quality in the services they provide.

The Malcolm Baldrige National Quality Award in Health Care

Although there are many methods to improve management performance, a recent innovative framework is presented by the Malcolm Baldrige National Quality Award in Health Care. The Baldrige

Award process offers an opportunity to improve public health organization management by addressing the principles of planning, organizing, directing, and controlling in a new context. The Malcolm Baldrige National Quality Award program was created by federal law in 1987. The findings and purposes section of the law states that poor quality costs companies, whereas improved quality of goods and services goes hand-in-hand with improved productivity, lower costs, and increased profitability. The legislation speaks to strategic planning for quality, worker involvement in quality, and a greater emphasis on statistical process control that can lead to dramatic improvements in both cost and quality. The findings also note that to be successful, quality improvement programs must be management led and customer oriented. This may require fundamental changes in the way companies and agencies do business in the public sector and private enterprise.

The Baldrige Criteria for Performance Excellence provide a systems perspective for understanding performance management, and are most relevant to public health organization management. The criteria reflect management best practices against which an organization can measure itself. The Baldrige criteria present a common language for communication among organizations for sharing best practices and serving as the Baldrige Award criteria.[14]

The Baldrige health care criteria are the basis for organizational self-assessments, for making awards, and for giving performance feedback to applicant organizations. In addition, the criteria have three important roles: (1) to help improve organizational performance practices, capabilities, and results; (2) to facilitate communication and sharing of best practice's information between health care organizations and among U.S. organizations of all types; and (3) to serve as a working tool for understanding and managing performance and for guiding planning and opportunities for learning.

The Baldrige health care criteria are designed to help organizations improve organizational performance and management that results in delivery of ever-improving value to patients and other customers, contributing to improved health care quality, improvement of overall organizational effectiveness and capabilities as a health care provider, and organizational and personal learning. One of the best ways to organize for Baldrige recognition is through the use of the planning, organizing, directing, and controlling functions of management. However these functions must be integrated into a broader management framework. The Baldrige model offers such a framework for improving management of public health organizations. The Baldrige health care core values and concepts are embodied in seven categories of organizational performance results (Figure 15.6):

1. Leadership
2. Strategic planning
3. Focus on patients, other customers, and markets
4. Information and analysis
5. Staff focus
6. Process management
7. Organizational performance results

The Baldrige health care criteria address a variety of topics including visionary leadership, patient-focused excellence, organizational and personal learning, valuing of staff and partners, agility, managing for innovation, managing by fact, public responsibility and community health, focus on results and creating value, systems perspective, and a focus on the future. To date, although there have been industrial, medical, and educational organizations recognized for excellence in quality, there has not been a public health entity acknowledged for quality by receiving the Baldrige Award.

There are a variety of tools in place for management control in health care and several are applicable to public health organizations. In addition, new models including the National Public Health Performance Standards Program and the Malcolm Baldrige National Quality Award in Health Care present exciting new opportunities for improved management in public health.

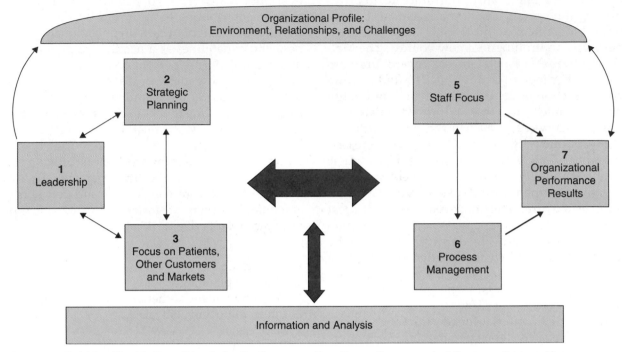

Figure 15.6. Baldrige Health Care Criteria for Performance Excellence Framework: A Systems Perspective

Source: Baldrige National Quality Program, 2001. *Health Care Criteria for Performance Excellence.* National Institute of Standards and Technology, U.S. Department of Commerce.

SUMMARY

In describing the Baldrige Quality Awards, the National Institute of Standards and Technology describes successful management:

Success in today's health care environment demands agility, a capacity for rapid change and flexibility. Health care providers face ever-shorter cycles for the introduction of new or improved health care services, and for faster and more flexible response to patients and other customers. All aspects of electronic communication and information transfer require and enable more rapid, flexible, and customized responses. Today's health care environment places a heavy burden on the timely design of health care delivery systems, disease prevention programs, health promotion programs, and effective and efficient diagnostic and treatment systems. Overall design must include the opportunity to learn for continuous organizational

improvement and must value the individual needs of patients. Design also must include effective means for gauging improvement of health status for patients and populations/communities. Beneficial changes must be introduced at the earliest appropriate opportunity. All aspects of time performance now are more critical, and cycle time has become a key process measure. Other important benefits can be derived from this focus on time; time improvements often drive simultaneous improvements in organization, quality, cost, patient focus, and productivity.

This chapter is designed as an overview of management concepts as a framework, and presentation of public health examples of these management tools. As previously noted, management is an extremely complex and interrelated set of activities. Management techniques will vary in the context of each public health organization's goals, and external environment. Application of the specific concepts associated with the four management functions of planning, organizing, directing, and controlling will contribute to the improved management of public health organizations. Effective application of management methods creates an opportunity to improve the efficiency and effectiveness of public health organizations in the pursuit of their mission and benefits the recipients of public health services.

References

1. Griffith JR. *The Well Managed Healthcare Organization.* Chicago, Ill: Health Administration Press; 1999.

2. Longest BB Jr, Rakich JS, Darr K. *Managing Health Services Organizations and Systems.* Baltimore, Md: Health Professions Press; 2000.

3. Novick LF, Mays GP. *Public Health Administration: Principles for Population-Based Management.* Gaithersburg, Md: Aspen Publishers; 2001.

4. Fleming ST, Scutchfield FD, Tucker TC. *Managerial Epidemiology.* Chicago, Ill: Health Administration Press; 2000.

5. MacStravic RE. *Marketing Health Care.* Germantown, Md: Aspen Publishers; 1977.

6. Seigel M, Doner L. *Marketing Public Health Strategies to Promote Social Change.* Gaithersburg, Md: Aspen Publishers, Inc; 1998.

7. Public Health Foundation. National Public Health Performance Standards Program. Available at: http://www.phf.org/performance.htm. Accessed 2001.

8. Gebbie C. *The Public Health Workforce: Enumeration 2000.* Washington, DC: US Dept of Health and Human Services, Bureau of Health Professions, National Center for Health Workforce Information and Analysis; 2001. (Also: available at: ftp://ftp.hrsa.gov//bhpr/nationalcenter/phworkforce2000.pdf.)

9. Public Health Leadership Society, Public Health Code of Ethics Work Group. *Public Health Code of Ethics.* Washington, DC: American Public Health Association; 2000. Available at: http://www.apha.org/codeofethics/background.pdf.

10. National Public Health Performance Standards Program. Atlanta, Ga: US Dept of Health and Human Services, Centers for Disease Control and Prevention; 2001. Available at: http://www.phppo.cdc.gov/nphpsp/.

11. Leebov W. *The Quality Quest: A Briefing for Health Care Professionals.* Chicago, Ill: American Hospital Publishing; 1991.

12. Nowicki M. *The Financial Management of Hospitals and Healthcare Organizations.* Chicago, Ill: Health Administration Press; 1998.

13. Seidel LF, Gorsky RD, Lewis JD. *Applied Quantitative Methods for Health Services Management.* Baltimore, Md: Health Professions Press; 1995.

14. Health Care Criteria for Performance Excellence, Baldrige National Quality Program/National Institute of Standards and Technology. Gaithersburg, Md: US Dept of Commerce, National Institute of Standards and Technology; 2001. Available at: http://www.quality.nist.gov/PDF_files/2001_HealthCare_Criteria.pdf.

CHAPTER 16

Public Health Workforce

Kristine M. Gebbie, Dr.P.H., R.N.
Hugh Tilson, M.D., Dr.P.H.

Effective public health practice is dependent upon the presence of a workforce that is well prepared and well matched to the specific community being served. The infrastructure of public health, that upon which all services and programs are built, has three components: accurate, timely data and information; effective systems and relationships; and a competent workforce. It may be true, however, to say that of these three apparent equals, workforce is the more important. This is because only people can gather the various bits of knowledge and interpret the data to develop meaningful descriptions of health and illness, and identify strategies for disease prevention and health promotion. Systems and relationships can only be built and maintained by individuals; thus a competent workforce is essential. If the connections made are to serve the health of the public, those making them must understand what public health is, and how it might be achieved.

This chapter will provide an overview of the public health workforce from the perspectives of what professions and skills they represent, the places they are employed, current issues regarding basic and life-long learning needs, emerging standards for public health practice, and areas of needed research. The reader already very familiar with the range of public health practitioners and public health practice may want to concentrate on the latter parts of the chapter; the reader coming new to the field should find the earlier portions helpful with an introduction to the complexities of the field.

WHO PRACTICES PUBLIC HEALTH?

Although often called a profession, public health is unusual because it is not a singular profession in the manner of dentistry or radiation technology. It is closer to a field of practice as might be described by

Table 16.1. Essential Public Health Services

- Monitor health status to identify community health problems
- Diagnose and investigate health problems and health hazards in the community
- Inform, educate, and empower people about health issues
- Mobilize community partnerships to identify and solve health problems
- Develop policies and plans that support individual and community health efforts
- Enforce laws and regulations that protect health and ensure safety
- Link people to needed personal health services and assure the provision of health care when otherwise unavailable
- Assure a competent public health and personal health care workforce
- Evaluate effectiveness, accessibility, and quality of personal and population-based health services
- Research for new insights and innovative solutions to health problems

someone saying "I work in education" or "I work in computers." That is, public health members often are defined by their commitment to the goal of disease prevention and health improvement for populations and communities. They do not focus on any one specific body of knowledge such as a specialized approach to diagnosis or treatment of individual problems. The description of public health provided in a 1988 report of the Institute of Medicine[1] has become well established: "assuring the conditions within which people can be healthy." This description has since been augmented by *Public Health in America*,[2] which identifies the specific responsibilities of public health as being to prevent epidemics and spread of disease, protect against environmental hazards, prevent injuries, promote and encourage healthy behaviors, respond to disasters and assist in recovery, and, finally, ensure the quality and accessibility of health services. Anyone whose major activities contribute to the fulfillment of these responsibilities of public health through one or more of the essential public health services (see table 16.1) can be considered a part of the public health workforce.[3] Not included in this discussion are those who coincidentally contribute to ensuring one or more of these services in the course of their work, such as those enforcing traffic safety laws and thus reducing injuries, or those delivering acute care in emergency rooms. Table 16.2 illustrates the range of workers encompassed in this scope.

WORKERS AND PROFESSIONALS

This chapter will concentrate on the workforce at the professional level, that is, those with at least a baccalaureate degree. Technical and support workers in public health should not be overlooked, however, by anyone wishing to achieve success in public health practice. These individuals are critical to achieving program goals, such as quality laboratory services. They are often the backbone of outreach and community development efforts in maternal and child health or chronic disease prevention, and can make or break relationships with the served community. The way in which telephones are answered, arriving citizens greeted, document requests processed, or the talk about work in the grocery checkout line influences others and shapes the community's understanding of and appreciation for public health. These workers, too, must be included in basic public health orientation and emergency response training, and should be incorporated into all thinking about public health improvement.

NUMBERS AND NAMES

Because public health is the vocation of professionals in many work settings, enumeration and assessment of the workforce is a complex endeavor. In the face of such complexities, a landmark report that enumerated the public health workforce was conducted in 2000. The findings indicated that in the year 2000 the

Table 16.2.   Range of Positions Engaged in Public Health Practice

Health Administrator	Public Health Laboratory	Health Information Systems/Data
Administrative/Business Professional	Professional	Analyst
Attorney/Hearing Officer	Public Health Nurse	Occupational Health and Safety
Biostatistician	Public Health Nutritionist	Technician
Clinical, Counseling, and School	Public Health Optometrist	Public Health Laboratory Specialist
Psychologist	Public Health Pharmacist	Other Public Health Technician
Environmental Engineer	Public Health Physical Therapist	Protective Service Workers
Environmental Scientist & Specialist	Public Health Physician	Investigations Specialist
Epidemiologist	Public Health Program Specialist	Other Protective Service Worker
Health Economist	Public Health Student	Paraprofessionals
Health Planner/Researcher/	Public Health Veterinarian/Animal	Community Outreach/Field Worker
Analyst	Control Specialist	Other Paraprofessional
Infection Control/Disease	Psychiatric Nurse	Support Workers
Investigator	Psychiatrist	Administrative Business Staff
Licensure/Inspection/Regulatory	Psychologist	Administrative Support Staff
Specialist	Public Relations/Media Specialist	Skilled Craft Workers
Marriage and Family Therapist	Substance Abuse & Behavioral	Food Services/Housekeeping
Medical & Public Health Social	Disorders Counselor	Patient Services
Worker	Other Public Health Professional	Other Service/Maintenance
Mental Health/Substance Abuse	Technicians	Volunteers
Social Worker	Computer specialist	Volunteer Health Administrator
Mental Health Counselor	Environmental Engineering	Volunteer Public Health Educator
Occupation Safety & Health	Technician	Volunteer Other Paraprofessional
Specialist	Environmental Science and	
Public Health Dental Worker	Protection Technician	
Public Health Educator		

public health workforce of the United States consisted of at least 448,254 paid individuals augmented by nearly 3 million volunteers.[4] The majority of the employed workers included in this estimated number work for local, state, or federal agencies. These include local and state health departments, state environmental agencies, and federal departments of health and human services, environmental protection, agriculture, labor, veterans affairs, and the military. The number of volunteers reported comes primarily from several of the larger community-based voluntary health organizations such as the March of Dimes and the American Cancer Society. The range of agencies and organizations, and the use of volunteers, has inhibited any regular inventory of public health workers. The enumeration cited above and completed in 2000 acknowledges a serious undercounting, particularly in environmental health and in community partner organizations.

Despite the daunting complexities of the field, and the difficulties arriving at exact numbers, the data indicate that there are but a few professional groups providing the vast majority of public health services. Rightly, these are getting the most attention[5] from those working to improve practice. These professionals usually work in interdisciplinary teams, to which each brings specific knowledge and a professional or technical worldview, but within which they share many skills. On a day-to-day basis it may not be possible to identify the exact professional background in which an individual public health worker was originally trained or to even specify the exact way in which these underlying professional disciplinary skills contribute to public health expression. That is, the process of doing an outbreak investigation, health facility inspection, or public education program for cancer prevention will be the same regardless if the person carrying out the task is a sanitarian, nurse, physician, health educator, nutritionist, or other professional. When individuals from these various fields gather to explore and interpret results of studies or relationships of findings to communities, each brings a distinct worldview that complements the others and enriches the analysis.

The largest number of professionals in the field of public health are nurses. Physicians are fewer, but are concentrated in leadership positions. Although undercounted, environmental health professionals are extremely important to public health practice, as are health educators. Administrators, both those with generic management skills and those with management responsibilities added to some other professional background, are essential to the organization and success of public health programs. Other professions found in public health practice include dentistry, nutrition, laboratory sciences, engineering, mental health specialties, law, and education.

Public Health Nurses

The title "public health nurse" at one time was bestowed only on those nurses who had completed a baccalaureate degree program that included public health nursing courses. Some states limit the use of the title to nurses who have verified their level of preparation to the nursing licensing board. The longstanding preference for nurses moving into senior roles within public health has been a master's degree in public health or nursing. Whereas these requirements remain the preference, the limited supply and uneven geographic distribution of public health-prepared nurses has meant that many agencies and programs employ nurses with diploma or associate degree preparation for many public health nursing jobs. These nurses have often performed well, particularly within specialized programs that require attention to individuals such as immunization programs, or directly observed therapy for tuberculosis. As public health has developed a larger repertoire of individual health programs in response to access problems and lack of insurance, the clinical skills of these nurses have been well used. As states develop improved health care financing mechanisms and move more care into private practice settings, the clinical skills of this group become less important and the lack of broader public health knowledge makes transition to other public health responsibilities difficult.

Public Health Physicians

Public health physicians have been described as an endangered species.[6] A part of this problem is the definition: most physicians practicing in public health do not have specialty training in preventive medicine, which is the only medical specialty area focused on population-based practice. Further, any physician who completes a required reportable disease notification to the local health department, immunizes a child or an adult, reinforces a public health message, or speaks up at the local civic club about the need for proper funding of environmental protection is acting as part of the public health workforce. There are some specialties often found in explicitly public health practices: obstetrics/gynecology and pediatrics (because of attention to maternal and child health) and internal medicine/infectious diseases (because of the epidemic control responsibilities). More recently, physicians have moved from the field of emergency medicine to public health due to an interest in injury prevention. Many of the physicians working in public health settings have been employed there in top leadership positions not because the jurisdiction understood what a physician brought to public health practice, but because state law or local ordinance required it, or because there is a perception that medical training carries with it knowledge of leadership and management. Services provided by public health agencies often may include prescribing and administering medications, as in tuberculosis and sexually transmitted disease or mental health programs, thus physicians may be seen as essential to these program areas for their prescribing authority. However, this need may be vanishing as advanced practice nurses have been granted prescribing authority and as "mainstreaming" and outsourcing initiatives have resulted in many official public health agencies substantially reducing their efforts at direct provision of personal health services. As is the experience of some nurses, public health physicians originally employed for a specific clinical program within public health may lack the broad understanding of public health's values and skills and encounter difficulty when making a transition to other public health practice areas.

Environmental Health

Environmental health professionals are the most difficult to describe because there is no single entry point for this group. Sanitarians are the largest of the environmental health occupations. However, the title may represent licensure under a state law, certification through the professional association, or simply a convenient job title. Sanitarians are usually prepared at the baccalaureate level in a science (e.g., biology or chemistry) and receive on-the-job training in public health concepts and applications. Many are employed to enforce public health ordinances such as restaurant codes, or drinking water standards. As with those nurses who lack formal public health education, they perform well in many specific program areas, but encounter difficulties when asked to change focus or develop new programs, due to limited knowledge of the broader theoretical underpinnings of public health practice. A particular challenge for many has been the move from the "command and control" approach of regulation enforcement to collaborative work with licensees to accomplish public health goals.[7] Within the environmental area are many types of engineers who bring knowledge of specific components of infrastructure and systems to bear on public health interests such as protection of water supplies, disposal of wastes, and development of safe environments. In addition, nuclear physics supplies professionals for radiation safety.

Health Educators

As with environmental health, the title "health educator" may represent completion of a specific course of study, professional certification program, or simply hiring into a position carrying that label. The title Certified Health Education Specialist is bestowed by the

major professional association of health educators (National Commission for Health Education Counseling) as a way of identifying those individuals who have demonstrated understanding of the role and work usually associated with this field. In actual practice, nurses, nutritionists, social workers, or teachers who have gravitated to health education and information distribution as meaningful work are also called health educators. Some of these have also sought certification as health educators. Historically, the use of health educators has been within specific programmatic areas working with individuals or groups, such as in the Women, Infants and Children's Nutrition Program (WIC) or well-child clinics. Increasingly, health educators are focused on shaping community-wide efforts to inform and shape public views of critical health issues and stimulate healthy behavior.

Administrators

Those assuming administrative roles within public health may be persons who have professional training or degrees in a medical or health discipline who have sought additional training in management and leadership (e.g., master's degrees in business, health administration, or public administration), persons with a career commitment to management but no formal health preparation, or individuals who rise to leadership positions by virtue of seniority, on-the-job training, and experience. The highest position in a governmental health agency is usually filled by the jurisdiction's chief elected official, who may or may not have restrictions imposed by law (i.e., must appoint a physician, or someone knowledgeable about public health) and may or may not understand the overall roles and responsibilities of the public health agency. In at least one state (New Jersey) only persons who meet licensing requirements as a health officer may be named to the leadership of a local health department. Any individual in a leadership position over an agency or a program, including those with no formal health professional background, must constantly assess the interests of the body politic as a counterpoint or adjunct to applying the best available public health knowledge. Although many decry the shifts in choices of leaders made today,[8] some of the newer appointees have understood the political nature of public health work and have facilitated the application of public health principles in difficult situations. For example, the state with the first Healthy People 2010 plan, developed using sound community participation, was led by a health director not formally trained in public health administration.

WHERE DO PUBLIC HEALTH WORKERS FIND EMPLOYMENT?

At a minimum, public health workers are found in 50 state public health agencies, nearly 3,000 local health departments, and the federal Department of Health and Human Services. This markedly understates the range of employment opportunities, however. Within all three levels of government public health workers are also found in programs that are concerned with energy, environmental protection, food safety, health insurance (including Medicaid), mental health, occupational health and safety, substance abuse, rural health, traffic safety, welfare, and zoning. The number of agencies housing these programs in any one state ranges from only one or two, to many, with some dedicated to individual programs. Many of these programs, originally part of a department or board of health, have since been relocated or combined as policy makers shift preferences for relating programs and people. For example, pesticide control programs now housed in agriculture were once part of health departments, and the function of assuring access to care for the poor encompassed by Medicaid may have been a part of the jurisdiction of a board of health. The Institute of Medicine report[1] described an ideal state health agency that encompasses all of these programs; however, no such agency exists, nor is one likely to rise. What is more important is that public health professionals work collaboratively across program and agency lines.

Nongovernmental Employment

Public health workers can be found in a range of settings beyond governmental public health agencies. For example, school districts and individual schools (public, private, and parochial) employ many public health nurses to ensure the health of school-aged children. They may also have nutrition and environmental health professionals working at a districtwide level to ensure the healthfulness and safety of school meal programs. Independent water, sewer, or waste management districts also employ public health professionals to ensure that standards for public health protection are met.

Hospitals and Health Care Organizations

Many hospitals and health care organizations (including staff-model and other health maintenance organizations) employ public health professionals. Many of the administrators of personal health care services have earned graduate degrees in administration from programs housed in schools of public health. Among the most common public health workers in these settings are health educators, outreach workers, and epidemiologists. A large system may have its own sanitarian, environmental engineer, and occupational health staff as well. Further, many localities expect that the clinical portion of public health services, such as immunizations or home-based education and outreach, will be housed with other care services rather than in the public health agency and often are incorporated seamlessly into daily practices such as a pediatrician's ongoing care. Conversely, it should be remembered that just providing a health-related service or activity outside the walls of a hospital does not make it a public health activity. The test for whether something should be considered part of public health is the presence of a focus on a population group and on a preventive outcome.[9]

Occupational Health

For workforce and other strategic considerations, occupational health is a subspecialty of public health practice that may take workers into almost any other field or endeavor as a part of the organization's infrastructure. These public health professionals include physicians (some board certified in occupational medicine), nurses, epidemiologists and industrial hygienists, and are involved primarily with protection of workers from hazardous working conditions. Some also develop workplace-based health promotion programs. Workers concerned about their health and safety may also employ public health expertise through unions or professional associations. For example, occupational health advocates on the staff of the American Nurses Association were leading activists in supporting legislation protecting health care workers from occupational exposure to blood-borne pathogens.

Voluntary Organizations

Voluntary health organizations provide another opportunity for public health employment. The American Red Cross is a special case of a voluntary agency, given the public health and caregiving role it plays during emergency response in coordination with local, state, and national officials. It also provides extensive public health education in many localities, for example, sponsorship of HIV/AIDS prevention training. Other voluntary organizations with a strong public health presence include the American Lung Association, the American Cancer Society, the American Heart Association, the American Diabetes Association, and Mothers Against Drunk Driving. Whereas each of these employ public health personnel, they also use extensive networks of volunteers, some of whom are also full-time public health workers. For their volunteers who are not public health workers, the training given for volunteer tasks results in expanding the public health knowledge within communities. To illustrate, few communities would be as strict in control of indoor tobacco smoke today were it not for the work of thousands of public health volunteers working through voluntary associations.

HOW DO PUBLIC HEALTH WORKERS KNOW WHAT THEY NEED TO KNOW?

What public health workers need to know is increasingly described in the language of competencies, rather than defined by a listing of relevant degrees. Core competencies for public health practice have been defined by the Council on Linkages between Academia and Public Health Practice (see table 16.3), and core areas of knowledge and skill needed by currently employed public health workers were identified through a series of meetings resulting in what has been called the Charleston Charter of needed knowledge (see table 16.4).

Basic Professional Training

As might be expected from the discussions of who are public health workers and where they work, there is no simple answer to explain how public health professionals gain the knowledge they need for practice. Basic professional training for every physician and baccalaureate nurse includes at least the core of population-based disease/injury prevention and community health knowledge. The accrediting bodies for medical schools and nursing schools have established this expectation, and courses have been offered for many years. However, in medical schools preventive medicine may no longer be taught by a separate department,[10] and the prevention curriculum is often taught by someone whose primary focus is on individual clinical preventive services rather than the population focus of public health. Although this knowledge is extremely important, it means that essential competencies such as interdisciplinary partnership activities with communities, and the application of epidemiology to problem analysis at the community level may be minimized. This means that only the physician going directly into a preventive medicine residency and accompanying masters of public health degree program is ensured of having full public health training prior to employment.

For the nursing student the problem is slightly different, although it has the same ultimate limitation on readiness to practice in public health. As some public health agencies have assumed a larger role in provision of direct personal health services (usually in response to the growing number of uninsured), the clinical experiences offered students during a public health nursing course may be limited to those associated with home care services. The competencies required differ little from those required to give the same care in a hospital or other facility, thus there is no opportunity to develop community assessment or partnership skills. Further, the associate degree in nursing curriculum does not include public health

Table 16.3. Core Competencies for Public Health Professionals (Council on Linkages between Academia and Public Health Practice, 2001)

Domain #1: Analytic Assessment Skills

1. Defines a problem
2. Determines appropriate uses and limitations of both quantitative and qualitative data
3. Selects and defines variables relevant to defined public health problems
4. Identifies relevant and appropriate data and information sources
5. Evaluates the integrity and comparability of data and identifies gaps in data sources
6. Applies ethical principles to the collection, maintenance, use, and dissemination of data and information
7. Partners with communities to attach meaning to collected quantitative and qualitative data
8. Makes relevant inferences from quantitative and qualitative data
9. Obtains and interprets information regarding risks and benefits to the community
10. Applies data collection processes, information technology applications, and computer systems storage/retrieval strategies
11. Recognizes how the data illuminates ethical, political, scientific, economic, and overall public health issues

Domain #2: Policy Development/Program Planning Skills

1. Collects, summarizes, and interprets information relevant to an issue
2. States policy options and writes clear and concise policy statements
3. Identifies, interprets, and implements public health laws, regulations, and policies related to specific programs
4. Articulates the health, fiscal, administrative, legal, social, and political implications of each policy option
5. States the feasibility and expected outcomes of each policy option
6. Utilizes current techniques in decision analysis and health planning
7. Decides on the appropriate course of action
8. Develops a plan to implement policy, including goals, outcome and process objectives, and implementation steps
9. Translates policy into organizational plans, structures, and programs
10. Prepares and implements emergency response plans
11. Develops mechanisms to monitor and evaluate programs for their effectiveness and quality

Domain #3: Communication Skills

1. Communicates effectively both in writing and orally, or in other ways
2. Solicits input from individuals and organizations
3. Advocates for public health programs and resources
4. Leads and participates in groups to address specific issues
5. Uses the media, advanced technologies, and community networks to communicate information
6. Effectively presents accurate demographic, statistical, programmatic, and scientific information for professional and lay audiences
7. **Attitudes**
   - Listens to others in an unbiased manner, respects points of view of others, and promotes the expression of diverse opinions and perspectives

Domain #4: Cultural Competency Skills

1. Utilizes appropriate methods for interacting sensitively, effectively, and professionally with persons from diverse cultural, socioeconomic, educational, racial, ethnic, and professional backgrounds, and persons of all ages and lifestyle preferences
2. Identifies the role of cultural, social, and behavioral factors in determining the delivery of public health services
3. Develops and adapts approaches to problems that take into account cultural differences

(continues)

Table 16.3. *(continued)*

4. **Attitudes**
   - Understands the dynamic forces contributing to cultural diversity
   - Understands the importance of a diverse public health workforce

Domain #5: Community Dimensions of Practice Skills

1. Establishes and maintains linkages with key stakeholders
2. Utilizes leadership, team building, negotiation, and conflict resolution skills to build community partnerships
3. Collaborates with community partners to promote the health of the population
4. Identifies how public and private organizations operate within a community
5. Accomplishes effective community engagements
6. Identifies community assets and available resources
7. Develops, implements, and evaluates a community public health assessment
8. Describes the role of government in the delivery of community health services

Domain #6: Basic Public Health Sciences Skills

1. Identifies the individual's and organization's responsibilities within the context of the Essential Public Health Services and core functions
2. Defines, assesses, and understands the health status of populations, determinants of health and illness, factors contributing to health promotion and disease prevention, and factors influencing the use of health services
3. Understands the historical development, structure, and interaction of public health and health care systems
4. Identifies and applies basic research methods used in public health
5. Applies the basic public health sciences including behavioral and social sciences, biostatistics, epidemiology, environmental public health, and prevention of chronic and infectious diseases and injuries
6. Identifies and retrieves current relevant scientific evidence
7. Identifies the limitations of research and the importance of observations and interrelationships
8. **Attitudes**
   - Develops a lifelong commitment to rigorous critical thinking

Domain #7: Financial Planning and Management Skills

1. Develops and presents a budget
2. Manages programs within budget constraints
3. Applies budget processes
4. Develops strategies for determining budget priorities
5. Monitors program performance
6. Prepares proposals for funding from external sources
7. Applies basic human relations skills to the management of organizations, motivation of personnel, and resolution of conflicts
8. Manages information systems for collection, retrieval, and use of data for decision making
9. Negotiates and develops contracts and other documents for the provision of population-based services
10. Conducts cost-effectiveness, cost-benefit, and cost-utility analyses

Domain #8: Leadership and Systems Thinking Skills

1. Creates a culture of ethical standards within organizations and communities
2. Helps create key values and shared vision and uses these principles to guide action
3. Identifies internal and external issues that may impact delivery of essential public health services (e.g., strategic planning)
4. Facilitates collaboration with internal and external groups to ensure participation of key stakeholders
5. Promotes team and organizational learning
6. Contributes to development, implementation, and monitoring of organizational performance standards
7. Uses the legal and political system to effect change
8. Applies theory of organizational structures to professional practice

Table 16.4. The Charleston Charter: What Currently Employed Public Health Professionals Need to Know

The nine core curriculum areas for currently employed public health workers are:
- Public health values and acculturation
- Epidemiology/quality assurance/economics
- Informatics
- Communication
- Cultural competency
- Team building/organizational effectiveness
- Strategic thinking and planning/visioning
- Advocacy/politics/policy development
- External coalition building/mobilization

Source: Adapted from Gebbie KM, Hwang I. *Preparing Currently Employed Public Health Professionals.* New York, NY: Columbia University School of Nursing, 1998.

theory or practice. In many parts of the country, nurses with associate degrees comprise the largest part of the workforce, and are hired by public health agencies because they are the only nurses available to fill vacancies.

Public Health Training

The master of public health degree (M.P.H.) is often described as the basic requirement for professional public health practice. It may be earned at a school of public health, or in one of the growing number of public health programs housed in other schools and departments. However, only a relatively small proportion of public health workers have this degree prior to beginning employment. Some others go on to earn an M.P.H. after initial exposure to a public health program area, having been employed either as an entry-level generalist, or because of some specialized advanced skill needed by a specific program. The M.P.H. does require minimum exposure to five content areas of public health practice: epidemiology, biostatistics, environmental health, social and behavioral science, and policy and management. However, there is no uniform requirement that students in

M.P.H. programs have field experience in public health practice, and many programs focus on narrow applications such as administration or biostatistics without addressing how such applications actually apply in communities. The student who adds the M.P.H. skills to an existing health profession should be well prepared to move from an individual focus to a population one, keeping overall population goals in mind even when working with individuals. The person who comes to the M.P.H. with a general science or liberal arts preparation will know a great deal about public health principals, but may still require significant coaching to become an effective public health professional.

Schools of public health also offer doctor of public health degrees for those interested in continuing to advance the practice field with an additional level of knowledge and research skills. Many schools also offer Ph.D. programs in some or all of the public health specialty areas, with the graduates of these programs usually going on to research careers in academic or other settings. In recent years there have been many efforts to increase the level of partnership between schools of public health and public health practice areas, such as establishing practice coordinators in all schools of public health.[11] This is encouraged to ensure that the curriculum is relevant to practice, students have learning experiences relevant to future employment, and for those already employed in the field, attainment of advanced education is facilitated. It also helps fulfill the broader community service mission of training initiatives.

Graduate degrees relevant to public health practice can also be obtained from other schools and departments. Many schools of nursing and medicine offer master's degree programs in public health and community health (a distinction that is often invisible to the observer, and may mean little in actual practice). Graduate degrees in environmental areas may be earned in schools of engineering, or planning. A narrow focus of the M.P.H. as "the" public health degree stereotypes education for practice and narrows the range of backgrounds from which well-prepared public health practitioners may be recruited.

Continuing Education

Given all that has been identified above, and coupled with the ever-changing nature of the challenges of the field, it should be no surprise that the field of public health is committed to development of a system of *lifelong learning* that can assure the newly employed person access to needed core knowledge about public health and facilitate rapid updates of practitioners when the science base for practice advances. Some continuing education comes from academic centers. In addition, many of the professional associations to which public health workers belong offer continuing education. This is done at regular meetings and special educational conferences and through selected sections in professional journals. The American Medical Association, American Nurses Association, American College of Preventive Medicine, National Environmental Association, and the American Public Health Association all make efforts to ensure that members can remain current in important areas of public health practice.

Through a collaborative effort involving the federal Centers for Disease Control and Prevention and the Health Resources and Services Administration; the Associations of Schools of Public Health, State and Territorial Health Officials, County and City Health Officials, Teachers of Preventive Medicine, and others, a strategic plan for the development of the public health workforce was designed and is being implemented.[12] Figure 16.1 illustrates the cycle of discovery and action needed to ensure a fully competent public health workforce.

The responsibility for becoming and remaining competent to perform job functions is one that should be shared by both the individual and the employing agency. That is, anyone who aspires to be recognized by society as a professional should understand that society expects, in return, that the professional is up to date on the full range of information required to deliver the promised level of services. In a complementary way, those employing public health professionals (actually, any employer) should recognize that it is of mutual benefit to make the process of lifelong learning possible without excessive time away from the job,

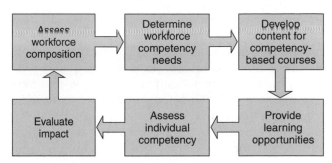

Figure 16.1. Toward an Integrated Lifelong Learning System for Public Health Practice

Source: Centers for Disease Control and Prevention. Strategic Plan for the Development of the Public Health Workforce. 2001.

and at reasonable cost. In pursuit of this joint goal, the workforce collaboration described in the previous paragraph has moved to make the competencies required for public health practice clear, and to encourage the development of a range of both in-person and distance-based learning opportunities available. A national network of funded centers for public health workforce development is working in partnership with practice agencies to ensure that this comprehensive approach to workforce preparation becomes a reality.[12] As a next step this developmental opportunity, which has been primarily built around official health agencies, could be extended to all engaged in public health practice, wherever that might be.

MAINTAINING PUBLIC HEALTH STANDARDS

Standards for public health practice have tended to take the form of performance expectations, tied to federal funding. However, this is not a solid basis because there is no equivalent of the Joint Commission on the Accreditation of Health Care Organizations for public health. Some states have had standards for local agencies; the enforcement of these standards has been variable. In developing standards, the traditional triumvirate of structure, process, and outcome has been invoked, with issues of worker preparation and ongoing education being a part of both structure and process. If workers with the requisite competencies are not employed, it is unlikely that the standards for programs or outcomes can be met. Likewise, because public health practice is based on an ever-enlarging science base, it is not possible that any staff member could continue to function effectively throughout a career without access to new information and new skills. Therefore, agencies must have in place some mechanism for determining whether or not staff are current in their competence, and facilitate the process for acquisition of new knowledge and skills.

There are specific standards of practice for public health nurses. These are the product of collaboration among the ANA (Community Health Nurse section), Association of State and Territorial Directors of Nursing, Association of Community Health Nursing Educators, and the National League for Nursing. Using this resource it is possible to assess the competency of individual nurses practicing in public health. Standards for individual workers do not, however, ensure that any group of public health professionals with a common purpose are meeting expectations in a mutually rewarding and effective manner.

This makes the roles of managers and leaders in public health extremely critical. Those placed in positions to make employment decisions, or to direct the work of others, should be knowledgeable about the required public health competencies associated with the program area and skills of employees under their direction. In applying this knowledge to the process of matching specific workers to specific tasks within the public health mission, attention should be paid to supporting the interdisciplinary collaboration that has always been a strength of public health. Although care must be paid to avoid asking any professional to practice outside his or her legal scope of practice, it is also important to make full use of all of the knowledge and skill each worker brings to the effort, without regard to historic prejudices about who does what best. As an example, in one southern health department, a public health nurse has established an exciting role as a troubleshooter and problem solver for environmental health enforcement problems.

There should be ongoing communication between anyone in a supervisory position and his or her staff to identify needed new competencies, or emerging science relevant to the practice field. The staff members need to identify ways to gain these new skills, and the supervisor should work to ensure that the required learning takes place in a timely way. For small agencies, collaboration with state or national groups serves to reduce the cost for development of training programs. In addition, distance-based learning approaches show much promise for making the achievement of lifelong learning a reality.

THE UNANSWERED QUESTIONS

This chapter has been written within the assumption that for a community to become healthier, essential public health services must be available, and for essential public health services to be delivered effectively, public health workers must be competent. Further, it is assumed that the competence is in the areas identified as core public health practice, and any of the specific public health practice areas relevant to the population and delivering agency. There is a further assumption that the preferred health outcomes will be achieved more quickly, and more effectively, as staff move from beginning levels of competence to mastery. Whereas these may be logical assumptions, the public health workforce research base is sufficiently thin that there will be no footnotes to research findings in this paragraph.

The public health community is actively pursuing support for the necessary research on infrastructure and its relationship to public health outcomes. Workforce is an essential element of infrastructure, and in some ways the most important third. Given the range of public health professions, and the variety of practice settings in which they are found, and the immense range of knowledge and skills they bring to bear on solving public health challenges, it is essential that this research be initiated quickly. The human capital of public health is a precious resource that must be developed strategically, deployed thoughtfully, and nurtured responsibly. Knowing more about the connections between who we are and what we can accomplish is critical if we are to deliver on the promises of public health security and a healthy America.

References

1. Institute of Medicine, Committee for the Study of the Future of Public Health. *The Future of Public Health.* Washington, DC: National Academy Press; 1988.
2. Public Health Functions Steering Committee. *Public Health in America.* Washington, DC: US Department of Health and Human Services; 1994.
3. Public Health Functions Steering Committee. *The Public Health Workforce: An Agenda for the 21st Century.* Washington, DC: US Department of Health and Human Services, Public Health Service; 1997.
4. Health Resources and Services Administration (HRSA), Bureau of Health Professions, National Center for Health Workforce Information and Analysis. *The Public Health Workforce, Enumeration 2000.* Washington, DC: HRSA; 2000.
5. Gebbie K. The public health workforce: Key to public health infrastructure [Editorial]. *Am J Public Health.* 1999; 89(5):660-661.
6. Tilson H, Gebbie K. Public health physicians: An endangered species. *Am J Preven Med;* in print, October 2001.
7. Bloom A, Gebbie K. *Preparing Currently Employed Public Health Environmental Professionals for Changes in the Health Systems.* New York, NY: Columbia University School of Nursing, Center for Health Policy and Health Services Research; 1998.
8. Gerzoff R, Richards T. The education of local health department top executives. *J Public Health Manage.* 1997; 3(4);50-56.
9. Gebbie K. Community-based health care: An introduction. In: Brennan P, Schneider S, Tornquist E, ed. *Information Networks for Community Health.* New York, NY: Springer-Verlag; 1997:3-14.
10. Dismuke S, Sherman L. Identifying population health faculty in U.S. medical schools. *Am J Preven Med.* 2001; 20(2):113-117.
11. Centers for Disease Control and Prevention. *Report from the Task Force on Public Health Workforce Development: CDC/ATSDR Strategic Plan for Public Health Workforce Development: Executive Summary and Recommendations.* Washington, DC: US Department of Health and Human Services, Center for Disease Control; 1999.
12. Gordon A K, Chung K, Handler, A, Turnock B J, Schieve L A, Ippoliti P. Final report on public health practice linkages between schools of public health and state health agencies: 1992-1996. *J Public Health Manage Pract.* 1999; 5(3):25-34.

PART

4

The Provision of
Public Health Services

CHAPTER
17

Prevention Effectiveness

Jeffrey R. Harris, M.D., M.P.H.
Stephanie Zaza, M.D., M.P.H.
Steven M. Teutsch, M.D., M.P.H.

Over the past several decades, the importance, effectiveness, and value of prevention have come into sharp focus. The decades-long fall in smoking prevalence and accompanying partially related drop in cardiovascular mortality rates are but two examples of the power of prevention. Nevertheless, public health practitioners, and other decision makers who seek to manage or improve the health of populations through prevention, frequently face constrained resources and must make decisions about how to allocate those resources. Over the last two decades, the field of prevention has paralleled the field of medicine in development of evidence-based information. The term "prevention effectiveness" has been coined to describe this body of evidence-based information. Prevention-effectiveness information helps decision makers choose among preventive interventions by answering three questions: "What is important?" "What works?" and "What offers the best value?" In this chapter, we address the methods and sources of information to answer each of these three questions, and end with examples of practical uses of prevention-effectiveness information.

WHAT IS IMPORTANT?

Answering the question "What is important?" starts with an assessment of the relative magnitude of the burden associated with a given disease or health problem. Various measures of disease burden are commonly used, and multiple measures of a single health problem may offer greater insight than a single measure. This section uses a framework for thinking about causation and health outcomes. The framework includes death, disease, and disability as the most distal health outcomes, preceded in a causal chain by behavioral risk factors, such as smoking and physical inactivity. Even more proximal in the chain of causation are social determinants of health, such as income and education. We begin with a discussion of health outcomes and move on to behavioral risk factors and social determinants of health.

Mortality

Death, or mortality, is a health outcome that has long been used as a measure of disease burden. Mortality has limitations as a measure of disease burden because death is a relatively rare health event. Compared to other measures, however, mortality has the advantage of being undeniably important, and easy to define and count. Common causes of mortality are important not only from an emotional standpoint but also because they frequently result in high health care costs.[1] Because mortality increases with age, simple mortality measures highlight causes of late-in-life death. In addition to these simple measures, recently, various measures have been developed to take into account life expectancy at death. These measures estimate the amount of potential life lost due to a death, and, therefore, tend to highlight causes of death at an early age. A commonly used measure is Years of Potential Life Lost before age 75 (YPLL-75). Chronic diseases, such as heart disease and cancer, are important causes of both mortality and YPLL-75, but injuries, which kill at an early age, rank higher as causes of YPLL-75 (Table 17.1).

Morbidity

Morbidity is another health outcome used to measure disease burden. Morbidity measures the incidence or prevalence of acute and chronic illness, by cause. A chief limitation of morbidity as a measure of disease burden is that illness is common and frequently brief, therefore difficult to count. Among the measures of morbidity, two that are particularly useful to policy makers and those purchasing health care are causes of health care expenditures[1] and of missed work days.[2] The leading causes of health care expenditures include injuries, major depression, arthritis, and chronic diseases of the major organs including the heart. The number of missed workdays, or absenteeism, is a common measure of health-related productivity of employees.[3] Particularly among employers, the connection between health and employee productivity is increasingly recognized as an important issue. In addition to missing work, employees who have health problems or have family members with health problems are often less productive while working.[3] The leading causes of missed workdays are acute illnesses, such as injuries, influenza, and other infections, particularly of the respiratory system.

An emerging concept related to morbidity is that of compression of morbidity. Fries has pointed out that

Table 17.1. Leading Causes of Death and of Years of Potential Life Lost Before Age 75, Ranked in Descending Order, United States, 1998

Causes of Death	Causes of Years of Potential Life Lost Before Age 75
Diseases of heart	Malignant neoplasms
Malignant neoplasms	Diseases of heart
Cerebrovascular diseases	Unintentional injuries
Chronic obstructive pulmonary diseases	Suicide
Unintentional injuries	Homicide and legal intervention
Pneumonia and influenza	Cerebrovascular diseases
Diabetes mellitus	Chronic obstructive pulmonary diseases
Suicide	Human immunodeficiency virus infection
Nephritis, nephrotic syndrome, and nephrosis	Diabetes mellitus
Chronic liver disease and cirrhosis	Chronic liver disease and cirrhosis

SOURCE: National Center for Health Statistics. *Health, United States, 2000 With Adolescent Health Chartbook.* Hyattsville, Md: National Center for Health Statistics; 2000.

recent gains in life expectancy have resulted in lengthening portions of life lived with chronic, disabling illness.[4] Further gains in life expectancy will be more meaningful if accompanied by shortening, or compression, of these periods of morbidity.

Combined Measures

Because mortality and morbidity each have limitations as measures of disease burden, there has been growing interest in developing measures that combine the two. For a given health problem, these combined measures quantify the amount of healthy life lost to morbidity, and add this to the amount of potential life lost to mortality. Measurement of the amount of healthy life lost to morbidity depends on measuring the quality of life lived with acute or chronic illness and disability. Measuring quality of life depends on surveying people about their impressions of the reduced quality of life for people with a specified cause of illness or disability. Although the methods for this measurement vary, and there are strong controversies about which method is best, the net result is a quality weight, or proportion less than one, that is multiplied by the number of years, or portion thereof, lived by a person with a specified cause of morbidity.

Two of the most commonly used combined measures of morbidity and mortality are the Quality Adjusted Life Year (QALY) and the Disability Adjusted Life Year (DALY).[5,6] A key difference between the two is that the DALY weights life according to productivity at different ages while the QALY does not. In this weighting, life lived by children and older adults is weighted lower than life lived by working-age adults. A listing of the most common causes of DALYs lost in the United States (Table 17.2) gives a different perspective on disease burden than does a listing of the most common causes of death (Table 17.1). Although chronic illnesses that cause mortality still predominate, also prominent are chronic illnesses, such as depression, arthritis, and dementia, that result in disability but not necessarily death.

Behavioral Risk Factors

Health outcomes provide a valuable but limited perspective on "What is important?" Knowing the distal causes of mortality and morbidity does not necessarily help with preventing illness before it occurs. In 1993, McGinnis and Foege[7] published an analysis that divided the causes of death into genetic and nongenetic. Their analysis showed that half of all deaths are nongenetic and could be prevented, or at least

Table 17.2. Leading Causes of Disability-Adjusted Life-Years Lost, for Men and Women, Ranked in Descending Order, United States, 1996

Men	Women
Ischemic heart disease	Ischemic heart disease
Road traffic collisions	Unipolar major depression
Lung, trachea, and bronchus cancers	Cerebrovascular disease
HIV/AIDS	Lung, trachea, and bronchus cancers
Alcohol abuse and dependence	Osteoarthritis
Cerebrovascular disease	Breast cancer
Homicide and violence	Chronic obstructive pulmonary disease
Chronic obstructive pulmonary disease	Dementia and other degenerative and hereditary central nervous system disorders
Self-inflicted	Diabetes mellitus
Unipolar major depression	Road traffic collisions

SOURCE: Michaud CM, Murray CJL, Bloom BR. Burden of disease—Implications for future research. *JAMA*. 2001;285:535-539.

delayed, through reduction of behavioral risk factors. Four risk factors account for 40 percent of all deaths: tobacco use, physical inactivity, poor nutrition, and alcohol misuse. All four are risk factors for some or all of the leading chronic illnesses, including heart disease, cancer, lung disease, diabetes, and liver disease. Behavioral risk factors have also been shown to be important causes of DALYs lost.[5] The behavioral risk factor perspective facilitates earlier intervention than does the health-outcome perspective. In addition, it highlights for public health agencies, and others, the importance of community-based and policy interventions that go beyond the clinical care system.

Social Determinants of Health

A third perspective on "What is important?" looks even further up the chain of causation of disease to "root" causes, or social determinants of health. Marmot and colleagues'[8] classic studies of mortality among British civil servants found a step-ladder increase in mortality at successively lower job classifications within the civil service. Major social determinants of health include social class as described by Marmot et al, and racism.[9] Social class includes both education and income. In America, race also tends to correlate with social class and health status, with members of several racial minorities more likely to be poorly educated, have low incomes, and be in poor health. Racism, however, adds an extra insult to health that goes beyond the effects of social class. This extra effect of racism may be related to racially motivated restriction of access to health care.[9] The biological mechanisms linking social determinants to health outcomes are incompletely understood, but include higher prevalence of behavioral risk factors and lower access to, and poorer use of, health care among the poorly educated and impoverished.[10]

WHAT WORKS?

In order to address the important causes of morbidity and mortality, risky health behaviors, and social determinants of health, public health practitioners need effective preventive interventions from which to choose. In 1992, the Centers for Disease Control and Prevention (CDC)[11] published a framework for assessing prevention effectiveness that included categorizing preventive interventions into three groups: clinical, behavioral (health promotion), and environmental (health protection) prevention strategies. We will combine and expand on this categorization to address the following types of interdependent and complementary preventive interventions:

- Clinical preventive interventions aim to change the health or risk of an individual during a face-to-face encounter with a clinician. These services include screening for early detection of illness, counseling about health risk behaviors, or providing chemoprophylaxis or vaccines. These interventions are usually delivered by a health care professional in a one-on-one setting with a patient or client in a traditional health care delivery system.
- Clinical system interventions, such as provider or client reminder systems, case management systems, standing orders, or provider education and feedback, attempt to increase or improve the delivery of clinical preventive interventions by health care providers by changing the health care system at the organizational level.
- Community-based preventive interventions aim to change the health or risk of a group. This large category is further grouped into large- or small-group education (e.g., mass media, targeted information campaigns, or classes), legislation and enforcement, organizational policies (e.g., worksite or school-based rules or programs), and environmental strategies. Included in this category are behavioral and health promotion interventions that might occur in a variety of settings, including health care settings.

The historically rigid line between clinical and community settings is eroding. For example, health care systems are increasingly taking population-based approaches to health promotion and disease prevention in their enrolled populations. Conversely, public health agencies are often involved in providing clinical care in community settings, such as schools, or in ensuring the delivery of clinical services. Although it is becoming harder to completely distinguish between clinical and community preventive services, the distinction is useful for thinking about assessing effectiveness of different strategies.

All of these types of interventions are important to public health practitioners. As part of the core public health functions of policy development and assurance, public health practitioners must be able to identify effective strategies from each of these groups in order to implement programs, advocate for funding, or partner with health care organizations, businesses, and schools. For example, in order to achieve Healthy People 2010 objectives for increasing rates of influenza vaccinations or cessation of tobacco use, a combination of clinical, clinical system, and community interventions can be employed (Table 17.3). In choosing interventions, public health practitioners must make accountable decisions based on intervention effectiveness, economic feasibility, acceptability of interventions to the local populations, and the political and other resource feasibility of interventions.

The focus of this section is on the first of those criteria: identifying effective preventive interventions. We will discuss why identifying effective preventive interventions will increasingly rely on systematic literature reviews, why it is critical to evaluate the quality of individual studies in the course of those reviews, and selected examples of systematic review-based guidelines for the three categories of preventive interventions.

Methods for Collecting and Summarizing Evidence of Effectiveness

In assessing an intervention strategy, we must know what it can realistically accomplish in terms of health outcomes. The first evidence usually comes from research on cause-and-effect relationships associated with health problems, in which the link between a risk factor and an outcome is identified (e.g., the relationship between hypertension and coronary artery disease).

Table 17.3. Healthy People Objectives and Corresponding Recommended Clinical, Clinical System, and Community Interventions for Tobacco Control and Influenza Vaccine

Healthy People 2010 Objective	Recommended Interventions		
	Clinical	Clinical System	Community
Increase the percentage of adult smokers stopping smoking for a day or longer from 43% to 75% (27–5).	Advise patients who use tobacco to quit.	Provider reminders—automated reminders to health care providers to advise patients to quit.	Patient telephone support, or quit lines, provide tobacco users with cessation counseling or assistance in attempting to quit and to maintain abstinence.
Increase to 90% the rate of [influenza and pneumococcal] immunization coverage among adults aged ≥ 65; 65% for high-risk adults aged 18–64 years (22–24).	Deliver influenza vaccine annually to patients aged ≥ 65 years.	Standing orders—nonphysician personnel prescribe or deliver vaccinations by protocol without direct physician involvement.	Policies that reduce a patient's out-of-pocket costs for vaccination, such as paying for vaccinations, providing insurance coverage, or reducing copayments.

SOURCES: Data from US Preventive Services Task Force. *Guide to Clinical Preventive Services.* 2nd ed. Alexandria, Va: International Medical Publishing; 1996.

The Task Force on Community Preventive Services. Recommendations regarding interventions to improve vaccination coverage in children, adolescents, and adults. *Am J Prev Med.* 2000;18(1S):92-96.

Task Force on Community Preventive Services. Recommendations regarding interventions to reduce tobacco use and exposure to environmental tobacco smoke. *Am J Prev Med.* 2001;20(2S):10-15.

US Department of Health and Human Services. *Healthy People 2010* (conference ed., 2 vols.). Washington, DC: US Dept of Health and Human Services; 2000.

The relative risk associated with the risk factor provides a traditional epidemiologic measure of the potential impact. However, the overall public health impact is based not only on the relative risk, but also on the frequency at which the condition occurs in the population. This impact is measured in terms of attributable risk. The attributable risk is a measure of the amount of disease or injury that could be eliminated if the risk factor never occurred in a given population. In contrast, the prevented fraction is a measure of the amount of a health problem that has actually been avoided by a prevention strategy, and reflects what can be achieved in a real-world setting.

Public health practitioners determine the effectiveness of different preventive interventions in a variety of ways and rely on different types of resources. Consultation with peers and experts has long been a means of gathering information. Many public health decision makers rely on the scientific literature.

In addition to individual studies, scientific literature also includes review articles. Historically, review articles were the domain of experts in the field under study. These "narrative reviews" are developed based on literature that has been collected over a number of years, often focusing on the review author's personal perspective about the issue. Systematic and a priori rules for collecting, evaluating, and summarizing the literature are not applied.

A more recent development, the systematic literature review, reflects an increasing understanding of the potential limitations of expert opinion and the narrative review. These limitations include: (1) errors and biases in how information is interpreted and combined; and (2) difficulties for readers in assessing how conclusions were drawn, how accurate those conclusions are, and whether they make sense from the reader's perspective. First developed to evaluate the effectiveness of psychotherapy and counseling,[12] systematic literature reviews are, by definition, based on an explicit, a priori set of rules to minimize bias on the part of the reviewer. Methods for conducting systematic reviews, or research syntheses, have been well established.[13] The Cochrane Collaboration, a worldwide network of reviewers, has advanced systematic review methods through its reviews on all types of clinical therapeutic and preventive interventions.[14,15]

Systematic literature reviews consist of four basic steps:

- Developing a conceptual approach to the study question. In evaluating the effectiveness of preventive interventions, we must determine which interventions will be reviewed; what is the likely mechanism of the effect of the intervention; and what outcomes are needed to demonstrate the effectiveness of the intervention. The answers determine which studies will be included in the review, and help define the search parameters for the next step.
- Searching for and collecting the body of evidence. Systematic reviews are based on thorough literature searches according to a priori inclusion criteria. Inclusion criteria often include the study designs to be allowed, the outcomes required for determining success of the intervention, the databases and years to search, the languages, and the countries in which the research was conducted. These inclusion criteria are based on the nature of the study question and the resources available to the reviewers.

For clinical preventive interventions and some clinical system interventions, easily accessible, comprehensive medical databases, such as Medline and Embase, are particularly useful. However, for community-based preventive strategies, it is often necessary to search multiple databases, including some that are difficult for public health practitioners to access, such as legal or educational databases. In addition, evaluation studies of community-based interventions are often carried out in state and local health departments for internal purposes and are not published in the literature that is included in such databases. Accessing this information can be extremely time-consuming and subject to bias on the part of the investigator.

- Evaluating the quality of the individual studies in the body of evidence. Both the suitability of the study design to evaluate effectiveness and the strength of the execution of that design can affect the validity of the study. The randomized controlled trial (RCT) has long been the gold standard for evaluating therapeutic and clinical preventive interventions. However, for population-based interventions (e.g., clinical system interventions and community-based interventions), RCTs might be infeasible, inappropriate, or in some cases, unethical. Although systematic reviews to evaluate intervention effectiveness do not have to rely on randomized controlled trials, establishing effectiveness does require that some kind of comparison to a nonexposed group be made in order to attribute the effect to the intervention. Case studies and focus groups, for example, are excellent methods to explore the reasons why a particular intervention succeeded or failed, but are unreliable designs for measuring the effectiveness of an intervention. In addition to randomized controlled trials, quasi-experimental designs and some observational designs can make use of comparison or control groups in a variety of ways in order to establish the effect of an intervention.[16,17] Thus, the systematic reviews conducted for the *Guide to Community Preventive Services,* a major Department of Health and Human Services initiative to evaluate the effectiveness of clinical system and community interventions, include a variety of study designs, all of which have comparison groups.[18]

The second element of evaluating the quality of individual studies in a systematic review is how well a particular study design was executed by the investigators. Limitations to internal (e.g., bias and confounding) validity in individual studies can affect the estimated summary effect. Important issues that must be evaluated for each individual study include the fidelity of the intervention to its underlying theoretical basis, selection and sampling of the study and comparison populations, outcome and exposure reliability and validity, response and follow-up rates, appropriateness and completeness of the data analysis, control of confounding, and limiting other biases.

Finally, the external validity (i.e., generalizability) of the studies should be assessed. It has been argued that the inclusion of a variety of study designs in systematic reviews of population-based preventive interventions might result in increased applicability of the review findings to broader populations and settings than would be allowed by tightly controlled RCTs.[18]

• Summarizing the effects across the body of evidence. Finally, the systematic review process involves summarizing what the body of evidence tells us about the effectiveness of the intervention. This summary can consist of a description of the studies without combining the results (e.g., when there are too few studies, or when results are conflicting), a "qualitative" combination of the results (e.g., when effect measures are varied and cannot be combined, but indicate change in the same direction), simple quantitative descriptive combination (e.g., providing the median effect size and range), graphical displays (e.g., scatterplots), or mathematical combination (e.g., meta-analysis). The type of summary often depends on the goals of the review, available resources, the number of studies in the body of evidence, and the data available. When a meta-analysis is done, each study in the model is weighted by a measure of precision of the effect-size estimate. Meta-analytic models can also include weighting of studies by other variables such as study quality.

Developing Guidelines Based on Systematic Reviews

Systematic reviews that are conducted for the purposes of developing guidelines (e.g., the *Guide to Clinical Preventive Services* or the *Guide to Community Preventive Services*) take the additional step of characterizing the strength of the body of evidence of effectiveness. Different sets of rules have been established, but often include similar elements, such as quality of studies in the body of evidence, and the consistency and size of the effect.[18,19] At least one guideline process also includes the number of studies in the body of evidence as a criterion.[18]

There are potential drawbacks to developing evidence-based guidelines using systematic review methods. First, it might be difficult to make recommendations about a given intervention because evidence may be altogether lacking, or of poor quality. Relevant outcomes to determine effectiveness can be difficult to measure or take years to develop, and emerging approaches might not have been evaluated. Second, systematic review methods might lead to recommending interventions too broadly or based on too little information.[18]

However, the advantages of using systematic review methods to develop practice guidelines far outweigh the drawbacks. Systematic methods reduce errors and biases in information collection and interpretation. They reduce the likelihood that the guidelines reflect only selected information. Systematic reviews provide a clear analytic rationale and explicit rules for each step. This allows the reader to assess the value of the guidelines from his own perspective.

Examples of Guidelines Developed Through Systematic Reviews

The most comprehensive set of systematic review-based clinical preventive guidelines is the *Guide to Clinical Preventive Services (Clinical Guide).*[20] Sponsored by the Department of Health and Human Services, today overseen by the Agency for Healthcare Research and Quality (AHRQ), the *Clinical Guide* was first released by the U.S. Preventive Services Task Force (USPSTF) in 1989, and described the effectiveness of 60 screening, counseling, chemoprophylaxis, and immunization interventions. A second edition, updating and expanding interventions reviewed to 70, was released in 1996. The USPSTF has begun to release reviews and recommendations from its third edition.[21]

Clinical preventive interventions are usually amenable to testing through the use of randomized trials and prospective cohort studies. For that reason, the systematic review methods employed by the task force weight these types of designs much more heavily than other comparative study designs. The first two editions of the *Clinical Guide* do not include information about the costs of the clinical preventive interventions that are reviewed; however, the USPSTF is including available economic information in the third edition.[22]

In addition to the *Clinical Guide,* AHRQ funds the development of systematic reviews for other preventive interventions. For example, AHRQ funded reviews of tobacco cessation interventions that included both clinical preventive and clinical system interventions. These systematic reviews provided the basis for the Public Health Service tobacco cessation guidelines.[23]

Based in part on the success of the *Clinical Guide,* the Department of Health and Human Services, through the Centers for Disease Control and Prevention, convened a second task force to develop systematic review-based guidelines focused on clinical system and community-based preventive interventions, the *Guide to Community Preventive Services (Community Guide).*[24] The Task Force on Community Preventive Services has already released several sets of systematic reviews, and recommended clinical system and community-based preventive interventions from the *Community Guide,* with plans to compile these and others in book form.[25–28]

The preventive interventions covered in the *Community Guide* are often not amenable to evaluation using randomized controlled trials. In order to expand the study designs included in the systematic reviews without compromising the validity of the review findings, study execution quality is carefully considered. In addition, economic information is routinely sought for each effective intervention.

Development of the *Community Guide* has highlighted the importance of evaluating effectiveness of community preventive interventions. This is particularly true of large, comprehensive, and often expensive interventions because they can be extremely difficult to implement and require enormous human and financial resources. Public health laws should also be subjected to the scrutiny of evaluation and synthesis of that information. Because legislators must be held accountable for their decisions, it will often be necessary to develop strong advocacy for public health laws based on how well they meet stated objectives and their cost-effectiveness.

Implementation of Evidence-Based Preventive Guidelines

Both the *Clinical* and *Community Guides* lack information on how to implement interventions. Companion materials to the *Clinical Guide, Put Prevention Into Practice (PPIP),* outline how to use the clinical recommendations and suggest some clinical system interventions that might increase the delivery of clinical preventive interventions.[29] However, *PPIP* is not based on systematic literature reviews. Together, the *Clinical* and *Community Guides* provide the range of information needed to determine which clinical, clinical system, and community preventive interventions can be packaged together to address a particular health issue. In the future, electronic materials that link these evidence-based preventive guidelines to existing implementation advice, such as protocols, implementation steps, questionnaires, and so on, will be available to assist local decision makers. One such electronic tool, Health Policy Coach provided by the Center for Health Improvement, is currently available at http://www.healthpolicycoach.org.

WHAT OFFERS THE BEST VALUE?

In addition to knowing which health problems are associated with the most morbidity and mortality, and which preventive interventions are most effective, public health practitioners need to know which interventions offer the greatest return on investment. Economic evaluations are divided into three types (cost-benefit, cost-effectiveness, and cost-utility analysis) and allow comparison of different intervention strategies based on the resources they consume and the outputs they generate. Each of the three types requires a careful cost analysis (i.e., identification of costs associated with a health intervention), and an assessment of outcomes, both harms and benefits (Table 17.4). The scope of an analysis and the intended audience usually determine the appropriate analytic method and range of costs and consequences to con-

sider. A brief discussion of each of the three types of economic evaluation follows.

Cost-benefit analysis includes all costs, benefits, and harms, and converts them into dollars. It therefore includes costs of programs, costs to patients and others in terms of direct out-of-pocket costs, productivity changes, and intangible costs (e.g., grief, pain, suffering). It requires that the value of health outcomes be converted to dollars. Cost-benefit analysis is particularly suited to comparisons with interventions that include cross-sectoral considerations; for example, housing, education, or transportation interventions that have significant nonhealth benefits or harms. Methods for valuing intangible costs, such as willingness-to-pay, are available, but different approaches may yield different valuations. Many in the health community have significant reservations about valuing health in dollar terms.

Cost-effectiveness analysis usually examines direct medical and nonmedical costs and productivity losses. It compares those costs with outcomes in standard natural units, such as cost per case averted or cost per life saved. It is most suitable when comparing interventions that have similar health outcomes. Standards for cost-effectiveness analysis and a guide to conducting such studies provide more details of these methods.[30,31]

Cost-utility analysis compares direct medical and nonmedical costs with health outcomes converted to a standard health index, often a QALY. Because it provides a general health measure, cost-utility analysis is often used to compare health interventions that have different types of health outcomes. Users should rec-

Table 17.4. Components of Economic Analyses

Analysis Type	Costs			Outcome Measure	Summary Measure
	Direct	Productivity	Intangible		
Cost Benefit	Yes	Yes	Yes	Dollars	Net Benefits or Net Present Value (Benefits—Costs)
Cost-Effectiveness	Yes	Yes	No	Natural Unit	Cost/Natural Unit
Cost Utility	Yes	No	No	Health Index	Cost/QALY or DALY

ognize that these analyses provide a great deal of information about interventions, and how they can be targeted, modified, or made more efficient. In evaluating clinical preventive services, for example, cost-utility analyses can assess the frequency of screening tests, populations that might be targeted, different test methods, and ages at which testing may have less value.

Using economic evaluations to identify strategies for enhancing the economic value of interventions can be as beneficial as simply comparing the bottom-line cost-effectiveness. Table 17.5 provides a list of factors that improve cost-effectiveness.

Table 17.5. Attributes of Cost-Effective Preventive Intervention Strategies

Natural History of the Disease or Injury
- Frequent health outcome
- Health outcome severe and/or of long duration
- Short time interval between the intervention and the improvement in the health outcome

Characteristics of Intervention
- Reduces a large proportion of the health outcome
- Service needs to be given once or infrequently
- Given to the population as a whole rather than one person at a time
- Targeted to those at greatest risk
- Safe
- Compliance is high
- For screening tests, has high sensitivity and specificity

Characteristics of the Population
- A high risk or particularly severely affected target population can be identified

Cost of the Disease
- The disease is costly to individuals, employers, and society

Cost of the Intervention
- Low cost of the preventive service and program
- Does not induce other costs

Current Level of Intervention
- Can significantly increase the use of the intervention

Other Considerations
- The intervention has secondary benefits

SOURCE: Teutsch SM, Murray JF. Dissecting cost-effectiveness analysis for preventive interventions: A guide for decision makers. *Am J Managed Care.* 1999;5:301-305.

Although great strides have been made in standardizing cost effectiveness and cost-utility analyses, readers should be aware of some critical factors. First, the perspective of the study determines the costs and outcomes of interest. In the societal perspective, which should always be presented, all the costs, benefits, and harms should be included, regardless of to whom they accrue. The societal perspective, of course, represents no one perspective in particular, so frequently other perspectives, such as the payer, government, or employer, are used. A payer's perspective, for example, would include the direct medical costs and the health outcomes, but the direct nonmedical costs (e.g., transportation, day care), indirect (e.g., work loss), and intangible costs would be excluded (Table 17.6).

Second, people prefer to receive benefits as quickly as possible, and delay harms. To more accurately value events that occur in the future, a discount rate is used. Currently 3 percent is the recommended discount rate, although other values are often used in sensitivity analyses. The higher the discount rate, the lower the value of events that occur in the future. A 0 percent discount rate implies that future events have the same value as they would if they occurred today. Although some suggest that costs should be discounted but health outcomes should not, current practice is to discount both at the same rate.

Third, economic evaluations should use a time horizon that includes the duration of the intervention, sometimes called the time frame, as well as the usually much longer time during which costs, benefits, and harms occur (often called the analytic horizon).

Fourth, economic evaluations compare two or more interventions. Analyses should compare reasonable alternative interventions. Usually at least one option includes current care or no intervention.

Fifth, an average cost-effectiveness ratio presents the net cost of an intervention divided by the net benefit. This ratio is useful if one is comparing an intervention to doing nothing or if one is interested in the value of an intervention that is already in place. In many cases, an intervention is already in place and the question for the decision maker is what are the additional costs and benefits of doing something more. An incremental cost-effectiveness analysis

Table 17.6. Examples of Costs Included in Typical Cost-Effectiveness Analyses Based on Perspective of the Analysis

Cost	Perspective			
	Societal	Payer	Employer	Patient
Direct Medical	Y	Y	Y	Out-of-pocket
Direct Nonmedical (e.g., transportation, day care)	Y	N	N	Y
Indirect (e.g., productivity)	Y (if not a denominator)	N	Y	Y (if not a denominator)
Intangibile (e.g., grief, pain, suffering)	Y (if not a denominator)	N	N	Y (if not a denominator)

assesses the additional benefits and costs of another intervention compared to the status quo. A marginal cost-effectiveness analysis compares the benefits and costs of two levels of intensity of the same intervention. The incremental or marginal cost-effectiveness is calculated as the ratio of the difference in the net costs and the net benefits between one intervention and another. In other words, it represents the additional benefit achieved with one intervention for the additional cost incurred compared to another intervention.

Economic evaluations can be conducted as part of a study evaluating an intervention. However, in practice, it is uncommon for studies to have all required information, reflect real-world implementation, and provide follow-up until all economic consequences are observed. For many interventions, this could be a lifetime. Hence, in practice, most economic evaluations are based on decision models that synthesize information from multiple sources. Depending on the study, the data required might include demographic information, characteristics of screening tests, adherence (patient, provider, community), effectiveness of the intervention, intermediate outcomes, health outcomes, and costs. The simplest model is a decision tree, whereby the sequence of events in the intervention is modeled from left to right graphically to depict the probability of events occurring, as well as their outcomes. More complex models, such as Markov models and Monte Carlo simulations, may be required for more complex situations.

One of the primary concerns in economic evaluations is how to deal with uncertainty and any assumptions that are made. These are usually handled through sensitivity analysis, which is a technique for examining how the results would differ under differing scenarios and assumptions. A one-way sensitivity analysis examines the effect of varying a single variable over a range of plausible values; multivariate sensitivity analysis examines scenarios when multiple variables are changed simultaneously. Often, best-case, worst-case, and most-likely-case scenarios are constructed to see how robust the models are (i.e., the likelihood that the interpretation of the results would change with different scenarios and assumptions).

PRACTICAL USES

Thus far, this chapter has described separately the types of information that allow us to effectively prevent illness and death. Taken together, prevention-effectiveness information (e.g., burden of illness, intervention effectiveness, and economic evaluation) is a powerful tool for setting priorities, developing accountability systems, and developing research agendas.

Setting Priorities

A primary use of prevention-effectiveness information is to provide data for decision making about resource allocation—setting priorities. Setting priorities is an extremely complex process that involves a number of important considerations; for example, scientific data, political constraints, community needs and perceptions, and acceptability of potential interventions. Prevention-effectiveness information should play a key role in setting priorities for health departments, employers, health care systems, and policy makers.

In any of these settings, prevention-effectiveness information allows us to determine what problems to address in an environment of high burden but constrained resources. In the clinical setting, physicians are regularly faced with having to decide which preventive services to offer to their patients in short visits that are often focused on addressing specific problems. Employers must make decisions about which preventive services to include in benefits packages. Likewise, health plans need to know which services to offer as part of those packages, and which to encourage their physicians to deliver more frequently. In public health departments, program managers must choose among numerous options for community-based preventive services. Legislators and other policy makers must determine how to allocate resources for health and the environment and what types of protective legislation to enact (e.g., safety belt laws).

Familiar to many public health and health care professionals is the concept of triage in the clinical setting. For example, in a disaster setting, numerous patients with varying severity of illness or injury flood into an emergency room. Clinicians triage the patients into those already dead, those unlikely to survive, and those for whom something can be done, and allocate human and material resources accordingly. For prevention, we "triage" our health problems according to those illnesses and injuries that pose the greatest burden on the population (measured in health and/or economic terms) and those with the greatest likelihood of being prevented (i.e., with higher preventable fractions). Once we determine which health issues to address, prevention-effectiveness information about specific interventions (e.g., intervention effectiveness and economic evaluation) allows us to determine what clinical, clinical system, and community interventions to use to begin to ameliorate those problems.

Several approaches have been developed to combine information about burden, effectiveness, and economics to set priorities among competing needs for clinical preventive interventions. For example, league tables rank interventions by their cost effectiveness ratio. Although there is no cutoff for what represents good value, a recent league-table review of the cost-effectiveness of preventive services found that most ratios are clustered in the range of $10,000 to $100,000 per QALY.[32] This approach was attempted by Oregon in establishing Medicaid spending priorities,[33] and other such rankings have appeared as well.[34,35]

A second example, the Clinical Preventive Services Priorities Project conducted by Partnership for Prevention in collaboration with the Centers for Disease Control and Prevention, applies a standard approach to all of the clinical preventive services recommended by the USPSTF[36,37] (Table 17.7). Two dimensions are used. The first is the clinically preventable burden for each service. This represents the amount of a disease (in QALYs) that could be prevented in actual practice by delivering a clinical preventive service (i.e., a combination of burden and intervention effectiveness information). The second dimension is the cost utility of each service. This method identifies those priority clinical preventive services that should be offered first to patients. Physicians, health-system managers, and benefits managers can use one or the other dimension, or a combination of both, to make decisions about which services to provide, encourage, and buy. The results of this analysis are useful for health care system managers to determine where to target effective clinical system changes (e.g., those recommended in the *Guide to Community Preventive Services*) to improve the delivery of priority services that are underutilized.

Similar combinations of prevention-effectiveness information could be used to set priorities among community-based preventive interventions (e.g., mass media, environmental changes, or laws and policies) to assist decision makers in public health departments and legislatures. A comprehensive examination of the effectiveness of community-based preventive interventions is under way (i.e., the *Guide to Community Preventive Services*) that includes information about the economic efficiency of effective interventions. Once a substantial number of effective

Table 17.7. Priorities Among Recommended Clinical Preventive Services

Vaccinate children: DTP/DTaP, MMR, Oral Polio/IPV, Hib, Hep B, Varicella	5	5	10
Assess adults for tobacco use and provide tobacco cessation counseling	5	4	9
Screen for vision impairment among adults 65+ years	4	5	9
Assess adolescents for drinking and drug use and counsel on alcohol and drug abstinence	3	5	8
Assess adolescents for tobacco use and provide an anti-tobacco message or advice to quit	4	4	8
Screen for cervical cancer among sexually active women or 18+ years	5	3	8
Screen for colorectal cancer (FOBT and/or sigmoidoscopy) among all persons 50+ years	5	3	8
Screen for hemoglobinopathies, PKU, and congenital hypothyroidism among newborns	3	5	8
Screen for hypertension among all persons	5	3	8
Vaccinate adults 65+ years against influenza	4	4	8
Screen for chlamydia among women 15–24 years	3	4	7
Screen for high blood cholesterol among men 35–65 years and women 45–65 years	5	2	7
Screen for problem drinking among adults and provide brief counseling	4	3	7
Vaccinate adults 65+ years against pneumococcal disease	2	5	7
Assess infant feeding practices and provide counseling on:			
Breastfeeding; use of iron-enriched foods; risk of baby bottle tooth decay	1	5	6
Assess risk of STDs (including HIV) and provide counseling on measures to reduce risk	3	3	6
Screen for breast cancer (mammography alone or with CBE) among women ages 50–69 years	4	2	6
Screen for vision impairment at age 3–4 years	2	4	6
Assess oral health practices and provide counseling on:			
Brushing and flossing daily; visiting a dental care provider regularly	3	2	5
Assess the safety practices of parents of children 0-4 years and provide counseling on:			
Child safety seats; window/stair guards; pool fence; poison control; hot water temp; bicycle helmet	1	4	5
Counsel on risks/benefits of hormone replacement among peri- and post-menopausal women	4	1	5
Assess calcium/vitamin D intake of adolescent and adult women and counsel on use of supplements	2	2	4
Assess folic acid intake among women of childbearing age and counsel on use of supplements	1	3	4
Assess physical activity patterns of all persons over age 2 and counsel on increasing activity levels	3	1	4
Provide newborns with ocular prophylaxis to protect against gonococcal eye disease	1	3	4
Screen for hearing impairment among persons 65+ years	2	2	4
Assess dietary patterns of persons over age 2 and provide counseling on:			
Intake of fat/cholesterol; caloric balance; intake of fruits, vegetables, grains	2	1	3
Assess the safety practices of all persons over age 4 and provide counseling on:			
Seat belt use; smoke detector use; firearm storage/removal from home; bicycle/motorcycle helmet use; dangers of alcohol use; protection against slip and fall hazards for older persons	2	1	3
Screen for rubella among women of childbearing age using serology and/or history and vaccinate	1	1	2
Vaccinate all persons against tetanus-diphtheria (Td boosters)	1	1	2

Note: Figures are based on clinical preventable burden and cost effectiveness. Each service was classified on a 1 (lowest preventable burden or most costly) to 5 (highest preventable burden or cost saving) scale.

SOURCE: Coffield AB, Maciosek MV, McGinnis JM, et al. Priorities among recommended clinical preventive services. *Am J Prev Med.* 2001;21:1-9.

interventions is identified, a process like that used for the Clinical Preventive Services Priorities Project could be applied to these community-based preventive services. In the meantime, program managers and policy makers can use the available information from the *Guide to Community Preventive Services* to inform decisions about intervention selection in these environments.

Designing Accountability Systems

Prevention-effectiveness information is also useful for the design of systems of accountability for the quality of health care and health-related services. Interest and activity in this area has grown in recent years for a number of reasons. First, managed care has emerged as the most common type of health insurance in the United States.[38] The 1990s saw a massive migration of Americans into some form of managed care, as employers purchasing health insurance sought to control soaring costs through either capitated prepayment via health maintenance organizations (HMOs), or discounted fee-for-service via preferred provider organizations (PPOs). To a lesser extent, governmental purchasers mirrored this movement in purchasing insurance for their own employees and beneficiaries of Medicaid and Medicare. With this growth in managed care came growth in anxiety about the quality of care, as capitation and discounted fee-for-service both provided incentives for providing less care. The growth in capitated HMOs also increased the feasibility and incentives for accountability within the systems themselves. HMOs care for defined populations and have information systems that account for the care provided to those populations, including those persons who do not actively seek care. Because HMOs receive a fixed annual prepayment for providing care, regardless of the amount and cost of care they actually end up providing, the HMOs have a strong incentive to find cost-effective interventions that keep populations healthy and to account for the delivery of those interventions.

A second reason for the increased interest in accountability has been a flood of new information on the variability, and generally low level, of quality of health care. Using health insurance claims data, Wennberg[39] pioneered efforts showing dramatic variations, from one geographic area to another, in the numbers of medical procedures performed. Because these variations were apparently without logic and because medical procedures universally carry risk of adverse events, Wennberg's work raised doubts about the quality of care. Millenson[40] documented the history of the measurement and management of quality of care in the United States and showed that, although strong concerns about quality are more than a century old, efforts to manage and improve the quality of care have been weak and intermittent. Most recently, the Institute of Medicine (IOM)[41–43] has published a series of reports documenting the high variability and poor quality of health care, and highlighting the importance of medical errors as a leading cause of death.

A third reason for the increased interest in accountability has been the growth of computing power and the accompanying growth in capability of health information systems. To cite two examples, neither the accountability systems in HMOs nor Wennberg's work would have been possible without the increased computing power of the past three decades.[39]

NCQA/HEDIS

Although a number of accountability systems for health care have been developed, the most widely used and important for prevention is HEDIS (Health Plan Employer Data and Information Set), which is used by more than 90 percent of HMOs to measure the quality of the care they provide.[44] Developed by the nonprofit National Committee for Quality Assurance (NCQA), HEDIS is also a part of the measurement system used by NCQA to accredit HMOs.[45] Because some purchasers of health care require that HMOs be accredited in order to be eligible for contracts, HEDIS receives a lot of attention from HMOs. The HEDIS performance measures are divided into 7 domains, but the 16 measures in the effectiveness-of-care domain receive most attention, at least partly because they are the measures incorporated into the

Table 17.8. HEDIS 2001 Effectiveness-of-Care Measures

Childhood Immunization Status
Adolescent Immunization Status
Breast Cancer Screening
Cervical Cancer Screening
Chlamydia Screening in Women
Controlling High Blood Pressure
Beta Blocker Treatment After a Heart Attack
Cholesterol Management After Acute Cardiovascular
  Events
Comprehensive Diabetes Care
Use of Appropriate Medications for People with Asthma
Follow-up After Hospitalization for Mental Illness
Antidepressant Medication
Advising Smokers to Quit
Flu Shots for Older Adults
Pneumonia Vaccination Status for Older Adults
Medicare Health Outcomes Survey

SOURCE: National Committee for Quality Assurance. *HEDIS® 2001, Volume 1: Narrative—What's in It and Why It Matters.* Washington, DC: National Committee for Quality Assurance; 2000.

accreditation scoring system (Table 17.8). NCQA has formally adopted Donabedian's structure-process-outcome framework[46] for measuring the quality of health care, and the HEDIS effectiveness-of-care domain almost exclusively measures health care processes, such as mammography, that have been shown to result in improved health outcomes, such as fewer breast cancer deaths. Of the 16 effectiveness-of-care measures, 5 measure the quality of primary, 3 the quality of secondary, and 3 the quality of tertiary preventive care.

To date, preventive care has dominated the HEDIS effectiveness-of-care measures because much preventive care readily meets NCQA's three sets of criteria for selecting HEDIS measures: relevance, feasibility, and scientific soundness. Criteria for relevance include proven effectiveness and cost-effectiveness. The *Guide to Clinical Preventive Services* and other prevention-effectiveness information cited in this chapter provide a strong evidence base for these relevance criteria. A key criterion for feasibility is the number of persons, within a given HMO, to which a potential HEDIS

measure applies. Primary prevention and the screening tests of secondary prevention apply to large populations and make prevention performance measurement highly feasible. A key criterion for scientific soundness is validity; in particular, because of cost of measurement issues, the validity of measurement via transactional codes in electronic information systems is important. Screening procedures, such as mammography or laboratory tests, usually have well-validated billing and other transaction-related codes that facilitate measurement. HEDIS has also relied heavily on patient surveys to measure care that may not be well documented in medical records. An example is the survey-based measurement of advice to quit smoking. The existence of well-validated prevention-related questions from the National Health Interview Survey and the Behavioral Risk Factor Surveillance System has facilitated the inclusion of prevention measures in HEDIS.

HEDIS is but one example of an accountability system for measuring the quality of preventive and other health care. HEDIS is exceptionally important, however, because it is so widely used and emulated, and it has undoubtedly increased the resources devoted to prevention in health care. HEDIS also demonstrates the importance of prevention-effectiveness information, which has been heavily used in the selection and development of HEDIS measures. Prevention-effectiveness information, such as the *Guide to Community Preventive Services'* information on the effectiveness of clinical systems, has also been key for HMOs as they have attempted to improve their HEDIS scores by improving the quality of preventive care they provide to their members.

Clinical accountability systems are relevant to public health practitioners for two reasons. First, many public health departments are responsible for providing, or ensuring the provision of, clinical services to poor populations. In their roles as health care system managers or purchasers of health care, public health officials must be aware of the issues of quality and accountability and provide services or purchase benefits packages accordingly. Second, accountability is not solely a clinical issue. Public health officials must be accountable to policy makers and constituents about the services they provide, whether they are clinical preventive services or community-based preventive services. For example, knowing that effective clinical and community-based programs for helping smokers quit are available, public health officials would be remiss if they implemented only less effective or unproven strategies. Although standardized and widely accepted accountability systems such as HEDIS do not yet exist for public health programs, accountability is nevertheless an important public service issue.

Guiding Research

Prevention-effectiveness information is also an important guide to future research. What questions need answering? What questions have been heavily researched, perhaps overly researched? The systematic reviews from the *Guide to Community Preventive Services* answer both of these questions in a section guiding future research at the end of each of its topic-specific reviews of intervention effectiveness. For example, in its review of the effectiveness of interventions to increase vaccination, it highlighted the questionable effectiveness of patient and family incentives for vaccination as an important area for further research.[28] On the other hand, it pointed out that a large body of literature clearly establishes the effectiveness of vaccination reminder-recall systems aimed at patients and providers and urged that future research be directed elsewhere.

SUMMARY

The past two decades have seen a revolution in the type of information available to practitioners of public health and other decision makers seeking to improve the public's health. Prevention-effectiveness information has been at the heart of this revolution. With this information, decision makers can make evidence-based choices about which health problems to address first, which interventions to use, and what returns to expect for a given investment. Information on clinical prevention was the first available and is still the most comprehensive, but development of information on clinical-systems and community-based interventions is following closely behind. Because this information has been systematically developed with explicit criteria, it serves well not only clinicians and public health practitioners, but also the employers, health-system managers, and legislators who play an increasingly important role as population-health managers.

References

1. Hodgson TA, Cohen AJ. Medical expenditures for major diseases, 1995. *Health Care Financing Rev.* 2000;21(2):119-64.

2. National Center for Health Statistics. Current estimates from the National Health Interview Survey, 1992. *Vital and Health Statistics 1994.* Hyattsville, Md: National Center for Health Statistics; 1994. Series 10, No. 189.

3. Riedel JE, Lynch W, Baase C, Hymel P, Peterson KW. The effect of disease prevention and health promotion on workplace productivity: Literature review. *Am J Health Promotion.* 2001;15:167-191.

4. Fries JF. Aging, natural death, and the compression of morbidity. *N Engl J Med.* 1980;303:130-135.

5. Michaud CM, Murray CJL, Bloom BR. Burden of disease—Implications for future research. *JAMA.* 2001; 285:535-539.

6. Torrance GW, Feeny D. Utilities and quality-adjusted life years. *Int J Technol Assess Health Care.* 1989; 5:559-575.

7. McGinnis JM, Foege WH. Actual causes of death in the United States. *JAMA.* 1993;270:2207-2212.

8. Marmot MG, Shipley MJ, Rose G. Inequalities in death—Specific explanations of a general pattern? *Lancet.* 1984;1:1003-1006.

9. Gornick ME, Eggers PW, Reilly TW, et al. Effects of race and income on mortality and use of services among Medicare beneficiaries. *N Engl J Med.* 1996;335:791-799.

10. Adler NE, Boyce WT, Chesney MA, Folkman S, Syme SL. Socioeconomic inequalities in health. *JAMA.* 1993;269:3140-3145.

11. Centers for Disease Control and Prevention. A framework for assessing the effectiveness of disease and injury prevention. *MMWR.* 1992;41(RR-3):1-14.

12. Glass GV. Primary, secondary, and meta-analysis of research. *Educ Res.* 1976;5:3-8.

13. Cooper H, Hedges LV, eds. *The Handbook of Research Synthesis.* New York, NY: Russell Sage Foundation; 1994.

14. Mulrow CD, Oxman AD, eds. Cochrane collaboration handbook. In: The Cochrane Library [CD-ROM, updated September 1997]. The Cochrane Collaboration. Oxford, England: Update Software; 1997: Issue 4.

15. The Cochrane Collaboration. The Cochrane database of systematic reviews, 1999, Vol. 2 [database online]. Available at: http://www.update-software.com/cochrane. Accessed June 1, 2001.

16. Cook TD, Campbell DT, eds. *Quasi-Experimentation: Design and Analysis Issues for Field Settings.* Boston, Mass: Houghton Mifflin Co; 1979.

17. Wholey JS, Hatry HP, Newcomer KE, eds. *Handbook of Practical Program Evaluation.* San Francisco, Calif: Jossey-Bass Publishers; 1994.

18. Briss PA, Zaza S, Pappaioanou M, et al. Developing an evidence-based *Guide to Community Preventive Services*—Methods. *Am J Prev Med.* 2000;19(1S):35-43.

19. Harris RP, Helfand M, Woolf SH, et al. Current methods of the US Preventive Services Task Force: A review of the process. *Am J Prev Med.* 2001;20(3s):21-35.

20. US Preventive Services Task Force. *Guide to Clinical Preventive Services.* 2nd ed. Alexandria, Va: International Medical Publishing; 1996.

21. Atkins D, Best D, Shapiro EN, eds. The Third US Preventive Services Task Force: Background, methods, and first recommendations. *Am J Prev Med.* 2001;20(3S):1-108.

22. Saha S, Hoerger TJ, Pignone MP, et al. The art and science of incorporating cost effectiveness into evidence-based recommendations for clinical preventive services. *Am J Prev Med.* 2001;20(3S):36-43.

23. Fiore MC, Bailey WC, Cohen SJ, et al. Treating tobacco use and dependence: Clinical practice guideline. Rockville, Md: US Dept of Health and Human Services, Public Health Service; 2000. Available at: http://www.surgeongeneral.gov/tobacco. Accessed June 1, 2001.

24. Task Force on Community Preventive Services. Introducing the *Guide to Community Preventive Services:* Methods, first recommendations, and expert commentary. *Am J Prev Med.* 2000;19(1S):1-142.

25. Task Force on Community Preventive Services. Recommendations regarding interventions to improve vaccination coverage in children, adolescents, and adults. *Am J Prev Med.* 2000;18(1S):92-96.

26. Task Force on Community Preventive Services. Recommendations regarding interventions to reduce tobacco use and exposure to environmental tobacco smoke. *Am J Prev Med.* 2001;20(2S):10-15.

27. Centers for Disease Control and Prevention. Motor-vehicle occupant injury: Strategies for increasing use of child safety seats, increasing use of safety belts, and reducing alcohol-impaired driving. A report on recommendations of the Task Force on Community Preventive Services. *MMWR.* 2001;50(RR-7):1-12.

28. Briss PA, Rodewald LE, Hinman AR, et al. Reviews of evidence regarding interventions to improve vaccination coverage in children, adolescents, and adults. *Am J Prev Med.* 2000;18(1S):97-140.

29. Agency for Healthcare Quality and Research. *Put Prevention Into Practice:* Available at: http://www.ahrq.gov/clinic/prevenix.htm. Accessed June 1, 2001.

30. Gold MR, Siegel JE, Russell LB, Weinstein MC. *Cost-Effectiveness in Health and Medicine.* New York, NY: Oxford University Press; 1996.

31. Haddix AC, Teutsch SM, Shaffer PA, Duñet DO, eds. *Prevention Effectiveness: A Guide to Decision Analysis and Economic Evaluation.* New York, NY: Oxford University Press; 1996.

32. Stone PW, Teutsch S, Chapman RH, Bell C, Goldie SJ, Neumann PJ. Cost-utility analyses of clinical preventive services: Published ratios, 1976-1997. *Am J Prev Med.* 2000;19:15-23.

33. Eddy DM. Oregon's methods: Did cost-effectiveness analysis fail? *JAMA.* 1991;266:2135-2141.

34. Tengs TO, Adams ME, Pliskin JS, et al. Five-hundred life-saving interventions and their cost-effectiveness. *Risk Anal.* 1995:369-390.

35. Chapman RH, Stone PW, Sandberg EA, Bell C, Neumann PJ. A comprehensive league table of cost-utility ratios and a sub-table of "panel-worthy" studies. *Med Decis Making.* 2000;20:451-467.

36. Coffield AB, Maciosek MV, McGinnis JM, et al. Priorities among recommended clinical preventive services. *Am J Prev Med.* 2001;21:1-9.

37. Maciosek MV, Coffield AB, McGinnis JM, et al. Methods for priority setting among clinical preventive services. *Am J Prev Med.* 2001;21:10-19.

38. Harris JR, Caldwell B, Cahill K. Measuring the public's health in an era of accountability: Lessons from HEDIS. *Am J Prev Med*. 1998;14(3S):9-13.

39. Wennberg JE, Cooper MM, eds. *The Dartmouth Atlas of Health Care 1998*. Chicago, Ill: American Hospital Publishing Inc; 1998.

40. Millenson ML. *Demanding Medical Excellence—Doctors and Accountability in the Information Age*. Chicago, Ill: University of Chicago Press; 1997.

41. Institute of Medicine. *Measuring the Quality of Health Care*. Donaldson MS, ed. Washington, DC: National Academy Press; 1999.

42. Institute of Medicine. *To Err Is Human: Building a Safer Health Care System*. Kohn LT, Corrigan JM, Donaldson MS, eds. Washington, DC: National Academy Press; 2000.

43. Institute of Medicine. *Crossing the Quality Chasm: A New Health System for the 21st Century*. Washington, DC: National Academy Press; 2001.

44. National Committee for Quality Assurance. *HEDIS®* 2001, Volume 1: Narrative—What's in It and Why It Matters. Washington, DC: National Committee for Quality Assurance; 2000.

45. National Committee for Quality Assurance. *2001 Standards for the Accreditation of Managed Care Organizations*. Washington, DC: National Committee for Quality Assurance; 2001.

46. Donabedian A. Evaluating the quality of medical care. *Milbank Memorial Fund Q*. 1966;44:166-203.

CHAPTER
18

Chronic Disease Control

David V. McQueen, Sc.D.
James S. Marks, M.D., M.P.H.

In this new century, heart disease, cancer, and other chronic diseases will place a huge burden on global health. By 1990, chronic diseases had already surpassed infectious diseases as the leading cause of death in all areas of the world except sub-Saharan Africa and the Middle East. By 2020, chronic diseases are expected to account for 7 of every 10 deaths in the world. These projections suggest that chronic diseases—and the death, illness, and disability they cause—will soon dominate health care costs and change the role of public health worldwide.[1,2]

In this chapter, we focus on the burden of chronic disease in the United States, the role of surveillance, the complex relationships between risk behaviors and chronic diseases, and public health approaches to chronic disease control. We also discuss emerging issues such as the obesity epidemic in America, global health issues, and mental health problems that are closely linked with chronic disease.

BURDEN OF CHRONIC DISEASE

Chronic disease trends in this country have followed the pattern of most advanced industrialized countries. Rates of cardiovascular disease deaths have declined steadily since the 1960s, and cancer survival rates have improved in recent decades.[3-5] Despite these improvements, more than 1.7 million people die of a chronic disease each year.[6,7] Cardiovascular disease is the leading cause of death in this country, accounting for more than 40 percent of all deaths.[3,4] Cancer is the second leading cause, accounting for about one-fourth of all deaths, and many cancers still have low survival rates. For example, only about 14 percent of people with lung cancer survive for more than five years.[5]

Many people who die of chronic diseases are older, but chronic diseases also take a heavy toll on adults who are in the prime of life. Many of the years of potential life lost before age 75 can be attributed to

Table 18.1. Years of Potential Life Lost before Age 78 for Selected Causes of Death, United States, 1990 and 1998*

	1990	1998
Heart disease	1,517.6	1,343.2
Cancer	1,863.4	1,715.9
Stroke	246.2	233.0
Chronic obstructive pulmonary diseases	182.5	187.5
Pneumonia and influenza	139.9	122.8
Chronic liver disease and cirrhosis	178.4	159.2
Diabetes mellitus	147.0	174.1
Human immunodeficiency virus infection	391.2	177.2
Unintentional injuries	1,221.2	1,051.6
Suicide	404.8	365.4
Homicide	446.5	301.0
All causes	8,997.0	7,733.3

*Crude number of years lost before age 75 per 100,000 people under 75 years of age. Italic type denotes chronic diseases.
SOURCE: Eberhardt MS, Ingram DD, Makuc DM, et al. *Urban and Rural Health Chartbook. Health, United States, 2001.* Hyattsville, Md: US Dept of Health and Human Services, Centers for Disease Control and Prevention, National Center for Health Statistics; 2001:170.

chronic disease (Table 18.1).[8,9] Moreover, chronic diseases cause the most premature deaths among minority racial and ethnic groups and disadvantaged populations. These conditions account for the largest part of the health gap between African Americans and whites.[6]

Chronic disease deaths often can be traced back to unhealthy behaviors, many that begin early in life. Nearly 40 percent of U.S. deaths can be attributed to smoking, physical inactivity, poor diet, and alcohol misuse—all risk factors for chronic diseases and all modifiable (Table 18.2).[10] Tobacco use alone has been described as the largest single factor resulting in early deaths in most of the developed world.[11–13] In the United States, more than 430,000 people die each year because of tobacco use. Smokers who die of a tobacco-related illness lose 12 years of expected life. An unhealthy diet and lack of physical activity account for at least 300,000 deaths each year in this country. Reducing the prevalence of these risk factors is essential to reducing the burden of chronic disease.[6]

Deaths alone do not give a complete picture of the chronic disease burden. Millions of people in the United States endure years of pain, disability, and lower quality of life because of chronic diseases such as arthritis and diabetes. Chronic disabling conditions cause major limitations in activity for more than 1 in every 10 Americans. This impact is expected to increase dramatically as baby boomers age. For example, by 2020, an estimated 60 million Americans—or 1 in every 5 persons—will be affected by arthritis, and nearly 12 million of these people will have activity limitations.[6]

Chronic diseases also place a tremendous financial burden on individuals and society. Each year in the United States, medical care and lost productivity costs total about $327 billion for cardiovascular disease, $107 billion for cancer, and $65 billion for arthritis. As the U.S. population ages and chronic diseases become more prevalent, these costs are projected to rise rapidly.[6]

PUBLIC HEALTH SURVEILLANCE

Public health surveillance has a critical role in chronic disease control because it allows us to monitor changes and trends over time and in different populations.[14] Surveillance gives us information that we need to develop more effective public health interventions and better target program efforts. In recent

Table 18.2.   Major External (Nongenetic) Factors That Contributed to Death in the United States, 1990

	Deaths	
Cause*	Estimated no.[†]	Percentage of total deaths
Tobacco use	400,000	19
Diet/activity patterns	300,000	14
Alcohol use	100,000	5
Microbial agents	90,000	4
Toxic agents	60,000	3
Firearms use	35,000	2
Sexual behavior	30,000	1
Motor vehicle crashes	25,000	1
Illicit use of drugs	20,000	<1
Total	1,060,000	50

*Italic type denotes risk factors related to chronic disease.

[†]Composite approximation drawn from studies that used different approaches to derive estimates, ranging from actual counts (for example, firearms use) to population-attributable risk calculations (for example, tobacco use). Numbers over 50,000 are rounded to the nearest 10,000, and those below 50,000 are rounded to the nearest 5,000.

SOURCE: McGinnis JM, Foege WH. Actual causes of death in the United States. *JAMA.* 1993;270:2207-2212.

years, chronic disease surveillance has expanded beyond the mere collection of data to also include analysis, interpretation, and use of the data. Surveillance is now viewed as a system of related actions ranging from recognizing the magnitude of a chronic disease problem in a particular population to analyzing and interpreting the data and using the findings to develop public health actions.

Criteria for Effective Surveillance

To be effective, surveillance approaches must meet the criteria for public health surveillance,[14,15] which include the following attributes:

1. Simplicity
2. Flexibility
3. Acceptability
4. Sensitivity
5. Specificity
6. Representativeness
7. Timeliness

Two major surveillance systems now in use in the United States—National Health Interview Survey (NHIS) and National Health and Nutrition Examina-

tion Survey (NHANES) are shown in Table 18.3 and share these attributes. These systems and the two other approaches shown also have the following characteristics in common:

1. A comprehensive approach to data collection
2. Modern methods of data collection
3. The potential to analyze multiple risk factors for chronic disease
4. Availability for public use

This comprehensive, systematic approach and the dynamic nature of data collection separate chronic disease surveillance from the mere collection of vital statistics and records. Chronic disease surveillance relates powerfully to the role of modern epidemiology, with its focus on the reasons why chronic disease patterns change in the population. The long-term goal of surveillance is to aid in identifying the factors that help prevent disease and promote health.

In the United States, we have numerous sources of chronic disease data and many types of surveillance systems. Disease notification systems, registries, medical records, and death certificates are among the various data sources used to monitor chronic diseases and deaths. Each of these sources has well-documented

Table 18.3. Four Major Survey-Based Chronic Disease Surveillance Approaches

	BRFSS*	NHIS†	NHANES§	YRBSS¶
Date established	1982	1957	1960	1990
Outcome	risk factor data for individual states	data on health status and risk factors in the United States	risk factor and disease data in the United States; focus on diet	risk factor data on children in schools
Scope	nationwide, state by state; adults >17 years of age	national sample; primarily adults >17 years of age	noninstitutionalized national sample; primarily adults >17 years of age	national, state, territorial, and local samples; primarily students in grades 9–12
Method	random-digit-dial household, computer-assisted telephone interview	household survey	household interview plus medical exam and lab work	written survey, self-administered in school
Strengths	timely, state-level data; monthly data points	depth of question areas; supplemental surveys	very comprehensive; objective lab work	in-depth look at health of schoolchildren
Weaknesses	lack of depth; telephone-dependent	self-reported data; data not local	complicated analytical challenges; not timely	limited to children in school
Comments	highly flexible system that allows states to add questions on numerous health topics	the standard for health status data in the United States	extensive information on chronic diseases	extensive information on risk factors that lead to chronic diseases

*Behavioral Risk Factor Surveillance System.
†National Health Interview Survey.
§National Health and Nutrition Examination Survey.
¶Youth Risk Behavior Surveillance System.

strengths and limitations that are familiar to every public health scientist. Unfortunately, few of these systems provide data that are timely enough to be useful for surveillance. Instead, these systems often record the failure of prevention activities because they chronicle the later and end stages of chronic disease. Although these systems are effective in establishing the magnitude of the problem and highlighting the overall importance of chronic disease in the population, the data arrive too late to be useful for early interventions. Risk factor surveys, on the other hand, are useful for early intervention planning. The sections below discuss three types of surveillance data that are tracked: mortality, morbidity, and risk factors for chronic disease.

Mortality Surveillance

Mortality surveillance is the systematic and ongoing collection of data on the causes of death for individuals. Mortality surveillance is perhaps the most basic type of surveillance, and has been practiced for hundreds of years.[16] Mortality data are one type of vital statistics. In most of the world, including the United States, mortality surveillance is routine. Classification of cause of death is standardized worldwide by using an internationally agreed upon system.[17] Mortality surveillance works best when measures are taken to ensure that the cause-of-death data are highly accurate. This is especially important for chronic disease deaths, which have a greater likelihood of being misclassified than infectious disease deaths. Every death that occurs outside the hospital, or where the cause is not patently clear, should be carefully assessed by a medical professional.

In addition, the place of death must be standardized if mortality records are to be of high quality. Generally, the place of death is recorded as at or near the site where the death actually happens (e.g., the death of a worker at a construction site in a city would be considered a death occurring in that city, not in the city where the worker lived). Increasingly, people who die of chronic diseases expire in a care facility, and generally these deaths are associated with multiple causes and comorbidity. Thus, medical professionals often have difficulty attributing the cause of death to a specific chronic disease.

Morbidity Surveillance

Morbidity surveillance is the tracking of illness, injury, disability, and other related complications. It often is far more complicated, expensive, and prone to error than mortality or risk factor surveillance. This is especially the case with chronic diseases. Many chronic diseases have no readily detectable signs or symptoms during the course of their development. This makes detection either difficult or costly. In addition, detection of many chronic diseases often offers only limited possibilities for primary prevention activities. Essentially, morbidity surveillance is a form of screening for diagnosis of chronic diseases. Nonetheless, morbidity surveillance can be used as an integrated part of monitoring very targeted public health interventions.

Morbidity is tracked by using data from disease registries (e.g., cancer incidence, by stage of diagnosis) and hospital discharge data (e.g., lower extremity amputations associated with diabetes). Despite the difficulties of tracking chronic disease morbidity, these data allow us to interlock health care expenditures with chronic conditions. Morbidity surveillance remains an important tool for persons concerned with medical care costs and chronic disease.

Behavioral Risk Factor Surveillance

The type of surveillance most salient to chronic disease prevention is behavioral risk factor surveillance. This type of surveillance is relatively easy to carry out and interrelates strongly with public health interventions. The role of behavioral risk factors in chronic disease is well documented. Given the weight of the scientific evidence, many arguments can be given for establishing health promotion and risk reduction programs directed at changing the prevalence of behavioral risk factors in the population to enhance the health of the public. By establishing a behavioral risk factor surveillance system, we can ensure that we will have appropriate and useful data to help us plan or guide these efforts. In Oregon, for example, recent survey findings indicate that 85 percent of residents think that breathing secondhand smoke is harmful to health, and 73 percent think smoking should be banned in the workplace. State health officials have used these findings to promote health policies such as bans on smoking in the workplace and in licensed child care facilities.[18]

Epidemiology tends to link chronic diseases with a variety of prior conditions. Thus, public health practitioners often look at chronic diseases and ask: What are the causal factors? What are the determinants? Can we do anything about them? Over the past 50 years, this approach has led us to focus on particular lifestyle behaviors: tobacco use, smoking, poor nutrition, physical inactivity, and alcohol and other substance abuse. In recent years, particularly with the advent of HIV and the AIDS epidemic, sexual behaviors have been added to this list.

McGinnis and Foege postulated that half of all deaths could be attributed to modifiable human behaviors.[10] The exact contribution of modifiable behaviors to chronic disease deaths and morbidity remains a research question. Nevertheless, we know that these behaviors have a considerable impact on public health in terms of not only death but also impaired quality of life, disability years, and premature morbidity.[9] Given the number of behaviors related to chronic disease, the magnitude of these behaviors and changes over time need to be assessed.

There are many detailed overviews of disease surveillance,[14] but this next discussion is limited to surveillance related to human behavior. The surveillance of human behavior is different from other types of surveillance, and some criteria imposed on disease surveillance are less appropriate for human behavior surveillance. We must be aware of this difference, particularly now, when there are calls for standardized, centralized systems for surveillance in public health.

Human Behavior and Risk

In public health surveillance, the complexity of human behavior is reduced to making associations between health risks and several key human behaviors or behavioral patterns. The foundation for this approach is based in both scientific knowledge and assertions that link specific behaviors to specific disease processes. Although the theoretical basis is sound, the science of exact risk determination is complex, and it is difficult to prove conclusively that a behavior—either alone or in concert with other factors—actually causes a disease. However, we can estimate the relationships between risk behaviors at the population level and disease patterns in the population.

Tracking behavioral risk factors in the population relies principally on the sample survey. When sample surveys are conducted in a continuous series over many years, such as in the Centers for Disease Control and Prevention (CDC)-supported Behavioral Risk Factor Surveillance System (BRFSS), they are considered a basic surveillance system. The BRFSS is a state-based, random-digit-dialed telephone survey of noninstitutionalized U.S. civilians aged 18 years and older. The survey collects state-level information on adults' health status, use of preventive services, and risk behaviors associated with many of the leading causes of illness and death. With surveillance systems such as the BRFSS, epidemiologic methods are enhanced by the social and behavioral sciences. Such surveys are not, however, effective in assessing the risk behaviors of hard-to-reach segments of the population.

Another survey-based system is the Youth Risk Behavior Surveillance System (YRBSS), which collects extensive data from schoolchildren on many of the risk factors that can lead to chronic diseases. The CDC-supported YRBSS includes a national survey as well as surveys conducted by state and local education and health agencies. The questionnaires are written and self-administered in classrooms at public and private schools.

Assessments of Multiple Risk Factors

Behind most surveillance systems, notably those that are survey-based, is the notion that individual risk factors cause disease. This has been both a strength and a limitation of surveillance in public health. Much research in chronic disease now stresses the interaction of multiple factors working together to cause chronic disease. Yet, traditional surveillance systems might treat risk factors as single entities. An extreme case of this limitation is seen in surveillance systems that are developed to assess changes and trends in a single risk factor or disease outcome. Data collection techniques now allow for more complicated data sets requiring the use of analytic techniques that take multiple risk factors into account. The success of chronic disease surveillance efforts undoubtedly will depend on the assessment of patterns of risk in populations.

Public health agencies that conduct behavioral surveillance must deal with complexities that can affect the logistics of operating the system, the quality and usefulness of the data, and how the data are translated into public health action. In the following sections, we explore some of these issues.

Ownership and Partnership

Who controls or "owns" surveillance systems that track human behaviors? The debate over ownership is couched in terms such as *national* versus *local* surveillance. The need for national surveillance has long been recognized. Many *Healthy People 2010* objectives require tracking of human behaviors at the national level. Although the national data argument is widely accepted, there is also a strong movement for behavioral data at a more local level. For example, the states rely heavily on their own BRFSS data for assessment of year 2010 and other objectives in their own states.[19]

Increasingly, the term *local* is used to refer to smaller geopolitical areas. Whereas some people argue that national data might not reflect state interests, others contend that state data, particularly from large states, might not reflect the perceived and real differences within the states. Perhaps the most notable examples come from those many states with wide disparities between highly populated urban and low-density rural areas. In planning and assessing public health programs, states want data considered meaningful by the affected residents. One of the truisms about behavioral data is that people seem to identify more with data that are from their area; that is, the reported information should be germane to where people live if we want it to lead to changes in behaviors or policies.

There is another dimension of ownership: public health researchers tend to think in geopolitical terms (e.g., federal, state, county, city). Increasingly, however, surveillance of human behavior is being conducted in communities of interest that do not fit neatly within geopolitical boundaries. For example, high-risk behaviors for HIV infection might be found among a population of individuals cutting across state lines, yet sharing a common community of interest. Similarly, a managed care organization may be interested in the behaviors of the group that has pockets of membership in several geopolitical areas.[20] In these two cases, a surveillance system based on a traditional geopolitical sample may be of limited use. The locus of current public health action is moving to health issues in these types of communities.

The ownership theme is closely tied to the concept of partnership. Partnership implies reciprocity, an equitable dialogue among parties. For example, in the BRFSS, there is an extensive and explicit cooperative agreement between the states and CDC on how to carry out the surveillance. States participate significantly in the design and format of the questionnaire and are in charge of collecting their data. It is because of this participation that states take on ownership of the BRFSS in their own states while partaking in the ownership of the whole.

Quality of Behavioral Data

Quality of data is always a prime concern in surveillance. With human behavior, the concern is fraught with complexity. The scientific notion that data should be readily interpretable in the same manner by any external observer has been questioned by many in the behavioral science community and by renowned philosophers of science. Behavioral data are different in many fundamental ways. For example, we attach meaning to behaviors, and we depend on those carrying out the behavior to report it and interpret it. The individuals collecting the data attach meanings to the behaviors about which they ask.

Questions of quality in behavioral data need to go well beyond the standard concerns with validity and reliability.[21] The concerns have moved onto notions of "total survey errors," which take into account errors arising from coverage, nonresponse, sampling, interviewers, respondents, instruments, mode, and other sources. Validity is now seen from many perspectives that include construct, theoretical, criterion, empirical, predictive, concurrent, discriminate, convergent, internal, external, and reliability, depending on your approach, which stems from the psychometric and/or statistical literature. The sheer size of this survey research literature is daunting. Nevertheless, some outstanding issues in surveillance can be seen within an error context. Three hotly debated issues in behavioral risk factor surveillance are questionnaire content, method of data collection, and standardization.

Questionnaire content cannot be separated from the theme of ownership. In earlier times questionnaire development may have been chiefly carried out by academics and government agencies, but now questionnaire development belongs to many different constituencies. Questions in surveillance systems are the product of competing interest groups with many different agendas. The present concern is often not what question to ask, but what the question is going to be used for and who will use it. Thus, good surveillance systems are by necessity responsive to arising needs and flexible enough to adapt quickly to questions dictated by policy needs and shifts in the topics of relevance to public health.

The role of cognition in asking behavioral questions is now a chief concern of questionnaire construction.[22] Understanding the psycholinguistics associated with the meaning of questions is an art. At both governmental levels and in academic practice, cognitive questionnaire design laboratories put potential and widely used questions in surveys through extensive qualitative testing. The interpretation of questions in surveillance systems is now viewed as often highly influenced by the social and cultural dynamics of the times and the cognitive characteristics of the respondents. Thus, one sees the growing recognition in the field that there are no perfect questions to assess human behavior, only approximations of the most appropriate questions.

Data collection methodology also has benefited greatly from more than two decades of experience with different data collection approaches. The once accepted belief in the gold standard of face-to-face interviewing has been replaced with a careful understanding, largely in terms of survey errors and survey costs, of the strengths and weaknesses of mail, telephone, and face-to-face strategies.[23] Telephone interviews became a highly useful method for behavioral surveillance with the coming of Computer Assisted Telephone Interviewing (CATI). Telephone interviews provided a data collection methodology that was accurate, cost-effective, and rapid, replacing the more ponderous, expensive series of cross-sectional surveys.

One characteristic of behavioral risk factor surveillance is that it relies on the vagaries of self-reported information. There are a number of reasons why this is a very important information source, however. First, self-reporting is the only logical and ethical way to obtain data on many behaviors, particularly with sexual behaviors related to HIV transmission. Second, we are genuinely interested in the answers people give to questions, many of which are concerned with attitudes, opinions, and beliefs that relate to behaviors. In these cases the "correct" re-

sponses can lie only within the volition of the respondents and their self-reports. Finally, we now have an extensive literature that has documented and assessed the validity of self-reporting many different behaviors.[21] Much of this literature documents research carried out in academic settings using appropriate methods to assess the validity of self-reporting. In addition, many comparisons have been made between self-reported health behaviors and measured or other documented evidence about these behaviors. As a result, we know much about the relative accuracy and inaccuracy of self-reporting in many contexts. Thus, it is possible to consider the levels and significance of measurement error in analyzing those behaviors affected by self-reporting, or more accurately termed, "respondent error."

Another controversial issue is standardization. In principle, standardization is a good thing. The physical sciences in particular have standardization as a goal. It would be a big problem if countries used different lengths for one meter. However, many health-related behaviors have relatively few agreed-upon standards for measurement. Quite often, this issue is simplified by standardizing individual questions on surveys and surveillance systems.

Standardizing these questions presents three dangers. First, almost all the evidence from survey research shows that the "true" values or answers can be imputed only by studying the convergence of responses through several alternative, but highly related questions where response variance is carefully assessed. Second, human behavior and the way it is reported may be highly affected by the context of that behavior. For example, the accuracy of self-reported alcohol use is affected by the amount of alcohol regularly consumed by the respondent. Thus, the standard question cannot be interpreted without knowing more contextual information that can vary with the population being sampled. In addition, many questionnaire items that appear weak on their own may function well in an index or when embedded in a questionnaire of related health topics. Therefore, one should not consider a standard question without considering standard indices and contextual questions at the same time. Finally, there is the real danger that a widely accepted standardized question could be wrong—that is, on a cognitive, epistemological basis. For example, a simple measure claiming to measure quality of life might produce consistent and reliable measurement over time but, in fact, not really tap the cognitive dimensions of quality of life.

Analysis and Use of Data

In the past, people working in surveillance concerned themselves chiefly with data collection, management, and archiving. With the rise and attention to health promotion as a central activity of public health, the emphasis is now on the analysis and use of surveillance data. Although the emphasis is changing, it will undoubtedly take many years before analysis and use of data are given the same resources as data collection activity. Often, use of the data still entails the routine preparation and distribution of extensive cross-tabulations of data.

In the analysis of risk behavior data, two areas need more attention. First, we need to be mindful that risk behaviors and surveillance systems change over time. Many behavioral surveillance systems have been collecting data for years, often with a relatively smooth series or interrupted series of data points. Nonetheless, most surveillance systems aggregate data annually and compare year-to-year data as if these were independent large cross-sectional surveys. Thus, the data become less dynamic. Second, considerable attention needs to be paid to the effects of questionnaire changes in surveillance systems over time and how these differences can be interpreted in terms of their effect on changes in the reported behaviors over time. There are now many techniques to analyze data in this manner.

Moreover, interpretation of surveillance data would benefit from analytic approaches that take into account that the sociocultural backgrounds of both the respondents and the designers of the surveillance system affect how the results are interpreted. There are many multivariate analytical methods available that examine behaviors in their broader context (e.g., socioeconomic status, ethnicity, gender, race). We now have an extensive two-decade history of developing approaches to models and methods that deal with behaviorally dynamic data. Many of these new approaches to analysis have only begun to be applied to the huge public data sets held by health agencies.[24,25]

Finally, and perhaps most important, is the need to examine the relationship between ongoing behavioral surveillance systems and their use in informing and tracking public health interventions. Increasingly, community-based interventions and health promotion activities seek information on the behavioral and contextual attributes of populations for decision making. Surveillance information is useful for identifying the target population and for tracking changes in behaviors before, during, and after interventions. In addition, surveillance systems can add components of relevance to interventions through a partnership, as previously discussed.

PUBLIC HEALTH APPROACHES TO CHRONIC DISEASE CONTROL

In the past, public health efforts to control chronic disease focused mainly on primary prevention and early detection. Early programs within state and local health departments were generally limited and had difficulty being sustained during tight budget times. As recently as the late 1980s, few states had programs of meaningful size to reduce the burden of cardiovascular disease, cancer, tobacco use, physical inactivity, or obesity. Fewer than half of the states had programs in diabetes control. Much of the activity that did exist was supported by the Preventive Health and Health Services Block Grant, which in 1981 combined a variety of existing grants for activities such as health education, hypertension control, and fluoridation.

In the last 20 years, however, we have seen substantial growth in the scope and scale of chronic disease control efforts. State health departments, which once relied almost exclusively on federal dollars to support their chronic disease control efforts, are garnering more funding from state legislatures and executive branches. States are increasingly aware that chronic diseases—as the leading causes of death and disability—are also the leading source of health care costs. These costs, particularly those related to long-term care, are often born by the states. The financial burden on states will only increase with the aging of the population. Also driving the expansion of chronic disease control efforts are scientific advances and a growing base of interventions that have been proven effective in preventing or substantially delaying illness.

The enormous number of people with well-established risk factors for chronic diseases or needing to be screened means that clinic-based interventions alone are not likely to reach many of those in need of the services. Thus, in recent years, public health approaches have emphasized more links with community organizations and coalition-building as fundamental strategies to leverage resources and, more important, to engage a wider segment of the population in chronic diseases control activities.

For example, the Prevention Research Center at Morehouse School of Medicine[26] has worked hard to solicit community input and support for its projects, which focus on risk reduction and early detection of diseases in African American and other minority populations in Atlanta. Neighborhood groups, schools, youth clubs, health agencies, and organizations serve as links to the target populations. The center has a Coalition Board that is active in setting research priorities and reviewing research projects. The board has defined community values and worked collaboratively to ensure the center's projects are based on these values. Another example is the Cambodian Community Health 2010 project,[27] which is targeting cardiovascular disease and diabetes among Cambodian refugees in Lowell, Massachusetts. The project established a Cambodian Elders' Council to give a voice to older refugees, who often are homebound and isolated and have limited English skills.

Public health has also placed a greater emphasis on policy and environmental changes to support individual behavioral changes or to reduce barriers for specific services. These changes have often led to increased work between public health agencies and managed care organizations to adopt policies related to preventive services. The rise of managed care over the last decade has changed the face of medical care from individual practitioners, each of whom had to be directly engaged to change their practice patterns, to networks that have regularly used policies of reimbursement and reporting to influence care patterns.

Under such a structure, organizational policies have become important levers to encourage more complete adherence to proven preventive practices.

Programs Targeting Diseases

In the sections that follow, we describe interventions that target specific chronic diseases and those that target risk factors. Also discussed are program settings and populations that are the focus of chronic disease control programs.

Heart Disease and Stroke

Although heart disease and stroke have been the first and third leading causes of death in the country for many years, there has been no nationwide, concerted public health program aimed at their prevention until just recently. In the late 1970s, many efforts were launched to screen people for high blood pressure since studies had shown that a large number of persons with elevated blood pressure were unaware of it and the risk it carried. Awareness increased substantially, as did treatment. However, public screening efforts in community settings as opposed to clinical settings came under attack because so often, there was no referral link for treatment.

Although nearly one million people still die of heart disease or stroke each year, overall the age-adjusted rates of heart disease and stroke deaths have declined by 50 percent since peaking in the early 1960s.[3] This progress is attributed to primary prevention, secondary prevention, and better treatment.[28] When conditions such as hypertension and elevated cholesterol are included, estimates are that about 60 million Americans have a cardiovascular disease.[4] Research has clearly shown that reduction in cholesterol, control of blood pressure, tobacco use cessation, and physical activity can substantially lower a person's risk for developing or dying of cardiovascular disease. Unfortunately, studies also have shown that many people with these conditions or risks are unable to sustain their therapy or make the behavioral changes needed to lower their risk. But, these same studies show that education and training can greatly improve people's likelihood of making long-term changes.

Since 1998, CDC has provided grants to states (initially those with the highest rates of mortality) to begin developing public health programs aimed at these conditions.[29] The programs focus on the broad spectrum of prevention from primary through treatment post illness. Most states have begun to look at the areas of community and societal changes that can support healthful personal behavioral choices. Examples include the development of walking trail networks, work site nutrition and exercise programs, school health education, and physical education. There is also increasing interaction with managed care organizations to encourage strong patient education programs and monitor quality of care for persons with identified cardiovascular illness.

An area of great need in the states is the ability to monitor rates of illness. New public health programs are beginning to look at ways of tracking incidence. This ability to track rates of chronic disease is especially important because congestive heart failure is now the leading cause of hospitalization among the Medicare-aged population, and more studies are showing that good patient management programs can substantially lower rates of hospitalization for congestive heart failure.

Cancer

In the early 1990s, CDC began providing support to state health departments, allowing them to pay for breast and cervical cancer screening,[30,31] illustrating the growth in chronic disease prevention and control efforts in public health. Breast cancer is the second leading cause of cancer death among women, with about 190,000 new cases and 40,000 deaths each year.[32] Mammography is the best available method of screening. Mammography is estimated to detect breast cancer about one to two years before a woman can feel the lump and thus, with adequate treatment, to prevent about 25–30 percent of these deaths.[33–35] Cervical cancer is a much smaller problem, in part because of the widespread use of Pap smears, but recent progress has been slow. Each year, 4,000–5,000 women die of cervical cancer, and about 12,000 new cases are diagnosed.[32,35,36] Most of the women who die of these cancers have not received regular screenings.

In the United States, the Breast and Cervical Cancer Mortality Prevention Act of 1990 established the National Breast and Cervical Cancer Early Detection Program (NBCCEDP).[30,31,37] The program pays for screening and diagnostic services for poor women who have no other source of health insurance, but does not pay for treatment of cancers detected. The program also gives state health agencies the resources to conduct public and provider education about screening for these cancers and to conduct outreach activities to identify women who have never or rarely been screened. Much of this outreach activity involves working with community-based organizations to get the information out to their constituencies regarding the importance of screening and the availability of financial support.

Another element of the program is tracking, follow-up, and case management of women enrolled in the system. Since the program was established, more than three million screening examinations have been provided and about 10,000 cancers detected. The program now operates in all 50 states, the District of Columbia, 6 territories, and 12 American Indian/Alaskan Native organizations. The state health agencies, through relationships with local providers of care, are required to ensure that women identified with cancer are able to obtain treatment, despite their limited financial means. Treatment is usually provided as charity care, deeply discounted care, or, in a few states, is supported by specific appropriations for indigent care. In late 2000, however, Congress expanded Medicaid coverage, permitting states to cover treatment provided to women found to have cancer through this program.[37]

Since the beginning of the NBCCEDP, mammography rates nationwide have climbed steadily and reached over 80 percent of women in some states.[38] There have been especially large increases in screening among women with incomes of less than $35,000 and a shrinking of disparities in screening rates nationwide (Figure 18.1). Especially noteworthy has been the success of community efforts in which many groups have become active in helping to find women and getting them into the program.[31] An interesting offshoot has been increasing support for efforts to screen these women also for cardiovascular risks and to provide counseling or help in finding treatment.

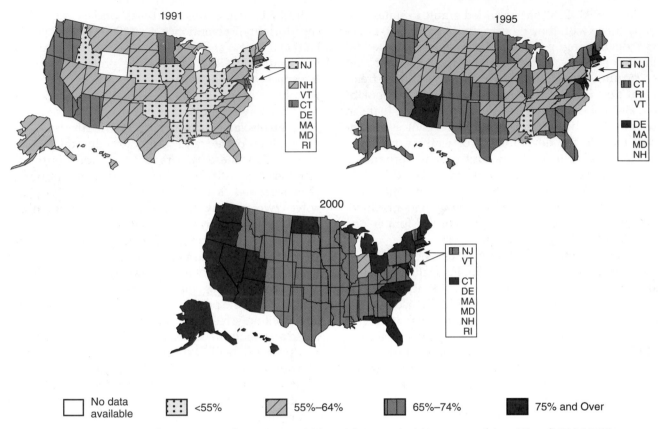

Figure 18.1. Percentage of Women Aged 50 Years or Older with Household Incomes of Less Than $35,000 Who Reported Having Had a Mammogram within the Previous 2 Years

Source: Centers for Disease Control and Prevention, Behavioral Risk Factor Surveillance System, 1991, 1995, and 2000.

Another new area of growth in public health is the establishment of populationwide cancer registries in all states. The National Program of Cancer Registries supports 45 states, allowing them to register all cancers by type, stage, and basic demographic information.[39] This new data system can serve as the base for assessing the quality of prevention and control programs. Before, with only mortality data, it was not possible to track trends in incidence or stage of cancer, so the impact of cancer control efforts that would be manifest by declines in breast and cervical cancer diagnosed in the late stages could not be assessed. The increasing use of data systems like the National Program of Cancer Registries is critical to the evaluation and improvement of public health control efforts.

Diabetes

The number of persons with diagnosed diabetes increased substantially during the 1990s, and recent BRFSS interviews indicate that 16 million Americans have diabetes.[40] This increase has been greatest among younger adults and minority populations. Although this increase in diagnosed cases has occurred, advancements in science have proven that interventions such as good foot care and retinal screening can prevent or delay the amputations and blindness that so often complicate diabetes. Further, good control of blood glucose can delay the renal disease that often comes with diabetes. Recent studies also have shown that moderate weight loss and physical activity can decrease the development of diabetes by about 60 percent.[41,42] Yet many of these advances are not being widely applied to persons at high risk.

For persons known to have diabetes, public health efforts have influenced systems of care to ensure appropriate services are provided that are known to delay complications. In some states, the public health agency has convened managed care organizations to agree on standards of care they would offer persons with diabetes. The cost of diabetes is so great on a day-to-day basis that efforts to upgrade quality of care would be problematic for any single health care organization lest even more persons with diabetes enroll, driving up costs. The use of a convening/consensus development process in some states has allowed all companies to upgrade care on an equivalent basis, not putting any one organization at a competitive disadvantage. This brokering could be possible only by a neutral other party, like the health department. Other states have established reminder systems and tracking programs, some of which have shown promising results, reducing hospitalizations and amputations by more than a third. Others have shown substantial improvement in measures of glucose control, retinal screening rates, and the use of influenza and pneumococcal vaccine among persons with diabetes.

Now that we know ways to delay the onset of diabetes for persons at high risk of developing the disease, we need to focus on providing the needed counseling and education to these persons regarding how they can modify their lifestyles to increase activity and to lose weight. Counseling and education will be important in both clinical and public health interventions. The successes being demonstrated in state pilot programs highlight the urgency to expand those programs to reduce and delay the complications among persons who already have diabetes. We also need to look beyond clinic-based activities. Programs that use churches and other community groups to help provide education to people with diabetes have helped these individuals improve their day-to-day management of the disease.

Arthritis

Arthritis is a relatively new area of emphasis in state public health control programs. It has many charac-

teristics that make it a good choice for intervention. Arthritis is very common, with estimates of more than 40 million Americans having one of the various forms. Arthritis affects people of all ages, and it is the leading cause of disability among adults.[43] Research has shown that some of the newer interventions can change the course of the illness, if begun early, and continued physical activity is vital to maintaining function.

Some people perceive that arthritis is an inevitable consequence of aging and that it is an irritation rather than a truly disabling condition. Such perceptions tremendously understate the importance of arthritis as a serious disease and can lead to delays in seeking care. States are now looking at what they can do to change these perceptions through public and provider education and to assess quality of care, with efforts focusing especially on racial and ethnic minorities and underserved populations.

Programs Targeting Risk Factors

One approach to analyzing risk factors is to determine how modifiable they are. Sex, age, and race are considered unchangeable. However, factors such as education, income, and levels of social support are moderately modifiable either at an individual or societal level. Other risk factors, such as diet, physical activity, smoking, and substance abuse, are highly modifiable. The revolution in what we know about genes and their relationship to different chronic diseases will lead to a new level of interplay between risk factors. We will be putting this new knowledge together to determine ultimately the outcomes for chronic diseases. When we talk about the idea of modifying risk factors, however, we usually think in terms of individual behavior change. Although we do try to modify group behavior and work at an organizational level, frequently, it comes down to an individual changing his or her routine behaviors.

How these various lifestyle factors relate to aging is another issue to consider. Lifestyle practices might not manifest themselves in terms of disease outcomes until years later. Moreover, the lifestyle factors themselves have different levels of prevalence over the course of any of our lifetimes. Therefore, it makes a much more complicated picture than the typical communicable disease relationship of a determinant of behavior, a risk that occurs relatively soon thereafter, and the consequences that occur soon after that. In the chronic disease field, we have latent periods between exposures and outcomes, and we have exposures that occur in varying amounts over long periods of time. Chronic disease control programs have targeted a variety of risk factors. The sections that follow focus on three risk factors: tobacco use, nutrition, and physical activity.

Tobacco Use

State health department activities to prevent and control tobacco use have increased markedly in recent years. This growth has resulted from a variety of factors:

- Rising public intolerance of environmental smoke as a health hazard and unpleasant annoyance
- State legislation to restrict indoor smoking
- Increased excise taxes on cigarettes, with funds going to support tobacco control programs
- Funding and support from the National Cancer Institute, the American Cancer Society, the CDC's Office on Smoking and Health, and nongovernment sources
- Master Settlement Agreement funds from the tobacco industry
- Activism by consumer groups

In addition, public health activities to prevent and control tobacco use include mass media campaigns, community efforts such as school-based interventions, tobacco use cessation services, and policies.[44] California had much success during the early years after passing Proposition 99, which raised the excise tax on a pack of cigarettes by 25 cents in 1989 and originally designated some of the revenues for tobacco control activities. In the first five years after the excise tax was raised, monthly cigarette consumption per person declined 52 percent, from 9.7 packs in 1989 to 6.5 packs in 1993.

The decline was significantly greater in California than in the rest of the United States. No significant declines in cigarette consumption occurred between 1994 and 1996, possibly because of reduced funding for the state's tobacco control program, increased funding for tobacco advertising and promotion, tobacco industry pricing, and political activities.[45,46] Since 1996, however, per capita cigarette consumption has continued to decline, dropping 11.5 percent between 1998 and 1999.[47] Because of the reductions in tobacco consumption observed in California, rates of new lung cancer cases and deaths from coronary heart disease have both declined significantly faster among California residents in recent years than in the rest of the country.[46,48]

Nutrition

Only in recent years have state nutrition programs expanded beyond their traditional maternal, infant, and childhood nutrition activities, which have focused primarily on undernutrition. Increasingly, overnutrition is being recognized as the major contemporary nutritional issue in the United States. Most Americans, including children, need to reduce their intake of calories, fat, salt, and sugar and to increase their intake of grains, fiber-containing foods, fruits, and vegetables. Such a healthful diet would help prevent many chronic diseases, including coronary heart disease, hypertension and stroke, noninsulin-dependent diabetes mellitus, and several types of cancer.

Such a diet also would help prevent overweight and obesity, which have increased in prevalence in recent decades.[8,49] The percentage of U.S. adults aged 20–74 years who were overweight (body mass index of 25 or more) increased from 46.4 percent in 1976–1980 to 55 percent in 1988–1994.[8] Public interest in weight loss is great, but few weight-loss programs have yielded sustainable results. Experts in the field generally agree that sustainable weight loss depends on a combination of balanced diet and increased physical activity.

Physical Activity

In 1996, the U.S. surgeon general reported that a majority of U.S. adults either were not active enough to achieve health benefits or were sedentary, engaging in no leisure-time physical activity.[50] This trend has not changed substantially. In 1998, nearly 46 percent of adults reported insufficient physical activity, and more than 28 percent reported no physical activity, according to BRFSS data.[51] An increasing body of evidence shows that being sedentary is unhealthy and that even moderate amounts of low-intensity physical activity improve health outcomes.

Increased physical activity is associated with better outcomes for such diverse conditions as coronary heart disease, diabetes, hypertension, colorectal cancer, depression, and osteoporosis. Despite such findings, limited public health attention and resources have been devoted to promoting physical activity. Public health interventions that have been tried include environmental approaches that encourage increased activity as a part of daily life, such as attractive and accessible stairwells and sidewalks, safe neighborhoods, and affordable neighborhood facilities for leisure-time exercise. Mass media campaigns, health provider incentives, school programs, and activities to increase strength and mobility among older Americans are also components of public health interventions to promote physical activity.

Program Settings

Risk behaviors, health status, and health outcomes are the product of their unique environments. By looking at cultural, community, and social settings, we can learn much about the context *within which* health occurs as well as the context *through which* health occurs. For instance, the places where people spend most of their time (e.g., family, workplace, school, leisure setting) provide an efficient way to analyze, understand, and influence the determinants of health. These settings also allow us to effectively reach and influence individuals and communities.

The settings where chronic disease control activities take place are diverse. For example, an intervention's setting could be a geopolitical area such as a city. It might be the local school or hospital. Programs can also be set in workplaces or in areas where people spend their leisure time, such as a recreation area or a restaurant. Setting might not refer to a place at all, but rather the relationships that people share—for example, people who belong to a social club or who are

part of an Internet group. In this chapter, four types of settings are discussed: families, schools, workplaces, and communities.

Families

The home is where many health behaviors are established. Family members influence, motivate, and reinforce each other's behaviors and decisions about nutrition, physical activity, health screenings, oral health, and use of tobacco, alcohol, and other substances. A family's health can be greatly affected by an intervention, even an activity that targets just one family member. However, health promotion programs can have even greater effectiveness when multiple family members are involved and when links are strengthened between families and other settings such as schools, workplaces, and health care systems.[52] Interventions targeting smoking and obesity among schoolchildren have been more effective when other family members have been involved.[53–56]

Schools

School-based interventions to promote health can be highly effective because schools are where children spend much of their time. In addition, schoolchildren are impressionable, and many lifelong habits—healthy and unhealthy—are formed during childhood and adolescence. Moreover, because schools are relatively controlled environments, they are ideal sites for environmental interventions such as no-smoking policies, healthy school lunch programs, and physical education classes that promote physical activity.[57]

Schools also offer resources that can aid in chronic disease control and health promotion efforts. For example, teachers can serve as role models to encourage children to adopt healthy habits, and they can incorporate health messages in their curricula. Numerous curricula for school health education are available, and some schools have integrated school health into physical education, science, and math curricula. More U.S. school health programs are placing greater emphasis on preventing tobacco use, pregnancy, violence, and suicide and on case management for students with chronic health conditions, according to findings from the School Health Policies and Programs Study 2000. In addition, more middle/junior and senior high schools are offering 1 percent milk, and fewer schools are offering whole milk to students.[58]

The Institute of Medicine and CDC recommend planned, sequential strategies that promote the physical development of children in grades K–12 as well as their emotional, social, and educational development.[59,60] The CDC approach includes eight components: (1) health education curricula; (2) physical education curricula; (3) health services that focus on prevention and early intervention; (4) nutrition services in the cafeteria and classrooms; (5) health promotion for school staff; (6) counseling, psychological, and social services for students; (7) a healthy school environment; and (8) activities that encourage parents and community members to support healthy behaviors among students and that link school and community health programs.

School settings also can pose barriers—such as overworked teachers, lack of school resources, lack of teacher training in health issues, and competing academic priorities—that impede the intervention's success.[57] These limitations must be considered when school-based health promotion programs are being planned.

Workplaces

From a public health perspective, the workplace provides many opportunities for promoting health and preventing disease. Such programs have the potential to influence social norms, establish health policies, promote healthy behaviors, improve employees' knowledge and skills, help them get necessary health screenings and follow-up care, and reduce their on-the-job exposure to substances that can cause chronic diseases.[61] From the employer's point of view, workplace health promotion programs offer the promise of lower health, life, and disability insurance costs; reduced workers' compensation costs; less absenteeism; increased productivity and morale; and less turnover.

For these reasons, most U.S. employers now provide some type of health promotion activities.[62] The scope of these activities varies according to the employer's size and resources. For example, a small business might give employees self-help materials on reducing stress or lowering cholesterol levels. A large corporation might have a full staff, on-site facilities, and classes promoting fitness, weight management, nutrition, blood pressure control, smoking cessation, and counseling about drug and alcohol abuse. Most employee health programs aim to change the behaviors of individual employees, but some employers have made policy and environmental changes—for example, by passing and enforcing no-smoking policies and providing healthy food choices in vending machines and at cafeterias. Community outreach is also a part of some workplace health promotion programs, which offer their services to employees' families and members of the community.

Unfortunately, few workplace interventions have undergone rigorous, long-term evaluation to determine their effects on employee health or costs. Moreover, measuring the effects of workplace programs is difficult. As Polanyi and colleagues point out, most health indicators used to measure employee health—such as absenteeism, sick leave, and use of benefits—also reflect factors outside the job.[63] The best studied and most cost-effective interventions are those providing work-based monitoring and treatment for high blood pressure. Workplace smoking-cessation programs also appear to be cost-effective.

Communities

There are many definitions for community. Some chronic disease control programs define community as a place, such as a neighborhood that has geographic boundaries. For other programs, the community setting might be a group of people who share a common bond—for example, a religious congregation or a sports league. Using a community setting for an intervention can have many benefits:

- The community can give health providers access to specific populations, particularly racial and ethnic groups that are at increased risk for chronic disease and populations that are underserved.
- People in the community have a chance to establish their own health priorities and agendas.

- Health messages are more likely to be effective when they are delivered by someone within the community, who is socially and culturally similar to community members and who speaks the same language.
- Communities provide the opportunity for social support for healthy behavioral changes.

Some of the drawbacks of community settings include concern about differential treatment and discrimination; arguments over who owns or controls the program; lack of trust; apathy or lack of interest; the economic costs of participating in the program; and cultural insensitivity and ignorance.

Several successful chronic disease control efforts have been set in a combination of community sites. These programs have reached more people at the multiple sites, but more important, they have reestablished norms on a widespread basis and significantly reduced risk behaviors, biological risk factors, as well as deaths and morbidity.[64–68]

Populations

Specific populations are the focus of public health programs for most chronic diseases.

Racial and Ethnic Groups

First are some racial and ethnic groups because they have a higher incidence of chronic diseases, poorer health outcomes, or both. Because chronic illnesses place such a burden on the population, these conditions contribute greatly to the overall disparity in health between these groups of people and the majority population. The Healthy People 2010 objectives of eliminating racial and ethnic disparities in health emphasize the importance of increased efforts in chronic disease prevention and control in minority populations with poor health indicators.[19]

Young People

The opportunities for successful intervention are great during youth because many of the behaviors that increase a person's risk for chronic disease are established in late childhood or adolescence. For example, about 80 percent of regular adult smokers began regular tobacco use by age 18.[69] Moreover, poor eating habits and low levels of physical activity among children and teenagers are contributing to increasing rates of obesity and diabetes. There is a growing science base indicating that programs aimed at children and teenagers can lessen the likelihood they will start using tobacco and improve their nutritional and physical activity choices.[12,50]

Older People

The aging of the population has led to increasing interest in programs that encourage older adults to engage in healthful behaviors, especially physical activity. In years past, we had a sense of futility, believing there would be little benefit if older adults changed their behaviors. We now know that quality of life and functioning are substantially improved when older people become physically active and quit smoking, even late in life. The cost of health care and the growing concern over the cost of long-term health care has led public health agencies to explore their role in fostering active lifestyles among older adults.

EMERGING ISSUES

The beginning of the new millennium was a time of appraisal for public health.[63] The twentieth century witnessed an extraordinary change in the health of the public, particularly in the economically developed world.[70, 71] A transition occurred as we became less worried about infectious diseases of the past and more focused on newly emerging health problems. In many cases, these new health problems are the fruits of successful public health actions, such as clean water systems and childhood immunizations. The simple fact that every day people live to an age when the simple biology of aging takes its toll is an impressive phenomenon.

The success of the past century has also made us painfully aware of the challenges still facing public health worldwide. Many of these challenges have direct and extraordinary implications for chronic disease prevention and control. Several areas of concern for public health that greatly affect chronic disease and health promotion include (1) war and terrorism; (2) migration and urbanization; (3) environmental degradation; (4) inequality related to economic, social, and gender differences; and (5) the role of genetic interventions. These are global phenomena, thus our approach to addressing them domestically will be limited.

It is impossible to fully cover each of these challenges in this chapter; however, we briefly touch on four critical areas for chronic disease in the context of the larger global concerns raised above. First, we will address immigration and border health, which have a high impact on the United States and illustrate keenly how dependent we are on our neighbors. Population movements play a key role in defining the epidemiological landscape for chronic disease. Second, we will cover this country's global connections and how the behaviors that increase people's risk for chronic diseases in the United States—for example, tobacco use and physical inactivity—are spreading to other parts of the world. Likewise, U.S. knowledge about effective interventions is being shared with other nations. A third topic, obesity, reflects a larger concern with malnutrition around the globe. Some countries suffer from undernutrition, some from overnutrition, and yet others from chronic conditions resulting from the fundamental lack of basic micronutrients such as vitamin A and iodine. Finally, we discuss mental health and mental disorders, which need to be rationally integrated into our understanding of chronic diseases and health promotion. Many mental disorders are chronic in their course, and many chronic diseases result in mental pathology as well as associated mental disability. A holistic view of chronic disease demands consideration of the whole person, physical and mental.

Immigration and Border Health

Immigration and migration across national boundaries are significant phenomena around the world.[72] One often thinks of such migration as an outcome of war or tragedy and associates it with disruptions of populations under duress. Although that is certainly true, the impact of immigration in the United States is largely and historically of a different type. It is the result of significant numbers of foreign nationals migrating to the United States to seek work and economic benefits from one of the wealthiest countries in the world. The magnitude of this migration has been most pronounced in the growth of the Hispanic population in the United States during the last decade of the twentieth century. Although this population growth has occurred in many large U.S. cities, the public health impact has been most notable along the border between the United States and Mexico.[73–77]

The United States–Mexico border region is defined as an area 62 miles (100 kilometers) north and south of the border, as established by the United States–Mexico Border Health Commission. Healthy Border 2010 is a binational initiative that contains characteristics of health programs in both the United States and Mexico.[73] From the United States, this initiative draws on this country's Healthy People 2010 program.[19] From Mexico, the initiative draws on the National Health Indicators *(Indicadores de Resultados)* Program, which tracks health measures at the national, state, and local levels in Mexico. These two programs share 20 objectives, which represent most of the priority areas for action on health issues in the border region. Several of these shared objectives address chronic diseases. Notable in particular are cancer (reducing breast cancer and cervical cancer deaths) and diabetes (reducing diabetes-related deaths and the need for hospitalization).

Studying chronic diseases in a defined border region undergoing enormous population change provides an important research opportunity. Health problems in the border region of Mexico are in an epidemiologic transition from infectious to chronic diseases.[75,77] For example, the cancer death rate in the border region of Mexico is higher than the rate for the rest of Mexico. People in this region are also hard hit by diabetes-related deaths. Age-adjusted mortality rates were 13.7 per 100,000 for U.S. border residents in 1998 but a striking 74.6 for Mexican border residents in the years 1995–1997. As years pass and the border possibly settles into a more stable area of transition, the U.S. rate might increase while the Mexico rate falls. But we have no way of knowing whether this will happen because so many variables come into play in this changing, dynamic population.

Global Connections

Global interest in the burden of chronic diseases and their risk factors has grown dramatically over the last several years, reflecting a confluence of factors. Several recent World Health Organization reports have noted that chronic diseases are now the leading causes of death and disability-adjusted life years worldwide, and their prevalence is growing rapidly.[1] Although chronic diseases make up a greater proportion of illnesses and deaths in developed countries, the aggregate greatest numbers of deaths and illnesses are occurring in the developing world.

Perhaps most compelling is the realization that the forces increasing risk—including the spread of tobacco use, reductions in physical activity, and increases in obesity—do not stop at any one nation's border. We have long known that infectious organisms easily cross borders, given extensive world travel, shipment of goods, and migration of peoples and animals. Thus, solutions have had to be global and nations have had to cooperate extensively and share responsibility to curtail the spread of infectious diseases. For the United States, self-interest requires that we provide global assistance for the control of chronic diseases as well as for infectious diseases. Through mass communications such as television and the Internet, patterns of behavior that increase or decrease risk (like the use of tobacco) are rapidly communicated across thousands of miles and to millions of people. One can easily make the case that these diseases are actually more communicable than those of infectious origin. Knowledge, attitudes, behaviors, and policies spread across borders with greater ease than ever before. These problems are global, and solutions will need to be as well.

Relatedly, much of the science regarding intervention comes from countries other than the United States. North Karelia, Finland, was the site of the most famous intervention effort to reduce cardiovascular disease through community-wide risk factor modification.[64,65] Some of the best data on the effectiveness of mammography come from Sweden. The first randomized studies of the prevention of diabetes come from Finland and China. The behavioral risk factor surveillance carried out in the United States is increasingly being used as a model by other countries around the world.

We must both learn from and share with others outside our borders to attend to our own best interests.

Obesity

Evidence from various sources has shown a startling increase in the prevalence of obesity in the U.S. population (Figure 18.2).[40,78] Since the late 1980s, this country has seen a 50 percent increase in the proportion of adults who are obese (they have a body mass index of 30 or more).[79] This increase has been greater among minority populations and younger adults. The obesity epidemic has spread even faster among children, with a doubling of their rate of overweight between the early 1980s and the early 1990s.[49] This increase is clearly the result of environmental changes that foster inactivity and overnutrition.

Genetics influences weight, but the human genome has not changed substantially in the last two decades. Rather, trends such as the loss of physical education in schools, increasing portion sizes, and the tendency to eat meals away from home are making it hard for people to maintain their appropriate weight. As would be expected with the increase in weight, we have seen a parallel increase in the prevalence of diabetes among adults, especially young adults.[40] Public health has been slow to address these issues, and most states have very rudimentary programs to support changes in communities or individuals. These twin epidemics represent a critical challenge facing public health in this next century, in part because of their scale, affecting so many millions of persons, and also because of their serious disease implications.

The causes of the obesity epidemic are society-wide, rather than individual, and the solutions will lie outside the usual purview of public health influence. To combat obesity, public health practitioners will need to be more advocacy-oriented than in the past. We also will require greater support from other sectors of our society—outside of public health—to reverse this epidemic.

Mental Health

In the United States, mental health has often been viewed as outside the realm of public health. Although it is readily apparent that many mental health

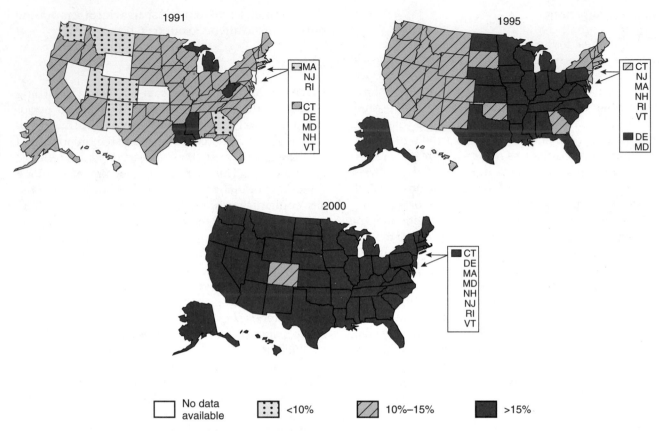

Figure 18.2. Percentage of Adults Who Are Obese (Approximately 30 Pounds Overweight or Body Mass Index of 30 or More)

Source: Centers for Disease Control and Prevention, Behavioral Risk Factor Surveillance System, 1991, 1995, and 2000.

problems such as unipolar and bipolar depression are often long term and chronic, they have seldom been considered one of the chronic diseases. Further, the public health approach, focusing on the population perspective, was not considered applicable to mental health issues. These views have changed dramatically in recent years. We are beginning to recognize the burden of mental illness, and organizations such as the Institute of Medicine are adding a public health and population prevention perspective to mental health.[80,81]

Neurological, psychological, and developmental disorders raise some interesting and new concerns for chronic disease prevention. Although certain chronic diseases such as cancer have historically been associated with the irrational shunning of afflicted individuals, the mental illnesses, ranging from epilepsy to schizophrenia, have long suffered from stigma. Thus, the general nature in which these disorders are treated and viewed has itself become a concern for public health activists.

One common aspect of mental health disorders and chronic diseases is the strong emphasis on behavior. Many of the same strategies for prevention that involve changing knowledge, attitudes, and behaviors in chronic disease apply equally to mental disorders and mental health. Equally appropriate is the core scientific approach of chronic disease epidemiology. Many mental health problems share a position of comorbidity and causation with chronic illnesses. For example, alcohol abuse can lead to any number of chronic diseases but also to neurological and psychological disorders as well as violence and injury. Thus, the strategies for defining mental health problems as well as the interventions must be integrated with well-established chronic disease and health promotion efforts at the individual, community, and population levels.

CONCLUSIONS

The rising prominence of chronic diseases to the point where they are now the leading causes of death can be thought of as one of the great success stories of public health during the twentieth century. This growth reflects our tremendous success in controlling infectious agents with sanitation, safe water, immunizations, and antibiotics. It also reflects improvements in nutrition, living conditions, and income and education and the fact that life expectancy has increased so remarkably that people now live long enough to develop and usually die of one of the major chronic illnesses. Just as seriously, the growth of chronic illnesses can be thought of as one of public health's greatest failures, especially of the late twentieth century. The principal known causes of premature chronic diseases are tobacco use, overnutrition, and physical inactivity. During the 1960s and 1970s, we made some progress in diminishing the toll that tobacco use has had on this country. Then in the 1990s, rates of tobacco use among children started to climb. Rates of overnutrition and physical inactivity continue to increase unabated.

On the hopeful side is that a generation of investment in research has led to much understanding about the causes of these diseases and how to intervene, especially clinically. However, the translation of science into widespread application has been neglected and, hence, is painfully slow. For example, the first recommendations that women should receive mammograms were announced in the late 1970s, and yet we are only now beginning to see more than 70 percent of women receiving regular screening. As a result, many thousands of women have died because of failure to receive mammograms after the science was clear that they should. Similar stories exist for diabetes, heart disease, stroke, and other chronic ill-

nesses. This issue becomes even more critical for the poor and underserved. The prevention, delay, and control of chronic diseases, without a doubt, will be one of the fundamental challenges for public health in the twenty-first century.

Although there are many ways we can respond to this challenge, three will be among the most prominent. First, we must shorten the time it takes to get the fruits of research widely applied, especially to those in great need. If we fail to do so, our whole research enterprise is undermined. Research, unapplied, is sterile, serving no purpose. Second, we must recognize that chronic illnesses will require more societal, environmental, and policy interventions. Individual-level interventions that might have been effective for one person will not be sufficient for the many millions who are at risk. People's attempts at individual behavioral change must be supported and fostered by societal cues and policies that help them more easily choose and sustain healthful behaviors. Last, arguably the greatest challenge to public health in the twenty-first century will be to eliminate health disparities between racial and ethnic groups, between rich and poor. Although we have made great strides overall in promoting health, we have made little progress in eliminating these disparities.

To effectively address these challenges, we in public health need to establish partnerships with many sectors of U.S. society that have not traditionally worked with us. We also will need to be more oriented to advocacy than ever before and persuade these nontraditional partners to embrace our mission and goals in chronic disease control.

ACKNOWLEDGMENTS

We are deeply indebted to Valerie R. Johnson for her editorial assistance, Deborah Holtzman and Karin Mack for verifying and updating BRFSS data for the U.S. maps, Herman Surles for graphics support, and Emma G. Stupp and Brenda W. Mazzocchi for assistance with the references. We also thank the following individuals for providing helpful feedback on the manuscript: Donna F. Stroup, Phyllis L. Moir, Terry F. Pechacek, William H. Dietz, Sue Lin Yee, Ralph J. Coates, Michael M. Engelgau, and Nancy A. Haynie-Mooney.

References

1. World Health Organization, World Bank. *The Global Burden of Disease.* Cambridge, Mass: Harvard University Press; 1996.
2. World Bank. *World Development Report 1993.* New York, NY: Oxford University Press; 1993.
3. Murphy SL. Deaths: Final data for 1998. *National Vital Statistics Reports.* Vol 48, No. 11. Hyattsville, Md: National Center for Health Statistics, Centers for Disease Control and Prevention; 2000. PHS Publication 2000-1120.
4. American Heart Association. *2001 Heart and Stroke Statistical Update.* Dallas, Tex: American Heart Association; 2000.
5. American Cancer Society. *Cancer Facts and Figures— 2000.* Atlanta, Ga: American Cancer Society; 2000.
6. Centers for Disease Control and Prevention. *Unrealized Prevention Opportunities: Reducing the Health and Economic Burden of Chronic Disease.* Atlanta, Ga: Centers for Disease Control and Prevention; 2000.
7. Centers for Disease Control and Prevention. *Chronic Diseases and Their Risk Factors: The Nation's Leading Causes of Death.* Atlanta, Ga: Centers for Disease Control and Prevention; 1999.
8. Eberhardt MS, Ingram DD, Makuc DM, et al. *Urban and Rural Health Chartbook. Health, United States, 2001.* Hyattsville, Md: US Dept of Health and Human Services; Centers for Disease Control and Prevention, National Center for Health Statistics; 2001.
9. Centers for Disease Control and Prevention. *Revised Final FY 1999 Performance Plan and FY 2000 Performance Plan.* Atlanta, Ga: Centers for Disease Control and Prevention; 2001. Available at: www.cdc.gov/od/perfplan/2000vii.htm. Accessed September 26, 2001.
10. McGinnis JM, Foege WH. Actual causes of death in the United States. *JAMA.* 1993;270:2207-2212.
11. Hahn RA, Teutsch SM, Rothenberg RB, Marks JS. Excess deaths from nine chronic diseases in the United States, 1986. *JAMA.* 1990;264:2654-2659.
12. US Department of Health and Human Services. *Reducing Tobacco Use: A Report of the Surgeon General.* Atlanta, Ga: US Dept of Health and Human Services, Centers for Disease Control and Prevention, National Center for Chronic Disease Prevention and Health Promotion; 2000.
13. Thun MJ, Apicella LF, Henley SJ. Smoking vs. other risk factors as the cause of smoking-attributable deaths. *JAMA.* 2000;284:706-712.
14. Teutsch SM, Churchill RE. *Principles and Practice of Public Health Surveillance.* New York, NY: Oxford University Press; 2000.
15. Centers for Disease Control and Prevention. Updated guidelines for evaluating public health surveillance systems: recommendations from the Guidelines Working Group. *MMWR.* 2001;50 (RR-13):1-35.
16. General bill of mortality for the year 1665. In: David FN. *Games, Gods, and Gambling.* London, England: Griffin; 1962:101.
17. Centers for Disease Control and Prevention. *International Classification of Diseases, Tenth Revision, Clinical Modification (ICD-10-CM).* Hyattsville, Md: US Dept of Health and Human Services, Centers for Disease Control and Prevention, National Center for Health Statistics; 2001. Available at: http://www.cdc.gov/nchs/about/otheract/icd9/abticd10.htm. Accessed October 4, 2001.
18. Oregon Department of Human Services. *Oregon's Tobacco Prevention and Education Program: Saving Lives and Saving Dollars.* Portland: Oregon Depart of Human Services; 2000.
19. US Department of Health and Human Services. *Healthy People 2010.* 2nd ed. Washington, DC: US Government Printing Office; November 2000.
20. Washington Business Group on Health. *WBGH/CDC Disease and Disability Prevention Resources.* Washington, DC: Washington Business Group on Health; 2001. Available at: http://www.wbgh.org/cdc. Accessed October 5, 2001.
21. Jessen RJ. *Statistical Survey Techniques.* New York, NY: John Wiley & Sons; 1978.
22. Forsyth BH, Lessler J. Cognitive laboratory methods: a taxonomy. In: Biemer PP, Groves RM, Lyberg LE, Mathiowetz NA, Sudman S, eds. *Measurement Errors in Surveys. Wiley Series in Probability and Mathematical Statistics.* New York, NY: John Wiley; 1991:393-48.
23. Lyberg L, Kasprzyk D. Data collection methods and measurement error: an overview. In: Biemer PP, Groves RM, Lyberg LE, Mathiowetz NA, Sudman S, eds. *Measurement Errors in Surveys. Wiley Series in Probability and Mathematical Statistics.* New York, NY: John Wiley & Sons; 1991:237-258.
24. Stroup DF, Teutsch SM. *Statistics in Public Health: Qualitative Approaches to Public Health Problems.* New York, NY: Oxford University Press; 1998.

25. Dean K, ed. *Population Health Research: Linking Theory and Methods*. London, England: Sage Publications; 1993.

26. Centers for Disease Control and Prevention. *Prevention Research Centers: Investing in the Nation's Health*. Atlanta, Ga: Centers for Disease Control and Prevention; 2001. Available at: http://www.cdc.gov/prc/glance.htm. Accessed October 5, 2001.

27. Centers for Disease Control and Prevention. *Racial and Ethnic Approaches to Community Health (REACH 2010): Addressing Disparities in Health*. Atlanta, Ga: Centers for Disease Control and Prevention; 2001. Available at: http://www.cdc.gov/reach2010/aag-reach.htm. Accessed October 5, 2001.

28. McKenna MT, Taylor WR, Marks JS, Koplan JP. Current issues and challenges in chronic disease control. In: Brownson RC, Remington, PL, Davis JR, eds. *Chronic Disease Epidemiology and Control*. Washington, DC: American Public Health Association; 1998.

29. Centers for Disease Control and Prevention. *Preventing Heart Disease and Stroke: Addressing the Nation's Leading Killers*. Atlanta, Ga: Centers for Disease Control and Prevention; 2001. Available at: http://www.cdc.gov/nccdphp/cvd/cvdaag.htm. Accessed October 5, 2001.

30. Henson RM, Wyatt SW, Lee NC. The National Breast and Cervical Cancer Early Detection Program: a comprehensive public health response to two major health issues for women. *J Public Health Manage Pract*. 1996;2(2):36-47.

31. Holt H. Progress report: the National Strategic Plan for the Early Detection and Control of Breast and Cervical Cancers. *J Womens Health*. 1998;7(4):411-413.

32. National Cancer Institute. *SEER Cancer Statistics Review, 1973-1998*. Bethesda, Md: National Cancer Institute; 2001.

33. Brekelmans C, Westers P, Faber J, Peeters P, Collette H. Age-specific sensitivity and sojourn time in a breast cancer screening programme (DOM) in the Netherlands: a comparison of different methods. *J Epidemiol Com Health*. 1996;50:68-71.

34. Duffy SW, Day NE, Tabar L, Chen H, Smith T. Markov models of breast tumor progression: some age-specific results. *J Natl Cancer Inst Mono*. 1997;22:93-97.

35. Rimer BK, Schildkraut J, Hiatt, RA. Cancer screening. In: DeVita VT, Hellman S, Rosenberg SA, eds. *Cancer Principles and Practice of Oncology*. 6th ed. Philadelphia, Pa: Lippincott-Williams & Wilkins; 2001.

36. US Preventive Services Task Force. *Guide to Clinical Preventive Services*. 2nd ed. Baltimore, Md: Williams & Wilkins; 1996.

37. 106th Congress. *Breast and Cervical Cancer Prevention and Treatment Act of 2000*. Pub L No. 106-354, 114 Stat 1381. H.R. 4386 (S. 662). Approved October 24, 2000.

38. Blackman DK, Bennett EM, Miller DS. Trends in self-reported use of mammograms (1989-1997) and Papanicolaou tests (1991-1997)—Behavioral Risk Factor Surveillance System. *CDC Surveillance Summaries. MMWR*. 1999;48(SS-6):1-22.

39. Hutton M, Simpson LD, Miller DS, Weir HK, McDavid K, Hall HI. Progress toward nationwide cancer surveillance: an evaluation of the National Program of Cancer Registries, 1994-1999. *J Registry Manage*. 2001;28(3):113-120.

40. Mokdad AH, Bowman BA, Ford ES, Vinicor F, Marks JS, Koplan JP. The continuing epidemics of obesity and diabetes in the United States. *JAMA*. 2001;286(10):1195-1200.

41. Tuomilehto J, Lindstrom J, Eriksson JG, et al. Prevention of Type 2 diabetes mellitus by changes in lifestyle among subjects with impaired glucose tolerance. *N Engl J Med*. 2001;344(18):1343-1350.

42. US Department of Health and Human Services. Diet and exercise dramatically delay Type 2 diabetes; diabetes medication Metformin also effective. *HHS News*. August 8, 2001.

43. Centers for Disease Control and Prevention. Prevalence of disabilities and associated health conditions among adults—United States, 1999. *MMWR*. 2001;50:120-125.

44. Centers for Disease Control and Prevention. *Best Practices for Comprehensive Tobacco Control Programs*. Atlanta, Ga: US Dept of Health and Human Services, Centers for Disease Control and Prevention; 1999.

45. Pierce JP, Gilpin EA, Emery SL, White MM, Rosbrook B, Berry CC. Has the California Tobacco Control Program reduced smoking? *JAMA*. 1998;280:893-899.

46. Centers for Disease Control and Prevention. Declines in lung cancer rates—California, 1988-1997. *MMWR*. 2000;49(47);1066-1069.

47. California Department of Health Services. *California Tobacco Control Update*. Sacramento, Calif: California Depart of Health Services; 2000.

48. Fichtenberg CM, Glantz SA. Association of the California Tobacco Control Program with declines in cigarette consumption and mortality from heart disease. *New Engl J Med*. 2000;343(24):1772-1777.

49. Troiano RP, Flegal KM. Overweight children and adolescents: description, epidemiology, and demographics. *Pediatrics*. 1998;101(3):497-504.

50. US Department of Health and Human Services. *Physical Activity and Health: A Report of the Surgeon General.* Atlanta, Ga: US Dept of Health and Human Services, Centers for Disease Control and Prevention, National Center for Chronic Disease Prevention and Health Promotion; 1996.

51. Centers for Disease Control and Prevention. Physical activity trends—United States, 1990-1998. *MMWR.* 2001;50(9):166-169.

52. Soubhi H, Potvin L. Homes and families as health promotion settings. In: Poland BD, Green LW, Rootman I, eds. *Settings for Health Promotion.* Thousand Oaks, Calif: Sage Publications; 2000.

53. Bonaguro EW, Bonaguro JA. Tobacco use among adolescents: directions for research. *Am J Health Promotion.* 1989;4(1):37-41.

54. Nader PR, Sellers DE, Johnson CC, et al. The effect of adult participation in a school-based family intervention to improve children's diet and physical activity: The Child and Adolescent Trial for Cardiovascular Health. *Prev Med.* 1996;25:455-464.

55. Epstein LH, Wing RR, Koeske R, Valoski A. Long-term effects of family-based treatment of childhood obesity. *J Consult Clin Psychol.* 1987;55:91-95.

56. Kirschenbaum DS, Harris ES, Tomarken AJ. Effects of parental involvement in behavioral weight loss therapy for preadolescents. *Behav Ther.* 1984;15:485-500.

57. Parcel GS, Kelder SH, Basen-Engquist K. The school as a setting for health promotion. In: Poland BD, Green LW, Rootman I, eds. *Settings for Health Promotion.* Thousand Oaks, Calif: Sage Publications; 2000.

58. Kolbe LJ, Kann L, Brener ND. Overview and summary of findings: School Health Policies and Programs Study 2000. *J School Health.* 2001;71(7):253-259.

59. Institute of Medicine. *Schools and Health: Our Nation's Investment.* Washington, DC: National Academy Press; 1997.

60. Allensworth DD, Kolbe LJ. The comprehensive school health program: exploring an expanded concept. *J School Health.* 1987;57(10):409-412.

61. Davis JR, Schwartz R, Wheeler F, Lancaster RB. Intervention methods for chronic disease control. In: Brownson RC, Remington PL, Davis JR. *Chronic Disease Epidemiology and Control.* 2nd ed. Washington, DC: American Public Health Association; 1998.

62. Biener L, DePue JD, Emmons KM, Linnan L, Abrams DB. Recruitment of work sites to a health promotion research trial: implications for generalizability. *J Occup Med.* 1994;36:631-636.

63. Polanyi MFD, Frank JW, Shannon HS, Sullivan TJ, Lavis JN. Promoting the determinants of good health in the workplace. In: Poland BD, Green LW, Rootman I, eds. *Settings for Health Promotion.* Thousand Oaks, Calif: Sage Publications; 2000.

64. Puska P, Tuomilehto J, Nissinen A, et al. The North Karelia Project: 15 years of community based prevention of coronary heart disease. *Ann Med.* 1989;21:169-173.

65. Farquhar JW, Fortmann SP, Flora JA, et al. Effects of communitywide education on cardiovascular disease risk factors. *JAMA.* 1990;264:359-365.

66. Blackburn H, Luepker RV, Kline FG, et al. The Minnesota Heart Health Program: a research and demonstration project in cardiovascular disease prevention. In: Matarazzo JD, Weiss SM, Herd JA, Miller NE, Weiss SM, eds. *Behavioral Health: A Handbook of Health Enhancement and Disease Prevention.* New York, NY: John Wiley & Sons; 1984:1171-1178.

67. Farquhar JW, Maccoby N, Wood PD, et al. Community education for cardiovascular health. *Lancet.* 1997;1:1192-1195.

68. Lasater T, Abrams D, Artz L, et al. Lay volunteer delivery of a community-based cardiovascular risk factor change program: the Pawtucket experience. In: Matarazzo JD, Weiss SM, Herd JA, Miller NE, Weiss SM, eds. *Behavioral Health: A Handbook of Health Enhancement and Disease Prevention.* New York, NY: John Wiley & Sons; 1984:1166-1170.

69. US Department of Health and Human Services. *Preventing Tobacco Use Among Young People: A Report of the Surgeon General.* Atlanta, Ga: US Dept of Health and Human Services, Centers for Disease Control and Prevention, National Center for Chronic Disease Prevention and Health Promotion; 1994.

70. Koop CE, Pearson CE, Schwarz MR, eds. *Critical Issues in Global Health.* San Francisco, Calif: Jossey-Bass; 2001.

71. Centers for Disease Control and Prevention. Ten great public health achievements—United States, 1900-1999. *MMWR.* 1999;48(12):241-243.

72. United Nations Population Division. *World Population Prospects: The 1998 Revision.* New York, NY: United Nations; 1999.

73. Office of International and Refugee Health. *Health on the US–Mexico Border: Past, Present and Future. A Preparatory Report to the Future United States–Mexico Border Health Commission.* Rockville, Md: US Dept of Health and Human Services; 1999.

74. Bruhn JG, Brandon JE, eds. *Border Health: Challenges for the United States and Mexico.* New York, NY: Garland; 1997

75. Pan American Health Organization. *Mortality Profiles of the Sister Communities on the United States–Mexico Border.* Washington, DC: Pan American Health Organization; 2000.

76. Power JG, Byrd T. *US-Mexico Border Health: Issues for Regional and Migrant Populations.* Thousand Oaks, Calif: Sage Publications; 1998.

77. Mitchell BD, Haffner SM, Hazuda HP, et al. Diabetes and coronary heart disease risk in Mexican Americans. *Ann Epidemiol.* 1992;2:101-106.

78. Mokdad AH, Serdula MK, Dietz WH, Bowman BA, Marks JS, Koplan JP. The spread of the obesity epidemic in the United States, 1991-1998. *JAMA.* 1999;282:1519 1522.

79. Flegal KM, Carroll MD, Kuczmarski RJ, Johnson CL. Overweight and obesity in the United States: prevalence and trends, 1960-1994. *Int J Obesity.* 1998;22:39-47.

80. Mraazek PJ, Haggerty RJ, eds. *Reducing Risks for Mental Disorders: Frontiers for Preventive Intervention Research.* Washington, DC: Institute of Medicine, National Academy Press; 1994.

81. US Department of Health and Human Services. *Mental Health: A Report of the Surgeon General.* Rockville, Md: US Dept of Health and Human Services, Substance Abuse and Mental Health Services Administration, Center for Mental Health Services, National Institutes of Health, National Institute of Mental Health; 1999.

CHAPTER
19

Progress and Next Steps in Reducing Tobacco Use in the United States

Michael P. Eriksen, Sc.D.
Lawrence W. Green, Dr.P.H.

Tobacco control in the last half of the twentieth century has been a study of contrasts. In the 1950s, smoking was riding high. Nearly half of adult men smoked, women were smoking at increasing rates, smoking was not only normative but completely accepted, and cigarette advertisements were everywhere, including on our favorite TV shows. There was virtually no investment in tobacco control and there was little in the way of regulatory or legislative protection. By the end of the twentieth century, smoking rates had been cut nearly in half, smoking was socially unacceptable and seen as a habit increasingly limited to lower socioeconomic populations. Smoke-free areas had become the norm, with most public places, private workplaces, and modes of transportation being smoke-free. Combined federal and state resources for tobacco control totaled nearly one billion dollars, and there was an intricate web of laws and regulations, primarily at the state level, protecting

children from becoming addicted to tobacco, and providing assurances of smoke-free air.

The job is far from complete, and about a quarter of the U.S. population continues to smoke,[1] with great variation in those at risk based on regional, racial, and socioeconomic characteristics. However, the progress has been undeniable and, in fact, has been considered one of the 10 greatest public health achievements of the twentieth century.[2]

Both to further accelerate achievements in tobacco control and to export successful lessons to other urgent public health challenges, it is important to understand how and why this transformation took place. This chapter will review the current status of tobacco control in the United States with particular emphasis on (1) the continuing harm caused by tobacco use, (2) the current levels and patterns of use, (3) the factors that contributed to the changing tobacco control environment, (4) effective interventions in reducing tobacco use, and (5) future challenges and directions.

TOBACCO USE CAUSES CONTINUING HARM

The harm caused by cigarette smoking is without precedent. The Centers for Disease Control and Prevention (CDC) estimates that since the time of the first Surgeon General's Report in 1964, 10 million Americans have died as a result of smoking.[3] If current trends continue, another 25 million Americans alive today will be killed by cigarette smoking, including 5 million children.[4] Although progress in the United States has been great, the continuing burden caused by tobacco is unacceptable.

Smoking is the leading preventable cause of death in the United States, responsible for over 1 in 5 deaths, over 430,000 deaths a year, with the annual loss of over 5 million years of life.[5,6] An estimated 1 out of 2 lifetime smokers will have their lives shortened as a result of smoking.[7] On average, a death caused by smoking reduces a person's life expectancy by about 12 years.[3] Although there is a decades-long lag time from the beginning of tobacco use to the manifestation of clinical illness, the harm caused by smoking is not limited to the elderly. Cigarette smoking is a major killer of the middle-aged (45 to 64) and 80 percent of coronary heart disease deaths in this age group is caused by smoking.[8]

In a perverse way, it is a marvel how many diseases are caused by smoking and how it affects nearly every organ system. Diseases of the pulmonary and cardiovascular systems predominate, with heart disease, lung cancer, and respiratory diseases being most common. Each year, smoking causes 155,000 cancer deaths, 122,000 cardiovascular deaths, and 72,000 chronic lung disease deaths, along with 81,000 deaths from other causes in the United States alone.[3]

Lung cancer provides an interesting illustration of the public health impact of cigarette smoking. Nearly 90 percent of lung cancer is caused by cigarette smoking[9] and at the beginning of the twentieth century, lung cancer was rare. As cigarette smoking became more popular, the incidence of lung cancer increased dramatically. For example, in 1930, the lung cancer death rate for men was 4.9 per 100,000; in 1990, the rate had increased to 75.6 per 100,000.[10] In 1964, on the basis of approximately 7,000 articles relating to smoking and disease, the Advisory Committee to the U.S. Surgeon General concluded that cigarette smoking is a cause of lung cancer in men, and a probable cause of lung cancer in women.[11] The committee stated that "Cigarette smoking is a health hazard of sufficient importance in the United States to warrant appropriate remedial action." Today, smokers die more frequently from lung cancer (123,000 deaths a year) than any other disease caused by smoking, and lung cancer is now the leading cause of cancer deaths. This is true for both men and women, with lung cancer surpassing breast cancer as the leading cause of cancer death among U.S. women in 1987.[12] In 2000, 27,000 more U.S. women died from lung cancer than from breast cancer.[13]

CURRENT LEVELS AND PATTERNS OF USE

The United States is fortunate to have multiple systems to measure and track tobacco use, both among adults and children. For adults, the National Health Interview Survey (NHIS) is the oldest and most continuous system for monitoring tobacco use, and other critical health behaviors and conditions. The NHIS provides annual national estimates of tobacco use by age, gender, region, and socioeconomic status, as well as providing the opportunity to investigate the relationship between tobacco use and other health behaviors.

The Behavioral Risk Factor Surveillance System (BRFSS) has provided state-specific data on behavioral risk factors, including tobacco use for the last 20 years, and is now operational in every state. Although only providing a median national value, the BRFSS provides valuable state-specific, and state-owned data that is valuable for local public health programming and policy setting. Somewhat surprisingly, the BRFSS data has shown consistently large differences in smoking and smokeless tobacco rates by state, nearly three times as high in tobacco-growing states such as Kentucky, compared to western states such as Utah or California. The National Household Survey on Drug Abuse (NHSDA) has recently been expanded, both in sample size and in depth of tobacco questions, as well as having improved computer methodology to obtain valid measures of illicit and private information during interviews in the home. The NHSDA provides valuable information on the incidence of initiation of smoking, the number of new smokers in a given year, and most recently, cigarette brand preference among adolescents.

Although tobacco surveillance systems for adults are strong, the systems in place to monitor tobacco use among young people are even more robust. In 2000, the NHSDA, mentioned above, surveyed over 70,000 Americans, 25,000 of whom were 12 to 17 years old. Thus, the NHSDA provides a large and valuable data source for better understanding tobacco use, particularly the initiation of use, and the combination of the use of tobacco with a variety of illicit drugs and alcohol. However, because the methodology has been changed many times during the past 10 years, it is not a good source of data for historical trend analysis. Fortunately, there are multiple sources for trend analysis, particularly from data collected in schools. Most notably, the Monitoring the Future (MTF) study, conducted by the University of Michigan, with support from the National Institute of Drug Abuse (NIDA), and the Youth Risk Behavior Survey (YRBS) conducted by the CDC provide valuable trend data on tobacco use rates among various age groups.

The MTF survey has been in operation since 1976, surveying the use of tobacco and other substances among high school seniors. In the early 1990s, MTF added 8th- and 10th-grade samples to its survey. The YRBS has been operating since 1990, providing national estimates and state-specific estimates in alternating years. Both of these surveys are school-based, providing valid and reliable estimates for those children in school. Because school dropouts are known to have higher smoking rates than children in school, the MTF and YRBS estimates should be considered as conservative estimates of overall smoking rates among young people.

In addition to these federal surveys, and as a result of increasing demand for in-depth data on tobacco control behaviors, attitudes, and perceptions of young people, a new school-based surveillance system has been developed, the Youth Tobacco Survey (YTS).[14] The YTS, as opposed to the NHSDA, MTF, and YRBS (which are all multirisk-factor surveillance systems) focuses just on tobacco use. The YTS was developed in response to requests from state health departments, which received early settlements from tobacco industry litigation. The YTS began in Florida, Texas, and Mississippi in 1998, providing valuable data for program planning and evaluation purposes, and is currently being used in over 40 states.

The need for in-depth tobacco data was recognized by the American Legacy Foundation, which sponsored a national version of the YTS, called the National Youth Tobacco Survey (NYTS),[15] and has repeated this survey for the last few years. Finally, because of the broad interest in preventing tobacco use among young people, in cooperation with the World Health Organization, the YTS was modified for global use. As of this writing, the Global Youth Tobacco Survey[16] (GYTS) has been completed in over 50 countries, with another 50 countries trained to use the system in the upcoming year. Thus, as an outgrowth of the original Youth Tobacco Survey conducted in a few states in 1998, a true global system of in-depth and comparable tobacco surveillance has evolved, with city and regional, state, national, and international data available for comparison and analysis.

Patterns of Use among Adults

Whereas early tobacco use was primarily ceremonial by Native Americans, with more widespread use of tobacco for pipes, hand-rolled cigarettes, cigars, and chewing, tobacco use today is a highly addicting and habituated behavior. The introduction of blended tobacco that allowed for inhalation, the invention of the safety match, the introduction of mass production of cigarettes, coupled with sophisticated distribution systems and creative marketing efforts led to the rapid adoption of cigarette smoking during the first half of the twentieth century, peaking in the mid-1960s. A major accomplishment of the last third of the twentieth century was the reduction in cigarette smoking from a per capita consumption of 4,345 cigarettes in 1963, to 2,136 in 1999,[17] a reduction of more than 50 percent since the first Surgeon General's Report in 1964.[11]

In addition to the reduction in per capita consumption, the United States has also experienced a reduction in adult smoking prevalence, decreasing from about 43 percent in 1965 to 25.5 percent in 1990.[18] Prevalence remained fairly flat until 1998,[19] but then declined to 23.5 percent in 1999, and 22.3 percent according to preliminary estimates for 2001. Also, the percentage of adults who never smoked increased from 44 percent in the mid-1960s to 55 percent in 2001.[20] The net effect resulted in tens of millions of fewer American smokers than would have been expected if earlier rates of smoking continued, although this progress has not been experienced equally by all U.S. population groups.

Smoking rates vary by demographic characteristics, such as race and ethnicity, level of education, age, poverty status, and region of the country of residence. However, there are relatively small differences in smoking prevalence based on gender. In 1999, there was a more than threefold difference in the likelihood of smoking by race and ethnicity, with the highest smoking rates found among American Indian and Alaska Native populations (40.8 percent), and the lowest among Asian and Pacific Islander groups (15.1 percent).[19] A similar difference was seen in terms of level of education, with high school dropouts about four times more likely to smoke than those with a graduate degree (37.7 percent vs. 8.5 percent, respectively).

Patterns of Use among Young People

The 1994 Surgeon General's Report, *Preventing Tobacco Use Among Young People*,[21] focused intense interest on smoking among youth and young adults. This report emphasized the fact that smoking onset, and nicotine addiction, almost always began in the teen years, and provided an early warning to an increased use of tobacco products among young adults. In fact, after more than a decade of relatively stable youth smoking rates in the 1980s,[22] cigarette smoking began increasing among high school students in the early 1990s, only to have peaked in 1996–1997.[23]

Overall, smoking among adolescents has tended to moderate over the last few years. According to the MTF project,[24] the prevalence of daily smoking by high school seniors peaked at a high of 28.8 percent in

1976, then dropped to a low of 17.2 percent in 1992. The 2000 rate for high school seniors is 20.6 percent, significantly lower than that of the late 1990s, but still showing that one out of five high school seniors smokes cigarettes every day. The prevalence of current smoking (defined as smoking within the past 30 days) among high school seniors is also showing a similar pattern, having peaked in 1997 at 36.5 percent, and lowering to 31.4 percent in 2000. The picture is similar for 8th- and 10th-grade students, with current and daily smoking having peaked in the mid-1990s, and with 2000 rates the lowest seen in a decade—except for 10th graders, who continue to have relatively high rates compared to the reductions seen among 8th and 12th graders.

The YRBS data suggest a more mixed picture in terms of smoking among high school students. For 9th graders, smoking appears to have clearly peaked in 1997 at 33.4 percent. In 1999, the 9th-grade current smoking rate dropped significantly to 27.6 percent. However, similar patterns have not been seen with either 10th or 11th graders, with their most recent data (1999) staying around the highest level of the decade—34.7 percent for 10th graders, and 36.0 percent for 11th graders. The picture for 12th graders is even more disturbing, with 1999 rates the highest recorded, 42.8 percent current smoking among high school seniors. The difference between the results from the MTF study and the YRBS survey requires additional analysis and research.

It is also instructive to look at the 1999 and 2000 Substance Abuse and Mental Health Services Administration (SAMHSA) estimates for young people. SAMHSA notes that there was a significant decline in smoking among teenagers (aged 12–17) and young adults (aged 18–25) between 1999 and 2000. Specifically, past-month use among teenagers declined from 14.9 percent in 1999 to 13.4 percent in 2000. Young adults declined from 39.7 percent in 1999 to 38.3 percent in 2000, with both reductions being statistically significant.

Youth smoking rates appear to differ greatly by race and ethnicity, and differently than do the rates for adults. In the late 1970s, there was virtually no difference between smoking rates among youth based on race. However, over the subsequent two decades, white youth continued relatively high smoking rates, even increasing, while smoking rates among black youth fell.[25] Unfortunately, the difference between black and white youth in high school is beginning to erode,[23] and there is now no difference in cigarette smoking rates between black and white middle school students.[26]

In addition to prevalence rates, it is important to analyze incidence of initiation rates of smoking. The incidence rate for cigarette use among youth aged 12 to 17 decreased between 1998 and 1999, from 141.4 to 120.0 persons per 1,000 potential new users. The numbers and rates among young adults aged 18 to 25 remained stable between 1998 and 1999. The overall annual number of persons who first tried a cigarette had increased between 1991 and 1996 from about 2.4 to 3.4 million, then decreased to 2.9 million in 1998.[27]

The incidence of initiation of smoking cigarettes daily has decreased since its recent peak in 1997 at 1.9 million new users. In 1998, the number of initiates dropped to about 1.7 million, and it dropped again in 1999 to about 1.4 million. Contributing to this decrease was the smaller number of new daily smokers among youths aged 12 to 17, falling from about 1,163,000 in 1997 to 783,000 in 1999. Translated to a per-day basis, the number decreased from 3,186 youths per day in 1997 to 2,145 per day in 1999.[27]

Data from government surveys clearly demonstrate that over three-quarters of adult smokers smoke their first cigarette before age 18.[21] About 90 percent of adult smokers first tried a cigarette before age 19. In the 1994 Surgeon General's report, the mean age at which people smoked their first cigarette was calculated to be 14.5. Although some estimates of mean age of first use are slightly higher and some are lower, in every case, the estimated mean age of first use is well below 18.

Surveys also clearly show that many smokers become daily smokers before age 18. Among adult smokers who have ever smoked daily, about half (53 percent) began smoking daily before age 18, 71 percent began at age 18 or younger, and 77 percent began before age 20. According to the latest data from the NHSDA,[27] the mean age of first daily smoking appears to be dropping, and was 17.7 in 1999, compared to 18.4 in 1998. Thus, whereas many measures suggest a reduction in smoking rates among young people, it appears that people are becoming daily smokers at younger ages.

FACTORS CONTRIBUTING TO THE CHANGING TOBACCO CONTROL ENVIRONMENT

The recent progress made in tobacco control, besides being noted as one of the 10 greatest public health achievements of the twentieth century,[2] is physically palpable to all Americans. Increasingly fewer people are smoking, we seemed to have turned the corner with youth smoking, and exposure to secondhand smoke has decreased dramatically. Despite these advances, the question needs to be asked, given the magnitude of harm caused by tobacco, the epidemiologic certainty that tobacco is the agent of harm, the fact that illnesses caused by tobacco are completely preventable, and the availability of extremely cost-effective interventions: Why has it taken so long for progress to be achieved, and what factors limit further progress?

To answer these questions, it is necessary to determine both the factors that have contributed to our progress, as well as the factors that have impeded progress, in what otherwise would have been a fairly simple resolution to a very serious public health problem. It is perhaps better to look at the second question first: Why is continuing progress so difficult? For those in the tobacco control movement, the answer is obvious—the tobacco industry. This logical deduction that the tobacco industry works in its economic self-interest to get as many people to smoke as many cigarettes as possible, is a simple economic conclusion. What has been most revealing, through a review of industry documents released in the discovery process during litigation, is the revelation of the lengths to which the tobacco industry went to mislead the public, and subvert public health, for the purposes of maximizing profits. It is reassuring and validating for the first major conclusion of the 2000 Surgeon General's Report to read as follows:

> Efforts to prevent the onset or continuance of tobacco use face the pervasive, countervailing influence of tobacco promotion by the tobacco industry, a promotion that takes place despite overwhelming evidence of adverse health effects from tobacco use. (p. 6)

Having acknowledged the factors that have and continue to impede public health progress in tobacco control, the next issue of importance is, despite these impediments, how have we been able to make the remarkable progress that we have? This question is more difficult to answer, but has major implications for future progress, and perhaps for other public health problems.

Progress in tobacco control has not been the result of any single event or policy, nor has it corresponded to a specific public health plan. Rather, progress has resulted from several factors: the scientific discovery of the harm caused by smoking and the broad dissemination of these findings; very large reductions in smoking rates among opinion leaders (physicians, attorneys, teachers, etc.); and aggressive advocacy by nonsmokers for smoke-free environments. All of these factors led to changes in the social acceptability and public perception of tobacco use. In the 1990s, these changes partially led to, and were also built upon by, litigation against the tobacco industry for the harm caused by tobacco use, particularly by state attorneys general. This litigation resulted in the disclosure of previously secret industry documents, which in turn led to an increased distrust of the tobacco industry, and a further erosion of the acceptability of tobacco use.

This blending of the scientific documentation of harm, media coverage, public advocacy, changing social norms, and litigation and associated disclosure of industry documents has contributed to the major decline of U.S. tobacco consumption. Although many of these trends are likely to continue, future progress in reducing tobacco use will only be accelerated by continued advocacy, as well as by the vigorous implementation of comprehensive and effective tobacco control programs.

EFFECTIVE INTERVENTIONS IN REDUCING TOBACCO USE

Substantial public health efforts to reduce the prevalence of tobacco use began shortly after the cancer risk was described in 1964. With the subsequent decline in smoking, there have been huge public health improvements. For example, the incidence of smoking-related cancers has declined, with the exception of lung cancer among women.[10] Age-adjusted death rates per 100,000 persons for heart disease have de-

creased from 307.4 in 1950 to 134.6 in 1996. Overall, it is estimated that between 1964 and 1992, approximately 1.6 million deaths caused by smoking were prevented.[28]

Overall, among the many interventions that have been found to be effective in reducing tobacco use and exposure to secondhand smoke are increasing the price of tobacco products, sustained media campaigns, decreasing the out-of-pocket costs for treating nicotine addiction, and restricting indoor smoking. Others have been shown to increase the use of tobacco products (e.g., tobacco advertising campaigns targeted to young people, decreases in the price of tobacco products), and yet others have little evidence, simply because they have yet to be tried (e.g., plain packaging, limits on tar and nicotine levels).

Reducing Tobacco Use: An Intervention Typology

To continue this reduction in tobacco use and to accelerate action, it is essential to know what works, and under what conditions, to reduce tobacco use. With this as an objective (and ultimately the title of the 2000 Surgeon General's Report), a multiyear effort was undertaken to identify effective interventions that have been shown to reduce tobacco use, and to organize these interventions conceptually to form an intervention typology. The result of this process was *Reducing Tobacco Use: A Report of the Surgeon General*[29] which was released in August 2000, at the 11th World Conference on Tobacco or Health in Chicago.

The report organized tobacco control interventions into five distinct categories: educational, clinical, regulatory, economic, and social or comprehensive, and reviewed the evidence in support of each category of intervention.

Educational

Educational interventions included both school-based curriculum and mass media or counteradvertising programs. The report concluded that both of these types of interventions have large spans of impact, but that the size of the impact was either moderate or small. Media campaigns are an effective strategy to change social norms around tobacco use.

Sustained media campaigns have been shown to decrease adolescent initiation and increase adults' cessation.[30] Of greatest importance, school programs should be conducted in conjunction with community- and media-based activities. When this is done, smoking onset can be postponed or prevented in 20 to 40 percent of adolescents. The 2000 report further noted that current levels of school tobacco prevention practice were not optimal and more consistent implementation was needed, especially in establishing multi-year prevention programs that were coordinated with community and media efforts.

Clinical

Clinical interventions reviewed both pharmacologic and behavioral approaches to help smokers quit smoking and concluded that the span of impact was quite small due to the one-on-one nature of the interventions, and that the size of the impact was moderate to very small for behavioral interventions alone. The report noted that combined pharmacologic and behavioral programs can have success rates of 20 to 25 percent at one-year post-treatment, for those smokers that participate in such programs. The problem, of course, is that although most smokers would like to quit smoking, most do not make serious attempts to quit involving health professionals. To improve the likelihood that clinical encounters are as successful as possible, in 2000, the Public Health Service (PHS) published an evidence-based guideline on effective clinical interventions to treat tobacco use and dependence.[31]

The importance of getting existing smokers to quit smoking cannot be overstated. Because many of the health impacts of smoking do not occur until middle age, even if smoking among adolescents could be completely eliminated tomorrow, the impact on morbidity and mortality would take 20–30 years to become evident. For example, the American Cancer Society has set goals for 2015 of a 25 percent reduction in cancer incidence and a 50 percent reduction in cancer mortality rates.[32] Approximately 50 percent of that goal can be achieved with a 40–50 percent reduction in smoking prevalence by 2005. This level of population change can be achieved only through massive changes in behavior among current smokers.

Fortunately there are numerous studies documenting the effectiveness of clinical interventions to enhance quitting, including the PHS guidelines, mentioned above. It is estimated that if half of the physicians in the United States advised their smoking patients to quit, more than two million more smokers would quit each year. These clinical interventions are also highly cost-effective.[33] A recent study that prioritized 30 recommended clinical preventive services based upon their impact and the effectiveness and cost-effectiveness of the service found that treating adult tobacco use ranked second (after childhood immunization).[34] The challenge, however, has been to integrate routine tobacco use treatment into the health care system and increase access to effective treatments.

The Task Force for Community Preventive Services examined health care system changes that foster effective clinical cessation treatment. This guideline found that reminder systems alone increase the provision of treatment services, and that reminder systems in conjunction with provider training were even more effective. Both use of effective treatments and cessation rates can also be increased by reducing the out-of-pocket costs of treatment and by making cessation counseling more convenient (such as by providing treatment through telephone cessation helplines).[30]

Regulatory

Regulatory interventions included product manufacture and sale, as well as smoking restrictions in public venues and in worksites. For each of these areas, the span of impact was viewed to be large, with the size of impact varying from very large for product manufacturing regulations to small for worksite restrictions. The 2000 report concluded that regulation of advertising and promotion, particularly that directed at young people, would very likely reduce smoking rates, and that clean air regulations and restrictions of minors' access to tobacco products contribute to changing social norms against tobacco, and may even reduce tobacco use directly.

Of particular importance is the need to establish meaningful regulation of tobacco products. Not only do tobacco products lack meaningful regulation, but they are also expressly exempted from regulation by various federal laws designed to protect consumers, such as the Consumer Product Safety Act.

Analysis of the tobacco product is essential to successful reduction of the harm caused by tobacco use. The cigarette itself has changed dramatically during the last half-century, and it is likely to change even more in the twenty-first century. When cigarettes were first associated with lung cancer in the early 1950s, most U.S. smokers smoked unfiltered cigarettes. With a growing awareness of the danger of smoking came the first filter, which was designed to reduce the tar inhaled in the smoke. Later, low-tar cigarettes were marketed; however, many smokers compensated by smoking more intensely and by blocking the filter's ventilation holes.[35] Research is needed to determine whether new "highly engineered" products can reduce exposure to toxins and carcinogens, decrease individual risk, or decrease the population harm of tobacco, or whether the mistakes associated with low-tar and nicotine cigarettes with smoke compensating for the product's engineering will be repeated.[36]

Meaningful product regulation will also restrict the promotion and marketing of tobacco products. Money spent by the tobacco industry to market and promote tobacco products contributes to continued usage by enhancing the appeal, access, and affordability of tobacco products. In 1999, the U.S. cigarette companies reported spending $8.24 billion on marketing and promoting cigarettes,[37] the most ever spent, and a 22 percent increase from expenditures in the preceding year. This amounts to an annual marketing expenditure of approximately $165 per smoker, or over 40 cents for every pack sold. This level of expenditure is particularly surprising, given the rapid decline in per capita consumption (15 percent since 1997) and at a time following the Master Settlement Agreement which, most have thought, would have reduced the total expenditures on cigarette marketing. Successful efforts to reduce tobacco use must restrict the form, content, and magnitude of tobacco advertising.

Economic

Economic interventions included efforts to modify taxation and tariffs and trade policy, and it was con-

cluded that both the span of impact, as well as the size of impact, was very large for both. One of the most effective means of reducing the population prevalence of tobacco use is increasing federal and state excise tax rates. A 10 percent increase in the price of cigarettes can lead to a 4 percent reduction in the demand for cigarettes. This reduction is the result of people smoking fewer cigarettes or quitting altogether. Studies show that low-income, adolescent, Hispanic, and non-Hispanic black smokers are more likely than others to stop smoking in response to a price increase.[38]

Social or Comprehensive

Under this heading, comprehensive statewide programs were determined to have a larger span and size of impact. The report further concluded that the true effect of the program components are likely to be underestimated, due to the synergistic effect of comprehensive efforts. Just as school-based programs are deemed to be more effective when coordinated with community and media efforts, a comprehensive approach that combines all of the interventions outlined in the report will be optimally effective in reducing tobacco use.

In fact, most practitioners and scholars recommend comprehensive approaches, where the different program elements work in concert to reinforce a specific tobacco control message. These program components should strive to reduce both the demand and the supply of tobacco products, although a recent review of the evidence strongly recommends that "demand" reduction strategies are more effective than those attempting to influence the "supply" of tobacco products.[39]

Targets for Tobacco Control: Leading Health Indicators and Healthy People 2010 Objectives

Although the United States does not have a formal strategy or plan to reduce tobacco use, it does have explicit objectives for the year 2010 (in fact, 467 of them) to guide the direction and activities, not only of the federal government, but also of states, communities, and voluntary organizations. It also has developed a series of 10 Leading Health Indicators that will guide the federal government in setting priorities and monitoring progress in improving the public health. The Leading Health Indicators reflect the major health concerns in the United States at the beginning of the twenty-first century. Within this Healthy People 2010 framework,[40] there are 21 tobacco objectives, 3 of which are also considered to be Leading Health Indicators. Specifically, two prevalence objectives, to reduce current smoking rates in half among adults and teenagers, as well as an objective to reduce exposure to secondhand smoke, are among the Leading Health Indicators, reinforcing the importance of tobacco control in our nation's overall public health improvement efforts.

Of the 21 tobacco objectives for the year 2010, four pertain to patterns of tobacco use, four to cessation and treatment, five to exposure to secondhand smoke, and eight to social and environmental changes. In terms of changes in patterns of tobacco use, the overriding objective is to reduce tobacco use in half—to 12 percent for cigarette smoking by adults (Objective 27-1) and 16 percent for past-month cigarette smoking for high school students (Objective 27-2)—for all population groups by 2010. Both of these are also Leading Health Indicators. The concept of "for all population groups" is critical because currently, there is great variation in tobacco use rates by race, ethnicity, and socioeconomic status. By adopting the position that all groups should benefit equally, the Healthy People 2010 process will go a long way to eliminating health disparities in the United States. Other objectives that pertain to the use of tobacco products include reducing the initiation of tobacco use among children (Objective 27-3), and increasing the age of first use from 12 to 14 for adolescents (Objective 27-4).

In terms of cessation and treatment of tobacco use, objectives have been set to increase smoking cessation attempts by adults from 41 to 75 percent (Objective 27-5), to increase smoking cessation by women during pregnancy from 14 to 30 percent (Objective 27-6), as well as to increase cessation attempts by adolescents (Objective 27-7) and to increase insurance coverage of evidence-based smoking cessation treatments (Objective 27-8). Regarding secondhand smoke, objectives include reducing the proportion of children who are regularly exposed to tobacco smoke at home from 27 to 10 percent (Ob-

jective 27-9) and to reduce the proportion of non-smokers exposed to secondhand smoke from 65 to 45 percent (Objective 27-10). Objective 27-10 is also one of the Leading Health Indicators. Additional secondhand smoke objectives include increasing smoke-free environments in schools (Objective 27-11) and in worksites (Objectives 27-12 and 13).

Regarding objectives focusing on social and environmental changes, there are objectives targeted at reducing the illegal sales of tobacco products to minors (Objectives 27-11 and 12), eliminating advertising that influences adolescents (Objective 27-16), increasing adolescents' disapproval of smoking (Objective 27-17), increasing comprehensive, evidence-based tobacco control programs (Objective 27-18), eliminating laws that preempt stronger tobacco control laws (Objective 27-19), reducing the toxicity of tobacco products (Objective 27-20), and last, but very important, increasing the average tax on cigarette products from 63 cents to two dollars (Objective 27-21).

As one can see from the preceding paragraphs, although there may not be an explicit or official tobacco control "strategy" for the United States, there is a very comprehensive plan of action embracing behavioral, social, environmental, and policy outcomes. The challenge becomes to develop feasible plans of action necessary to achieve each of the objectives. Although ambitious, achievement of each of the 21 objectives, and simply putting in place what we know works, will allow us to reach our overall goal of reducing smoking rates in half, for *everybody*, to no more than 12 percent by the end of the decade.[41]

State Successes and Tobacco Control Funding

If the evidence-based interventions that already exist were applied, the Healthy People 2010 objective of reducing tobacco use in half could be achieved. If smoking rates are reduced in half, millions of lives will be saved, and the expenditure of billions of dollars on treating diseases caused by smoking can be averted. Preliminary evidence from California is already demonstrating that sustained implementation of effective tobacco control interventions not only reduces smoking rates, but also saves lives and dollars.[42,43]

The United States is fortunate to have models of successful tobacco control programs. Because of citizen initiative and political leadership, the United States enjoys a number of well-funded, evidence-based tobacco control programs, all originally emanating from an earmarked portion of an increase in the cigarette excise tax, followed in some states by a dedicated and purposeful use of tobacco industry settlement funds to reduce tobacco use. California was the first state to launch a concerted effort to raise the cigarette excise tax and devote a substantial portion to tobacco control, followed most notably by Massachusetts, Arizona, and Oregon. Among states that used their tobacco settlement dollars for tobacco control, and have already demonstrated the effectiveness of their program, are Florida and Mississippi. As more states launch comprehensive, evidence-based tobacco control programs, we expect even more examples of success.

In terms of the first model of increasing cigarette or tobacco excise taxes and earmarking a portion for tobacco prevention programs, data from both California and Massachusetts have indicated that increasing excise taxes on cigarettes is one of the most cost-effective short-term strategies to reduce tobacco consumption, and the ability to sustain lower consumption increases when the tax increase is combined with an antismoking campaign.[44] In terms of states that have used their settlement with the tobacco industry to fund aggressive tobacco control programs, Florida had the first program and was the first to demonstrate success. Data from Florida indicate that past-month smoking decreased significantly among public middle school students (19 to 15 percent) and high school students (27 to 25 percent) from 1998 to 1999 following implementation of their program, which has subsequently become a model for the country.[45]

Whereas a number of states have had successful comprehensive campaigns, and much has been published about their impact, Oregon is a state that has had a very successful program, but has not received the national attention it deserves. By looking at results from states such as Oregon, as well as from better-known programs in states such as California, Massachusetts, and Florida, there will be a greater number of models of success for other states to emulate. In Oregon, following its tax increase and the establishment of a comprehensive tobacco prevention and education program, per capita consumption declined

11.3% between 1996 and 1998, while it only declined 1 percent in the United States overall.[46] The net effect of this was 25 million fewer packs of cigarettes being sold in Oregon in 1998 than were sold in 1996. One part of Oregon's efforts was to implement CDC's guidelines for tobacco prevention in schools, and Oregon recently reported that smoking rates dropped by 20 percent in participating schools.[47] The Oregon experience also showed that the schools with the most comprehensive programs had the greatest decline in smoking rates. A school program is considered to be comprehensive if it includes not only an effective tobacco prevention curriculum, but also has a tobacco-free policy, cessation services for students, staff, and faculty, as well as coordination with community tobacco control activities.

Based on the experience of these states, as well as the literature, CDC published *Best Practices for Comprehensive Tobacco Control Programs*[48] to guide states in their tobacco control efforts following the implementation of the Master Settlement Agreement between state attorney's general and the tobacco industry. *Best Practices* provides the research and scientific evidence in support of nine elements that should comprise a comprehensive tobacco control program. Because *Best Practices* focused on providing guidance to states on the scientific evidence on public health programs, it did not include policy recommendations on product regulation, pricing, or other nonprogrammatic activities.

Most recently, the Task Force on Community Preventive Services[30] established rules of evidence to review the published literature on a variety of tobacco control strategies, including efforts to reduce exposure to secondhand smoke, to increase tobacco use cessation, and prevent initiation. Additional reviews will be forthcoming on pricing, minor's access to tobacco products, and media campaigns.

FUTURE CHALLENGES AND CONCLUSIONS

The 2000 Surgeon General's Report, besides reviewing the evidence base for tobacco control, also identified a number of future challenges that include:

• Continuing to build the science base of tobacco control

- Understanding the changing tobacco industry
- Implementing a comprehensive approach to tobacco control
- Identifying and eliminating disparities
- Improving the dissemination of state-of-the-art interventions
- Addressing global tobacco use

For continued progress to be achieved, these issues, and perhaps other emerging challenges, must compose our future agenda.

Despite the achievements of the last third of the twentieth century, much still remains to be done. Over 60 million Americans reported current use of a tobacco product in 2000.[27] Cigarette smoking is responsible for approximately 430,000 deaths each year—one of every five, and, if current trends continue, approximately 25 million Americans alive today, including 5 million of today's children, will die as a result of smoking.[4] But current trends do not need to continue, and tobacco use rates can be halved simply by putting in place those actions known to reduce tobacco use. The 2000 Surgeon General's Report[29] documented the scientific

evidence of what works, and concluded that if we implement what we know works, we can reduce smoking rates in half, for all population groups, in a decade. Surgeon General David Satcher said:

> If the recommendations in this report were fully implemented, the Healthy People 2010 objectives related to tobacco use could be met, including cutting in half the rates of tobacco use among young people and adults. It is clear that the major barrier to more rapid reductions in tobacco use is the effort of the tobacco industry to promote the use of tobacco products. Our lack of greater progress in tobacco control is more the result of failure to implement proven strategies than it is the lack of knowledge about what to do. As a result, each year, more than 1 million young people continue to become regular smokers and more than 400,000 adults die from tobacco-related diseases. Tobacco use will remain the leading cause of preventable illness and death in this nation and a growing number of other countries until tobacco prevention and control efforts are commensurate with the harm caused by tobacco use.[29]

References

1. Centers for Disease Control and Prevention. Cigarette smoking among adults—United States, 1999. *MMWR.* 2001;50:869-873.
2. Centers for Disease Control and Prevention. Achievements in public health 1900-1999: Tobacco use—United States, 1900-1999. *MMWR.* 1999;48:986-993.
3. Centers for Disease Control and Prevention. Smoking-attributable mortality and years of potential life lost—United States, 1984. *MMWR.* 1997;46:444-451.
4. Centers for Disease Control and Prevention. Projected smoking-related deaths among youth—United States, 1996. *MMWR.* 45:971-974.
5. Centers for Disease Control and Prevention. Cigarette smoking attributable mortality and years of potential life lost—United States, 1990. *MMWR.* 1993;42:645-649.
6. McGinnis M, Foege W. Actual causes of death in the United States. *JAMA.* 1993;270:207-212.
7. Doll R, Peto R, Wheatlet K, Gary R, Sutherland I. Mortality in relation to smoking: 40 years' observations on male British doctors. *BMJ.* 1994;309:901-911.

8. Peto R, Lopez AD, Boreham J, Thun M, Heath C. *Mortality from Smoking in Developed Countries 1950-2000.* Oxford, England: Oxford University Press; 1994.
9. American Cancer Society. *Cancer Facts and Figures—1999.* Atlanta, Ga: American Cancer Society; 1999.
10. Wingo PA, Ries LA, Giovino GA, et al. Annual report to the nation on the status of cancer, 1973-1996, with a special section on lung cancer and tobacco smoking. *J Natl Cancer Inst.* 1999;91:675-690.
11. US Public Health Service. *Smoking and Health. Report of the Advisory Committee to the Surgeon General of the Public Health Service.* Washington, DC: US Dept of Health, Education and Welfare, Public Health Service, Centers for Disease Control and Prevention; 1964. PHS Publication 1103.
12. Centers for Disease Control and Prevention. Mortality trends for selected smoking-related cancers and breast cancer—United States, 1950-1990. *MMWR.* 1993;42:863-868.
13. US Department of Health and Human Services. *Women and Smoking: A Report of the Surgeon General.* Rockville,

Md: Public Health Service, Office of the Surgeon General; US Dept of Health and Human Services, Washington DC; 2001.

14. Centers for Disease Control and Prevention. Youth tobacco surveillance—United States, 1998-1999. *MMWR.* 2000;Vol 49, No. SS-10.

15. American Legacy Foundation. Cigarette smoking among youth: Results from the 1999 National Youth Tobacco Survey. *Legacy First Look Report 1.* June 2000.

16. Warren CW, Riley L, Asma S, et al. Tobacco Use by Youth: A Surveillance Report from the Global Youth Tobacco Survey Project. *BullWHO.* 2000;78(7):868-876.

17. US Department of Agriculture. *Agriculture Outlook/January-February 2001.* Washington, DC: Economic Research Service, US Dept of Agriculture; 2001.

18. Giovino GA, Schooley MW, Zhu BP, et al. Surveillance for selected tobacco-use behaviors—United States, 1900-1994. In: *CDC Surveillance Summaries. MMWR.* 1994;43:1-43.

19. Centers for Disease Control and Prevention. Cigarette smoking among adults—United States, 1998. *MMWR.* 2000;49:881-884.

20. National Center for Health Statistics. Available at: http://www.cdc.gov/nchs/nhis.htm#New.

21. US Department of Health and Human Services. *Preventing Tobacco Use Among Young People: Report of the Surgeon General.* Atlanta, Ga: US Dept of Health and Human Services, Centers for Disease Control and Prevention, National Center for Chronic Disease Prevention and Health Promotion, Office on Smoking and Health; 1994.

22. Johnston LD, O'Malley PM, Bachman JG. *National Survey Results on Drug Use from the Monitoring the Future Study, 1975-1998.* Vol 1, *Secondary School Students.* Rockville, Md: National Institutes of Health, National Institute of Drug Abuse; 1999. NIH Publication 99-4660.

23. Centers for Disease Control and Prevention. Trends in cigarette smoking among high school students—United States, 1991-1999. *MMWR.* 2000;49:755-758.

24. University of Michigan. Cigarette use and smokeless tobacco use decline substantially among teens [press release]. Ann Arbor: University of Michigan News and Information Services; December 14, 2000.

25. US Department of Health and Human Services. *Tobacco Use Among U.S. Racial/Ethnic Minority Groups—African Americans, American Indians and Alaska Natives, Asian Americans and Pacific Islanders, and Hispanics: Report of the Surgeon General.* Atlanta, Ga: US Dept of Health and Human Services, Centers for Disease Control and Prevention, National Center for Chronic Disease

Prevention and Health Promotion, Office on Smoking and Health; 1998.

26. Centers for Disease Control and Prevention. Tobacco use among middle and high school students—United States, 1999. *MMWR.* 2000;49:49-53.

27. Substance Abuse and Mental Health Services Administration. *Summary of Findings from the 2000 National Household Survey on Drug Abuse.* Rockville, Md: Office of Applied Studies; 2001. HDHHS Publication (SMA) 01-3549.

28. Centers for Disease Control and Prevention. Decline in deaths from heart disease and stroke—United States, 1900-1999. *MMWR.* 1999;48:649-656.

29. US Department of Health and Human Services. *Reducing Tobacco Use. A Report of the Surgeon General.* Atlanta, Ga: US Dept of Health and Human Services, Centers for Disease Control and Prevention, National Center for Chronic Disease Prevention and Health Promotion, Office on Smoking and Health; 2000.

30. Centers for Disease Control and Prevention. Strategies for reducing exposure to environmental tobacco smoke, increasing tobacco use cessation, and reducing initiation in communities and health-care systems. A report on recommendations of the Task Force on Community Preventive Services. *MMWR.* 2000; (RR-12):1-11.

31. Fiore MC, Bailey WC, Cohen SJ, et al. *Treating Tobacco Use and Dependence. Clinical Practice Guidelines.* US Dept of Health and Human Services, Public Health Service; Washington,DC: 2000.

32. Byers R, Mouchawa J, Marks J, et al. The American Cancer Society challenge goals: How far can cancer rates decline in the U.S. by the year 2015? *Cancer.* 1999;86:715-727.

33. US Department of Health and Human Services. How to help your patients stop smoking: A National Cancer Institute manual for physicians. Rockville, Md: US Dept of Health and Human Services, National Institutes of Health, National Cancer Institute; 1993. NIH Publication 93-3064.

34. Coffield AB, Maciosek MV, McGinnis M, et al. Priorities among recommended clinical preventive services. *Am J Prev Med.* 2001;21(1):1-9.

35. Fielding JF, Husten CG, Eriksen MP. Tobacco: health effects and control. In: Wallace RB, Doebbeling BN, Last JM, eds. *Public Health and Preventive Medicine.* 14th ed. Stamford, Conn: Appleton & Lange; 1998.

36. Warner KE, Slade J, Sweanor DT. The emerging market for long-term nicotine maintenance. *JAMA.* 1997;278:1087-1092.

37. Federal Trade Commission. *Cigarette Report for 1999.* Washington, DC: Federal Trade Commission; 2001.

38. Chaloupka FJ, Warner KE. The economics of smoking. In: Newhouse J, Culyer A, eds. *The Handbook of Health Economics.* Amsterdam, The Netherlands: Elsevier Science; 1999.

39. Jha P, Chaloupka FJ, eds. *Tobacco Control in Developing Countries.* New York, NY: Oxford University Press; 2000.

40. US Department of Health and Human Services. *Healthy People 2010: Understanding and Improving Health.* 2nd ed. Washington, DC: US Government Printing Office; November 2000.

41. Green LW, Eriksen MP, Bailey L, Husten C. Achieving the implausible in the next decade: tobacco control objectives. *Am J Public Health.* 2000;90:337-339.

42. Centers for Disease Control and Prevention. Declines in lung cancer rates—California, 1988-1997. *MMWR.* 2000;49:1066-1069.

43. Fichtenberg CM, Glantz SA. Association of the California tobacco control program with declines in cigarette consumption and mortality from heart disease. *N Engl J Med.* 2000;343:1772-1777

44. Centers for Disease Control and Prevention. Cigarette smoking before and after an excise tax increase and an antismoking campaign. *MMWR.* 1996;45:966-970.

45. Centers for Disease Control and Prevention. Tobacco use among middle and high school students—Florida, 1998 and 1999. *MMWR.* 1999;48:248-253.

46. Centers for Disease Control and Prevention. Decline in cigarette consumption following implementation of a comprehensive tobacco prevention and education program—Oregon, 1996-1999. *MMWR.* 48:140-143.

47. Centers for Disease Control and Prevention. Effectiveness of school-based programs as a component of a statewide tobacco control initiative—Oregon, 1999-2000. *MMWR.* 2001;50:663-666.

48. Centers for Disease Control and Prevention. *Best Practices for Comprehensive Tobacco Control Programs—August 1999.* Atlanta, Ga: US Dept of Health and Human Services; 1999.

CHAPTER
20

A Public Health Approach to Alcohol and Other Drug Problems: Theory and Practice

James F. Mosher, J.D.
Traci L. Toomey, M.P.H., Ph.D.

This chapter seeks to lay the groundwork for building a citizen-based public health agenda for addressing alcohol and other drug problems. It addresses both policy and practice issues. In keeping with public health theory, it focuses particularly on prevention as a primary goal of public health policy.

Specifically, a theoretical perspective for addressing alcohol and other drug problems is presented, followed by an examination of the legal-illegal dichotomy that dominates current policies. Next, available data on the prevalence of alcohol and other drug use and their related problems are reviewed. Then public health prevention strategies are outlined, and the chapter concludes with implications of the previous sections for public health practice and policy development.

Some caveats should be mentioned first, however. The phrase *alcohol and other drugs* is used in this chapter to emphasize alcohol's status as a psychoactive drug. Tobacco should be included in the phrase and is omitted here only because a separate chapter in this volume discusses tobacco problems and policies. Due to space limitations, the chapter does not address inappropriate uses of prescription drugs.

BACKGROUND

In 1993, the new Clinton administration issued its *1993 Interim National Drug Control Strategy,*[1] which questioned the strategies and tactics of the war on drugs initiated by President Reagan in 1986. The report concluded that the dominant focus of the previous administration's policies on international drug interdiction had failed to stem the flow of drugs in this country and that federal policy should shift its focus to domestic law enforcement and demand reduction. The findings came as no surprise to public health professionals, researchers, and citizen activists seeking effective strategies for preventing alcohol and other drug problems. Numerous studies have documented the failure of strategies that rely on the drug interdiction and incarceration of drug users, which have been the cornerstones of the drug war.[2,3]

Eight years later, the essential components of President Reagan's drug policy remain intact. The Clinton administration changed the rhetoric, dropping the term *drug war,* but it continued the heavy reliance on drug interdiction, incarceration, and other criminal justice strategies. It increased the drug strategy budget 57 percent, from $11.5 billion in 1992 to $18.1 billion in 2001, but funding for demand reduction strategies (treatment and prevention) remained static, at 32 percent of the total.[4] Clinton's final major drug initiative—Plan Colombia—fit the classic drug war mold: a $1.3 billion drug interdiction effort in Colombia that includes heavy expenditures on military equipment and crop defoliants. Critics argue this new campaign is a thinly veiled antiguerrilla campaign that will have little or no effect on drug availability in the United States and potentially devastating effects on civilian populations.[5] The new Bush administration has made clear its intention to continue the drug war for the foreseeable future in essentially the same form as it began 15 years ago.

This country has witnessed a whole series of drug wars during the last 100 years with striking resemblances and consequences: excess reliance on criminal law and drug interdiction; definition of the problem as one of morality rather than public health; focus on drug use among disenfranchised groups, usually communities of color; deflection of policy focus from economic, social, and public health issues underlying the drug use; lack of attention to legal drugs; and, ultimately, failure of the drug war to address drug problems effectively.[6–8]

Perhaps most striking from the perspective of this volume is that public health theory and practice have played only a marginal role in defining federal alcohol and other drug policies in this country. This has been particularly true during the drug wars, when public attention has been at its height. During the early 1980s, for example, funding for public health prevention and treatment programs was cut at the same time that funding was increased dramatically for criminal justice and drug interdiction efforts.[7] As a result, treatment was significantly less available in 1987 than in 1976.[9]

Recent developments, particularly at the community level, bring hopes of changing this troubling picture of federal drug policy. Various citizen and professional groups have become increasingly effective at promoting public health strategies for addressing alcohol and other drug problems. These include: a shift of the policy focus away from criminal justice and interdiction strategies to public health strategies; increased attention to the legal drugs, alcohol and tobacco; greater accountability from the legal drug industries; and increased prevention and treatment services, particularly for low-income groups and communities of color.[10–12] This activism began to have an impact during the waning years of the Bush-Reagan drug war and provided the public health field an important opportunity, not only to influence drug policy, but also to build a citizen base for action in wider public health arenas.

A PUBLIC HEALTH PARADIGM FOR ALCOHOL AND OTHER DRUG PROBLEMS

Alcohol and other drug problems are best understood by examining the interaction of three key components of any public health problem: environment, agent, and host. In general, the **host** is the individual suffering the public health problem and the **agent** (or vector) is that which is necessary or sufficient to cause harm to the host. The **environment** consists of the social, economic, physical, political, and cultural settings in which the host and agent interact.[7]

Drugs, including alcohol, can play differing roles within this public health paradigm. For drug-related illnesses such as alcoholic cirrhosis, for example, the agent can be viewed as alcohol. In the case of alcohol-related trauma, on the other hand, the agent or vector is energy (the impact of an automobile hitting a tree), and alcohol is a significant environmental factor increasing the likelihood that an injurious energy exchange will occur.

The Role of Environmental Factors

Environmental factors—the forces that bring the agent into injurious contact with the host—are critical in this model. A high-risk environment creates myriad opportunities for public health harm. Focusing solely on the host requires as many separate interventions as there are individuals, whereas a single change in the environment may provide protection to large numbers of people by preventing the agent and host from interacting. A comprehensive public health strategy focuses on all three factors within the paradigm, providing care to those who suffer disease or injury, reducing the harmfulness and availability of particular agents, and addressing dangerous conditions or environments that put people at risk for harm.

The Need for a Systems Approach

At the heart of the host-agent-environment triad is the interaction of various causal factors within and between each point of the triangle. These interactions can best be viewed as a system, since changes at one point inevitably alter the other points and the model as a whole. Because the classic triangle model suggests a static rather than dynamic structure, Wallack and Holder[13] have argued for a systems approach that focuses on the dynamic interactions of all factors affecting alcohol and other drug problems.[14,15]

Using a systems model, an individual can be viewed as surrounded by a series of concentric circles representing various forces that impact the individual's drinking and drug-taking decisions. Family, school, workplace, media, community, and economic conditions, among other factors, interact with the individual and with each other in a dynamic system. Shifting individual behavior involves an understanding of the entire system. Similarly, strategies that address risk factors must consider the entire system and not just promote changes in the individual host.

Relationship to Alcohol Policy

Until recently, these public health principles had little impact on society's understanding of alcohol and other drug problems. The field has traditionally focused its attention instead on host and agent factors to the exclusion of an examination of environmental risk factors.

Historical Perspective

During the first part of this century, prior to the repeal of Prohibition in 1933, alcohol policy was dominated by a focus on the individual immorality of drinkers and the need to restrict and eventually prohibit the availability of "demon" alcohol.[16] This perspective continues today in policies addressing many illegal drugs.

Following the repeal, policy shifted to a medical and predominantly host perspective. The predominant focus was on identifying and treating alcoholics. Alcohol problems were considered to rest solely with a limited portion of the population, persons who were predisposed to alcoholism, the disease. With this perspective, policies to address environmental risk factors and controls on alcohol were irrelevant. In fact, they were potentially harmful because they could lead to increased criminal activities and create a "forbidden fruit" status for alcohol.

Recent Trends

In the last 25 years, application of a public health perspective to the alcohol field has brought a dramatic shift in these assumptions.[11,17] In part the shift was occasioned by epidemiologic findings that showed alcohol problems were not experienced by a small, discrete subpopulation of alcoholics but by many others as well. In fact, alcohol problems were reported by those who clearly did not exhibit drinking patterns associated with alcoholism. It was also discovered that individuals may drastically change their problematic drinking patterns over time without alcoholism treatment intervention.[18]

At the same time, researchers became more sensitive to the wide array of health problems associated with alcohol in addition to alcoholism: trauma, alcohol-related birth defects, sexual assaults and other violence, cirrhosis of the liver and other long-term health problems, and workplace and school problems, among others.[17-19] Although alcoholics were more likely to report these problems, the problems were also experienced more broadly across the entire society. The recognition of the diversity of problems associated with alcohol also led to a realization of their complexity. It became apparent that alcohol interacts with and contributes to a wide array of social and health problems; the problems occur in the context of a complex system; and strategies for addressing them must take into account the interaction of a diverse set of factors that put people at risk.

As a result of these shifts in perspective, the field has a new and intense concern with alcohol availability, drinking environments, and environmental risk factors. The focus now is on population-based rather than individual-based strategies. In contrast to Prohibition policies, the aim today is to reduce the harm associated with alcohol use rather than reduce use per se. These topics are explored in more detail later in the chapter.

Relationship to Illegal Drug Policy

Current policies regarding illegal drugs are still dominated by the Prohibition perspective that was applied to alcohol prior to the repeal. The focus has been on individual deviance and immorality and the need to abolish the illegal drug trade. As discussed by Zimring and Hawkins[20] and others,[7] the drug policies of the first Bush administration, as developed by the drug czar William Bennett, were based on four key assumptions:

1. Illegal drug use is fundamentally a moral problem.
2. Illegal drug policy should focus on deterring use, not on reducing associated health problems.
3. All illegal drugs should be treated as the same and different from legal drugs.
4. Punitive measures to stem use and supply should dominate illegal drug policy.

These assumptions are most apparent in the priorities set for the war-on-drugs budget. Between 1986 and 2001, the budget increased sixfold, from approximately $2.8 billion to $18.1 billion.[4] About 70 percent of the funds have been dedicated to law enforcement costs, primarily prison construction, criminal justice costs, drug interdiction programs, and other Department of Justice programs.

Environmental Approach to Drug Policy

An environmental approach to drug policy challenges each of these assumptions. It can be expressed in four basic principles for guiding the development of illegal drug policies:[7,10]

1. Drug use should be treated primarily as a public health issue rather than an issue of individual morality or deviance. Policy should focus on community and societal environments in which individual problems occur.
2. The primary purpose of drug policy should be to reduce drug-related problems. Reducing drug use may be one strategy to reduce drug harm, but it should not be an aim in itself. (Current policies designed to reduce use may actually increase drug-related problems due to the violence they foster.)
3. Priority should be given to those drugs that create the most risk of harm in society. On this basis primary attention needs to be given to alcohol and tobacco, the legal drugs. Drugs that carry a high risk for addiction and/or violent behavior also should receive a higher priority in drug policy than drugs with lower risks of such harm.
4. Prevention, treatment, and recovery measures should dominate drug policy. Punitive measures targeting drug users should be reserved primarily for drug-related behavior associated with other criminal acts.

As with alcohol policy, an environmental approach to preventing illegal drug problems focuses on two basic risk factors: the availability of illegal drugs and the broader family, community, social, cultural, and political contexts in which illegal drug problems occur. These risk factors are addressed by the specific prevention strategies discussed later in the chapter.

The Legal-Illegal Drug Policy Dichotomy

As the above summary suggests, the legality or illegality of a given drug dominates current and past drug availability policies. The legal-illegal dichotomy creates different responses that have little or no relationship to the relative risks to public health the drugs pose.[14,21] If a drug is legal, it is generally widely available at relatively low prices. Powerful economic interests push for ever-increasing markets and lower prices. In response to these economic pressures, legal drug policies generally focus on individual deviance. If a drug is illegal, criminal justice strategies dominate availability policy, with primary attention given to controlling the distribution network and punishing illegal drug users, who are treated as morally weak.

Although they are different, illegal and legal drug policies share basic assumptions: drug problems rest primarily in the individual drug user, either because of moral weakness, disease, or immorality; and environmental risk factors are only marginally addressed. An employee in a workplace with an alcohol or illegal drug problem, for example, may face dismissal or criminal sanctions (more likely with illegal drugs) or be offered treatment through an Employee Assistance Program (more likely with alcohol). In either case, the primary or exclusive focus will be on the individual's deviant behavior, and little or no attention is likely to be placed on workplace environmental factors that may put all employees at risk. For example, alcohol consumption may be implicitly required as part of the job, or difficult work shifts or other factors may increase stress levels, which in turn increase the risk of alcohol or drug use.[22,23]

The dominance of the dichotomy in availability policy has resulted in a basic weakness: our experience with strategies that do not fall within the two extremes is limited. A drug is either a scourge that must be eradicated and its users imprisoned, or a relatively benign substance (except for those few who need to be treated for addiction), with the regulation of its availability and marketing considered unnecessary.

Public support for the current drug war and its focus on criminal justice strategies appears to be waning. Numerous individuals and organizations, including respected public officials, have called for decriminalization or legalization of illegal drugs, arguing many of the principles cited above. Voters in several states have passed by large majorities initiatives that legalize medical marijuana and mandate drug treatment instead of incarceration for first-time drug offenders.[24]

Public health principles do indeed suggest a fundamental shift in focus, from criminal justice to public health strategies. Yet, calls for decriminalization or legalization may be premature or ill-advised. Given the lack of experience in effective control of legal drugs and our historical failure to address underlying environmental factors, deliberate planning and caution will be needed in shifting from a criminal justice focus if the public health consequences of drug use are to be minimized.

THE PREVALENCE OF ALCOHOL AND OTHER DRUG PROBLEMS

Alcohol and other drug use is present throughout society among all social and economic classes, ethnic and racial groups, and geographic regions. Rural areas and the southern region of the country in general have lower use rates. Rates of use vary by type of drug, with alcohol by far the most commonly used drug among all groups. Preferences for illegal drugs vary by type of drug, with some groups favoring one drug over another.

Significance of Alcohol

According to the 1998 National Household Survey (NHS), the most recent survey for which data are available, nearly 52 percent of the population over 12 years of age use alcohol at least once a month, compared to 6.2 percent for those who use any illegal drug. These data are shown in Table 20.1 Most illegal drug use can be attributed to marijuana, which is used by 5.0 percent of the population at least once a month. Cocaine, crack, heroin, and other illegal drug use rates are extremely low.[25]

These higher levels of alcohol use persist when comparing heavy use of drugs. Nearly 6 percent of those aged 12 and older report heavy drinking of five drinks or more on five or more occasions per month, and 15.1 percent report high-risk drinking (defined as five or more drinks on at least one occasion in the past month).[25] Heavy illegal drug use is defined by the Substance Abuse and Mental Health Services Administration (SAMHSA) as use on at least a weekly basis, except for marijuana. Heavy marijuana use is defined as daily use.[26] These contrasting definitions of use may reflect political rather than public health concerns. Even with its stricter definition, however, heavy alcohol use is higher than heavy use of illegal drugs: only 3.1 percent of respondents 12 and older in

Table 20.1. Household Population: Illegal Drug and Alcohol Use (Past Month) 1985, 1990, 1995, 1998

| | Percent of Population | | | |
	1985	1990	1995	1998
Any illegal drug	11.3	6.4	6.1	6.2
Cocaine use	3.0	0.8	0.7	0.8
Crack use	*	0.2	0.2	0.2
Marijuana use	9.4	5.1	4.7	5.0
Alcohol use[†]	59.1	51.2	52.2	51.7
Heavy alcohol use[§]	6.5	5.0	5.5	5.9

*Comparable data not available.
[†]Once a month.
[§]Five or more drinks on the same occasion, five or more times in the last 30 days.
SOURCE: National Household Survey on Drug Abuse, 1975–1998. Substance and Mental Health Data Archive, Data Analysis System. Office of Applied Studies, Substance Abuse and Mental Health Services Administration, US Depart of Health and Human Services. Available at: http://www.icpsr.umich.edu/SAMHDA.

the (NHS) in 1998 reported daily use of marijuana, and just 0.3 percent of respondents reported a weekly or more frequent rate of cocaine use.[25]

Prevalence in Young Adults

Young adults aged 18 to 25 are by far the most likely group to use alcohol and other drugs, with rates decreasing rapidly with age. For example, 16.1 percent of 18- to 25-year-olds used any illegal drug in the previous month as compared with just 3.3 percent of those over 35 years of age.[27] Men are more likely to report alcohol and other drug use than women, with gender differences being most pronounced among those reporting heavy alcohol use.

Between the late 1970s and early 1990s, illegal drug use rates among young adults declined steadily but have risen over the past 10 years (in contrast to the general population; Figure 20.1). Alcohol use rates also declined in this age group until the 1990s, but have been stable since then. Alcohol remains the drug of choice among young people.[28] Interestingly, high-risk drinking among college students has not declined and remains at an alarmingly high rate (over 40 percent). This contrasts with drinking rates of those in the same age group who do not attend college (35 percent), suggesting that college environments may put young people at risk for heavy drinking.[27,28]

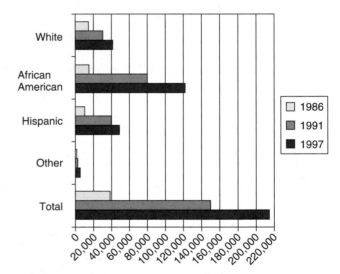

Figure 20.1. State Prison Incarcerations for Illegal Drug Offenses 1986, 1991, 1997.

Sources: *Survey of Prison Inmates,* US Department of Justice, Bureau of Justice Statistics. *Correctional Populations in the United States, 1997.* Washington, DC: US Dept of Justice, Bureau of Justice Statistics; November 2000. NCJ 177613.

Ethnic and Racial Group Variations

Table 20.2 shows rates of drug use by race and income level. Whites are more likely to use alcohol than either blacks or Hispanics. These data also suggest that in-

Table 20.2.   Prevalence of Alcohol and Illegal Drug Use among Full-Time Employed Persons Ages 18 to 40 by Selected Type of Drug, Personal Income, and Ethnicity, 1998

Personal Income by Race/Ethnicity	Percent of Population		
	Past-Month Use of Any Illegal Drug	Past-Month Use of Cocaine*	Past-Month Use of Alcohol
All Respondents			
White	10.0	1.8	69.7
Black	9.3	0.9	54.6
Hispanic	6.4	1.8	52.7
Total	9.1	1.5	65.3
Less than $12,000			
White	18.4	2.7	65.9
Black	12.2	1.6	49.1
Hispanic	8.5	1.9	47.4
Total†	14.9	2.3	58.6
$12,000-19,999			
White	8.7	1.6	61.8
Black	11.6	1.4	57.0
Hispanic	5.9	1.8	54.6
Total†	8.4	1.6	59.2
$20,000-29,999			
White	10.4	1.4	69.1
Black	7.6	0.4	52.1
Hispanic	5.2	1.6	57.7
Total†	9.2	1.2	65.4
$30,000 or over			
White	8.0	1.8	74.6
Black	6.4	0.5	58.7
Hispanic	5.8	2.1	75.0
Total†	7.2	1.6	71.8

*Includes crack.
†Prevalence data of "Other Ethnicities" not reported separately but included in "Total."
SOURCE: National Household Survey on Drug Abuse, 1998. Substance and Mental Health Data Archive, Data Analysis System. Office of Applied Studies, Substance Abuse and Mental Health Services Administration, US Depart of Health and Human Services. Available at: http://www.icpsr.umich.edu/SAMHDA.

come level may be a better predictor of illegal drug use than racial or ethnic background. Those with lower incomes may be more likely to use illegal drugs, including cocaine, and less likely to use alcohol than those with higher incomes, regardless of racial or ethnic background.[25] Employment status also serves as an important predictor of illegal drug use.[29] Unemployed respondents are more than twice as likely to report illegal drug use than those who have full-time employment, regardless of race.[27]

A recent study[30] of crack cocaine use reinforces the importance of looking beyond racial and ethnic factors in assessing drug use data. In the study, crack cocaine users from the 1988 NHS were grouped into neighborhood clusters, in effect holding constant shared characteristics such as drug availability and social conditions. Certain neighborhoods had higher rates of crack cocaine use, but the rates of use within the neighborhood clusters did not vary by race or ethnic background. In fact, the only statistically significant racial or ethnic association involved teenage African Americans, who were less likely to smoke crack cocaine than their white counterparts living in similar neighborhood clusters. The authors concluded, "Given similar social conditions, crack cocaine smoking does not depend strongly on race per se as a personal characteristic of individuals."[30] They urged greater attention to the social environments in which drug use takes place.

Excluded Populations

The NHS and high school and young adult surveys are the primary source for data on alcohol and other drug use in the United States, as the above discussion suggests. Unfortunately, these data sources are incomplete because they do not reflect the entire population. The NHS does not include individuals who reside in hotels, hospitals, and jails or who are homeless. The school-based surveys do not include young people who have dropped out of school before graduation or who are absent the day of the survey.

Various fragmentary studies suggest that alcohol and other drug use within these populations is significantly higher than in the general population.[7] Accurate estimates of drug use in these high-risk populations are impossible. The Office of Drug Control Policy estimated in that there were more than twice as many "hard-core" (at least weekly) cocaine users in the 2 percent nonhousehold-resident population than in the 98 percent household-resident population.[31]

Public Health Consequences of Alcohol and Other Drug Use

Differences in the rates of alcohol and other drug use are reflected in data reporting public health and societal problems, with alcohol problems far more prevalent than illegal drug problems. The nature and definition of the problems also differ, reflecting in part the social responses that emerge from their legal or illegal status. These differences make accurate comparisons between problems associated with alcohol and problems associated with other drugs difficult or impossible. In general, illegal drug use itself is defined as a problem, while alcohol use is usually defined as problematic only when it leads to specific behavioral or physical harm.

Mortality and Traumatic Injury

The federal government estimates that alcohol is a direct or indirect cause of approximately 110,000 deaths per year.[32] Alcohol-related traffic fatalities and cirrhosis of the liver comprise the largest groups of deaths, totaling 16,000 and 26,000 deaths, respectively.[33,34] Alcohol is also implicated in other forms of traumatic deaths, including homicide, suicide, burns, poisoning, drowning, and falls as well as other forms of alcohol-related disease, such as cancers of the liver and stomach.[33]

In addition, alcohol is a major contributor to traumatic injury. Alcohol-related motor vehicle injuries are by far the largest category of these, causing approximately 300,000 serious injuries each year.[35] In general, the higher the blood alcohol content of the person causing the injury, the more serious the injury. Tragically, alcohol-related injuries and deaths are most likely to impact young people. In fact, alcohol-related motor vehicle crashes constitute the leading cause of death for those between the ages of 1 and 24 years.[34] It is estimated that those dying from alcohol-related causes lose 26 years from their normal life expectancy, far higher than other major causes of death in the United States.[36]

Data regarding illegal drug-related deaths are not nearly as reliable or precise as those available for alcohol. The U.S. National Center for Health Statistics estimates that in 1997 there were approximately 15,973 deaths that were directly attributable to all illegal drug use.[37] The Office of National Drug Control Policy estimated that in 1995 there were 52,624 drug-related deaths, using a methodology that included other drug-related deaths such as HIV/AIDS, tuberculosis, hepatitis, and motor vehicle crashes.[38] The Drug Abuse Warning Network's (DAWN) medical examiner reports[39] provide data regarding drug-related deaths from 40 major metropolitan areas. In 1999, 9,684 deaths were reported to be related to heroin, morphine, or cocaine. By comparison, marijuana was mentioned in only 670 deaths.

DAWN also provides data regarding illegal drug episodes reported in emergency room (ER) visits.[40] Approximately 544,193 emergency room episodes involving drugs other than alcohol (including prescription and over-the-counter drugs) were reported in 2000. Among illegal drugs, cocaine was mentioned 174,896 times, heroin and morphine were mentioned 97,287 times and marijuana was mentioned 94,446 times. There are increases in illegal drug mentions in the DAWN reports between 1990 and 2000 after reductions in the late 1980s. DAWN does not provide a means to compare these data with data on alcohol-related ER episodes but does report 196,277 mentions of use of both illicit drugs and alcohol. Based on estimates of alcohol-related traumatic events, it is probable that alcohol accounts for several times the already alarming numbers reported for illegal drugs.

The relationship of alcohol and other drugs to violent episodes has become an increasing concern, reflecting the high rates of violence in our society. Available studies suggest that illegal drug-related violence is concentrated in African-American and Latino inner-city communities, with young people in these communities having, by far, the highest rates of homicide.[5] Drug-related violence is closely associated with the illegal drug trade.[38] Domestic violence, sexual violence, and child abuse and neglect are all closely associated with alcohol consumption.[41,42]

Alcohol and Drug Dependence

The 1998 NHS found that nearly 4.1 million individuals were dependent on illicit drugs.[27] Those with low incomes are more likely to be in need of drug treatment in part because of poorer social advantages and supports available to them.[9] A minority of those people who need drug treatment receive it. For the entire year of 1998, only 963,000 persons, or about 20 percent of those needing treatment, were actually enrolled in a drug treatment program.[27]

The federal government estimates that in 1998, 9.7 million adults were dependent on alcohol, more than two times the estimates of those needing drug treatment. Only 1.7 million (17 percent) persons requiring alcohol treatment were actually enrolled in alcohol treatment units in 1998.[27] There has been a long-term shift from publicly funded to privately funded treatment programs, which has led to long waiting lists for low-income individuals who cannot afford the privately funded programs.[7]

Other Public Health Problems

Alcohol and other drug use is associated with a wide array of other public health problems. Alcohol is a leading preventable cause of birth defects in the United States, and fetal exposures to maternal illegal drug consumption is a serious and growing concern.[43,44] Although illegal drug use is common in all racial and socioeconomic groups, the impact on infant health appears to be concentrated among women of color and those with lower incomes. This is due to their lack of other basic health and social support systems and the higher likelihood that their illegal drug use will be reported to authorities.[7,33]

The use of injection to administer illegal drugs has become a significant factor in the spread of AIDS. Alcohol use has been shown to increase the likelihood of unsafe sexual practices, thus contributing to the spread of AIDS.[7,33,45]

Alcohol, Other Drugs, and the Criminal Justice System

Alcohol and other drug use has an enormous impact on the criminal justice system. In 1999, over 1.9 million arrests were made for alcohol-related crimes (including, driving under the influence, liquor law violations, and public drunkenness), and another one million arrests were made for illegal drug crimes.[46] More than three-quarters (80 percent) of illegal drug arrests involve drug possession, with 40 percent involving marijuana possession. The remainder of drug arrests (20 percent) involve the manufacture and sale of drugs. Alcohol and other drug arrests constituted more than 31 percent of all arrests made in 1999.

Alcohol and other drugs also contribute to other crimes. Surveys suggest that 35 percent of those committing crimes were under the influence of alcohol.[40] Rates of alcohol involvement may vary by the type of crime committed. For example, among crimes between intimates, associated rates of alcohol use are higher.[47] In three out of four incidents of spousal abuse, the offender had been drinking alcohol. Studies

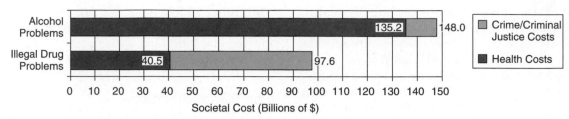

Figure 20.2. Economic Costs of Alcohol and Illegal Drug Problems.
Source: Harwood HJ, Fountain D, Livermore G. The economic costs of alcohol and drug abuse in the United States. *Addiction*. 1999; 94(5), 631–635.

also suggest a high level of association between crimes and other drug use, with 27 to 30 percent of jail and prison inmates reported being under the influence of illegal drugs at the time of the offense.[47]

Although alcohol offenses account for a greater number of arrests than illegal drug offenses, there are striking differences in both the trends and the consequences of the two types of offenses. Arrests for alcohol offenses decreased over 20 percent between 1990 and 1999, while arrests for illegal drug offenses increased by 36 percent, even though during that same period illegal drug use declined.[40]

Incarceration rates for drug offenders increased during this same period. As shown in Figure 20.1, in state prisons incarcerations for drug offenses increased from approximately 38,100 to 216,000 between 1986 and 1999, which is nearly a sixfold increase.[48,49] Drug offenders now account for 21 percent of all state inmates in 1997 (up from 9 percent in 1986) and for 58 percent of all federal inmates.[48–50] By contrast, public order offenses, which include all alcohol offenses, only total about 10 percent of all incarcerations. Among juvenile offenders in state prisons, admissions for drug offenses increased from 70 (2 percent of admissions) to 840 (14 percent of admissions) between 1985 and 1997.[51]

Perhaps most disturbing is the racial and ethnic makeup of those in prison for illegal drug offenses. As shown in Figure 20.1, African Americans and Latinos are more likely to be incarcerated for illegal drug offenses, a trend that has accelerated dramatically since 1986. Approximately 85 percent of the increase in state incarcerations for illegal drug crimes between 1986 and 1991 involved African Americans, Latinos, or other people of color.

Economic Costs of Alcohol and Other Drug Problems

As the data in this section suggest, alcohol and other drug problems create staggering costs for society in terms of human suffering. The impact is enormous for individuals, families, communities, and institutions within communities, as well as for society as a whole. The suffering associated with these problems also produces economic costs. As shown in Figure 20.2, in 1992 alcohol problems caused $148 billion and illegal drug abuse caused $97.6 billion in societal costs, including the costs of treatment, medical care, criminal justice, and prevention.[52] Nearly two-thirds of drug problem costs are related to crime and criminal justice, with only one-third of the costs related to health. By comparison, core health-related costs account for more than 90 percent of the costs associated with alcohol problems.[52] In other words, alcohol problems result in over three times more core health costs than illegal drug problems ($135.2 billion compared to $40.5 billion), and the bulk of economic costs ($57.1 billion) associated with illegal drugs are the direct result of the criminal justice response to the problems.

A PUBLIC HEALTH AGENDA FOR ADDRESSING ALCOHOL AND OTHER DRUG PROBLEMS

The preceding sections paint a distressing picture regarding the state of alcohol and other drug problems and related policy in the United States today.

Alcohol and other drugs are widely used throughout society, and problems resulting from their use are causing enormous suffering and economic costs, ranking among the most serious societal health problems. Society's response to the problems, however, has not been effective and in some cases has served to exacerbate underlying social, political, and economic injustices.

Although alcohol and other drug use rates are spread throughout all demographic groups in society, problems associated with that use are concentrated disproportionately among those with the least resources. This reflects, in part, underlying environmental factors (for example, racism, poverty, lack of employment, and neighborhood deterioration), which increase the prevalence and severity of alcohol and other drug problems.

Societal responses have focused primarily on illegal drugs despite the fact that alcohol problems are far more serious in terms of human suffering and economic costs than the problems associated with all illegal drugs combined. Individual based strategies focusing on punishing individuals have predominated in social policy, with environmental risk factors virtually ignored. This societal response to illegal drugs has created its own costs.

The war on drugs has dramatically increased the likelihood of incarceration, particularly for young African-American and Latino men. At the same time it has reduced the availability of treatment programs to those with low income. In general, someone who is Euro-American and middle or upper class and suffers an alcohol or other drug problem will probably receive treatment; someone of color and poor is much less likely to have access to treatment and much more likely to be imprisoned.

In short, current policy has largely ignored the public health priorities for both alcohol and other drugs discussed above. Both Republican and Democratic administrations have supported these policy priorities, and the new Bush administration has signaled in its 2001 national drug control strategy that there will be no change of direction for at least the next four years.

Specific policy reform agendas that need to be incorporated into the nation's agenda regarding alcohol and other drug problems are presented next. The discussion focuses on environmental prevention strategies. They should be viewed as complementing other strategies that address individual risk factors, such as educational campaigns and treatment/recovery programs, which are beyond the scope of this chapter.

Alcohol Availability

As previously mentioned, alcohol and other drug availability is a critical policy variable, with striking contrasts between drugs that are illegal and those that are legal. In general, alcohol is widely and increasingly available, the result of public policy measures supported by the alcohol industry.[11,14] Increasing availability increases the risk of alcohol problems. The following policy measures relating to availability have been shown to be effective in reducing alcohol problems.

Increase Alcohol Taxes

The relative price of alcohol has decreased steadily during the last four decades, primarily because state and federal alcohol taxes have been eroded by inflation. Research suggests that substantially increasing alcohol taxes (to levels reflecting the impact of inflation since 1967) will reduce alcohol consumption and alcohol problems, particularly among young people.[53–58]

Regulate the Number, Concentration, and Types of Alcohol Outlets

Alcohol outlets come in various forms—bars, liquor stores, and public arenas, among others. Recent research suggests that a high concentration of outlets within neighborhoods or blocks is associated with elevated rates of alcohol-related problems such as sexually transmitted diseases, crime, and violence.[59–62] Alcohol outlets are often concentrated in low-income communities,[63] thus increasing the risk of problems in these communities and adversely affecting their quality of life. Studies have also shown that a sudden increase in the number of outlets selling alcohol within a state (e.g., through introduction of alcohol into a new type of outlet such as grocery stores or through privatization of state monopoly systems) may increase alcohol consumption.[64,65] Control on retail availability involves both state and community action.

Encourage Responsible Practices among Alcohol Retailers

The serving practices of alcohol retailers often contribute to the risk of alcohol problems. Studies show that, prior to any intervention, retailers are likely to illegally sell alcohol to minors and intoxicated customers and may promote high-risk drinking through drink promotions such as happy hours.[66–71] Approximately 50 percent of drinking-while-driving events originate from licensed establishments.[72,73] To promote responsible service of alcohol, many communities and states have encouraged or mandated training for alcohol servers.[74] Although training alcohol servers on responsible service of alcohol may increase knowledge and change attitudes, server training by itself is unlikely to significantly reduce rates of illegal alcohol service.[75,76] Manager training is also necessary to provide managers with skills to develop establishment policies that will clearly communicate establishment expectations about responsible alcohol service.[75,77]

Whereas server and manager training is a promising approach for preventing overservice of alcohol and cutting off alcohol service to obviously intoxicated patrons, training by itself is less promising for preventing illegal alcohol sales to minors.[78] However, enforcement campaigns where law enforcement conduct compliance checks (e.g., underage person attempts to purchase alcohol under the supervision of a law enforcement agent; penalties are applied to the server and/or the license holder) is promising for preventing sales to minors.[79,80] Civil liability statutes (so-called "dram shop laws") can also provide incentives for the implementation of responsible serving practices.[81,82]

Increase the Minimum Drinking Age

Following Prohibition, most states had an age 21 minimum legal drinking age (MLDA). During the 1970s, many states lowered their MLDA to ages 18, 19, or 20. As a result of grassroots pressure, most of these states raised the MLDA back to age 21 by the 1980s.[83,84] In 1984, the federal government increased pressure on states that had not raised their MLDA,

threatening to take away federal highway funds.[85] By 1988, all states had established an age 21 MLDA. The preponderance of research findings indicates that increases in the MLDA resulted in less alcohol consumption and fewer traffic crash deaths among youth.[83,86]

The National Highway Traffic Safety Administration estimates that the age 21 MLDA has saved over 19,000 lives since 1975 through prevention of traffic crashes.[87] Recent studies suggest that the age 21 MLDA may also be preventing other alcohol-related problems among youth such as suicides and vandalism.[83,86] Despite the age 21 MLDA, many youth continue to drink alcohol, no doubt in part because the MLDA has not been well enforced across most states.[88,89] As a result, youth have had easy access to alcohol from commercial (e.g., bars, restaurants, convenience and liquor stores) and social (e.g., friends, family, coworkers) sources.[90] To increase effectiveness of the age 21 MLDA, many communities and states are developing and enforcing policies targeting specific sources of alcohol (e.g., compliance checks to prevent illegal sales to minors).

Regulate the Types of Alcoholic Beverages on the Market

The alcohol industry is continuously developing new types of beverages as well as new packaging for existing products. Some new products have raised serious public health concerns, particularly when young people appear to be targeted. African-American communities, for example, have protested the marketing of malt liquor products because the marketing appears to target young people and saturates their communities.[91] Young people are purchasing these products in 40-ounce bottles and drinking them as single servings, thereby increasing the risk of intoxication.[91] Other high-alcohol content products, often called alcopops, are sweetly flavored (e.g., watermelon or lemonade) and are packaged in ways that are appealing to youth (e.g., in test tubes, with cartoonlike characters on the package).[92] Alcopops are more popular among youth than adults and may be a gateway to use of other alcoholic beverages. Regulations at the state and/or federal level can control these marketing practices.

Regulate Alcohol Availability in Institutional and Public Settings

Alcohol service is not limited to commercial alcohol establishments. Drinking occurs in a wide variety of public and private settings—community fairs, public parks, sports stadia, private clubs, and churches, among others. Every community institution has a policy regarding alcohol service, although in many cases that policy is unwritten and unspoken. A community-based prevention strategy should include the development of alcohol policies in these settings and institutions. It should address such questions as: Is alcohol service appropriate in the given setting? If so, how should it be made available? What steps will be taken to reduce the risk of intoxication and service to minors?[93]

Implement Alcohol Production Reforms

Several state and federal policies actively encourage and subsidize alcohol production and marketing. For example, special tax incentives have encouraged the replanting of agricultural lands with wine grapes in California and the production of rum in the Virgin Islands.[14] A variety of production reforms should be instituted to end subsidies to the alcohol industry, encourage nonalcohol-producing crops, and lessen the profitability of alcohol production.

Promote Enforcement of Alcohol Availability Laws and Impose Administrative Sanctions When Violations Are Detected

Enforcement and the resulting penalty are the two key components for creating *deterrence:* a credible threat that a significant, relatively swift, penalty will be imposed when violations occur.[94] Laws prohibiting sales to minors and intoxicated persons, for example, are routinely violated, increasing the risk of underage drinking, public intoxication, and drinking while driving. Research shows that increased enforcement substantially reduces violations of these laws.[95] In general, administrative sanctions, such as fines, license suspensions, and license revocations, are preferable to criminal penalties because they are

easier and cheaper to enforce, are more quickly imposed, and do not carry the moral overtones inherent in criminal justice proceedings.[14,96] Reforming state Alcoholic Beverage Control agency licensing and enforcement practices is therefore a high priority in the alcohol policy prevention field.[96]

Many or most of these proposed reforms were included in the recommendations of former Surgeon General C. Everett Koop in his workshop on preventing drunk driving.[97] The philosophy underlying the reforms and many of the recommendations themselves are incorporated into other policy documents, including reports by the American Assembly,[98] the National Academy of Sciences,[19] and the American Public Health Association.[10]

Illegal Drug Availability

Much of the enforcement action taken to cut off the supply of illegal drugs has focused on border interdiction, with little success. Future efforts to reduce availability of illegal drugs may be best served by focusing on controls at the local level—a strategy that has been used successfully for alcohol control.[99,100] However, only limited options are available for addressing the availability of illegal drugs as long as they remain illegal.[14] Four policy reforms are outlined here, but implementation should be instituted with caution, with the impact carefully assessed. A shift from a predominantly criminal justice focus to a public health focus could unintentionally increase drug availability, thereby potentially increasing the risk of drug problems.

Discontinue the Heavy Reliance on Border Interdiction and Incarceration of Drug Users

These strategies have created enormous economic and social costs and have not been effective in reducing the availability and use of drugs. Their use should be greatly limited or discontinued and the resources they use redirected to public health reforms. Treatment should be readily available for those in need without regard to income, and treatment availability should be a high priority for those who are incarcerated. Alternatives to incarceration, such as fines and community service, should be investigated.

Redirect Drug Eradication and Control Efforts

Drug eradication and control efforts should focus on the violence associated with the drug trade, on large producers and retailers, and on those drugs causing the greatest public health harm, such as cocaine and heroin. As discussed above, the reduction of harm should be the primary goal of a public health drug policy.

Promote Drug Control Programs That Limit Availability at the Community Level and Address Community Safety

Illegal drugs create unsafe community environments. Drug sales and drug use may concentrate in public areas (for example, parks, liquor stores, sidewalks), adversely affecting the quality of life of the neighborhood and community and increasing the risk of violence. Drug sales and use at private residences may have a similar impact. Various programs have organized community action to address these problems, thereby building a constituency for broader public health reforms.[101,102] This in turn supports environmental interventions, which are discussed below.

Promote the Use of Various Civil Sanctions as Possible Alternatives to Criminal Sanctions

As with administrative penalties (discussed above), civil sanctions are preferable to criminal sanctions because they are easier to administer and enforce, they are cheaper, and they do not carry the moral overtones inherent in criminal justice proceedings.[14] For example, public nuisance statutes can be used to close down crack houses; forfeiture, civil liability, and tax laws can deter drug production; and local zoning ordinances can deter businesses from allowing loitering and drug dealing in and around their premises.[102–104]

Addressing Other Environmental Factors

As discussed above, an individual's environment affects his or her alcohol and other drug use behavior. The environment can be conceptualized as expanding levels of influence over individual behavior, with each level interacting with the others. Prevention efforts will be more effective if they operate across differing environmental levels. The availability of alcohol and other drugs at each level is a critical environmental factor, and it interacts with each of these other major aspects of the environment: family systems; school, peer, and neighborhood environment; workplace environment; community environment; alcohol marketing and mass media; and social, economic, and political environments.

Family Systems

Family experience with and parental attitudes towards alcohol and other drug use and their related problems affect a child's likelihood of developing alcohol and other drug problems.[105,106] Poor family management, lack of family bonding, poor monitoring of a child's behavior, and physical abuse or neglect have all been identified as risk factors.[107]

School, Peer, and Neighborhood Environment

Schools that maintain and enforce clear, strict policies toward alcohol and other drug use report less use among students.[105,108] Peer use of alcohol and other drugs has consistently been found to be a strong predictor of use among young people. Neighborhoods with high-density housing, high residential mobility, physical deterioration, and high unemployment rates have high rates of juvenile crime and illegal drug trafficking.[7,105,109]

Workplace Environment

Workplaces and occupations with high availability of alcohol, unclear rules and expectations regarding drinking on the job, high stress, and limited supervision create high risks for alcohol problems among workers.[110]

Community Environment

The above factors interact and are included in the community environment. Current prevention planning stresses the need to plan and implement programs at the community level. This permits programs to address the multiplicity of factors in a coordinated fashion.[7,101]

Two recent community trials were designed to influence and evaluate effects of multiple environmental changes occurring within communities: (1) the Communities Trial Project (CTP), and (2) Communities Mobilizing for Change on Alcohol (CMCA). The goal of CTP was to reduce injuries and deaths related to alcohol among the general population.[111] Community mobilization was used to implement a multicomponent intervention that included media to increase awareness, training of alcohol establishments, compliance checks conducted by law enforcement to reduce illegal alcohol sales to underage individuals, increased enforcement of drunk-driving laws, and reduction of alcohol availability through regulation of alcohol outlets. The intervention was implemented in three communities, selected based on readiness to address alcohol-related issues. The overall intervention of CTP resulted in decreases in self-reported consumption, drinking and driving, injury-producing crashes, assaults, and injuries.[99]

The goal of CMCA was to reduce alcohol consumption and related problems among youth by reducing youth access to alcohol from commercial (e.g., liquor stores, bars, restaurants) and social (e.g., parents, friends) sources through local and institutional policy changes.[112] Organizers were hired for each of the seven intervention communities to develop strategies and support for changes in community policies. The overall intervention across the communities resulted in statistically significant improvements in the serving practices at bars and restaurants (including increased age identification checking and decreases in their propensity to sell alcohol to underage individuals).[100] Additionally, reductions were also observed for drinking rates among 18- to 20-year-olds (but not 12th graders), the number of 18- to 20-year-olds providing to other underage youth, and arrest and traffic crash indicators among youth.[113]

Alcohol Marketing and the Mass Media

Industry marketing programs play a major role in shaping the alcohol environment, in turn, affecting children's beliefs, attitudes, and intentions to drink.[114,115]

Wallack describes alcohol advertising as the single most important source of alcohol education in our society today.[116] The alcohol industry spends over $1 billion annually in mass media advertising and three or more times that amount on promotional and sponsorship campaigns.[117] The mass media also play a major role in shaping the alcohol and other drug environment. Portrayals of alcohol and other drug use in entertainment programming and the presentation of alcohol and other drug issues in public affairs programming are all important environmental factors.[118,119] Several prevention strategies, including media advocacy and counteradvertising campaigns, seek to shift the role of mass media so that they support, rather than undercut, environmental strategies.[120]

Social, Economic, and Political Environments

Social, economic, and political forces interact and share the more immediate environments surrounding individual behavior. Economic and political conditions and social norms have a dramatic effect on all other environmental levels.[7,121]

These broader forces have their most dramatic impact in poor communities, which face multiple risk factors for alcohol and other drug problems. Many inner-city communities, for example, have high levels of alcohol and other drug availability; lack basic educational, housing, health care, child care, and employment opportunities; and face institutional racism.[122] These circumstances have put communities, neighborhoods, and families in stress and established the crack cocaine trade as an attractive economic alternative.[7,123] In short, these communities face a set of conditions identified in the literature as creating a high-risk environment for violence and alcohol and other drug problems.

Addressing these environmental concerns requires attention to broad economic, political, and social forces, including the development of a viable social support system, an economic base that is community controlled, and an end to institutional racism. Ironically, funds for some of these purposes were diverted to the war on drugs during the late 1980s, thereby exacerbating the very problems the war on drugs was attempting to address.

IMPLICATIONS FOR PUBLIC HEALTH PRACTICE

The ambitious public health agenda just outlined calls for fundamental changes in current alcohol and other drug policies. This call for reform is based on careful examination of data regarding use and problems and the application of a public health model of prevention. The proposed reforms are not new; indeed, as documented in previous sections, numerous authors and public policy officials are now calling for basic public health reforms. Why, then, has the public health field had so little impact on the public policy debate?

Addressing environmental risk factors, including availability, requires a fundamental shift in orientation in the field of public health, which has traditionally addressed alcohol and other drug problems primarily at the individual level and developed programs to be delivered to those at risk. The recommendations here, however, require changes in public policy. This requires very different skills. For success, the lobbying power of the alcohol industry must be neutralized. The powerful coalition that views the war on drugs as only one aspect of a broader social agenda must also be confronted. These goals require political and policy skills in addition to the program skills traditionally associated with the public health field. Three sets of skills are particularly important in this endeavor: community organizing, coalition building and political advocacy, and media advocacy skills.

Community Organizing

Public health's strength lies in its service to masses of citizens. Building a grassroots network of citizens to advocate for and support new alcohol and other drug policies must be a top agenda for the field. Only democratic action by large numbers of people can be effective in changing the current balance of power.[7,124] Community organizing begins at the neighborhood and community level. This serves to emphasize the need to address problems at these levels.

Coalition Building and Political Advocacy

Bridges across communities and among diverse groups within a community are needed to reform public policies at all levels—local, regional, state, and federal. Coalition building complements community organizing, stimulating community involvement and building on the power of numbers and diversity in a community.[11] Political advocacy and policy analysis skills involve learning to operate effectively within the policy arena. Public health data need to be presented effectively to policy makers, and arguments for reform need to be presented concisely and powerfully. A keen sense of political timing must also be developed.

Media Advocacy Skills

Public health professionals also need to become effective in the mass media, reframing issues and advancing alternative solutions.

CONCLUSION

The public health field provides a unique and powerful set of tools for conceptualizing and addressing alcohol and other drug problems in our society. These problems constitute a crisis for our society, causing untold tragedies in the lives of individuals, families, and communities. Their solution requires confronting some of the basic inequities and injustices afflicting our nation. Public health provides a foundation for action. It is up to those in the field to build on that foundation.

ACKNOWLEDGMENTS

Preparation of this manuscript was supported in part by grants from the Beryl Buck Memorial Trust and the California Wellness Foundation.

Special thanks to Kathleen Lenk for help with preparation of this document.

References

1. Office of National Drug Control Policy. *Breaking the Cycle of Drug Abuse: 1993 Interim National Drug Control Strategy.* Washington, DC: Office of National Drug Control Policy, US Executive Office of the President; September 1993.

2. Reuter P, Crawford G, Cave J. *Sealing the Borders.* Santa Monica, Calif: RAND Co; 1988.

3. Nadelmann E. U.S. drug policy: a bad export. *Foreign Pol.* 1988;70:83-108.

4. Office of National Drug Control Policy. *Summary: FY 2002 National Drug Control Budget.* Washington, DC: Office of National Drug Control Policy, US Executive Office of the President; 2001.

5. Vaicuis I, Isacson A. *"Plan Columbia": The Debate in Congress, 2000.* Washington, DC: Center for International Policy; December 2000.

6. Morgan P, Wallack L, Buchanan D. Waging drug wars: prevention strategy or politics as usual. *Drugs Soc.* 1989;3/4: 99-124.

7. Mosher J, Yanagisako K. Public health, not social warfare: a public health approach to illegal drug policy. *J. Public Health Pol.* 1991;12:278-323.

8. Musto D. *The American Disease: Origins of Narcotic Control.* New York, NY: Oxford University Press; 1973.

9. Gerstein D, Harwood H, eds. *Treating Drug Problems.* Institute of Medicine, Committee for the Substance Abuse Coverage Study, Division of Health Care Services. Washington, DC: National Academy Press; 1990.

10. American Public Health Association. *A Public Health Response to the War on Drugs: Reducing Alcohol, Tobacco and Other Drug Problems Among the Nation's Youth.* APHA Position Paper 8817: Am. J. Public Health. 1989;79:360-364.

11. Center for Substance Abuse Prevention. *Environmental Prevention Strategies: Putting Theory into Practice. Training and Resource Guide.* Rockville, Md: Center for Substance Abuse Prevention, Substance Abuse and Mental Health Services Administration; 2000.

12. Streicker J, ed. *Case Histories in Alcohol Policy.* San Francisco, Calif: Trauma Foundation; 2000.

13. Wallack L, Holder H. The prevention of alcohol-related problems: a systems approach. In: Holder H, ed. *Control Issues in Alcohol Abuse Prevention: Strategies for States and Communities.* Greenich, Conn: JAI Press; 1987.

14. Mosher J. Drug availability in a public health perspective. In: Resnik H, ed. *Youth and Drugs: Society's Mixed Messages.* OSAP Prevention Monograph 6. Rockville, Md: Office of Substance Abuse Prevention; 1990:129-168.

15. Mosher J. Alcohol and poverty: analyzing the link between alcohol-related problems and social policy. In: Samuels S, Smith M, eds. *Improving the Health of the Poor: Strategies for Prevention.* Menlo Park, Calif: Henry J. Kaiser Family Foundation; 1992:97-121.

16. Levine HG. The alcohol problem in America: From temperance to alcoholism. *Br J Addict.* 1984;79:109-119.

17. Room R. Alcohol control and public health. *Annu Rev Public Health.* 1984;5:293-317.

18. Cahalan D. *Problem Drinkers: A National Survey.* San Francisco, Calif: Jossey-Bass; 1970.

19. Moore M, Gerstein D, eds. *Alcohol and Public Policy: Beyond the Shadow of Prohibition.* Washington, DC: National Academy Press; 1981.

20. Zimring R, Hawkins G. *What Kind of Drug War?* Working Paper No. 16. Berkeley, Calif: Earl Warren Legal Institute; 1990.

21. Himmelstein J. *The Strange Career of Marihuana: Politics and Ideology of Drug Control in America.* Westport, Conn: Greenwood Press; 1983.

22. Mosher J. Preventing drinking-driving in the employment setting: Toward an environmental perspective. In: *Automobile Club of Southern California, Drinking and Driving Prevention Symposium: Proceedings.* Ontario: Automobile Club of Southern California; 1992:229-242.

23. Ames G. Research and strategies for the primary prevention of workplace alcohol problems. *Alcohol Health Res World.* 1993;17:19-25.

24. Lindesmith Center. Election yields largest-ever repudiation of nation's war on drugs [press release]. Washington, DC: Lindesmith Center; November 8, 2000.

25. *National Household Surveys on Drug Abuse 1975-1998.* Rockville, Md: Substance Abuse and Mental Health Services Administration, Office of Applied Studies, Substance and Mental Health Data Archive, Data Analysis System; 2001. Available at: http://www.icpsr.umich.edu/SAMHDA.

26. Epstein J, Gfroerer J. *Estimating Substance Abuse Treatment Need From a National Household Survey 1994-96.* Analyses of Substance Abuse and Treatment

Need Issues, Analytic Series Report A-7. Rockville, Md: Substance Abuse and Mental Health Services Administration, Office of Applied Studies; 2001. Available at: http://www.samhsa.gov/oas/oas.html.

27. *Summary of Findings From the 1998 National Household Survey on Drug Abuse.* Rockville, Md: Substance Abuse and Mental Health Services Administration, Office of Applied Studies; 2001. Available at: http://www.samhsa.gov/hhsurvey/hhsurvey.html.

28. Johnston LD, O'Malley PM, Bachman JG. *National Survey Results on Drug Use From the Monitoring the Future Study, 1975-1998.* Rockville, Md: National Institute on Drug Abuse; 1999.

29. Parker KD, Weaver G, Calhoun T. Predictors of alcohol and drug use: A multi-ethnic comparison. *J Soc Psychol.* 1995;135(5):581-590.

30. Lillie-Blanton M, Anthony J, Schuster C. Probing the meaning of racial/ethnic group comparisons in crack cocaine smoking. *JAMA.* 1993;69:993-998.

31. White House *National Drug Control Strategy.* Washington, DC: Office of National Drug Control Policy; 1990, 1991, 1992, 1993.

32. *National Institute on Alcohol Abuse and Alcoholism Databases: Quick Facts 1996.* Rockville, Md: US Depart of Health and Human Services, National Institute on Alcohol Abuse and Alcoholism; 2001. Available at: http://www.niaaa.nih.gov/databases/armort01.txt.

33. *Ninth Special Report to the US Congress on Alcohol and Health.* Rockville, Md: US Depart of Health and Human Services, National Institute on Alcohol Abuse and Alcoholism; 1997. NIH Publication 97-4017.

34. *Injury Facts, 1999 Edition.* Itasca, Ill: National Safety Council; 1999.

35. *Traffic Safety Facts 1999: Alcohol.* Washington, DC: US Depart of Transportation, National Highway Traffic Safety Administration; 1999. DOT Report HS 809 086.

36. Perspectives in disease prevention and health promotion. Alcohol-related mortality and years of potential life lost—United States, 1987. *MMWR.* 1990;39(11):173-178.

37. Hoyert DL, Kochanek KD, Smith BL, Murphy SL. Deaths: Final data for 1997. *National Vital Statistics Reports.* Vol 47, No. 19. Hyattsville, Md: National Center for Health Statistics; 1999. Available at: http://www.cdc.gov/nchs/nvss.htm.

38. *The National Drug Control Strategy 2000 Annual Report.* Washington, DC: Office of National Drug Control Policy; 2001.

39. *Drug Abuse Warning Network Annual Medical Examiner Data 1999.* Rockville, Md: Substance Abuse and Mental Health Services Administration, Office of

Applied Studies; 2000. Available at: http://www.samhsa.gov/oas/oas.html.

40. *Year-End 2000 Emergency Department Data from the Drug Abuse Warning Network.* Rockville, Md: Substance Abuse and Mental Health Services Administration, Office of Applied Studies; 2001. DAWN Series D-18 DHHA Publication (SMA) 013532. Available at: http://www.samhsa.gov/oas/oas.html.

41. *Alcohol and Crime.* Washington, DC: US Dept of Justice, Bureau of Justice Statistics; 1998. Available at: http://www.ojp.usdoj.gov/bjs/abstract/ac.htm.

42. *National Institute on Alcohol Abuse and Alcoholism. Tenth Special Report to the U.S. Congress on Alcohol and Health.* Rockville, Md: US Depart of Health and Human Services, National Institute on Alcohol Abuse and Alcoholism; 2000. NIH Publication 00-1583.

43. Jacobs EA, Copperman SM, Joffe A, et al. Fetal alcohol syndrome and alcohol-related neurodevelopmental disorders. *Pediatrics.* 2000;106(2):358-361.

44. McGinnis JM, Foege WH. *Mortality and Morbidity Attributable to Use of Addictive Substances in the United States.* Proceedings of the Association of American Physicians. Mar-Apr, 1999;111(2):109-118.

45. Cooper M. Alcohol and increased behavioral risk for AIDS. *Alcohol Health Res World.* 1992;16:64-71.

46. *Crime in the United States, 1999: Uniform Crime Reports.* Washington, DC: Federal Bureau of Investigation, US Dept of Justice; 1999. Available at: http://www.fbi.gov/ucr/ucr.htm.

47. *Drugs and Crime Facts, 1994.* Washington, DC: US Dept of Justice, Bureau of Justice Statistics; 1995. NCJ Publication 154043. Available at: http://www.ojp.usdoj.gov/bjs.

48. US Depart of Justice. *Survey of State Prison Inmates, 1991.* Washington, DC: Bureau of Justice Statistics; 1993.

49. *Correctional Populations in the United States, 1997.* Washington, DC: US Depart of Justice, Bureau of Justice Statistics; November 2000. NCJ Publication 177613. Available at: http://www.ojp.usdoj.gov/bjs/abstract/cpus97.htm.

50. US Depart of Justice, *Drugs, Crime and the Justice System.* Washington, DC: Bureau of Justice Statistics; 1992.

51. *Profile of State Prisoners Under Age 18, 1985–97.* Washington, DC: US Dept of Justice, Bureau of Justice Statistics; 2000. NCJ Publication 176989. Available at: http://www.ojp.usdoj.gov/bjs/abstract/pspa1897.htm.

52. Harwood HJ, Fountain D, Livermore G. The economic costs of alcohol and drug abuse in the United States. *Addiction.* 1999;94(5):631-635.

53. Chaloupka F. Effects of price on alcohol-related problems. *Alcohol Health Res World.* 1993;17:46-53.

54. Kenkel D, Manning W. Perspectives on alcohol taxation. *Alcohol Health Res World.* 1996;20(4):230-238.

55. Lockhart SJ, Beck KH, Summons TG. Impact of higher alcohol prices on alcohol-related attitudes and perceptions of suburban, middle-class youth. *J Youth Adolescence.* 1993;22(4):441-453.

56. Grossman M, Chaloupka FJ, Sirtalan I. An empirical analysis of alcohol addiction: Results from the monitoring the future panels. *Econ Inquiry,* 1998;36(January):39-48.

57. Saffer H, Grossman M. Beer taxes, the legal drinking age, and youth motor vehicle fatalities. *J Leg Stud.* 1987;16(2):351-374.

58. Smart RG, Mann RE. Treatment, Alcoholics Anonymous and alcohol controls during the decrease in alcohol problems in Alberta: 1975-1993. *Alcohol Alcohol.* 1998;33(3):265-272.

59. Alaniz ML, Cartmill RS, Parker RN. Immigrants and violence: The importance of neighborhood context. *Hispanic J Behav Sci.* 1998;20(2):155-174.

60. Scribner RA, MacKinnon DP, Dwyer JH. The risk of assaultive violence and alcohol availability in Los Angeles County. *Am J Public Health.* 1995;85(3):335-340.

61. Scribner RA, Cohen DA, Farley TA. A geographic relation between alcohol availability and gonorrhea rates. *Sex Transm Dis.* 1998;25(10):544-548.

62. Scribner R, Cohen D, Kaplan S, Allen SH. Alcohol availability and homicide in New Orleans: Conceptual considerations for small area analysis of the effect of alcohol outlet density. *J Stud Alcohol.* 1999;60(3):310-316.

63. Gorman DM, Speer PW. Concentration of liquor outlets in an economically disadvantaged city in the northeastern United States. *Subst Use and Misuse.* 1997;32(14):2033-2046.

64. Wagenaar AC, Holder HD. Changes in alcohol consumption resulting from the elimination of retail wine monopolies: Results from five U.S. states. *J Stud Alcohol.* 1995;56:566-572.

65. Wagenaar AC, Langley JD. Alcohol licensing system changes and alcohol consumption: introduction of wine into New Zealand grocery stores. *Addiction.* 1995;90:773-783.

66. Babor TF, Mendelson JH, Greenberg I, Kuehnle J. Experimental analysis of the "happy hour": effects of purchase price on alcohol consumption. *Psychopharmacology.* 1978;58:35-41.

67. Center for Science in the Public Interest. *Advertising and Marketing to the College Student.* Available at: http://www.health.org/pubs/lastcall/chapter2.htm. Accessed September 2000.

68. McKnight AJ, Streff FM. The effect of enforcement upon service of alcohol to intoxicated patrons of bars and restaurants. *Accident Analysis Prev.* 1994;26(1): 79-88.

69. Forster JL, Murray DM, Wolfson M, Wagenaar AC. Commercial availability of alcohol to young people: results of alcohol purchase attempts. *Prev Med.* 1995;24:342-347.

70. Preusser, DF, Williams AF. Sales of alcohol to underage purchasers in three New York counties and Washington, DC *J Public Health Pol.* 1992;13(3):306-317.

71. Toomey TL, Wagenaar AC, Kilian GR, Fitch OB, Rothstein C, Fletcher L. Alcohol sales to pseudo-intoxicated bar patrons. *Public Health Rep.* 1999;114(4):337-342.

72. O'Donnell, M. Research on drinking locations of alcohol-impaired drivers: implication for prevention policies. *J Public Health Pol.* 1985;6:510-525.

73. Wood LJ, McLean S, Davidson J, Montgomery IM. One for the road: On the utility of citation data for identifying problem hotels. *Drug Alcohol Rev.* 1995;14(1):115-124.

74. Toomey TL, Kilian GR, Gehan JP, Wagenaar AC, Perry CL, Jones-Webb R. Qualitative assessment of responsible alcohol service training programs. *Public Health Rep.* 1998;113(2):162-169.

75. Howard-Pitney B, Johnson MD, Altman DG, Hopkins R, Hammond N. Responsible alcohol service: A study of server, manager, and environmental impact. *Am J Public Health.* 1991;81(2):197-199.

76. McKnight J. Factors influencing the effectiveness of server-intervention education. *J Stud Alcohol.* 1991;52(5):389-397.

77. Saltz RF. Research needs and opportunities in server intervention programs. *Health Educ Q.* 1989;16(3):429-438.

78. Toomey TL, Wagenaar AC, Gehan JP, Kilian G, Murray D, Perry CL. Project ARM: Alcohol risk management to prevent sales to underage and intoxicated patrons. *Health Educ Behav.* 2001;28(2):186-199.

79. Grube JW. Preventing sales of alcohol to minors: results from a community trial. *Addiction.* 1997;92(suppl Jun)2;251-260.

80. Preusser DF, Williams AF, Weinstein HN. Policing underage alcohol sales. *J Safety Res.* 1994;25(3): 127-133.

81. Mosher J. Legal liabilities of licensed alcoholic beverage establishments: recent developments in the United States. In: Single E, Storm T, eds. *Public Drinking and Public Policy.* Toronto, Canada: Addiction Research Foundation; 1985.

82. Holder HD, Janes K, Mosher J, Saltz R, Spurr S, Wagenaar AC. Alcoholic beverage server liability and the reduction of alcohol-involved problems. *J Stud Alcohol.* 1993;54:23-36.

83. Toomey TL, Rosenfeld C, Wagenaar AC. The minimum legal drinking age: History, effectiveness, and ongoing debate. *Alcohol Health Res World.* 1996;20(4):213-218.

84. Wolfson M. The legislative impact of social movement organizations: The anti-drunken driving movement and the 21-year-old drinking age. *Soc Sci Q.* 1995;76(2):311-327.

85. King RF. The politics of denial: The use of funding penalties as an implementation device for social policy. *Pol Sci.* 1987;20:307-337.

86. Wagenaar AC, Toomey TL. Effects of minimum drinking age laws: Review and analyses of the literature. *J Stud Alcohol.* In press.

87. National Center for Statistics and Analysis. *Traffic Safety Facts 1999—Alcohol.* Washington, DC: US Dept of Transportation; 2000.

88. Wagenaar AC, Wolfson M. Enforcement of the legal minimum drinking age in the United States. *J Public Health Pol.* 1994;15:37-53.

89. Wagenaar AC, Wolfson M. Deterring sales and provision of alcohol to minors: A study of enforcement in 295 counties in four states. *Public Health Rep.* 1995;110:419-427.

90. Wagenaar AC, Toomey TL, Murray DM, Short BJ, Wolfson M, Jones-Webb R. Sources of alcohol for underage drinkers. *J Stud Alcohol.* 1996;57:325-333.

91. Marriott M. Cheap high lures youths to malt liquor "40s." *New York Times.* April 16, 1993:A1, A12.

92. Penn, Schoen, and Berland Associates, Inc. *What Teens and Adults Are Saying About Alcopops: Major Findings of a National Poll.* Washington, DC: Center for Science and the Public Interest; 2001.

93. Mosher J. *Responsible Beverage Service: An Implementation Handbook for Communities.* Palo Alto, Calif: Health Promotion Resource Center, Stanford University; 1991.

94. Gibbs JP. *Crime, Punishment, and Deterrence.* New York, NY: Elsevier; 1975.

95. Ross H. *Confronting Drunk Driving: Social Policy for Saving Lives.* New Haven, Conn: Yale University Press; 1992.

96. Mosher J, Stewart K. *Regulatory Strategies for Preventing Youth Access to Alcohol: Best Practices.* Prepared for the Office of Juvenile Justice and Delinquency Prevention National Leadership Conference July 11-14, 1999. Rockville, Md: Pacific Institute for Research and Evaluation.

97. US Depart of Health and Human Services. *Surgeon General's Workshop on Drunk Driving: Proceedings.* Washington, DC: Office of the Surgeon General; 1988.

98. The American Assembly. Alcoholism and Related Problems: Issues for the American Public. Englewood Cliffs, NJ: Prentice Hall Inc; 1984.

99. Holder HD, Gruenewald PJ, Ponicki WR, et al. Effect of community-based interventions on high-risk drinking and alcohol-related injuries. *JAMA.* 2000;284(18):2341-2347.

100. Wagenaar AC, Murray DM, Gehan JP, et al. Communities mobilizing for change on alcohol: Outcomes from a randomized community trial. *J Stud Alcohol.* 2000;61(1):85-94.

101. Gerstein D, Green L. *Preventing Drug Abuse: What Do We Know?* Committee on Drug Abuse Prevention Research, National Research Council. Washington, DC: National Academy Press; 1993.

102. Rosenbaum D, Bennett S, Lindsay B, Wilkinson D. *Community Responses to Drug Abuse: A Program Evaluation.* Washington, DC: National Institute of Justice; 1994. NCJ Publication 145945.

103. Davis R. Curbing the sale of illegal drugs through environmental strategies. Paper presented at the 11th Annual National Prevention Network Research Conference, San Antonio, Texas, August 1998.

104. Davis R, Smith B, Lurigio A, Skogan W. Community responses to crack: Grassroots anti-drug programs. New York, NY: Victim Services Research Department; 1991.

105. Hawkins JD, Catalano RF, Miller JY. Risk and protective factors for alcohol and other drug problems in adolescence and early adulthood: Implications for substance abuse prevention. *Psychol Bull.* 1992;112(1):64-105.

106. Bry BH, Catalano RF, Kumpfer KL, Lochman JE, Szapocznik J. Scientific findings from family prevention intervention research. In: Ashery R, Robertson E, Kumpfer K. *Drug Abuse Prevention Through Family Interventions.* National Institute on Drug Abuse Research Monograph 177, Publication 99-4135. Rockville, Md: US Depart of Health and Human Services, National Institutes of Health, National Institute on Drug Abuse; 1998.

107. Dishion TJ, McMahon RJ. Parental monitoring and the prevention of problem behavior: A conceptual and empirical reformulation. In: Ashery R, Robertson E, Kumpfer K. *Drug Abuse Prevention Through Family*

Interventions. National Institute on Drug Abuse Research Monograph Number 177, Publication 99-4135. Rockville, Md: US Depart of Health and Human Services, National Institutes of Health, National Institute on Drug Abuse; 1998.

108. Moskowitz J, Jones R. Alcohol and drug problems in the schools: results of a national survey of school administrators. *J Stud Alcohol.* 1988;49:299-305.

109. Bowser B. Bayview-Hunter's Point: San Francisco's black ghetto revisited. *Urban Anthropol.* 1988;17:383-400.

110. Ames G. Research and strategies for the primary prevention of workplace alcohol problems. *Alcohol Health Res World.* 1993;17:19-27.

111. Holder HD, Saltz RF, Grube JW, Voas RB, Gruenewald PJ, Treno AJ. A community prevention trial to reduce alcohol-involved accidental injury and death: overview. *Addiction.* 1997;92(2).

112. Wagenaar AC, Murray DM, Wolfson M, Forster JL, Finnegan JR. Communities mobilizing for change on alcohol: Design of a randomized community trial. *J Community Psychol.* 1994;(CSAP Special Issue):79-101.

113. Wagenaar AC, Murray DM, Toomey TL. Communities mobilizing for change on alcohol: Effect of a randomized trial on arrests and traffic crashes. *Addiction.* 2000;95(2):209-217.

114. Grube J, Wallack L. Television beer advertising and drinking knowledge, beliefs, and intentions among schoolchildren. *Am J Public Health.* 1994;84:254-260.

115. Casswell S, Zang J. Impact of liking for advertising and brand allegiance on drinking and alcohol-related aggression: A longitudinal study. *Addiction.* 1998;93:1209-1217.

116. Wallack L. Drinking and driving: Toward a broader understanding of the role of mass media. *J Public Health Pol.* 1984;5:471-496.

117. Federal Trade Commission. *Self-Regulation in the Alcohol Industry. A Review of Industry Efforts to Avoid Promoting Alcohol to Underage Consumers.* Washington, DC: Federal Trade Commission; September 1999: Appendix B.

118. Gitlin T. On drugs and mass media in America's consumer society. In: Resnik H, ed. *Youth and Drugs: Society's Mixed Messages.* Rockville, Md: Office of Substance Abuse Prevention; 1990:31-52. OSAP Prevention Monograph 6.

119. Gerbner G. Stories that hurt: Tobacco, alcohol and other drugs in the mass media. In: Resnik H, ed. *Youth and Drugs: Society's Mixed Messages.* Rockville, Md: Office of Substance Abuse Prevention; 1990:53-128. OSAP Prevention Monograph 6.

120. Wallack L, Dorfman L, Jernigan D, Themba M. *Media Advocacy and Public Health: Power for Prevention.* Newbury Park, Calif: Sage Publications; 1993.

121. Wagenaar AC, Perry CL. Community strategies for the reduction of youth drinking: Theory and application. *J Res Adolesc.* 1994;4:319-345.

122. Lee M. *Drowning in Alcohol: Retail Outlet Density, Economic Decline, and Revitalization in South LA.* San Rafael, Calif: Marin Institute for the Prevention of Alcohol and Other Drug Problems; 1998.

123. Bourgois P. In search of Horatio Alger: culture and ideology in the crack economy. *Contemp Drug Problems.* 1989;16:619-650.

124. Wechsler R. Community organizing principles and local prevention of alcohol and drug abuse. In Mecca A, ed. *Prevention 2000—A Public/Private Partnership.* San Rafael, Calif: California Health Research Foundation; 1988:41-52.

CHAPTER
21

Oral Diseases: The Neglected Epidemic

Myron Allukian Jr., D.D.S., M.P.H.

You're not healthy without good oral health.

C. Everett Koop, M.D.
former United States Surgeon General

Oral diseases are a neglected epidemic for millions of Americans who suffer unnecessarily from them, even though many oral diseases are preventable.[1] The combination of high prevalence, high morbidity, and relative inattention from the health community makes oral diseases a significant public health problem in need of a public health solution.

Public health practitioners have the responsibility and opportunity to include oral health as an integral component of health in the development of policies and programs. Oral health is an essential component of health and well-being.[2] When a needs assessment is done of a community or group of individuals, oral health must be included.

This chapter explains why oral health is a neglected epidemic, why oral health is important, and how public health can help promote good oral health. It also describes the epidemiology of oral disease and discusses the preventive programs that can improve oral health. It concludes with a discussion of dental personnel in the United States.

BACKGROUND

Unfortunately, beginning in the early 1800s and due to a variety of factors, the mouth was disconnected from the rest of the body in health sciences, education, and practice. After the first dental school in the world, the Baltimore College of Dental Surgery, was founded in 1840, dentistry became a separate health profession from medicine with separate schools, organizations, institutions, and programs. As dentistry evolved, many physicians, nurses, and even public health professionals were left without an understanding or appreciation of the impact oral diseases have on individuals and society.

When public health practitioners properly assess the major health needs of a target population, they usually find that the need for better oral health is a significant public health problem from the perspectives of both prevention and treatment. Major oral diseases and conditions include:

- dental caries (tooth decay)
- periodontal diseases (gum diseases)
- malocclusion (crooked teeth)
- edentulism (complete tooth loss)
- oral and pharyngeal cancer
- craniofacial anomalies including cleft lip/cleft palate
- soft tissue lesions
- orofacial injuries
- temporomandibular dysfunction (TMD)

Dental expertise is also of value in promoting and protecting the general health of communities. Examples of health concerns in which dental public health expertise has been invaluable to society are infection control, mercury toxicity, tobacco control, school-based programs, maternal and child health, primary care, AIDS, hepatitis B, tuberculosis, occupational health, needs assessment, policy development, quality assessment, community organization, and prevention on both the individual and community levels.

THE NEGLECTED EPIDEMIC

Although there has been substantial improvement in oral health on a national level in the last 20–30 years due to water fluoridation, topical fluorides, and an emphasis on prevention, oral diseases are still pandemic in the United States, as the following statistics show:

- Twenty-nine percent of adolescents have severe or very severe malocclusion.[3]
- Sixty percent of adolescents experience gum infections.[4]
- Eighty-four percent of 17-year-old school children have had tooth decay, with an average of eight affected surfaces.[5]
- Ninety-nine percent of adults aged 40 to 44 have had tooth decay, with an average of 30 affected surfaces.[6]

- Thirty percent of those aged 65 and older have no teeth at all.[7]
- Over 30,000 Americans are diagnosed with oral and pharyngeal cancer each year and about 7,800 die annually.[8]
- One out of 700 Americans are born with cleft lip/cleft palate.[9]

For vulnerable populations, such as children, minorities, the elderly, and those with low incomes, oral diseases are especially problematic. Selected studies have shown that up to 97 percent of the homeless need dental care.[10] Over half of some Head Start children have had early childhood caries.[11] Almost half of abused children have orofacial trauma.[12] Sixteen percent of emergency room visits are for orofacial injuries.[13] Low-income seniors aged 65 to 74 are almost four times as likely to be edentulous than high-income seniors.[14] African-American, low-income, and American Indian and Alaska Native children aged 2–4 years have about two to six times more untreated tooth decay than their peers.[7,15] More than 50 percent of the homebound elderly have not seen a dentist for 10 years.[16] Finally, people *without* health insurance have four times the rate of unmet dental needs as those *with* private insurance.[17]

Fortunately, most oral diseases can be prevented. Unfortunately, once they occur they usually do not resolve themselves without the physical intervention of a dental provider. Two exceptions to this are an incipient carious lesion that is reversible when exposed to fluoride and mild gingivitis.

Untreated dental caries usually progresses to an infection of the nerve and blood supply to the involved tooth, which may result in an abscess, cellulitis (an infection of the soft tissue), and sometimes even death. When dental caries is treated, a dentist must physically remove the bacterial infection, reshape the infected area of the tooth, and then restore the tooth with an artificial substance to retain its function. Restored teeth are weaker than intact healthy teeth and subject to fracture and additional caries attack.

IMPORTANCE OF ORAL HEALTH

Oral health is an integral component of total health. The maintenance of good oral health is important for:

- freedom from pain, infection, and suffering
- ability to eat and chew food, thus for proper digestion and nutrition
- ability to speak properly
- social mobility
- employability
- self-image and self-esteem
- quality of life and well-being

Studies have shown associations between periodontal disease and premature low-birth-weight babies, and between oral infections and heart disease and stroke.[18–24] Poor oral health may also compromise individuals in school, work, or daily living.[2,25] People with poor oral health may suffer unnecessarily with pain, have difficulty in interpersonal relationships, and have diminished job opportunities. One study estimated that about 20 percent of Americans experience orofacial pain in a six-month period.[26] For the young, elderly, and medically compromised, good oral health is even more important to function and thrive.

Social Cost of Oral Disease

The social cost of oral diseases to the individual and society are great. For example, in 1989 over 51 million hours of school were lost due to oral health problems, almost 1.2 hours per school child.[27] Also in 1989, over 164 million hours were missed from work, an average of 1.48 hours per employed adult.[27] In 1991, school-age children had almost 4.8 million restricted activity days and 2.2 million bed days.[28] In 1994, low-income children had almost 12 times more days of missed school due to dental problems than higher income children.[29] In 1996, employed persons 18 years and over had over 9.7 million restricted activity days and over 4.6 million bed days.[2]

Economic Cost of Oral Disease

The economic cost of oral diseases is also significant. Dental services consumed about $65.4 billion, or 4.6 percent of all health expenditures, in 2001.[30] Dental expenditures are expected to reach $108.9 billion by the year 2010, or about 4.1 percent of personal expenditures.[30] Most dental expenditures are from private sources, such as private insurance, or out-of-pocket.

Only about 51.6 percent of the U.S. population have some form of dental insurance/benefit plan.[31] Of the enrolled individuals, 43 percent are in indemnity plans, 17.9 percent in dental HMOs, 31.2 percent in PPOs, and 7.5 percent in other types of plans. About 30.7 percent of all dental patients are self-payors and 5.4 percent are on public assistance.[31]

Public programs providing dental insurance are few. Medicaid includes dental services, primarily for children as part of the Early Periodic Screening Diagnosis and Treatment (EPSDT) Program. In 1998, dental Medicaid expenditures were about $2 billion, or 1.25 percent of the $159.6 billion spent for all Medicaid personal health care expenditures.[2] Fewer than 20 percent of Medicaid eligible recipients actually received dental care.[32] In addition, many Medicaid programs do not adequately reimburse for effective preventive procedures such as dental sealants. Dentistry is an optional service for adults under Medicaid, and many states provide only limited services to adults. Unfortunately, Medicare, which provides health care to individuals over age 65, does not include dental services at all unless they are related to trauma or oral cancer.

AN OVERVIEW OF ORAL HEALTH PROBLEMS

Major oral health problems include dental caries, periodontal diseases, and oral/pharyngeal cancer. The prevalence and public health significance of these problems are addressed next.

Dental Caries

Dental caries, or tooth decay, is the most prevalent oral disease in the United States. It is a bacterial infection that is influenced by a variety of factors in the host, agent, and environment.

Prevalence

Prevalence of dental caries increases progressively with age throughout life, especially during the first two decades, as shown in Table 21.1. At age six when the 32 permanent teeth usually begin erupting, only about 5.6 percent of school children have had tooth decay in their permanent teeth.[5] Not only does the

Table 21.1. Prevalence of Tooth Decay and Mean Number of Permanent Tooth Surfaces Affected, United States School Children, 5 to 17 Years of Age, 1986 to 1987

Age	% Prevalence	Mean Number Affected Tooth Surfaces
5	2.7	0.07
6	5.6	0.13
7	15.8	0.40
8	25.0	0.71
9	34.5	1.14
10	44.3	1.69
11	55.0	2.33
12	58.3	2.66
13	66.0	3.76
14	72.3	4.68
15	78.2	5.71
16	80.0	6.68
17	84.4	8.04
all ages (5 to 17)	49.9	3.07

SOURCE: National Institute of Dental Research. *Oral Health of United States Children. The National Survey of Dental Caries in US School Children, 1986–1987.* Bathesda, Md: US Dept of Health and Human Services; 1989. DHHS publication NIH 89-2247.

prevalence of the disease increase with age, but the number of affected tooth surfaces also increases. By age 17, 84 percent of 17-year-olds have had tooth decay, with an average of 8 affected tooth surfaces, and by age 40 to 44, almost 99 percent of adults have had tooth decay, with an average of 30 affected tooth surfaces.[5,6] For all children in the United States, 75 percent of the dental caries actually occur in only about 25 percent of children.[5]

Types of Caries

There are three general types of tooth decay: coronal, which occurs on the crowns of teeth; root surface, which occurs on the roots of teeth; and recurrent, which is reoccurring tooth decay. Root surface decay usually occurs in older individuals. A study of New England elders showed that 52 percent of individuals over age 70 years had root caries. For 22 percent of them, the disease was untreated.[33] In a national study of individuals over age 75 years, almost 60 percent had root caries with 3.1 affected tooth surfaces.[34] The level of untreated dental caries is much higher among minorities and those with low income and less education. People who have lived in fluoridated communities since birth experience much lower rates of dental caries.

Early Childhood Caries (ECC)

The 20 primary teeth begin erupting at about six to nine months of age, and by about two years of age they have all erupted. *Early childhood caries,* also called baby bottle tooth decay, is tooth decay that occurs primarily in the upper anterior primary teeth when a baby is given a bottle at bedtime or nap time with sugar added to the contents. Juices or milk alone can cause ECC if they are given over extended periods of time.

About 8.3 percent of children in the United States aged two to five years still use a baby bottle, and of these 48.3 percent were reported as having gone to bed with a bottle containing something other than water.[35] The prevalence of ECC has averaged as high as 53 percent for Head Start children who were rural Native Americans or Alaskan Natives, and up to 11 percent for children in urban areas. ECC is higher in preterm, low-birth-weight infants and those that are malnourished. This may be due to poor tooth development of the fetus in utero when the mother is malnourished. Other possible causes include bacteria transferred from the caregiver after birth and improper baby feeding practices.

ECC may be painful and expensive. The treatment may cost about $2,200 to $6,000 per child because general anesthesia and therefore the use of an operating room are often required. It is much more cost effective to prevent it. ECC can be prevented by educating parents and caretakers about the dangers of giving infants bottles for prolonged periods of time unless they are filled with plain water. Bottle-fed infants should not be given bottles with juices, milk, or sweetened fluids when they are going to bed or otherwise using the bottle as a pacifier. Once a child has been fed by bottle, the teeth should be wiped clean. In general, breast-feeding should be encouraged over bottle-feeding, and parents should be taught to wean from the breast to the cup, rather than the bottle, at around age one year. If ECC is prevalent in a given population, widespread prevention requires the development of a comprehensive, multidisciplinary, community-oriented education program.[11]

Periodontal Diseases

There are essentially two types of infections of the soft tissues (gums) surrounding a tooth: gingivitis and periodontitis. Both are quite common.

Gingivitis

Gingivitis is a localized infection or inflammation of the soft tissues surrounding a tooth that results in swelling and bleeding of the gums. It may or may not be self-limiting. Poor oral hygiene is the major contributing factor to gingivitis; therefore, good self-care is important in its prevention. Some forms of gingivitis, such as acute necrotizing ulcerative gingivitis (ANUG), or trench mouth, can be extremely painful. ANUG is often associated with stress, lack of sleep, poor nutrition, and poor oral hygiene.

Gingivitis occurs in about 60 percent of adolescents and about 48 percent of adults.[7,4] Among certain high-risk populations, the prevalence is even higher. For Native American and Alaskan Natives, as many as 98 percent may have the disease, and it is found in up to 64 percent of Mexican Americans and 50 percent of low-income individuals.[7]

Periodontitis

Periodontitis is an infection or inflammation of the soft tissues *and* of the supporting alveolar bone around teeth with loss of periodontal attachment. When left untreated, periodontitis usually results in teeth becoming loose, necessitating extensive treatment and possible removal. For persons with AIDS or HIV infection, periodontitis can progress quite rapidly.

The prevalence of periodontitis increases with age. About 22 percent of people aged 35 to 44 have periodontitis, with the prevalence higher in high-risk populations such as minorities and low-income individuals.[7]

Prevention

Successful prevention of periodontal disease is oriented more to the individual than to the community. Prevention measures are similar for gingivitis and periodontitis, but gingivitis responds better to preventive measures. Patient compliance with proper oral hygiene procedures and regular mechanical removal of dental plaque with a toothbrush and floss helps prevent periodontal disease. It also usually responds well to a thorough professional cleaning, prophylaxis, scaling, and root planing performed by a dentist or dental hygienist.

Educational programs need to be developed as part of comprehensive health education for school children to reinforce the importance of good oral hygiene. Public awareness also needs to be increased so that individual compliance is improved in the use of proper oral hygiene practices and periodic dental visits.

Oral and Pharyngeal Cancer

Over 30,000 new cases of oral and pharyngeal cancer and 7,800 deaths from oral and pharyngeal cancer were estimated for the United States for 2001.[8] It is the seventh most common cancer for men who are more than two times more at risk than women. More Americans die from oral cancer than from cervical cancer. Tobacco and alcohol use are associated with over 70 percent of oral cancers, and they occur most often in men over the age of 40.[36] The increase in the use of spit (smokeless) tobacco, especially among teenagers, may result in more individuals with oral cancer in the future. The five-year oral and pharnygeal cancer survival rate for Euro-Americans is 56 percent compared with 36 percent for African-Americans. Of all cancer it shows the largest discrepancy in survival between these two races.[8]

Early detection and treatment of oral cancer results in higher survival rates. In 1998 only 13 percent of adults over age 40 in a national survey reported that they had ever been examined for oral cancer.[7] One study showed that for the two years prior to being diagnosed with oral cancer, patients had a median of 7.5 to 10.5 health care visits, yet 77 percent of the eventual diagnoses were for late-stage cancer.[37] Most of these visits were with physicians considered to be their regular source of care.

It is apparent that physicians and other health care providers need to be motivated and trained in early recognition of oral cancer. Health education programs for children and adults should emphasize the dangers of (smokeless) spit tobacco, cigarette smoking, and alcohol use. Policies should be implemented to discourage youth from tobacco and alcohol use. For example, in 1994 the National Collegiate Athletic Association (NCAA) banned student athletes and coaches from using smokeless or any other tobacco product during practices and games.[38] Periodic dental visits should also be promoted for early detection and treatment.

THE UTILIZATION OF DENTAL SERVICES

The utilization of dental care varies with age, income, and race,[14] as shown in Table 21.2. It also varies by in-

Table 21.2. Percent of Persons Two Years of Age and Over with Dental Visits in the Past Year and Number of Visits Per Person Per Year, by Age, Race, and Income: United States, 1989

Characteristics	Persons With Visit in Past Year	Visits per Person Per Year
Age	Percent	Number
All ages	57.2	2.1
2–4 years	32.1	0.9
5–17 years	69.0	2.4
18–34 years	57.0	1.8
35–54 years	57.4	2.3
55–64 years	54.0	2.4
65 years and over	43.2	2.0
Race		
African-American	44.5	1.2
Euro-American	59.3	2.2
Family income		
Less than $10,000	40.9	1.3
$10,000–$19,999	43.4	1.5
$20,000–$34,999	58.3	2.0
$35,000 and over	73.0	2.8

SOURCE: Bloom B, Gift HC, Jack SS. Dental services and oral health; United States, 1989. *Vital Health Stat.* 1992;10:183.

surance status.[14] In 1989 approximately 57 percent of the population in the United States over age two years had seen a dentist in the past year, for an average of 2.1 visits per year. For 5- to 17-year-olds, 69 percent had been to a dentist in the last year, as compared with only 43 percent of persons over age 65. For individuals with a family income of over $35,000 a year, 73 percent had visited a dentist in the last year compared with 40 percent with family incomes of less than $10,000. About 59 percent of Euro-Americans saw a dentist in the past year, with 2.2 visits on average, as compared with 44 percent of African-Americans, with an average of 1.2 visits.[14]

Dental utilization is the lowest for those over age 65 years, but this age group has been increasing its visits to the dentist over the years. For those over age 65 in nursing homes, the unmet needs are even greater, and access to care is limited. The Omnibus Budget Reconciliation Act (OBRA) of 1989 has regulations requiring an oral examination of patients in long-term-care facilities within 14 days of admission and annually thereafter. These regulations became effective in 1992. The extent of the impact this will have for this neglected population remains to be seen.

THE PUBLIC HEALTH APPROACH TO ORAL DISEASES

The oral disease epidemic presents a unique challenge to the public health professional, who has the responsibility to prevent as much disease as possible and to improve access to care for those least able to obtain such services. A population-based approach centered on the three core functions—assessment of dental needs, policy development for dental disease prevention and treatment, and assurance of access to needed services—is most likely to make an impact on oral disease.[39]

Every local, state, and federal health agency and department should have a dental public health program with properly trained staff to address this neglected epidemic. The national oral health objectives for the year 2010 as defined in *Healthy People 2010* can be achieved more easily with dental public health expertise and the appropriate resources.[7] Smaller local health departments should also utilize such dental expertise. Schools of public health and dental, medical, and nursing schools should also include dental public health expertise to help educate health profession students about oral health needs and programs from the public health perspective.

Dental Public Health

Expertise in dental public health is essential to respond to the oral disease epidemic in a meaningful and effective way. Dental public health has been defined by the American Board of Dental Public Health as:

> . . . the science and art of preventing and controlling dental diseases and promoting dental health through organized community efforts. It is that form of dental practice which serves the community as a patient rather than the individual. It is concerned with the dental health education of the public, with applied dental research, and with the administration of group dental programs, as well as the prevention and control of dental diseases on a community basis.[10]

Dental public health is the second smallest of the nine dental specialties recognized by the American Dental Association. Public health dentists are trained in program and policy development, management and administration, research methods, health promotion, disease prevention, and delivery of care systems. The competency objectives and competencies for dental public health have been delineated,[41,42] and this expertise is unique in dentistry because of its population-based approach.

Public health dentists have improved the oral health of millions of Americans by their initiatives. There are about 1,600 dentists in the United States who work in public health roles, of which about 1,000 have at least one year of advanced education and over 600 have two years.[43] In 2001, 145 dentists were board-certified in dental public health (American Board of Dental Public Health personal communication, September 2001).

The American Board of Dental Public Health is the certifying board for this specialty, which requires a dental degree, a master's degree in public health, a one-year residency, two years' experience in dental public health, and then successful completion of a comprehensive three-day examination.

The five major national dental public health associations are:

1. American Association of Public Health Dentistry
2. American Board of Dental Public Health
3. American Public Health Association, Oral Health Section
4. American Association of Community Dental Programs
5. Association of State and Territorial Dental Directors

The American Association of Public Health Dentistry and the Oral Health Section of the American Public Health Association are the two major dental public health membership organizations. The Association of State and Territorial Dental Directors (ASTDD) is made up of state dental directors, and the American Association of Community Dental Programs consists of local dental directors. In addition, the National Network for Oral Health Access (NNOHA), the Community and Preventive Dentistry Section of the American Dental Education Association (ADEA), and the Behavioral Sciences and Health Services Research Group of the American Association of Dental Research (AADR) have strong community orientations. NNOHA membership is primarily made up of community and migrant health center dentists; the ADEA section consists primarily of educators, and the AADR researchers. Some dental hygienists also have training in public health and are an important resource for improving the oral health of the public.

Individuals trained in dental public health have the knowledge and education to respond to the oral disease epidemic. Public health leaders and programs can utilize these national public health associations as well as the U.S. Public Health Service for assistance if they do not have access locally to the expertise of public health-trained dentists or hygienists.

Healthy People 2010

Healthy People 2010 includes oral health as one of 28 priority areas. This area contains 17 objectives and numerous subobjectives.[7] The goal of the oral health objectives is to prevent and control oral and craniofacial diseases, conditions, and injuries, and improve access to related services. The 17 objectives cover the following:

- Dental caries experience
- Untreated dental decay
- No permanent tooth loss
- Complete tooth loss
- Periodontal diseases
- Early detection of oral and pharyngeal cancers
- Annual examinations for oral and pharyngeal cancers
- Dental sealants
- Community water fluoridation
- Use of oral health care system
- Use of oral health care system by residents in long-term-care facilities
- Dental services for low-income children
- School-based health centers with oral health component
- Health centers with oral health service components
- Referral for cleft lip/cleft palate
- Oral and craniofacial state-based surveillance system
- Tribal, state, and local dental programs

Examples of complete objectives for the year 2010 are as follows:

1. Increase the proportion of children who have received dental sealants on their permanent teeth (target, 50 percent; baseline, children age eight, 23 percent; adolescents aged 14, 15 percent)
2. Increase the proportion of the U.S. population served by community water systems with optimally fluoridated water (target, 75 percent; 1992 baseline, 62 percent)
3. Increase the proportion of long-term-care residents who use the oral health care system each year (target, 25 percent; 1992 baseline, 19 percent)
4. Increase the proportion of low-income children and adolescents who received any preventive dental service during the past year (target, 57 percent; baseline, 20 percent)
5. Increase the proportion of local health departments and community-based health centers, including

community, migrant, and homeless health centers, that have an oral health component (target, 75 percent; baseline, 34 percent of local jurisdictions and health centers had oral health components in 1997).
6. (Developmental) Increase the number of tribal, state (including the District of Columbia), and local health agencies that serve jurisdictions of 250,000 or more persons that have in place an effective public dental health program directed by a dental professional with public health training.

Surgeon General's Report

The first-ever U.S. Surgeon General's Report on Oral Health was released in the year 2000.[2] This report raised the visibility of the oral health crisis in the United States and delineated the importance of oral health. It also discussed the status of oral health in the United States, the relationship between oral health and general health, how oral disease is prevented, and the needs and opportunities to enhance oral health. The report called the oral health crisis "a silent epidemic" and highlighted the disparities of oral health between the haves and the have-nots. The report also called for action on the national level to prevent oral diseases, improve access to services, and reduce oral health disparities among different population groups.

The major findings of the report were as follows:

1. Oral diseases and disorders in and of themselves affect health and well-being throughout life.
2. Safe and effective measures exist to prevent the most common dental diseases—dental caries and periodontal diseases.
3. Lifestyle behaviors that affect general health such as tobacco use, excessive alcohol use, and poor dietary choices affect oral and craniofacial health as well.
4. There are profound and consequential oral health disparities within the U.S. population.
5. More information is needed to improve America's oral health and eliminate health disparities.
6. The mouth reflects general health and well-being.
7. Oral diseases and conditions are associated with other health problems.
8. Scientific research is key to further reduction in the burden of diseases and disorders that affect the face, mouth, and teeth.

A framework for action was outlined by the Surgeon General's Report as follows:

1. Change perceptions regarding oral health and disease so that oral health becomes an accepted component of general health.
2. Accelerate the building of the science and evidence base and apply science effectively to improve oral health.
3. Build an effective health infrastructure that meets the oral health needs of all Americans and integrates oral health effectively into overall health.
4. Remove known barriers between people and oral health services.
5. Use public-private partnerships to improve the oral health of those who still suffer disproportionately from oral diseases.

Guide to Community Preventive Services

Chapter 17 discusses the *Guide to Community Preventive Services* and the work of an independent nonfederal Task Force on Community Preventive Services. The *Community Guide* is being developed with the support of the U.S. Department of Health and Human Services working with private and public parties. This publication includes an oral health component that delineates

effective population-based preventive measures. It will be helpful to local and state health departments as well as other health personnel who wish to improve the oral health of a community or population group.

PREVENTION

Many oral disease prevention measures prevent the disease before it occurs, which is called primary prevention, as well as control or respond to the disease after it occurs, which is called secondary or tertiary prevention. Because dental caries is the most common oral disease, and because the prevention methods for caries have such a well-documented scientific basis and are cost effective, the focus here is on dental caries prevention.

Community and Individual Preventive Measures

Dental caries can be prevented on the community or individual level, as shown in Table 21.3. Community prevention programs are more effective than individual prevention programs because they are population based.

The most effective, economical, and practical preventive measure for dental caries is community water fluoridation.[44,45] The most significant contribution a public health professional can make to improve the

Table 21.3. Effective Community and Individual Preventive Measures for Dental Caries

Measure	Method of Application	Target	Period of Use
Community Programs			
Community water fluoridation	Systemic	Entire population	Lifetime
School water fluoridation	Systemic	School children	School years
School fluoride tablet program	Systemic	School children	Age 5-16 yrs
School fluoride rinse program	Topical	School children	Age 5-16 yrs
School sealant program (professionally applied)	Topical	School children	Age 6-8, 12-14 yrs
Individual Approach			
Prescribed fluoride tablets or drops	Systemic	Children	Age 6 months-16 yrs
Professionally applied fluoride treatment	Topical	Individual need	High-risk populations
Over-the-counter fluoride rinse	Topical	Individual need	High-risk populations
Fluoride toothpaste	Topical	Entire population	Lifetime
Professionally applied dental sealants	Topical	Children	Age 6-8 and 12-14 yrs

SOURCE: Allukian, Jr, M. and Horowitz, A. M., Effective Community Prevention Programs for Oral Diseases, Chapter in Jong's Community Dental Health, fifth ed., Gluck, G., and Morganstein, W. ed. Mosby Press, St. Louis, (to be published).

oral health of a community is to help that community become fluoridated if natural fluoride levels are too low to be effective. Individual prevention measures are not as effective as community prevention measures in general because they rely on the individual to carry them out, decreasing the effectiveness of these measures on a population or group basis. However, individual prevention measures should be continuously recommended and reinforced in all programs to improve individual compliance.

Systemic and Topical Fluorides

Fluoride may be provided systemically or topically as shown in Table 21.3. Preventive measures that provide fluoride to the teeth systemically by ingestion, such as water fluoridation or fluoride tablets, strengthen the teeth *while they are developing* and protect the teeth after they have erupted into the oral cavity throughout life. Continued exposure to fluoridated water and fluorides after tooth eruption are also beneficial.

Children who live in communities that do not have fluoridation should be given a daily dietary fluoride supplement beginning at six months of age. In 1989 about 15.1 percent of children under the age of two used a fluoride supplement in the United States.[46] There are major differences in dietary fluoride supplement use by race, income, and education as shown in Table 21.4. About 16.6 percent of Euro-American children use fluoride supplements as compared with 6.5 percent of African-American children and 12.9 percent of Hispanic children. Only 6.4 percent of children below the poverty level use fluoride supplements compared with 18.2 percent at or above the poverty level. Some of the geographic variation in fluoride supplement use may be due to water fluoridation status.

Professionally applied fluoride treatments, school and over-the-counter fluoride rinses, and fluoride toothpaste protect the teeth by providing fluoride to the teeth topically after they have erupted into the oral cavity. These fluorides provide an additional benefit to systemic fluoride, especially for high-risk individuals. The direct application of fluoride helps in the remineralization, or repair, of tooth enamel that is in the early stages of tooth decay. Professionally applied fluoride treatments need to be done periodically as long as the individual is at high risk for den-

Table 21.4. Percent of U.S. Children Under Two Years of Age by Selected Characteristics Who Use a Dietary Fluoride Supplement, 1989

	%		%
All children	15.1	Parents' Education:	
		Some college	19.8
Race/Ethnicity:		High school or less	10.8
African-American	6.5		
Euro-American	16.6	Region:	
Hispanic	12.9	North	20.6
Non-Hispanic	15.5	Midwest	7.9
SES Status:		South	10.4
At/above poverty level	18.2	West	20.6
Below poverty level	6.4		

SOURCE: Wagener DK, Nourjah P, Horowitz A. *Trends in Childhood Use of Dental Care Products Containing Fluoride: U.S. 1983–1989.* Hyattsville, Md: National Center for Health Statistics; 1992. Advance data from Vital and Health Statistics no. 219.

tal caries. Fluoride toothpaste should be used by people of all ages at least twice a day, after breakfast and before going to sleep at night. About 93.7 percent of school-age children 5 to 17 years of age in the United States use a fluoride-containing toothpaste.[46]

Due to the widespread use of fluorides in water supplies, dental offices, and over-the-counter dental products, there has been a national decline in tooth decay in the last 20-30 years.

Dental Sealants

Because fluorides prevent dental caries most effectively on the smooth surfaces of the teeth, now almost two-thirds of tooth decay occurs on the chewing surfaces of teeth.[5] Dental sealants effectively prevent tooth decay on the chewing surfaces of the teeth. Dental sealants are thin plastic coatings placed as liquid plastics on the pits and fissures of the chewing surfaces of teeth and then polymerized. Ideally, susceptible tooth surfaces should be sealed soon after the tooth has erupted. This painless and noninvasive procedure does not require anesthesia or the cutting of tooth structure. A good school-based prevention program should use both fluorides and sealants.

Dental Fluorosis

With the increasing use of fluorides there has been an increase in dental fluorosis. This is a chronic, fluoride-induced condition, in which enamel development is disrupted and the enamel is hypomineralized.[47] It occurs when the teeth are forming, primarily from birth to six years of age, due to excessive fluoride intake. A confirmed history of fluoride exposure is needed to validate this diagnosis. In the 1980s, a series of studies showed that the prevalence of fluorosis had increased in both fluoridated and nonfluoridated communities.[47] Fluorosis appears clinically as a bilateral chalky white appearance of the teeth. In severe forms the teeth may be discolored or pitted. Most of the increase in fluorosis is of a very mild or mild form that would probably only be noticed by a dentist. Fluorosis is not a health problem, but may be considered an individual cosmetic problem in its more severe forms. It is correctable with dental treatment.

Individuals and populations with varying levels of dental fluorosis have less decay than those without fluorosis. Fluorosis may be due to inappropriate prescriptions of dietary fluoride supplements, ingestion of fluoride toothpaste by children under six years of age, infant formula reconstituted with fluoridated water, and communities fluoridated naturally at higher than the recommended level. In 1978, manufacturers of infant formulas, cereals, and juices voluntarily began processing their baby food products with water containing minimal amounts of fluoride. In 1979 a revised lower fluoride supplement schedule was adopted for children under two years of age by the American Academy of Pediatrics following the guidelines of the American Dental Association. In 1994 the recommended fluoride supplement schedule was revised again lowering the dosage for children under six years of age.[48] To prevent fluorosis, health professionals and their patients need to be educated about the proper use of fluoride-containing products, particularly for children six years of age and under.

Community Water Fluoridation

Community water fluoridation should be the foundation for improving the oral health of every community. Community water fluoridation is defined as the upward adjustment of the fluoride content of a community water supply for optimal oral health. It is the most cost-effective preventive measure for preventing tooth decay.[11] Fluoridation is safe, economical, and practical.[44,45,47,49–51] It has been estimated that for each dollar spent on fluoridation, there is a $25–$80 savings in dental treatment costs.[52,53] Today, fluoridation can be expected to prevent tooth decay in both primary and permanent teeth by up to 40 percent. Before the widespread use of fluorides, fluoridation prevented tooth decay by 50 to 60 percent. It is still a public health bargain, however. Because it has demonstrated benefits for adults, everyone reared in a fluoridated community benefits, regardless of age and also regardless of income, education, race, gender, or access to dental care.

All water supplies contain some fluoride naturally but generally not enough to prevent dental caries. The recommended fluoride level is 0.7 to 1.2 parts per million (ppm), depending on the mean maximum daily air temperature over a five year period.[54] Most water supplies in the United States are fluoridated at about 1.0 ppm. At the recommended level in the water supply, fluoride is odorless, colorless, and tasteless. The mean national weighted cost of fluoridation in 1989 was $0.51 per capita with a range of $0.12 to $5.41, depending on the size of the community and the complexity of its water distribution system.[44] In 1999 dollars, the range was $0.17–$7.62, with an average of $0.72 a person (CDC). In 1999 dollars, for communities with more than 10,000 persons, the range is $0.29 to $1.05 per capita, and for communities with less than 10,000 persons, it is $0.84 to $7.62. Once a community is fluoridated, fluoride levels in the water supply must be monitored on a regular basis so that the population served receives the maximum health and economic benefits at little or no risk.[54]

Historical Perspective

Fluoridation's effectiveness was first demonstrated in the United States, and the history of its discovery is one of the great public health success stories. For generations, millions of Americans lived in communities that were naturally fluoridated, though not necessarily at the recommended level. Communities then sought to duplicate the benefits that had been demonstrated by nature. In 1945, the first communities implemented *adjusted fluoridation* on a study basis, and in 1950, adjusted fluoridation was endorsed by the U.S. Public Health Service and then the American

Dental Association as a public health measure. Fluoridation is now recognized as one of the great public health achievements of the twentieth century.[55]

Fluoridation in the United States Today

By 1992, 10,567 community water systems serving 134.6 million Americans in 8,572 communities had adjusted fluoridation.[56] Another 10 million people live in communities that are fluoridated naturally at the recommended level. Indeed, the United States has the largest number of people in the world living in fluoridated communities. Consider the following statistics:

• In 1992, of the 232 million people on public water supplies, about 144.6 million were served by fluoridated water. This is about 62.2 percent of the U.S. population on public water systems and 55.9 percent of the total U.S. population.
• Water supplies of 42 of the 50 largest cities in the United States are fluoridated.

Variation in Fluoridation Rates by State and City

Table 21.5 shows for each state the percentage of the public water supply population that uses fluoridated water. The 8 cities of the largest 50 that are *not* fluori-

Table 21.5. Percentage of U.S. Population on Public Water Supply Systems Receiving Fluoridated Water

Location	1992[1]	2000[2]	Location	1992[1]	2000[2]
United States	62.1	65.8	Missouri	71.4	80.5[4]
Alabama	82.6	89.2[4]	Montana	25.9[6]	22.2
Alaska	61.2[6]	55.2	Nebraska	62.1	77.7[3]
Arizona	49.9	55.5	Nevada	2.1[5]	65.9[3]
Arkansas	58.7[5,6]	59.9[3]	New Hampshire	24.0	43.0
California	15.7[5,6]	28.7	New Jersey	16.2[6]	15.5
Colorado	81.7	76.9[3]	New Mexico	66.2	76.7
Connecticut	85.9[6]	88.8	New York	69.7[6]	67.8[3]
Delaware	67.4[6]	80.9	North Carolina	78.5	83.3
DC	100.0[5]	100.0	North Dakota	96.4	95.4
Florida	58.3[5]	62.6	Ohio	87.9	87.6
Georgia	92.1	92.9	Oklahoma	58.0[5,6]	74.6[3]
Hawaii	13.0[5]	9.0[4]	Oregon	24.8[6]	22.7[3]
Idaho	48.3	45.4	Pennsylvania	50.9[6]	54.2
Illinois	95.2	93.4	Rhode Island	100.0[5]	85.1
Indiana	98.6	95.3	South Carolina	90.0[6]	91.2
Iowa	91.4	91.3	South Dakota	100.0	88.4[3]
Kansas	58.4	62.5	Tennessee	92.0	94.5
Kentucky	100.0	96.1	Texas	64.0[6]	65.7
Louisiana	55.7[5]	53.2[4]	Utah	3.1[5]	2.0[3,4]
Maine	55.8[6]	75.4	Vermont	57.4	54.2
Maryland	85.8[6]	90.7[3]	Virginia	72.1[6]	93.3
Massachusetts	57.0[5]	55.8[3,4]	Washington	53.2	57.8[3]
Michigan	88.5	90.7	West Virginia	82.1	87.0[3]
Minnesota	93.4[6]	98.2	Wisconsin	93.0	89.3
Mississippi	48.4	46.0	Wyoming	35.7	30.3[4]

[1]Data Source: 1992 CDC Fluoridation Census.
[2]Data Source: 2000 Water Fluoridation Reporting System.
[3]Complete data not available from WFRS; additional information obtained from states.
[4]Reported 2000 PWS population exceeded total 2000 state population, thus PWS population set to U.S. Census 2000 state population.
[5]Federal Reporting Data System PWS service populations exceeded the Bureau of Census total state population, thus PWS population set to Bureau of Census population.
[6]Data for these states based on EPA data with no update of new systems.

Table 21.6. The 8 Cities of the 50 Largest Cities in the United States That Are Not Fluoridated, 2001

City	Rank in Size	Population (1,000s)
San Diego, CA*	6	1,238
San Antonio, TX*	8	1,147
San Jose, CA	11	867
Portland, OR	26	503
Tucson, AZ**	31	466
Fresno, CA*	39	404
Honolulu, HI	41	395
Wichita, KS	50	335
		5,355

*Approved fluoridation in 2000.

**Voted for fluoridation in 1992.

SOURCE: Easely, MW. National Center for Fluoridation Policy and Research, March 3, 2001.

dated have a total of about 5.3 million people. They are listed in Table 21.6. Los Angeles, the second largest city in the United States became fluoridated in 1999. The Tucson City Council voted for fluoridation in 1992 and the San Diego City Council approved fluoridation in 2000.

Fluoridation Laws

Eight states have laws that require fluoridation, and these laws vary from state to state. The eight states and their national rank for percent of the population with a public water supply that is fluoridated are given in Table 21.7.

Illinois and Minnesota have the most comprehensive legislation requiring fluoridation. In the fall of 1995 the California legislature passed a law requiring fluoridation of all public water systems with at least 10,000 service connections, depending on funding. Fluoridation laws usually help facilitate public health policy to implement fluoridation, depending on the nature of the law and whether or not it is enforced. On the other hand, a referendum is required by the public in the following five states before fluoridation can be initiated: Delaware, Maine, Nevada, New Hampshire, and Utah. These states rank from 25 to 52 in terms of the percent of population with fluoridated public water.

Table 21.7. States With Fluoridation Laws

State	National Rank	State	National Rank
Connecticut	16	Nebraska	28
Georgia	10	Ohio	15
Illinois	7	S. Dakota	1
Minnesota	8	Michigan	14

SOURCE: *Fluoridation Census, 1992.* Atlanta, Ga: Centers for Disease Control and Prevention, US Public Health Service; 1993.

Mandatory referenda shift the responsibility for public health policy from the legislature or board of health to the voting public. This is an ineffective way to determine public health policy as shown by the low ranks of these states. It is essential that legislators, community leaders, and health policy makers are educated about the benefits of fluoridation.[57]

Comparison of Effective Community Prevention Programs

Community prevention programs are difficult to compare due to wide variation in the studies done. Table 21.8 compares five different community programs that have been shown to be effective. Most of the information (except the data on practicality) comes from the Michigan Conference on Cost Effectiveness on Caries Prevention in Dental Public Health.[44]

Due to the widespread use of fluoridation and fluorides, and the halo or diffusion effect through processed foods and beverages, all of which result in overlapping benefits and a national decline in dental caries in children, it is difficult to determine the absolute effectiveness of specific fluoride programs.[58] For any given community, a thorough analysis of the literature, consultation with a dental public health expert, and review of the community's needs and resources should be done to determine which type of program is best for that community. As shown in Table 21.8, community fluoridation is the most effective and economical of the five effective community prevention programs for dental caries.[44] It is also the most practical.

For communities without a public water supply, a school water supply fluoridation program or a school

Table 21.8. Comparison of Five Effective Community Prevention Programs for Dental Caries*

Program	Effectiveness (percent)	Adult Benefits	Cost per Year	Practicality
Community Fluoridation	20–40	demonstrated	$0.72 per capita[a]	excellent; most practical; no individual effort necessary
School Fluoridation	20–30[b]	expected but not demonstrated	$1.19–13.83 per child	good, if there is no central community water supply; no individual effort necessary
School Dietary Fluoride Daily Supplement Program	30	expected but not demonstrated	$1.13–7.56 per child	fair; continued school regimen required for 8–10 years
School Fluoride Mouth Rinse Program	25–28[b]	not expected	$0.73–2.49[c] per child	fair; continued daily or weekly school regimen required
School Sealant Program	51–67[d]	expected but not demonstrated	$18.30–39.72 per child	good; primarily done for children age 6–8 and 12–14 years

*This table is a simplified comparison of these prevention programs. A thorough analysis of the literature should be done to understand the relative merits of these programs.
[a]In 1999 dollars, see text for range.
[b]This range may now be high; no recent studies.
[c]Includes using volunteer personnel.
[d]First molar chewing surfaces only over a five-year period.
SOURCE: Burt B. Proceedings of the workshop: Cost effectiveness of caries prevention in dental public health. *J Public Health Dent.* 1989; 49:5. Special issue.

dietary fluoride supplement program would probably be the fluoride preventive measure of choice, depending on the dental health of school children and the community's resources. School-based dental disease prevention programs and clinics are effective because they work with population groups who have not yet had the disease, are readily accessible, and can be reached on a group basis with proven prevention programs. School prevention programs also reinforce the importance of good, regular oral hygiene.

School Fluoridation

School fluoridation is the adjustment of the fluoride content of a school's water supply to prevent dental caries. The school water supply is fluoridated at 4.5 times the level recommended for community fluoridation because children are in school only for a limited amount of time during the year. Studies have shown that school fluoridation prevents tooth decay by 20 to 30 percent over 12 years

for children aged 5 to 17.[44] This figure may now be too high, as there have been no recent studies since the national decline in dental caries due to the impact of more widely available fluorides. In 1992 there were 117,430 children in 330 schools and 12 states in the United States receiving the benefits of school fluoridation.[56]

School Dietary Fluoride Supplements

School dietary fluoride supplement programs, such as fluoride tablet programs, are done on a daily basis during the school year only for children who live in nonfluoridated communities. School dietary fluoride supplements are effective because children are assured of receiving fluoride on a regular basis. These programs should begin at the earliest age possible and continue until the age of 12 to 14 years. The programs are easy to implement and require little classroom time, although achieving compliance in the middle school years can be a challenge.

School Fluoride Mouth Rinses

Topical fluoride programs such as school rinse programs can be done in nonfluoridated communities, those recently fluoridated, or those with children at high risk for dental caries. The effectiveness of school fluoride rinse programs is no longer clear in communities where the amount of new tooth decay is already low due to the widespread use of fluorides in general.

School rinse programs are usually carried out weekly for ease of administration. Nondental personnel may supervise both fluoride tablet and rinse programs. They are easy to carry out and require little classroom time, about three to five minutes per procedure. About one in ten school children, 5 to 17 years of age, participate in a school-based fluoride mouth rinse program.[46]

School Sealant Programs

School sealant programs are recommended in both fluoridated communities and nonfluoridated communities for children age 6 to 8 and 12 to 14 years. School sealant programs are important because they target the 6- and 12 year molars, which are highly susceptible to decay. The 6-year molars are the most important teeth for maintaining the dental arch.

These programs are more cost-effective when sealants are placed by dental hygienists or dental assistants rather than dentists. In 1991, 48 states allowed dental hygienists to place sealants, and 15 states allowed dental assistants to place sealants, under various degrees of supervision by a dentist. About 43 percent of state dental practice acts did not require a dentist to be physically present at all when sealants were placed by auxiliaries in public programs, and 29 states reported having a community-based sealant program. In addition, Medicaid reimbursement for sealants was provided in 42 states.[59] In 2001, all states allowed dental hygienists to place sealants and in 2000, 24 states allowed dental assistants to do so.[60] (American Dental Hygienists Association personal communication, October 2001)

Sealants are generally applied to a tooth surface only once, but sometimes they need to be replaced, so they should be checked periodically. Five-year studies show a 51 to 67 percent reduction in tooth decay of the chewing surfaces of first molars to which sealants have been applied.[11] Targeted, school-based dental sealant programs have been shown to reduce racial and economic disparities in caries prevalence among schoolchildren.[61] School sealant programs should be done in conjunction with fluoride prevention programs to obtain the maximum protection for children.

Oral Health Education

Oral health education should be incorporated into the school curriculum beginning in kindergarten to reinforce in children the importance of individual and community dental preventive measures and the need for periodic dental visits. Parents, teachers, health professionals, community leaders, and the public in general also need to be informed about dental disease prevention and the significance of oral health.

Physicians, nurses, and other health providers, in addition to dental health providers, play an important role in educating the public about oral health. The United States Clinical Preventive Services Task Force included counseling to prevent dental disease and screening for oral cancer in its recommendations to physicians.[62] It recommended that all patients be encouraged to visit a dental care provider on a regular basis. In addition, primary care clinicians should counsel patients regarding daily tooth brushing and dental flossing, the appropriate use of fluoride for caries prevention, the importance of avoiding sugary foods, and risk factors for developing early childhood tooth decay. For children living in communities with inadequate water fluoridation, dietary fluoride supplements should be prescribed. While examining the mouth, clinicians should be alert for obvious signs of oral disease.

Screening for Oral and Pharyngeal Cancer

Although routine screening of asymptomatic persons for oral cancer by primary care clinicians is not recommended, it may be prudent for clinicians to perform careful examinations for cancerous lesions of the oral cavity in patients who are over age 40 years or who use tobacco or excessive amounts of alcohol, as well as those with suspicious symptoms or lesions detected through self-examination. All patients should also be counseled to receive regular dental examinations, discontinue the use of all forms of tobacco, and limit consumption of alcohol. In addition, persons with increased exposure to sunlight should be advised to take protective measures to protect their lips and skin from the harmful effects of ultraviolet rays.[62]

From the community-wide perspective, strategies for action to prevent oral and pharyngeal cancer have been recommended in five major areas:[63,64]

- Advocacy, Collaboration, and Coalition Building
- Public Health Policy
- Public Education
- Professional Education and Practice
- Data Collection, Education, and Research

Other Prevention Programs

It is beyond the scope of this chapter to discuss the full range of prevention programs related to oral health. Other examples of successful programs range from mouth guard programs for high school athletes in contact sports[65] to programs to educate dentists about children suffering from abuse or neglect[66] or how dental care providers may help the users of cigarettes and spit (smokeless) tobacco quit.[67] Clearly, there are a range of oral health programs to improve oral health that can be utilized in any community depending on their needs and resources.[68–73]

ORAL HEALTH—AN ESSENTIAL COMPONENT OF HEALTH AND PRIMARY CARE

Oral health is an essential component of total health and primary care.[74] Dental and oral diseases may well be the most prevalent and preventable conditions affecting Americans.[2,7,73,75] When any type of health or primary care program is being considered or developed there should be an oral health component. As oral diseases affect most of the population, community-based prevention should always be a very high priority.[2,7,73] Unfortunately, the United States does not have national disease prevention or treatment programs, or national health insurance. Regardless of whether an evolving health care system emphasizes oral health services, public health professionals have the responsibility and

opportunity to make meaningful contributions to the public's health by including oral health in health programs.

Vulnerable populations, such as those of low income, minorities, migrants, persons with HIV, and the institutionalized, homeless, homebound, elderly, and medically compromised, have the greatest dental needs as well as the least access to dental services. Health programs targeted to vulnerable and high-risk populations must have an oral health component. Although there are some dental programs provided by local, state, and federal agencies for vulnerable populations, they are usually inadequate.

Low-income groups and minorities suffer a disproportionate share of untreated oral diseases.[2,7,76] Community-based prevention, health care reform, and primary care dentistry can help address inequities and access issues for vulnerable populations.[77] In response to the Surgeon General's Report on Oral Health, a call to action includes the following six recommendations:[1]

1. Oral health must become a much higher priority at the local, state, and national levels, so that oral health disparities can be improved and resolved.
2. The federal government must be a role model and set the example that oral health is an integral and important component of all health programs.
3. Promotion and use of effective individual and population-based prevention services and programs must become a much higher priority at the local, state, and national levels, especially for children and high-risk populations.
4. The oral health component of Medicaid and the Child Health Insurance Program must be upgraded and improved.
5. All communities with a central water supply must have fluoridation.
6. The oral health workforce needs to be modified and augmented.

Examples of such initiatives have also been suggested. They include:[1]

a. Funding and development of an effective dental public health infrastructure at the local, state, and national levels to provide guidance in responding to these needs.

b. The oral health needs of the underserved must be more effectively met by community and migrant health centers, the National Health Service Corps, Head Start, maternal and child health agencies, Healthy Start, the Special Supplemental Nutrition Program for Women, Infants, and Children, area health education centers, school-based health centers, and other such programs.

c. Tobacco settlement funds must also be used to develop and institutionalize effective prevention programs because of the relationship between tobacco use and oral diseases. These services and programs can include school, community, or institutional prevention initiatives that provide fluorides, dental sealants, early childhood caries prevention, and oral and pharyngeal cancer examinations.

d. The accountability of state officials involved in dental Medicaid and the Child Health Insurance Program must be increased.

e. An effective statewide distribution of safety-net providers must be available in every state.

f. The U.S. Department of Health and Human Services must play a much stronger leadership role, working with local and state agencies and organizations to promote and support community water fluoridation.

g. More dentists, including those of minority backgrounds, should be trained in dental public health.

h. State practice acts must also be less restrictive and more responsive to the needs of the public in such areas as national reciprocity for licensees and delegation of duties for dental hygienists and assistants.

DENTAL PERSONNEL

The total number of dental personnel is adequate to meet the current demand for oral health services but not the need. There is also a maldistribution of dental personnel in certain parts of the United States, with many inner-city and rural areas left underserved. According to a 1994 personal written communication with J. Rossetti of the Health Resources and Service Administration, in FY 1993 there were 1,069 designated dental health professional shortage areas (HP-SAs) in the United States, requiring 2,087 dentists to fill the identified gaps. This increased to 1,480 dental shortage areas in 2001, requiring 4,650 dentists for about 31.4 million people.[31]

If there were health care reform in our country that included reimbursement for oral health needs, the demand for service would increase and stress the capacity of the existing dental care delivery system. The best response to the growing need would be to increase the use of dental auxiliaries and incorporate oral health services into existing programs for vulnerable populations. The public health professional, as a leader and policy maker, can play a key role in helping to meet oral health needs by drawing upon four categories of dental personnel for assistance: dentists, dental hygienists, dental assistants, and dental laboratory technicians.

Dentists

Dentists have a minimum of two years of college before going to dental school, and most have a college degree. In 2001, there were 54 dental schools in the United States, all but 1 of which had four-year curricula.[31] Two additional schools will open in Arizona and Nevada. Dentists receive a doctor of dental surgery (D.D.S.) or the equivalent doctor of dental medicine (D.M.D.) degree.

There were 148,800 dentists in the United States in 1990, for an active dentist-to-population ratio of 59.5 per 100,000.[78] In the year 2000, there were an estimated 154,460 professionally active dentists, of which 142,150 were in private practice.[31] Due to the closure of seven dental schools since 1985, a decrease in the applicant pool, and the increasing cost of a dental education, the number of dental school graduates dropped from 5,550 in 1980 to about 4,075 in 2000.[78,31] By the year 2000, the ratio of active dentists to population was 58.3 per 100,000 and this is expected to drop to 52.7 per 100,000 by 2020.[31] Most dentists in the United States are general practitioners who work in private practice. Only 21 percent of dentists are active specialists. Only about 14.1 percent of professionally active dentists are women and 14 percent are people of color, of which 7 percent are Asian/Pacific Islander,

3.4 percent African American, 3.3 percent Hispanic/Latino and 0.1 percent Native American.[31] The nine dental specialties are dental public health, endodontics, oral and maxillofacial surgery, oral pathology, orthodontics, pediatric dentistry, periodontics, prosthodontics and radiology.

Dental Hygienists

Dental hygienists primarily provide preventive services to patients, usually including screening, prophylaxis (cleaning), scaling, root planing, taking radiographs, health education, and topical fluoride and dental sealant application. Most hygienists have two years of education and training after high school. In 1998 there were 237 dental hygiene schools in the United States with 6,087 first-year students.[31] Once hygienists are licensed by the state, they are known as registered dental hygienists (RDHs). Some hygienists have four or more years of education. Hygienists who work in public health policy or administration usually have a master's or doctoral degree in public health or health sciences.

In 1990, there were about 98,000 hygienists with active licenses in the United States of which about 81,000 were in active practice.[80] In 1998 there were about 140,750 RDHs.[79] Dental hygienists are an excellent resource for public health initiatives for promoting and implementing prevention programs, health education, screening and referral, school-based programs, community outreach, and improved access to the underserved. Some state dental practice acts unnecessarily restrict what hygienists may do, resulting in access problems, lower efficiency, and higher costs for providing oral health services.

Dental Assistants

A formally trained dental assistant usually has one year of training after high school. Many dentists have trained their assistants on the job, but this is not recommended given the technological advances and challenges in dentistry, including the need for following the Centers for Disease Control and Prevention's guidelines for infection control. Dental assistants usually assist the dentist or hygienist when treatment is provided to the patient. Their duties include but are not limited to history taking, selecting and sterilizing instruments, mixing dental materials, and taking and developing radiographs.

Studies have shown that the productivity of dentists can be improved dramatically by the proper use of dental assistants. When dental assistants are allowed to perform expanded duties, the productivity of dentists increases even more.[80,81] Many state practice acts unnecessarily restrict what dental assistants are allowed to do, thus constraining dental productivity. In 1990, there were about 201,400 active dental assistants in the United States, for a ratio of 1.35 active assistants per active dentist.[78] In 1998 there were about 231,380 dental assistants and 248 dental assisting schools with 6,162 graduates.[79,31]

Dental Laboratory Technicians

Upon receiving a prescription from a dentist, dental laboratory technicians construct prostheses for the dentist to provide to the patient. These include but are not limited to dentures, crowns, bridges, and space maintainers. Lab technicians usually do not have direct contact with patients. In a few states, such as Oregon, dental laboratory technicians, known as denturists, are allowed to make dentures directly for the public. Lab technicians may have a one- to two-year training period after high school, but many are trained on-the-job. In 1990, there were about 70,000 laboratory technicians in the United States.[78] In 1996 there were about 53,000 technicians and in 1998, there were 34 schools for laboratory technicians with 487 graduates.[82,31]

CONCLUSION

Oral diseases are a neglected epidemic in our country. The public health professional has the responsibility and opportunity to respond to this epidemic. Oral health is an essential component of total health for both the individual and the community. The challenges to the public health professional for the future have been clearly delineated.[1,2,7,83] Oral health has 17 objectives in the year 2010 national health objectives and must be included in the three public health core functions of assessment, policy development, and assurance.

Most oral diseases can be readily assessed and prevented. Cost-effective individual and community preventive measures are available. Every local, state, and federal health department and agency should have dental public health expertise to respond effectively to this epidemic. Every health initiative or program should include an oral health component, from targeted programs for infants, pregnant women, persons with HIV, or the homeless, to health centers, managed care, and local, state, and national programs, including health care reform. The oral health needs of the American people must be addressed by the public health professional for healthier communities and a healthier nation.

ACKNOWLEDGMENT

The author would like to thank Dr. Stephen B. Corbin, formerly the Chief Dental Officer of the U.S. Public Health Service, and Dr. Alice M. Horowitz of the National Institute of Dental and Craniofacial Research for their assistance with this chapter in the first edition of this book.

References

1. Allukian M. The neglected epidemic and the Surgeon General's Report: A call to action for better oral health (editorial). *Am J Public Health.* 2000;90(6):843-845.
2. US Department of Health and Human Services. *Oral Health in America: A Report of the Surgeon General.* Rockville, Md: US Dept of Health and Human Services, National Institute of Dental and Craniofacial Research, National Institutes of Health; 2000.
3. National Center for Health Statistics. *An Assessment of the Occlusion of the Teeth of Youths, 12-17 Years, United States. Vital and Health Statistics.* Washington, DC: US Government Printing Office; 1977. DHEW publication HRA 77-1644. Series 11, no. 162.
4. Bhat M. Periodontal health of 14-17 year old U.S. school children. *J Public Health Dent.* Winter 1991;51(1):5-11.
5. National Institute of Dental Research. *Oral Health of United States Children. The National Survey of Dental Caries in U.S. School Children, 1986-1987.* Bethesda, Md: US Dept of Health and Human Services; 1989. DHHS publication NIH 89-2247.
6. National Institute of Dental Research. *The National Survey of Oral Health in U.S. Employed Adults and Seniors: 1985-1986.* Bethesda, Md: US Dept of Health and Human Services; 1987. DHHS publication NIH 87-2868.
7. US Department of Health and Human Services. *Healthy People 2010, With Understanding and Improving Health Objectives for Improving Health.* 2nd ed. Washington, DC: US Government Printing Office; 2000.
8. Greenlee RT, Hill-Harmon MB, Murray T, Thun M. Cancer statistics, 2001. *CA Cancer J Clin.* 2001;51:15-36.
9. Edmonds LD, James LM. Temporal trends in the prevalence of congenital malformations at birth based on the Birth Defects Monitoring Program, United States, 1979-1987. *MMWR.* 1993;39:19-23.
10. Allukian M, Kazmi I, Foulds SH, Horgan W. The unmet dental needs of the homeless in Boston. Presented at the 112th Annual Meeting of the American Public Health Association; November 13, 1984; Anaheim, California.
11. Kelly M, Bruerd B. The prevalence of nursing bottle decay among two Native American populations. *J Public Health Dent.* 1987;47:94-97.
12. Becker DB, Needleman HL, Kotelchuck M. Child abuse and dentistry: Orofacial trauma and its recognition by dentists. *J Am Dent Assoc.* 1978;97(1):24-28.
13. Flanders R. Orofacial injuries: Prevalence and prevention in Illinois. *Ill Dent J.* May/June 1992:211-216.
14. Bloom B, Gift HC, Jack SS. *Dental Services and Oral Health; United States, 1989. Vital Health Stat.* 1992;10:183.
15. *Healthy People 2000: National Health Promotion and Disease Prevention Objectives.* Washington, DC: US Public Health Service; 1990. PHS publication no. 91-50212.
16. Kaste LW, Marcus P, Monopoli M, Allukian M, Douglass CW. Oral health status of homebound elders in Boston. Paper presented at the 18th Annual Meeting of the American Association for Dental Research; March 15-18, 1989; San Francisco, California.
17. Mueller CD, Schur CL, Paramore C. Access to dental care in the United States. *J Am Dent Assoc.* 1998;129:429-437.
18. Dasanayake AP. Poor periodontal health of the pregnant woman as a risk factor for low birth weight. *Ann Periodontol.* 1998;70:206-211.

19. Offenbacher S, Katz V, Fertik G, et al. Periodontal infection as a possible factor for preterm low birth weight. *Ann Periodontol.* 1995;67(suppl 10):1103-1113.

20. Davenport ES, Willias CE, Sterne JA, et al. The East London study of maternal chronic periodontal disease and preterm low birth weight infants: Study design and prevalence data. *Ann Periodontol.* 1998;70:213-221.

21. Beck JD, Offenbacher S, Williams R, Gibbs P, Garcia R. Periodontitis: A risk factor for coronary heart disease? *Ann Periodontol.* 1998;70:127-141.

22. Genco RJ. Periodontal disease and risk for myocardial infarction and cardiovascular disease. *Cardiovasc Rev Rep.* 1998;19:34-40.

23. Slavkin HC. Does the mouth put the heart at risk? *J Am Dent Assoc.* 1999;130:109-113.

24. Jeffcoat MK, Geurs NC, Reddy MS, Cliver SL, Goldenberg RL, Hauth JC. Periodontal infection and preterm birth. *J Am Dent Assoc.* July 2001;132:875-880.

25. Hollister MC, Weintraub JA. The association of oral status and systemic health, quality of life, and economic productivity. *J Dent Educ.* 1993;57(12):901-912.

26. Lipton JS, Ship JA, Larach-Robinson D. Estimated prevalence and distribution of reported orofacial pain in the United States. *J Am Dent Assoc.* 1993;124(10):115-121.

27. Gift HC, Reisine ST, Larach DC. The social impact of dental problems and visits. *Am J Public Health.* 1992;82(12): 1663-1668.

28. Adams PF, Benson V. Current Estimates from the National Health Interview Survey, 1991. Vital Health Stat. 1992;10(184):46-47,54.

29. Adams PF, Marano MA. 1995. *Current Estimates from the National Health Interview Survey, 1994. Vital and Health Statistics.* Hyattsville, Md: US Dept of Health and Human Services, National Center for Health Statistics. Series 10, no. 193.

30. Health Care Financing Administration, Office of Actuary. *National Health Expenditure Amounts and Average Change by Type of Expenditure: Selected Calendar Years 1980-2010.* Available at: http://www.hcfa.gov/stats/NHE-Proj/Proj.2000/tables/t2.htm. Accessed June 14, 2001.

31. Valachovic RW, Weaver RG, Sinkford JC, Haden NK. Trends in dentistry and dental education. *J Dent Educ.* June 2001:539-561.

32. Office of Inspector General. *Children's Dental Services Under Medicaid: Access and Utilization.* Washington, DC: US Dept of Health and Human Services; 1996. OBI-09-93-00240.

33. Joshi A, Douglass CW, Jette A, Feldman H. The distribution of root caries in community-dwelling elders in New England. *J Public Health Dent.* Winter 1994:15-23.

34. Winn DM, et al. Coronal and root caries in the dentition of adults in the United States, 1988-1991. *J Dent Res.* 1996;75:642-651. Special issue.

35. Kaste LM, Gift HC. Baby bottle feeding behavior in children ages 2-5. *J Dent Res.* 1994;33(2):580.

36. *Cancers of the Oral Cavity and Pharynx: A Statistics Review Monograph, 1973-1987.* Atlanta, Ga: Centers for Disease Control and the National Institutes of Health; 1991.

37. Prout MN, Heeren TC, Barber CE, et al. Use of health services before the diagnosis of head and neck cancer among Boston residents. *Am J Prev Med.* 1990;6:77-83.

38. Palmer C. NCAA forbids tobacco usage. *ADA News.* 1994;25:4.

39. Institute of Medicine, Committee for the Study of the Future of Public Health. *The Future of Public Health.* Washington, DC: National Academy Press; 1988.

40. Executive summary: Application for continued recognition of dental public health as a dental specialty. *J Public Health Dent.* 1986;46(1):35-37.

41. Rozier RG. Competency objectives for dental public health. *J Public Health Dent.* 1990;50(5):338-344.

42. Dental public health competencies. *J Public Health Dept.* 1998;58 (suppl 1):121-122.

43. *Application for Continued Recognition of Dental Public Health as a Specialty.* Richmond, Va: American Association of Public Health Dentistry; December 1985.

44. Burt B. Proceedings of the workshop: Cost effectiveness of caries prevention in dental public health. *J Public Health Dent.* 1989; 49:5. Special issue.

45. Centers for Disease Control and Prevention. Recommendations for using fluoride to prevent and control dental caries in the United States. *MMWR.* 2001;50:1-42.

46. Wagener DK, Nourjah P, Horowitz A. *Trends in Childhood Use of Dental Care Products Containing Fluoride: U.S. 1983-1989.* Hyattsville, Md: National Center for Health Statistics; 1992. Advance data from Vital and Health Statistics no. 219.

47. *Review of Fluoride: Benefits and Risks.* Washington, DC: US Public Health Service; February 1991.

48. American Dental Association. Caries diagnosis and risk assessment. A review of preventive strategies and management. *J Am Dent Assoc.* 1995;126 (suppl).

49. Kaminsky LS, Mahoney MC, Leach JF, Melius JM, Miller MJ. Fluoride: Benefits and risk of exposure. *Crit Rev Oral Biol Med.* 1990;1(4):261.

50. National Research Council. *Health Effects of Ingested Fluoride.* Washington, DC: National Academy Press; 1993.
51. Institute of Medicine Food and Nutrition Board. *Dietary Reference Intakes: Calcium, Phosphorus, Magnesium, Vitamin D and Fluoride.* Washington National Academy Press; 1997.
52. Centers for Disease Control and Prevention. Public health focus: Fluoridation of community water systems. *MMWR.* 1992;2(41):372-375, 381.
53. Griffins S, Jones K, Tomar S. An economic evaluation of community water fluoridation. *J Public Health Dept.* 2001; 61:38-86.
54. Centers for Disease Control. *Water Fluoridation: A Manual for Engineers and Technicians.* Atlanta, Ga: US Public Health Service; 1986:19.
55. Centers for Disease Control and Prevention. Fluoridation of drinking water to prevent dental caries. *MMWR.* 1999;48:933-940.
56. *Fluoridation Census, 1992.* Atlanta, Ga: Centers for Disease Control and Prevention, US Public Health Service; 1993.
57. Allukian M, Ackerman J, Steinhurst J. Factors that influence the attitudes of first-term Massachusetts legislators toward fluoridation. *J Am Dent Assoc.* 1981;104(4):494.
58. Griffin SO, Gooch BF, Lockwood SA, Tomar SL. Quantifying the diffused benefit from water fluoridation in the United States. *Community Dent Oral Epidemiol.* 2001;29:120-129.
59. Cohen LA, Horowitz AM. Community-based sealant programs in the United States: Results of a survey. *J Public Health Dent.* Fall 1993;53:4.
60. American Dental Association. *2000 Survey of Legal Provisions for Delegating Intraoral Functions to Chairside Assistants and Dental Hygienists.* Survey Center; June 2001.
61. Impact of targeted, school-based dental sealant programs in reducing racial and economic disparities in sealant prevalence among school children—Ohio, United States, 1998-1999. *MMWR.* 2001;50(34):736-738.
62. US Preventive Services Task Force Report. *Guide to Clinical Preventive Services.* 2nd ed. Baltimore, Md: Williams and Wilkins; 1996.
63. Centers for Disease Control and Prevention. Proceedings from the National Strategic Planning Conference for the Prevention and Control of Oral and Pharyngeal Cancer, August 7-9, 1996, Atlanta. Bethesda, Md: 1997.
64. Centers for Disease Control and Prevention. Presenting and Controlling Oral and Pharyngeal Cancer. Recommendations from a National Strategic Planning Conference. *MMWR.* Morb Mortal Wkly Rep 1998;47(RR 1-14):1-12.
65. Flanders R. Mouthguards and sports injuries. *Ill Dent J.* Jan/Feb 1993:13-16.
66. Missouri Dental Association. Child abuse update 1994. Reprinted from the *Missouri Dent J.* 1994;1-101.
67. National Cancer Institute. *How to Help Your Patients Stop Using Tobacco: Manual for the Oral Health Team.* Washington, DC: National Institutes of Health; 1991. PHS publication no. 91-3191.
68. Allukian M. Effective community prevention program. In: Depoala DP, Cheney JG, eds. *Handbook of Preventive Dentistry.* Littleton, Mass: Publishing Services Group Inc; 1979.
69. Horowitz AM. Community-oriented preventive dentistry programs that work. *Health Values.* 1984;8(1):121-129.
70. Allukian M. Community oral health programs. In: Clark JW, ed. *Clinical Dentistry, II.* Philadelphia, Pa: Harper & Row; 1987.
71. Association of State and Territorial Dental Directors. *Guidelines for State Dental Public Health Programs.* 1985.
72. Association of State and Territorial Dental Directors. *Public Health Core Functions: Strategies for Addressing the Oral Health of the Nation.* March 1994. Discussion paper.
73. Allukian M Jr, Horowitz AM. Effective community prevention programs for oral diseases. In: Gluck G, Morganstein W, eds. *Jong's Community Dental Health.* 4th ed. St. Louis, Mo: Mosby Press; 1997:144-176.
74. Isman RE. Integrating primary oral health care into primary care. *J Dent Educ.* 1993;47(12):846-852.
75. Oral Health Coordinating Committee, Public Health Service. Toward improving the oral health of Americans: An overview of oral health status, resources, and care delivery. *Public Health Rep.* 1993;108(6):657-672.
76. Mouradian WE, Wehr E, Crall JJ. Disparities in children's oral health and access to dental care. *J Am Med Assoc.* 2000;284:2625-2631.
77. Bolden AJ, Henry JL, Allukian M. Implications of access, utilization and need for oral health care by low income groups and minorities on the dental delivery system. *J Dent Educ.* 1993; 57(12):888-900.
78. US Department of Health and Human Services. *Health Personnel in the United States, Eighth Report to Congress. Allied Health, 1991.* Washington, DC: HRSA/Bureau of Health Professions; September 1992.

79. Health Resources and Services Administration (HRSA) Bureau of Health Professions. *HRSA State Health Workforce Profile.* Rockville, Md: HRSA/Bureau of Health Professions; December 2000.

80. *Comptroller General: Increased Use of Expanded Function Dental Auxiliaries Would Benefit Consumers, Dentists and Taxpayers. Report to the Congress.* Washington, DC: General Accounting Office; March 7, 1980. Publication HRD-80-51.

81. Liang JN, Ogur JD. *Restrictions on Dental Auxiliaries; An Economic Policy Analysis.* Washington, DC: Federal Trade Commission; May 1987.

82. Health Resources and Services Administration (HRSA) Bureau of Health Professions. *Factbook, United States Health Workforce Personnel.* Rockville, Md: HRSA/Bureau of Health Professions; 1999.

83. Corbin SB, Mecklenburg RE. The future of dental public health report: Preparing dental public health to meet the challenges and opportunities of the 21st century. *J Public Health Dent.* 1994;54(2):80-91.

CHAPTER
22

Infectious Disease Control

Alan R. Hinman, M.D., M.P.H.

Historically, infectious diseases have been the major killers of humans. It is only within the last century that they have been replaced by chronic diseases and injuries as primary killers in the United States. Worldwide, however, infectious diseases still account for 25 percent of all deaths.[1] The major advances in infectious disease control to date have been through protection of food and water and through immunizations. This chapter begins with general considerations of infectious disease transmission, surveillance, and investigation, and then considers specific topics of immunization, sexually transmitted diseases (STDs, including human immunodeficiency virus [HIV] infection), tuberculosis (TB), foodborne and waterborne diseases, emerging/reemerging diseases and antibiotic resistance, and bioterrorism.

GENERAL CONSIDERATIONS

This section introduces general principles of infectious disease transmission. It also discusses how surveillance and outbreak investigation help control the spread of infectious diseases.

Transmission

The four means by which infectious diseases are transmitted are direct transmission, indirect transmission (vehicle or vector), and airborne transmission.[2] Direct transmission may occur as a result of touching, biting, kissing, or sexual intercourse, or as a result of inhaling large droplets of infected respiratory secretions generated by coughing, sneezing, talking, or singing. The latter type of direct transmission typically takes place over short distances (usually less than 3–6 feet [1–2 meters]). Sexually transmitted diseases and measles are conditions spread by direct transmission. Indirect transmission may occur as a result of contamination of inanimate vehicles such as needles, water, food, blood, and so on, or as a result of contact with vectors, living creatures (usually arthropods) that may serve as passive carriers of the organism (e.g., plague, Lyme disease) or play an integral part of the life cycle of the infectious agent (e.g., malaria). Airborne transmission occurs when infectious droplets form droplet nuclei that may remain suspended in the air for minutes to hours and be dispersed widely. For example, patients in a hospital several rooms away from a patient with varicella have become infected,[3] and measles has been transmitted to a patient visiting a physician's office approximately one hour after the source case had left the office.[4]

Surveillance

Surveillance is key to understanding the epidemiology of infectious diseases. Surveillance is "the continuing scrutiny of all aspects of occurrence and spread of a disease that are pertinent to effective control . . . [including] . . . systematic collection and evaluation of morbidity and mortality reports, special reports of field investigations . . . , isolation and identification of infectious agents . . . , data concerning the availability, use and untoward effects of vaccines . . . and other substances used in control, information regarding immunity levels in segments of the population, and other relevant data."[2] A simple definition of surveillance is "information for action."[5] Surveillance information is used to develop and modify interventions and monitor their success. In addition, surveillance may identify clusters of cases or outbreaks that warrant further investigation.

Outbreak Investigation

Outbreak investigation involves seven major steps, many of which may be carried out simultaneously:

1. Confirm whether there truly is an epidemic. The definition of an epidemic is "the occurrence in a community or region of cases of an illness (or an outbreak) with a frequency clearly in excess of normal expectancy."[2] Obviously, it is necessary to know not only how many cases there are, but how many are expected. A single case of paralysis due to wild poliovirus occurring in the United States, for example, would be considered a potential epidemic because there have been no such cases reported since 1979.[6] Two cases associated in time and place would be sufficient evidence of transmission to be considered an epidemic.
2. Identify the illness involved, often by establishing a clinical case definition if a definitive diagnosis has not been established.
3. Enumerate all cases and characterize them according to time, place, and person. Characterization as to time typically involves construction of an epidemic curve depicting the number of cases by time of onset (by hour, day, week, or month, as appropriate). A common vehicle outbreak with a point contamination of the vehicle typically has an epidemic curve with a single sharp peak centered on the median incubation period following exposure (typically a few hours to a few days). Person-to-person direct transmission is generally accompanied by an epidemic curve in which there is a gradual buildup of cases, often with a typical incubation period between "generations" of cases, and a gradual decline as susceptibles are exhausted, in the absence of measures to interrupt transmission. Characterization by place often involves constructing a map showing residence (or worksite) of individual cases in order to identify any geographic localization. Characterization by person involves the obvious—age and gender—but may also entail race/ethnicity, occupation, behavioral characteristic, or other variables.
4. Confirm the diagnosis in the laboratory or by other means.
5. Formulate a hypothesis about the cause of the epidemic and the means of transmission and test that hypothesis through further investigation or interview of cases, culture of suspected vehicle, or other means.
6. Take control measures to end the epidemic.
7. Prepare and disseminate a report about the epidemic, either through formal publication in the literature or through an administratively circulated report. This last step, which is the one most often ignored, is essential in order to learn from the current situation and prevent recurrences.

IMMUNIZATION

Immunization is one of the most important interventions for the control and prevention of infectious diseases. This section addresses vaccines, their impact, immunization coverage, immunization schedules, the immunization infrastructure in the United States, and vaccine safety and effectiveness

Vaccines

Vaccines are suspensions of attenuated live or killed microorganisms (bacteria, viruses, or rickettsiae) or fractions thereof that are administered to induce immunity and thereby prevent infectious disease. Live, attenuated vaccines consist of living organisms that have been adapted in the laboratory to reduce their ability to cause disease while still stimulating an immune response. They are believed to induce an immunologic response more similar to that resulting from natural infection than do inactivated vaccines. Inactivated or killed vaccines may consist of:

- Inactivated whole organisms (e.g., cholera, influenza)
- Soluble capsular material alone (e.g., pneumococcal polysaccharide)
- Soluble capsular material covalently linked to carrier proteins (e.g., *Haemophilus influenzae* type b [Hib] conjugate)
- Purified extracts of some component or components of the organism (e.g., hepatitis B, acellular pertussis)

Toxoids are modified bacterial toxins (e.g., diphtheria, tetanus) that have been rendered nontoxic but retain the ability to stimulate the formation of antitoxin. They are often included in the general category of vaccines.[7]

Impact of Vaccines

Introduction and widespread use of childhood vaccines have had a dramatic effect on the reported incidence of infectious diseases in the United States. The United States is currently enjoying historic low levels of disease incidence and historic high levels of vaccine coverage. Table 22.1 shows the maximum number of cases reported of childhood vaccine-preventable diseases and the provisional number of cases of those diseases reported in 2000.[8] There has been a reduction in excess of 95 percent in virtually every one of the conditions. Some of the reductions are quite recent— Hib conjugate vaccine was introduced in the United States for use in infants in 1990, but its widespread use led to virtual elimination of HiB disease in this country within a period of less than 10 years.[9]

Immunization Coverage

Table 22.2 shows the 1999 nationwide levels of vaccine coverage in 19 to 35-month-old children.[10] The levels are not uniform throughout the country. For example, in 1998, state-specific levels of measles vaccination ranged from 85.9 percent (New Mexico) to 96.6 percent (Connecticut). In addition there is racial and

Table 22.1. Maximum and Current Morbidity from Vaccine-Preventable Diseases, USA

Disease	Maximum	2000 (prov.)	Percentage decline
Diphtheria	206,939	2	−99.99
Hib (< 5)	20,000	~80	−99.60
Measles	894,134	80	−99.99
Mumps	152,209	323	−99.78
Pertussis	265,269	6,755	−97.45
Polio (paralytic)	21,269	0	−100.00
Rubella	57,686	152	−99.73
CRS	20,000	7	−99.96
Tetanus	1,733	26	−98.49

Table 22.2. Vaccination Coverage Levels among Children Aged 19–35 Months

United States, 1999

Vaccine/dose	Coverage (%)
DTP — 3	95.9
DTP — 4	83.3
Polio — 3	89.6
Hib — 3	93.5
MMR — 1	91.5
Hepatitis B — 3	88.1
Varicella	59.4
Combined series	
4 DTP/3 Polio/I MMR	79.9
4 DTP/3 Polio/1 MMR/3 Hib	78.4

socioeconomic variation in coverage rates, with blacks having lower rates than whites (88.9 and 93.3 percent, respectively), and children living in poverty having lower rates than the national average (90.2 and 92.1 percent, respectively).[11]

Immunization rates in adults are not as high as those in children. For example, in 1997, only 66 percent of adults 65 years of age or older had received influenza vaccine in the preceding year and only 46 percent had ever received pneumococcal vaccine.[12] Both vaccines have been recommended for all persons 65 or older (and for younger persons with certain conditions) for decades.

Immunization Schedules

Recommendations for immunization of children in the United States are developed principally by the Public Health Service's Advisory Committee on Immunization Practices (ACIP)[7] and the American Academy of Pediatrics' (AAP) Committee on Infectious Diseases ("Red Book Committee").[13,14] Along with the American Academy of Family Physicians (AAFP), these committees develop harmonized immunization schedules for infants and children (Figure 22.1). Immunization of all infants and children in the United States is currently recommended against 11 diseases:

diphtheria (D), hepatitis B, Hib, measles, mumps, pertussis (P), pneumococcal disease, poliomyelitis, rubella, tetanus (T), and varicella. In areas of high incidence, hepatitis A vaccine is also recommended.

Table 22.3 shows immunization recommendations for adolescents and adults, who may have special needs for vaccines because of increased risk of illness or death resulting from age, occupation, behavior, or chronic illness.[15,16] Recommendations have also been developed for health care workers.[17]

Immunization Infrastructure

Most children in the United States currently receive their immunizations in the private sector, from pediatricians or family physicians. A significant minority receive immunizations in the public sector, typically from local health departments. There is considerable variation around the country.[18]

Since 1962, the federal government has supported childhood immunization programs through a grant program administered by the Centers for Disease Control and Prevention (CDC). The grants support purchase of vaccine for free administration at local health departments and also support immunization delivery, surveillance, and communication/education.

At current prices, the cost for vaccines alone (irrespective of physician fees) is approximately $600 in the private sector (CDC, unpublished data). Most employer-based insurance plans now cover childhood immunizations. Children who are covered by Medicaid or the Children's Health Plan can receive vaccines free of charge through the Vaccines for Children program enacted in 1993.[19] Others may receive the vaccines free at health departments.

Immunization efforts in the United States have been significantly aided by the enactment and enforcement of laws in each state that require immunization before first entry into school. Since 1980 all states have had such laws in place. As a result, at least 96 percent of children entering school are fully immunized.[20]

Although immunization levels are currently at record high levels and vaccine-preventable disease incidence is at record low levels, there is continuing cause for concern about immunizations in the United States:

Recommended Childhood Immunization Schedule
United States, 2002

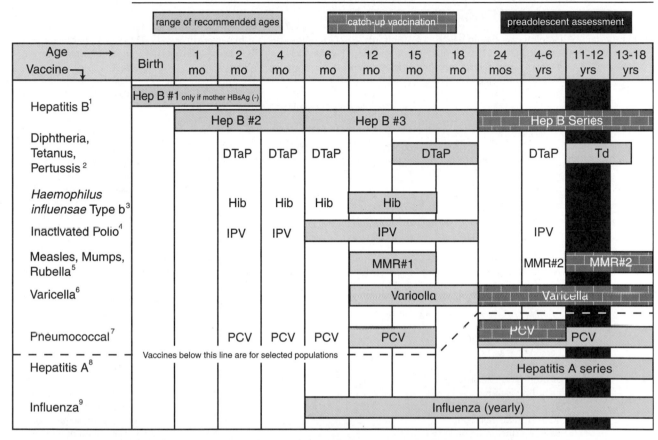

Figure 22.1. Recommended Childhood Immunization Schedule United States, 2002

Source: Centers for Disease Control and Prevention. Available www.cdc.gov/nip.

- There are approximately four million births each year (11,000 per day) and each of these children requires immunization.
- The population is quite mobile. Approximately 16 percent of Americans change address in any given year and at least 25 percent of children receive immunizations from more than one provider. This mobility creates problems in record keeping.
- The immunization schedule is increasingly complex as new vaccines or additional doses are recommended.
- Both parents and providers overestimate the immunization levels of their children/patients. Most parents

Table 22.3. Summary of Adolescent/Adult Immunization Recommendations

Agent	Indications	Primary Schedule	Contrain-dications	Comments
Tetanus and Diphtheria Toxoids Combined (Td)	All adults All adolescents should be assessed at 11–12 or 14–16 years of age and immunized if no dose was receive during the previous 5 years.	Two doses 4–8 weeks apart, third dose 6–12 months after the second. No need to repeat doses if the schedule is interrupted. Dose: 0.5 mL intramuscular (IM) Booster: At 10 year intervals throughout life.	Neurologic or severe hypersensitivity reaction to prior dose.	Wound Management: Patients with three or more previous tetanus toxoid doses: (1) give Td for clean, minor wounds only if more than 10 years since last dose; (b) for other wounds, give Td if over 5 years since last dose. Patients with less than 3 or unknown number of prior tetanus toxoid doses; give Td for clean, minor wounds and Td and TIG (Tetanus Immune Globulin) for other wounds.
Influenza Vaccine	a. Adults 50 years of age and older. b. Residents of nursing homes or other facilities for patients with chronic medical conditions. c. Persons ≥6 months of age with chronic cardiovascular or pulmonary disorders, including asthma. d. Persons ≥6 months of age with chronic metabolic diseases (including diabetes), renal dysfunction, hemoglobinopathies, immunosuppressive or immunodeficiency disorders. e. Women in their 2nd or 3rd trimester of pregnancy during influenza season. f. Persons 6 mo.–18 years of age receiving long-term aspirin therapy. g. Groups, including household members and care givers, who can infect high risk persons.	Dose: 0.5 mL intramuscular (IM) Given annually each fall and winter.	Anaphylactic allergy to eggs. Acute febrile illness.	Depending on season and destination, persons traveling to foreign countries should consider vaccination. Any person ≥6 months of age who wishes to reduce the likelihood of becoming ill with influenza should be vaccinated. Avoiding subsequent vaccination of persons known to have developed GBS within 6 weeks of a previous vaccination seems prudent; however, for most persons with a GBS history who are at high risk for severe complications, many experts believe the established benefits of vaccination justify yearly vaccination.

Table 22.3.   Summary of Adolescent/Adult Immunization Recommendations *(Continued)*

Agent	Indications	Primary Schedule	Contrain-dications	Comments
Pneumococcal Poly-saccharide Vaccine (PPV)	a. Adults 65 years of age and older. b. Persons ≥2 years with chronic cardiovascular or pulmonary disorders including congestive heart failure, diabetes mellitus, chronic liver disease, alcoholism, CSF leaks, cardiomyopathy, COPD or emphysema. c. Persons ≥2 years with splenic dysfunction or asplenia, hematologic malignancy, multiple myeloma, renal failure, organ transplantation or immunosuppressive conditions, including HIV infection. d. Alaskan Natives and certain American Indian populations.	One dose for most people* Dose: 0.5 mL intramuscular (IM) or subcutaneous (SC) *Persons vaccinated prior to age 65 should be vaccinated at age 65 if 5 or more years have passed since the first dose. For all persons with functional or anatomic asplenia, transplant patients, patients with chronic kidney disease, immunosuppressed or immunodeficient persons, and others at highest risk of fatal infection, a second dose should be given—at least 5 years after first dose.	The safety of PPV during the first trimester of pregnancy has not been evaluated. The manufacturer's package insert should be reviewed for additional information.	If elective splenectomy or immunosuppressive therapy is planned, give vaccine 2 weeks ahead, if possible. When indicated, vaccine should be administered to patients with unknown vaccination status. All residents of nursing homes and other long-term care facilities should have their vaccination status assessed and documented.
Measles and Mumps Vaccines**	a. Adults born after 1956 without written documentation of immunization on or after the first birthday. b. Health care personnel born after 1956 who are at risk of exposure to patients with measles should have documentation of two doses of vaccine on or after the first birthday or of measles seropositivity. c. HIV-infected persons without severe immunosuppression. d. Travelers to foreign countries. e. Persons entering post-secondary educational institutions (e.g., college).	At least one dose. (Two doses of measles—containing vaccine if in college, in health care profession or traveling to a foreign country with second dose at least 1 month after the first). Dose: 0.5 mL subcutaneous (SC)	a. Immuno-suppressive therapy or immunodeficiency including HIV-infected persons with severe immunosuppres-sion. b. Anaphylactic allergy to neomycin. c. Pregnancy. d. Immune globulin preparation of blood/blood product received in preceding 3–11 months. e. Untreated, active TB.	Women should be asked if they are pregnant before receiving vaccine, and advised to avoid pregnancy for 28 days after immunization.

Table 22.3. Summary of Adolescent/Adult Immunization Recommendations *(Continued)*

Agent	Indications	Primary Schedule	Contrain-dications	Comments
Rubella Vaccine**	a. Persons (especially women) without written documentation of immunization on or after the first birthday or of seropositivity. b. Health care personnel who are at risk of exposure to patients with rubella and who may have contact with pregnant patients should have at least one dose.	One dose. Dose: 0.5 mL subcutaneous (SC)	Same as for measles and mumps vaccines.	Women should be asked if they are pregnant before receiving vaccine, and advised to avoid pregnancy for 28 days after immunization.
Hepatitis B Vaccine	a. Persons with occupational risk of exposure to blood or blood-contaminated body fluids. b. Clients and staff of institutions for the developmentally disabled. c. Hemodialysis patients. d. Recipients of clotting-factor concentrates. e. Household contacts and sex partners of those chronically infected with HBV. f. Family members of adoptees from countries where HBV infection is endemic, if adoptees are HBsAg+. g. Certain international travelers. h. Injecting drug users. i. Men who have sex with men. j. Heterosexual men and women with multiple sex partners or recent episode of a sexually transmitted disease. k. Inmates of long-term correctional facilities. l. All unvaccinated adolescents.	Three doses: second dose 1–2 months after the first, third dose 4–6 months after the first. No need to start series over if schedule interrupted. Can start series with one manufacturer's vaccine and finish with another. Dose (*Adult*): intramuscular (IM) Recombivax HB®: 10 μg/1.0 mL (green cap) Engerix-B®: 20 μg/1.0 mL (orange cap) Dose (*Adolescents 11–19 years*): intramuscular (IM) Recombivax HB®: 5 μg/0.5 mL (yellow cap) Engerix-B®: 10 μg/0.5 mL (light blue cap) Two doses (*Only for Adolescents 11–15 years*): intramuscular (IM), 4–6 months apart. Restricted to Recombivax HB®: 10 μg/1.0 mL (green cap) Booster: None presently recommended.	Anaphylactic allergy to yeast.	a. Persons with serologic markets of prior or continuing hepatitis B virus infection do not need immunization. b. For hemodialysis patients and other immunodeficient or immunosuppressed patients, vaccine dosage is doubled or special preparation is used. c. *Pregnant women should be sero-screened for HBsAg and, if positive, their infants should be given post-exposure prophylaxis beginning at birth.* d. Post-exposure prophylaxis: consult ACIP recommendations, or state or local immunization program.

Table 22.3. Summary of Adolescent/Adult Immunization Recommendations *(Continued)*

Agent	Indications	Primary Schedule	Contrain-dications	Comments
Poliovirus Vaccine: IPV—Inactivated Vaccine;	Routine vaccination of those ≥18 years of age residing in the U.S. is not necessary. Vaccination is recommended for the following high-risk adults:	Unimmunized adolescents/adults: IPV is recommended—two doses at 4–8 week intervals, third dose 6–12 months after second (can be as soon as 2 months) Dose: 0.5 mL subcutaneous (SC) or intramuscular (IM).	*IPV:* Anaphylactic reaction following previous dose or to streptomycin, polymyxin B, or neomycin.	In instances of potential exposure to wild poliovirus, adults who have had a primary series of OPV or IPV may be given 1 more dose of IPV.
OPV—Oral (live) Vaccine	a. Travelers to areas or countries where poliomyelitis is epidemic or endemic. b. Members of communities or specific population groups with disease caused by wild polioviruses. c. Laboratory workers who handle specimens that may contain polioviruses. d. Health care workers who have close contact with patients who may be excreting wild polioviruses. e. Unvaccinated adults whose children will be receiving OPV.	Partially immunized adolescents/adults: Complete primary series with IPV (IPV schedule shown above). OPV is no longer recommended for use in the United States.		Although no adverse effects have been documented, vaccination of pregnant women should be avoided. However, if immediate protection is required, pregnant women may be given IPV in accordance with the recommended schedule for adults.
Varicella Vaccine	a. Persons of any age without a reliable history of varicella disease or vaccination, or who are seronegative for varicella. b. Susceptible adolescents and adults living in households with children. c. All susceptible health care workers. d. Susceptible family contacts of immunocompromised persons. e. Susceptible persons in the following groups who are at high risk for exposure: • persons who live or work in environments in which transmission of varicella is	For persons <13 years of age, one dose. For persons 13 years of age and older, two doses separated by 4–8 weeks. If >8 weeks elapse following the first dose, the second dose can be administered without restarting the schedule. Dose: 0.5 mL subcutaneous (SC)	a. Anaphylactic allergy to gelatin or neomycin. b. Untreated, active TB. c. Immunosuppressive therapy or immunodeficiency (including HIV infection). d. Family history of congenital or hereditary immuno-deficiency in first-degree relatives, unless the immune competence of the recipient has been clinically substantiated or verified by a laboratory.	Women should be asked if they are pregnant before receiving varicella vaccine, and advised to avoid pregnancy for one month following each dose of vaccine.

Table 22.3. Summary of Adolescent/Adult Immunization Recommendations *(Continued)*

Agent	Indications	Primary Schedule	Contrain-dications	Comments
Varicella Vaccine *(continued)*	likely (e.g., teachers of young children, day care employees, residents and staff in institutional settings) or can occur (e.g., college students, inmates and staff of correctional institutions, military personnel) • nonpregnant women of childbearing age • international travelers		e. Immune globulin preparation or blood/blood product received in preceding 5 months. f. Pregnancy.	
Hepatitis A Vaccine	a. Persons traveling to or working in countries with high or intermediate endemicity of infection. b. Men who have sex with men. c. Injecting and non-injecting illegal drug users. d. Persons who work with HAV-infected primates or with HAV in a research laboratory setting. e. Persons with chronic liver disease. f. Persons with clotting factor disorders. g. Consider food handlers, where determined to be cost-effective by health authorities or employers.	HAVRIX®: Two doses, separated by 6–12 months. Adults (19 years of age and older)—Dose: 1.0 mL intramuscular (IM); Persons 2–18 years of age: Dose: 0.5 mL (IM). VAQTA®: Adults (19 years of age and older): Two doses, separated by 6 months. Dose: 1.0 mL intramuscular (IM); Persons 2–18 years of age: Two doses, separated by 6–18 months; Dose: 0.5 mL (IM)	A history of hypersensitivity to alum or the preservative 2 phenoxyethanol	The safety of hepatitis A vaccine during pregnancy has not been determined, though the theoretical risk to the developing fetus is expected to be low. The risk of vaccination should be weighed against the risk of hepatitis A in women who may be at high risk of exposure to HAV.

Adapted from the recommendations of the Advisory Committee on Immunization Practices (ACIP).
Foreign travel and less commonly used vaccines such as typhoid, rabies, and meningococcal are not included.
**These vaccines can be given in the combined form measles-mumps-rubella (MMR). Persons already immune to one or more components can still receive MMR.

feel their children are fully immunized and so do physicians. However, several studies have demonstrated that pediatricians typically overestimate coverage in their patients by 20 percent or more.

• Few physicians use reminder or recall systems to notify their patients of immunizations due (reminder) or overdue (recall).[21]

All of these factors support the need for automated mechanisms to keep track of children's immunization status and notify parents and providers about needed immunizations. The National Vaccine Advisory Committee (NVAC) has called for a nationwide network of population-based immunization registries, and the Healthy People 2010 objectives call for 95 percent of children 0–6 to be enrolled in population-based immunization registries by 2010.[22]

The Institute of Medicine has recently released a report "Calling the Shots" discussing the appropriate role of the federal government in supporting immunization programs.[23] It called for an increase in both federal and state support for immunization programs and greater stability in that funding as well as an increased level of support for global immunization programs.

Vaccine Safety and Efficacy

Modern vaccines are safe and effective; however, they are neither perfectly safe nor perfectly effective. Some individuals who receive vaccine will not be protected against disease and some will suffer adverse consequences. Adverse events may range from minor inconvenience such as discomfort at the injection site or fever to serious conditions such as paralysis associated with oral poliovirus vaccine (OPV). The goal is to achieve maximum safety and maximum efficacy.

The fact that vaccines are not perfectly effective means that some vaccinated individuals will develop disease on exposure. A common situation in the United States in recent years has been that approximately half of the people who develop a disease (e.g., measles) give a history of vaccination. This leads many persons to question the efficacy of the vaccine.

A simple formula exists to determine *vaccine efficacy* (VE):

$$VE = (ARU - ARV)/ARU \times 100$$

where *ARU* is the attack rate of disease in unvaccinated individuals and *ARV* is the attack rate in vaccinated individuals.[24] A nomogram has been constructed, as shown in Figure 22.2, to demonstrate the relationship between the proportion of cases with a history of vaccination (*PCV*) and the proportion of the population vaccinated (*PPV*) at varying levels of vaccine efficacy (*VE*). Simply put, if 90 percent of the population has been vaccinated with a 90 percent effective vaccine, one would expect approximately half the cases to give a history of vaccination, thus supporting a continued high efficacy for the vaccine.

Decisions about use of vaccines are based on relative balance of risks and benefits. This balance may change over time. For example, recipients of oral polio vaccine (OPV), and their close contacts, have a risk of developing paralysis associated with the vaccine of 1 in approximately every 2.4 million doses of vaccine distributed. This risk is quite small and was certainly outweighed by the much larger risk of paralysis due to wild polioviruses at the time they were circulating in the United States. However, since wild polioviruses no longer circulate in the United States and the risk of importation of wild viruses has been greatly reduced by the global effort to eradicate polio, the balance has shifted.

There has not been a case of paralysis in the United States due to indigenously acquired wild poliovirus since 1979 and the entire Western Hemisphere has been free of wild poliovirus circulation since 1991.[25] The ACIP recommended, in 1997, that children receive a sequential schedule with two doses of inactivated polio vaccine (IPV, which carries no risk of paralysis) followed by two doses of OPV. In 2000, the recommendation was made to switch to an all-IPV regimen.[26]

It is often difficult to ascertain whether an adverse event that occurs after immunization was caused by the vaccine or was merely temporally related and caused by some totally independent (and often unknown or unidentified) factor. This is particularly a problem during infancy, when a number of conditions may occur spontaneously. In a given instance it may be impossible to determine whether vaccine was responsible.[27] Particularly when dealing with rare events, it may be necessary to carry out large-scale case-control studies or review comprehensive records of large numbers of infants to ascertain whether those who received a vaccine had a higher incidence of the event than those who did not. The CDC operates a large linked database involving several large health maintenance organizations. This Vaccine Safety Datalink project includes more than six million persons (approximately 2 percent of the U.S. population) and has proved to be an invaluable resource in attempting to determine causality.[28]

One result of the extraordinary success of immunization efforts has been the fact that today's young parents (and young physicians) have never seen

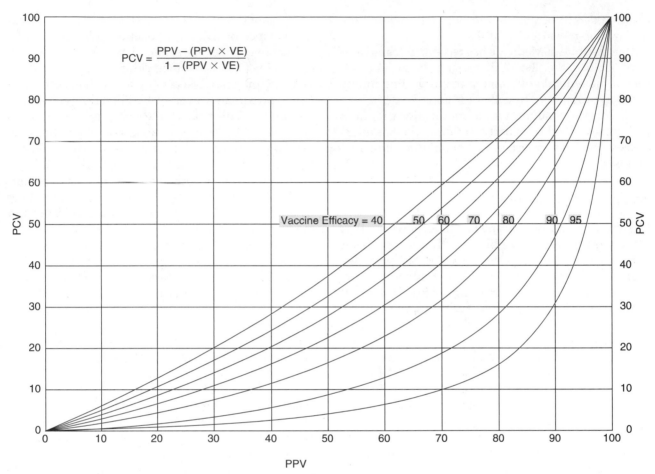

$$PCV = \frac{PPV - (PPV \times VE)}{1 - (PPV \times VE)}$$

Figure 22.2. Percentage of Cases Vaccinated (PCV) by Percentage of Population Vaccinated (PPV), for 7 Values of Vaccine Efficacy (VE).

Source: Orenstein WA, Bernier RH, Dondero TJ, et al. Field evaluation of vaccine efficacy. *Bull WHO.* 1985; 63:1055–1068.

many of the diseases against which they are being urged to have their children vaccinated. Consequently, they may not be as motivated as were parents and physicians in the past. In the absence of disease, the infrequent known (or alleged) adverse events associated with vaccines assume greater prominence. This imbalance has led some parents (and even some physicians) to question whether use of some (or all) vaccines is still warranted. The rise of the Internet has made it easier for opinions about vaccines to be disseminated, whether based in science or fact. This increases the obligation on public health authorities to explain fully the risks and benefits of vaccines. The occasional occurrence of previously unrecognized adverse events actually caused by vaccine (as with intestinal intussusception and rotavirus vaccine) adds to the complexity of the explanation.[29]

SEXUALLY TRANSMITTED DISEASES (STDS)

All sexually transmitted diseases (STDs), including human immunodeficiency virus (HIV) infection, are historically, biologically, behaviorally, economically, and programmatically related.[30] Intimate sexual contact is the common (but not exclusive) mode of transmission of the causative organisms. Several dozen bacterial, viral, parasitic, and fungal infections are now recognized as being commonly (or predominantly) transmitted by sexual contact. In general, they share the characteristic that women suffer disproportionately from their effects. This is a result of a variety of factors, including the fact that women are generally less able to prevent exposure to STDs than men because of the relative lack of safe, effective, female-controlled preventive measures. Women also are frequently unable to negotiate the conditions under which sexual intercourse occurs. In addition, complications of STDs in women are likely to be more severe: pelvic inflammatory disease (PID), infertility, ectopic pregnancy (the leading cause of maternal mortality in the United States), and cancer.[31]

Efforts to control STDs have been guided by both the magnitude of the problem and the availability of diagnostic and therapeutic measures. The United States began the twentieth century focusing on one dominant STD—syphilis—which could be diagnosed with newly developed serologic techniques and treated with a suppressive (but not, at the time, curative) therapy. Subsequent improvements in the ability to detect and treat syphilis led to a striking decline in its incidence. In 1999, CDC, in collaboration with other partners, launched a National Plan to Eliminate Syphilis from the United States.[32] Elimination is defined as the absence of sustained transmission (i.e., no transmission more than 90 days after the report of an imported index case). National targets for 2005 include reducing primary and secondary (P & S) syphilis incidence to fewer than 1,000 cases (0.4 cases per 100,000 population) and increase the number of syphilis-free counties to 90 percent. In 1999, there were 6,675 cases of P & S syphilis reported (2.5 cases per 100,000) and 79.4 percent of counties reported no cases of P & S syphilis.[33] The South had the highest rates in the country. The incidence rate in blacks (15.2 per 100,000) was 30 times the reported rate in whites (0.5).

Growing awareness of the serious individual and social implications of gonorrhea, accompanied by improvements in diagnostic techniques, led the United States to embark on a major program to control gonorrhea in the 1970s. Reported gonorrhea incidence reached an all-time high in 1975 and progressively declined, reaching record low levels in 1997 (325, 861 cases reported, 121.8 cases per 100,000 population). There was a 9 percent increase in cases reported in 1998, at least part of which may have been a result of changes in gonorrhea screening and surveillance practices.[34]

In the early 1980s, the spectrum of STDs expanded with recognition of the acute syndromes (and long-term consequences) caused by a number of other conditions, including *Chlamydia trachomatis, Trichomonas vaginalis*, herpes simplex virus, and human papillomavirus. These were all overshadowed by the discovery of a new STD, acquired immunodeficiency syndrome (AIDS), in 1981.[35]

The United States began the twenty-first century focusing on a new dominant STD, HIV/AIDS, for which there was an effective serologic diagnostic technique and suppressive but not curative therapy. It is hoped that advances in development of preventive and therapeutic measures will enable major progress to be made against this STD in the current century as occurred with syphilis in the twentieth century.[36]

Following the first report of AIDS cases in June 1981, there was a rapid increase in the number of cases and deaths reported during the 1980s followed by substantial declines in new cases and deaths in the late 1990s.[37] The decline in new cases represents the effect of HIV prevention efforts and increases in societal awareness of, and response to, the AIDS epidemic. The decline in numbers of deaths reflects both the decline in incidence as well as the impact of antiretroviral therapies. As of December 31, 2000, 774,467 persons had been reported with AIDS in the United States, at least 57 percent of whom had died. Approximately one-half of the cases in the United States have occurred in men who have sex with other men, and one-quarter have been associated with injection drug use. This is to be contrasted with the situation in the developing world, where the vast majority of cases are associated with heterosexual contact. Nearly all transmission of HIV through transfusion of blood or blood products occurred before screening of the blood supply for HIV antibody was initiated in 1985.

Model of STD Transmission

Anderson and May have developed a simple and very useful model of transmission of STDs based on earlier work by themselves and by Yorke and Hethcote.[38] It is based on the assumption that a disease can sustain itself only when the reproduction rate is greater than one, that is, when each infected person on average transmits the disease to at least one other person. If the reproduction rate is less than one, transmission of the disease cannot be sustained and it will die out. The formula for the reproduction rate is

$$R = B \times c \times D$$

where R is the reproduction rate (the number of new infections produced, on average, by an infected individual); B is a measure of transmissibility (the average probability that an infected individual will infect a susceptible partner given exposure); c represents the average number of different partners the infected individual has per unit time; and D represents the duration of infectiousness of the disease. These three determinants of the reproductive rate are influenced by the interplay of biological and behavioral variables for each STD.

The values for each parameter may vary depending on the STD and the type of sexual contact; estimates have been made for several of them. For example, for gonorrhea the overall estimate for B is 50 percent (50–90 percent for male-to-female transmission and 20–50 percent for female-to-male transmission). For syphilis, B is estimated at 20–30 percent and for HIV at 1–10 percent.[39] Additionally, HIV transmissibility is apparently higher for penile-anal intercourse than for penile-vaginal intercourse.

Because not all members of a given population have the same number of sex partners, a refinement can be made in the formula for variable c, using the median number of sex partners and the variance in the number of sex partners instead of a simple average. It appears that a core population of highly sexually active persons (with many different partners) plays a major role in the continued transmission of STDs.

The duration of the infectious period, D, is also quite different for the different STDs, ranging from a few days for gonorrhea (in men), to a lifetime for HIV

infection. There are other biological and behavioral factors affecting D, such as health care-seeking behavior, and compliance with treatment, among others.

Elements of STD Control Programs

Control strategies may aim to modify any of the factors in the equation of transmissibility. In general, control programs include public information and education, professional education and training, screening, prompt diagnosis and therapy, counseling, partner notification, and surveillance. No approach by itself is likely to prevent the spread of STDs, but each contributes to the overall effort.

The aim of public information and education, counseling, and partner notification is to reduce factors B, c, and D by encouraging changes in sexual and health care-related behaviors. Given the differential importance to overall STD transmission of those who have few and those who have many sex partners, targeted behavior change among core group members may have much greater impact on transmission than would behavior changes in noncore group members.

Through partner notification, the sex (and needle-sharing) partners of persons with STDs are contacted, notified of their risk of exposure (without disclosing the identity of the original patient), educated about risky practices and prevention methods, and encouraged to come in for examination and possible treatment. This activity can affect all three factors in the equation: persons can reduce transmissibility *(B)*, for example, by eliminating receptive anal intercourse or insisting on the use of condoms in all sexual activity; they can reduce the number of their sexual partners *(c)*; or they can be diagnosed and treated early in the progression of their own infection *(D)*.

Surveillance is essential to assess the magnitude of the problem, identify groups at particular risk, monitor trends, and evaluate the impact of control programs. It is (or should be) a major determinant of program direction.

With particular regard to HIV, it must be recognized that the HIV epidemic is not a monolithic event. Rather, it is a number of epidemics with varying primary means of transmission and different rates of spread in different areas and in different segments of society.[40] These may call for different approaches. Freedom from discrimination and guaranteed confidentiality are essential. Current HIV prevention efforts focus on preventing initiation of the behaviors and conditions that put individuals at risk of acquiring or spreading the virus (e.g., delaying onset of sexual activity, not starting to use drugs) and modifying behaviors to reduce the likelihood of transmission if exposure occurs (e.g., condom use, ensurance of clean needles and syringes). Other specific approaches include screening donated blood, treating HIV-infected pregnant women to prevent mother-to-child transmission, treating other STDs, treating tuberculosis, providing contraceptive services, and using highly active antiretroviral drugs in HIV-infected individuals to maintain their health and to reduce the levels of circulating virus (thereby reducing the likelihood of transmission). Another important component is the education of health care workers in the use of universal precautions to reduce the risk of nosocomial transmission.

TUBERCULOSIS (TB)

Tuberculosis (TB) is caused by *Mycobacterium tuberculosis*, a bacterium primarily transmitted through inhalation of airborne bacilli or droplet nuclei. Initial infection is usually not noticed but is accompanied by an immune response manifested by development of a positive reaction to purified protein derivative (PPD) applied intradermally.

Only 5–10 percent of immunocompetent persons infected with TB ultimately go on to develop TB disease at any time in their lives. However, for those with impaired immune systems the risk of developing active TB is much higher (on the order of 7–10 percent per year for those with HIV infection).[41] Clinical manifestations of TB commonly involve fever, weight loss, and cough, reflecting pulmonary infection. Persons with pulmonary TB may develop cavitary lesions visible on a chest x-ray and may excrete large numbers of organisms when they cough or sneeze.

For those excreting large numbers of bacilli (who are presumably most infectious), it may be possible to visualize characteristic acid-fast bacilli (AFB) on direct smear of the sputum. For others, however, diagnosis of TB is made difficult by the fact that the causative organisms are slow growing. Even with newer techniques, it may take more than one week for a culture to become positive and then another week or more to determine antibiotic susceptibility. Using older techniques, this period could extend to two or three months. During this time the patient may remain infectious if not started on appropriate therapy.

TB Prevention and Control

The approach to TB prevention and control in the United States has two major components. One is the identification and treatment of persons with TB disease. This both cures their infection and prevents transmission to others. The other is the identification and treatment of those with TB infection to prevent their subsequent development of TB disease.

Management of TB disease (or latent infection) is made difficult by the fact that treatment (either for infection or disease) involves six months or more of medication. Consequently, patient adherence to therapy is a major problem, and inconsistent adherence to therapy may result in the emergence of organisms resistant to the drugs being administered. Fortunately, directly observed therapy (DOT), in which a health worker personally gives each dose of medication to the patient and observes that it is taken, has been shown to be a highly effective way of ensuring completion of therapy.[42]

TB in the United States

At the beginning of the twentieth century, tuberculosis (TB) was the leading cause of death in the United States. Reported mortality from TB declined steadily during the first half of the century, in the absence of specific therapy, as a result of improvements in nutrition and housing and the isolation of infected individuals in sanatoriums. TB first became reportable on a nationwide basis in 1952, and from that time until 1985, there was a steady decline in reported incidence, averaging 4–5 percent per year (Figure 22.3). The overall decline from 1953 to 1985 was 74 percent. In 1985 there were 22,201 cases reported (9.3 cases per 100,000 population). The decline was so impressive

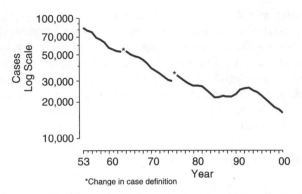

Figure 22.3. Reported Tuberculosis Cases in the United States, 1953–2000

*Reflects change in case definition.

that it was believed that TB could be eliminated from the United States and in 1989, CDC and the Advisory Council for the Elimination of Tuberculosis (ACET) issued "A Strategic Plan for the Elimination of Tuberculosis in the United States."[43] The plan established a national goal of TB elimination by 2010, defined as a case rate of less than 1 per 1,000,000 population. The plan described three components: (1) more effective use of existing prevention and control methods; (2) development and evaluation of new prevention, diagnostic, and treatment technologies; and (3) rapid transfer of newly developed technologies into clinical and public health practice.

The plan was widely endorsed and increased resources were made available to TB control programs, although not in the amounts necessary to fully implement the elimination program. In the late 1980s the incidence of TB began to rise, reaching a peak in 1992, when 26,673 cases were reported. There was a 20 percent increase in reported numbers of cases between 1985 and 1992. Assuming that the reported incidence should have continued to decline at the rate it did from 1980 to 1985, it is estimated that more than 63,000 excess cases of TB occurred during the period 1986–1992.

The increase during the period 1986–1992 was ascribed to at least four factors: (1) deterioration of the public health infrastructure; (2) immigration of persons from countries with high prevalence of TB; (3) the HIV epidemic; and (4) outbreaks of TB (particularly multidrug-resistant TB [MDR-TB]) in con-

gregative settings such as hospitals, correctional facilities, and shelters for the homeless, among others.[44]

In response to the outbreaks of MDR-TB, a national task force was formed and developed the *National Action Plan to Combat Multidrug-Resistant Tuberculosis,* first released in April 1992.[45] Commitment of significant federal, state, and local resources to combat TB and implement the MDR-TB plan resulted in a rapid turn-around in incidence and the number of reported TB cases in the United States has decreased each year since 1992, reaching a record low of 17,531 in 1999, representing a 34 percent decline since 1992.[46] The reduction is attributed to more effective implementation of "standard" TB control strategies.[47] However, TB in immigrants remains an important issue, as does TB and HIV. In 1998, 42 percent of all cases occurred in persons born in another country; a high proportion occurred within five years of arrival, indicating they probably arrived in this country infected with TB. In addition, CDC estimates that in 1998, 21 percent of cases of TB in persons aged 25–44 years occurred in HIV-infected individuals.[48]

Given the resurgence of TB in the late 1980s and the return to control in the 1990s, the ACET revisited the prospects for TB elimination and reaffirmed its call for the elimination of TB in the United States.[49] The Institute of Medicine examined issues relating to TB control in the United States and issued a report *Ending Neglect,*[50] which endorsed the prospects for eliminating TB in the United States if sustained commitment to resources could be provided and if the United States increased its involvement in global TB control (to reduce the threat of imported TB).

FOODBORNE AND WATERBORNE DISEASES

A variety of parasitic, bacterial, and viral diseases can be transmitted through food and water. Disease results either from infection or from intoxication. Some diseases, such as giardiasis and typhoid fever, result from ingestion of small numbers of microorganisms that subsequently multiply and cause disease, either local or invasive. Others, such as cholera and diarrhea caused by enterotoxigenic *Escherichia coli,* result from ingestion of living bacteria that multiply and elaborate toxins, which act on intestinal mucosa to cause diarrhea. Some conditions such as botulism or *Clostridium perfringens* food poisoning result from ingestion of toxins formed by organisms multiplying in the food before it is eaten. Finally, some fish and shellfish may contain toxins that cause neuromuscular symptoms. Food and water can also carry natural or synthetic toxins (e.g., metals, plant toxins, and insecticides).

These illnesses may vary greatly in symptoms. Some are characterized by mild nausea, vomiting, and diarrhea (e.g., most *Salmonella* infections). Others may be associated with life-threatening profuse diarrhea (cholera), hemorrhagic diarrhea with hemolytic-uremic syndrome (*E. coli* 0157:H7), sepsis (typhoid), infectious hepatitis (hepatitis A), miscarriage (*Listeria monocytogenes*), or cranial nerve and respiratory paralysis (botulism).

Waterborne Diseases

Waterborne illness is now relatively uncommon in the United States as a result of the protection of water supplies, prevention of cross-connections between water and sewage systems, and chlorination. If municipal water supplies become contaminated, large numbers of persons may become ill. During a 1965 outbreak of waterborne salmonellosis in Riverside, California, an estimated 16,000 persons became ill.[51] More than 400,000 persons became ill with waterborne cryptosporidiosis in Milwaukee in 1993.[52]

During 1997–1998, CDC received reports on 17 outbreaks (from 13 states) associated with drinking water, causing more than two thousand persons to become ill. The causative agent was identified for 12 (70 percent) of the outbreaks—4 were caused by *Giardia*, 3 by *E. coli* 0157:H7, 2 by *Cryptosporidium*, 1 by *Shigella sonnei*, and 2 by copper poisoning. Additionally, there were 32 outbreaks (from 18 states) attributed to recreational water exposure, also affecting more than two thousand persons. Eighteen of these were outbreaks of gastroenteritis (nine caused by parasites, four by bacteria, two by viruses, and three unknown). Eight outbreaks were of dermatitis (seven caused by *Pseudomonas aeruginosa*), four represented single (fatal) cases of meningoencephalitis caused by *Naegleria fowleri*, and there were single outbreaks of leptospirosis and Pontiac fever.[53]

Foodborne Diseases

Prevention of foodborne illness involves preventing initial contamination; cooking foods properly to destroy organisms that are present; preventing cross-contamination or recontamination (as can occur when cooked foods are sliced with a knife or on a cutting board contaminated by raw food or are placed back in containers from which they came before cooking); preventing incubation of microorganisms by keeping cold foods cold and hot foods hot; and ensuring other appropriate food-handling practices.

Foodborne illness remains common and has been estimated to cause 6.5 million cases of human illness and 9,000 deaths annually in the United States.[54] However, only a small proportion of the outbreaks estimated to occur are actually reported. During 1993–1997, a total of 2,751 outbreaks of foodborne disease were reported to the CDC, causing 86,058 persons to become ill.[55] The etiology was known for only 32 percent of the reported outbreaks; these accounted for 59 percent of reported illnesses. Of the outbreaks with known etiology, 75 percent were caused by bacterial pathogens, 17 percent by chemical agents, 6 percent by viruses, and 2 percent by parasites.

During the period 1993–1997, several different types of outbreaks were reported, including multistate outbreaks caused by ground beef contaminated with *E. coli* 0157:H7; fresh produce contaminated with *Salmonella* or *E. coli* 0157:H7; commercially distributed ice cream contaminated with *Salmonella*; alfalfa sprouts contaminated with *Salmonella*; and unpasteurized apple juice and orange juice contaminated with *E. coli* 0157:H7 and *Salmonella*, respectively. The factors most commonly reported as contributing to the outbreaks included improper holding temperatures of foods and inadequate cooking of food. Several outbreaks were associated with imported food items.

EMERGING/REEMERGING DISEASES AND ANTIBIOTIC RESISTANCE

Although we are making progress against many infectious diseases, we continue to recognize new diseases or discover infectious causes for already known conditions. Table 22.4 shows the year of recognition of selected new diseases or etiologic agents over the past 30 years. In 1973 rotaviruses were recognized as major causes of childhood diarrhea. Ebola virus was first recognized in the late 1970s, as were *Legionella pneumophila* (causative agent of Legionnaire's disease and Pontiac fever) and toxin-producing *Staphylococcus aureus* (causative agent of toxic shock syndrome). *E. coli* 0157:H7 (cause of hemorrhagic colitis and hemolytic-uremic syndrome) was first recognized in 1982 and HIV was first identified in 1983. It has only been in the past 20 years that we have learned that *Helicobacter pylori* is the primary cause of duodenal ulcer disease.[56]

Diseases known to occur in one part of the world may be introduced to other parts of the world, with devastating consequences, as occurred during the European colonization of the Americas, when significant proportions of the indigenous population were killed by smallpox and measles. Modern means of transportation mean that virtually any infectious disease is only an airplane ride away. Other diseases may be introduced from other countries by means which are yet unknown, e.g., West Nile virus.[57]

In addition to the recognition of new diseases, diseases once under control have an ability to reemerge. This happened in the United States with TB in the late 1980s as a result of lack of continued application of effective control measures. Changing ecological circumstances can also favor increases in new or old infectious diseases. Some of these factors include population growth, crowding, migration, urbanization, changes in behavior, changes in ecology, and modern travel and trade.

Development of resistance to antibiotics has led to the reemergence of some previously controlled conditions. Major factors leading to resistance are the indiscriminate, inappropriate, inadequate, incomplete, and inconsistent use of antibiotics. Each of these factors can result in selection of strains of microorganisms that are resistant to the drugs being used. *Streptococcus pneumoniae*, the causative agent of pneumococcal pneumonia and pneumococcal meningitis, was initially exquisitely sensitive to penicillin. However, a study of U.S. medical centers in 1997–1998 found that 29.5 percent of strains were at least partially resistant to penicillin and 12.1 percent were fully resistant.[58]

Prevention of the emergence of additional strains of antimicrobial-resistant microorganisms will require concerted action to ensure that antibiotics are used appropriately.

BIOTERRORISM

Biological agents have long been used in warfare, and their use has presumably come to an end as a result of international accords. As concerns about biological warfare have decreased, concerns about bioterrorism have come to the fore. The prospect exists that individuals or groups could use biological agents as political weapons and there have been isolated incidents in which this has been documented.[59] CDC convened a workgroup that developed a strategic plan for preparedness and response to biological and chemical terrorism.[60] The plan outlines a series of steps to prepare public health agencies for biological attacks, focusing on surveillance, education, and communication. De-

Table 22.4. Examples of New Disease/Organism Recognition

Year	Condition
1973	Rotavirus
1975	Parvovirus
1976	*Cryptosporidium parvum*
1977	Ebola virus
1977	*Legionella pneumophila*
1977	Hantaan virus
1980	HTLV-1
1981	Toxin-producing *S. aureus*
1982	*E. coli* 0157:H7
1982	*Borrelia burgdorferi*
1983	HIV
1983	*Helicobacter pylori*
1988	HHV-6
1989	Hepatitis C
1992	Bartonella henselae
1993	Sin nombre virus
1995	HHV-8

velopment of new diagnostic tests and stockpiling appropriate vaccines and drugs were also recommended. The agents/diseases thought most likely to be used as bioterrorism weapons included smallpox, anthrax, plague, botulism, tularemia, and viral hemorrhagic fevers (e.g., Ebola, Lassa). The purposeful spread of anthrax through the mail on the east coast of the United States in the Fall of 2001 verified the necessity for improving capacities at all levels to identify and respond to biologic agents dispersed as weapons of terror. (See chapters 3, 13, and 29)

CONCLUSION

Voltaire's phrase "the best is the enemy of the good"[61] applies to HIV prevention and to other infectious disease prevention and control measures. In some situations, the insistence on only the "best" solution to a given health problem may interfere with the incremental, partially effective steps that are collectively necessary in mounting effective (but not perfect) prevention programs. In fact, if the imperfect approach is more acceptable to the target population than the perfect one, it may ultimately have a greater effect on the occurrence of disease.

The HIV epidemic and other major infectious disease health problems do not happen in the same way or at the same rate in all groups. Nor are they uniformly susceptible to any single intervention. Controlling the HIV epidemic and solving other problems will require different, mutually reinforcing techniques to reach the myriad groups in this pluralistic society. Until more effective (or even "perfect") approaches are available, partially effective approaches should be more fully implemented. The world is not a perfect place, and the quest for solutions must reflect that fact.[62]

Infectious diseases remain significant causes of morbidity and mortality in the United States and are even greater problems in developing countries. The current favorable situation in the United States is a reflection of the active control measures that have been applied. However, it must be remembered that infectious diseases are merely being kept at bay. Unless they are eradicated, relaxation of control efforts can and will lead to a resurgence of disease. In addition, new infectious diseases are being recognized that pose new threats to health and necessitate maintenance of surveillance and response capability.[63]

References

1. World Health Organization. Health systems: Improving performance. *World Health Report 2000*. Geneva, Switzerland: WHO; 2000.
2. Chin J, ed. *Control of Communicable Diseases Manual*. 17th ed. Washington, DC: American Public Health Association; 2000.
3. Gustafson TL, Lavely GB, Brawner ER Jr, et al. An outbreak of airborne nosocomial varicella. *Pediatrics* 1982;70:550-556.
4. Bloch A, Orenstein WA, Ewing WM, et al. Measles outbreak in a pediatric practice: Airborne transmission in an office setting. *Pediatrics* 1985;75:676-683.
5. Orenstein WA, Bernier RH. Surveillance: Information for action. *Pediatr Clin North Am*. 1990;37:709-734.
6. Strebel PM, Sutter RW, Cochi SL, et al. Epidemiology of poliomyelitis in the United States one decade after the last reported case of indigenous wild virus-associated disease. *Clin Infect Dis*. 1992;14:568-579.
7. Centers for Disease Control and Prevention. General recommendations on immunization: Recommendations of the Advisory Committee on Immunization Practices (ACIP). *MMWR*. 1994;43(RR-1):1-38.
8. Centers for Disease Control and Prevention. Provisional cases of selected notifiable diseases, week ending December 23, 2000. *MMWR*. 2001;49:1164, 1167, 1173.
9. Centers for Disease Control and Prevention. Progress toward eliminating *Haemophilus influenzae* type b disease among infants and children—United States, 1987-1997. *MMWR*. 1998;47:993-998.
10. Centers for Disease Control and Prevention. National, state, and urban vaccination coverage levels among children aged 19-35 months—United States, 1999. *MMWR*. 2000;49:585-589.
11. Centers for Disease Control and Prevention. Surveillance for vaccination coverage among children and adults—United States. *MMWR*. 2000;49(SS09):1-65.

12. Singleton JA, Greby SM, Wooten KG, et al. Influenza, pneumococcal, and tetanus toxoid vaccination of adults—United States, 1993-1997. *MMWR*. 2000;49(SS09):39-62.

13. American Academy of Pediatrics. *Report of the Committee on Infectious Diseases*. 25th ed. Elk Grove Village, Ill: American Academy of Pediatrics; 2000.

14. Centers for Disease Control and Prevention. Combination Vaccines for Childhood Immunization: Recommendations of the Advisory Committee on Immunization Practices (ACIP), the American Academy of Pediatrics (AAP), and the American Academy of Family Physicians (AAFP). *MMWR*. 1999;48(RR05):1-15.

15. Centers for Disease Control and Prevention. Immunization of adolescents: Recommendations of the Advisory Committee on Immunization Practices, the American Academy of Pediatrics, the American Academy of Family Physicians, and the American Medical Association. *MMWR*. 1996;45(RR13):1-16.

16. Centers for Disease Control and Prevention. Update on adult immunization: Recommendations of the Immunization Practices Advisory Committee (ACIP). *MMWR*. 1991;40(RR12):1-52.

17. Centers for Disease Control and Prevention. Immunization of health-care workers: Recommendations of the Advisory Committee on Immunization Practices (ACIP) and the Hospital Infection Control Practices Advisory Committee (HIC-PAC). *MMWR*. 1997;46(RR18):1-42.

18. Orenstein WA, Hinman AR, Rodewald LE. Public Health Considerations—United States. In: Plotkin SA, Orenstein WA, eds. *Vaccines*. 3d ed. (pp. 1006-1032). Philadelphia, Penn: WB Saunders.

19. Centers for Disease Control and Prevention. Vaccines for Children program, 1994. *MMWR*. 1994;43:705.

20. Orenstein WA, Hinman AR. The immunization system in the United States—the role of school immunization laws. *Vaccine*. 1999;17:S19-S24.

21. National Vaccine Advisory Committee. Development of community and state-based immunization registries, January 12, 1999. Available at: http://www.cdc.gov/nip/registry/nvac.htm.

22. US Department of Health and Human Services. *Healthy People 2010*, Objective 14-26. Washington, DC; US Dept of Health and Human Services; 2000.

23. Institute of Medicine. *Calling the Shots: Immunization Finance Policies and Practices*. Washington, DC; National Academy Press; 2000.

24. Orenstein WA, Bernier RH, Dondero TJ, et al. Field evaluation of vaccine efficacy. *Bull WHO*. 1985;63:1055-1068.

25. Robbins FC, de Quadros CA. Certification of the eradication of indigenous transmission of wild poliovirus in the Americas. *J Infect Dis*. 1997;175(suppl 1):S281-S285.

26. Centers for Disease Control and Prevention. Poliomyelitis prevention in the United States: Updated recommendations of the Advisory Committee on Immunization Practices (ACIP). *MMWR*. 2000;49(RR05):1-22.

27. Centers for Disease Control and Prevention. Update: Vaccine side effects, adverse reactions, contraindications, and precautions. Recommendations of the Advisory Committee on Immunization Practices (ACIP). *MMWR*. 1996;45(RR12):1-35.

28. Chen RT, DeStefano F, Davis RL, et al. The Vaccine Safety Datalink: Immunization research in health maintenance organizations in the USA. *Bull WHO*. 2000;78:186-194.

29. Centers for Disease Control and Prevention. Intussusception among recipients of rotavirus vaccine—United States, 1998-1999. *MMWR*. 1999;48:577-581.

30. Cates W Jr, Hinman AR. Sexually transmitted diseases in the 1990s. *N Engl J Med*. 1991;325:1368-1370.

31. Hinman AR, Wasserheit HN, Kamb MI. Potential impact of STD prevention programmes. In: Rashad H, Gray R, Boerna T, eds. *Evaluation of the Impact of Health Interventions*. Liège, Belgium: International Union for the Scientific Study of Population; 1995.

32. Centers for Disease Control and Prevention. *The National Plan to Eliminate Syphilis from the United States*. Atlanta, Ga: US Dept of Health and Human Services, CDC, National Center for HIV, STD, and TB Prevention; 1999:1-84.

33. Centers for Disease Control and Prevention. Primary and secondary syphilis—United States, 1999. *MMWR*. 2001;50:113-117.

34. Centers for Disease Control and Prevention. Gonorrhea—United States, 1998. *MMWR*. 2000;49:538-542.

35. Centers for Disease Control and Prevention. Pneumocystis pneumonia—Los Angeles. *MMWR*. 1981;30:250-252.

36. Sepkowitz KA. AIDS—the first 20 years. *N Engl J Med*. 2001;344:1764-1772.

37. Centers for Disease Control and Prevention. HIV and AIDS—United States, 1981-2000. *MMWR*. 2001;20:430-434.

38. Anderson RM. The transmission dynamics of sexually transmitted diseases: The behavioral component. In: Wasserheit JN, Aral SO, Holmes KK, Hitchcock PJ, eds. *Research Issues in Human Behavior and Sexually Transmitted Diseases in the AIDS Era.* Washington, DC: American Society of Microbiology; 1992:61-80.

39. Brunham RC, Ronal AR. Epidemiology of sexually transmitted diseases in developing countries. In: Wasserheit JN, Aral SO, Holmes KK, Hitchcock PJ, eds. *Research Issues in Human Behavior and Sexually Transmitted Diseases in the AIDS Era.* Washington, DC: American Society of Microbiology; 1991:38-60.

40. Hinman AR. Strategies to prevent HIV infection in the United States. *Am J Public Health.* 1991;81:1557-1559.

41. Selwyn PA, Hartel D, Lewis VA, et al. A prospective study of the risk of tuberculosis among intravenous drug users with human immunodeficiency virus infection. *N Engl J Med.* 1989;320:545-550.

42. American Thoracic Society. Intermittent chemotherapy for adults with tuberculosis. *Am Rev Respir Dis.* 1974;110:374-375.

43. Centers for Disease Control and Prevention. A strategic plan for the elimination of tuberculosis in the United States. *MMWR.* 1989;38(S-3):1-25.

44. Cantwell MF, Snider DE, Cauthen GM, Onorato IM. Epidemiology of tuberculosis in the United States, 1985 through 1992. *JAMA.* 1994;272:535-539.

45. Centers for Disease Control and Prevention. National action plan to combat multidrug-resistant tuberculosis. *MMWR.* 1992;41(RR-11):1-48.

46. Centers for Disease Control and Prevention. Reported tuberculosis in the United States, 1999. Available at: http://www.cdc.gov/nchstp/tb/surv/surv99/surv99.htm.

47. McKenna MT, McCray E, Jones JL, et al. The fall after the rise: Tuberculosis in the United States, 1992 through 1994. *Am J Public Health.* 1998;88:1059-1063.

48. Centers for Disease Control and Prevention. Progress toward the elimination of tuberculosis—United States, 1998. *MMWR.* 1999;48:732-736.

49. Advisory Council for the Elimination of Tuberculosis (ACET). Tuberculosis elimination revisited: Obstacles, opportunities, and a renewed commitment. *MMWR.* 1999;48(RR09):1-13.

50. Institute of Medicine. *Ending Neglect: The Elimination of Tuberculosis in the United States.* Washington, DC; National Academy Press; 2000.

51. Collaborative Report: A waterborne epidemic of salmonellosis in Riverside, California, 1965. *Am J Epidemiol.* 1971;93:33.

52. MacKenzie W, Hoxie N, Proctor M, et al. A massive outbreak in Milwaukee of *Cryptosporidium* infection transmitted through the public water supply. *N Engl J Med.* 1994;331:161-167.

53. Centers for Disease Control and Prevention. Surveillance for waterborne-disease outbreaks— United States, 1997-1998. *MMWR.* 2000;49(SS-4):1-36.

54. Bennett JV, Holmberg SD, Rogers MF, Solomon SL. Infectious and parasitic diseases. In: Amler RW, Dull HB, eds. Closing the gap: the burden of unnecessary illness. *Am J Prev Med.* 1987;3(suppl):102-114.

55. Olsen SJ, MacKinnon LC, Goulding JS, et al. Surveillance for foodborne-disease outbreaks—United States, 1993-1997. *MMWR.* 2000;49(SS-1):1-63.

56. Committee on International Science, Engineering, and Technology. Infectious Disease—A global health threat. Washington, DC: US Government Printing Office; 1995.

57. Nash D, Mostashari F, Fine A, et al. The outbreak of West Nile virus infection in the New York City area in 1999. *N Engl J Med.* 2001;344:1807-1814.

58. Doem GV, Brueggemann AB, Huynh H, et al. Antimicrobial resistance with *Streptococcus pneumoniae* in the United States, 1997-1998. *Emerg Infect Dis.* 1999;5:757-765.

59. Torok TJ, Tauxe RV, Wise RP, et al. Large community outbreak of salmonellosis caused by intentional contamination of restaurant salad bars. *JAMA.* 1997;278:389-395.

60. Centers for Disease Control and Prevention. Biological and chemical terrorism: Strategic plan for preparedness and response. Recommendations of the CDC Strategic Planning Workgroup. *MMWR.* 2000;49(RR-4):1-5.

61. Kaplan J, ed. *Bartlett's Familiar Quotations.* 16th ed. Boston: Little Brown & Co; 1992:306.

62. Cates W Jr, Hinman AR. AIDS and absolutism: The demand for perfection in prevention. *N Engl J Med.* 1992;327:492-494.

63. Lederberg J, Shope RE, Oaks SC Jr, eds. *Emerging Infections: Microbial Threats to Health in the United States.* Washington, DC: National Academy Press; 1992.

CHAPTER
23

Environmental Health in Public Health

Darryl B. Barnett, Dr. P.H.
Joe E. Beck
Worley Johnson, Jr.
R. Steven Konkel, Ph.D.

A most intriguing question, and one that leads to many debates both inside and outside of the environmental health field, is a definition of *environmental health.* The answer given is often tempered by one's political slant (i.e., liberal, moderate, or conservative) and by one's professional training (e.g., public health sanitation, chemistry, nursing, ecology, planning, public administration, etc.). Although agreement is needed to effectively address the challenges in the field, disagreement often centers on what constitutes environmental health and even on the name or nickname that should be applied to individuals whose primary focus is on one or many aspects of environmental health. Unfortunately, this disagreement has caused confusion and splintering in the field itself. It is important to accurately define and understand what comprises environmental health, and to answer the question, "Is environmental health a profession or

a discipline, or is it merely a loosely joined group of activities with an eclectic army of individuals working in it?" The reader should be able to understand environmental health's role in the public health arena; more important, the reader should not be confused with the many evolving terms and "satellite" professions that are part of the greater field of environmental health.

This chapter will define environmental health and introduce or clarify how environmental health fits into public health. It will discuss, historically, what areas environmental health programs typically have addressed, new areas that are additions to the greater arena, and how this fits within the traditional public health field. Finally, it will discuss who the professionals are that perform these environmental health duties, where and how they are trained, and future challenges for environmental health in the public and private sectors.

THE DEFINITION DEBATE

It is often easier to begin defining a subject by what it is not rather than what it is. Over the past 35 years it has become trendy to add the term *environmental* or *environment* to almost every conceivable job. Accompanying this trend has been the elevation of the terms *ecology* and *ecosystem*. Additionally, terms such as *environmental science* and *environmental protection* have crept into the realm of environmental health, with the danger that the latter is being supplanted by the former in definition and in the focus of the general public, as well as public health organizations. These fields of study are important, often overlap, and are arguably partially included in environmental health, but are not the same as environmental health. This confusion of terms and roles can lead to a dichotomy of direction, as now seen in the work of the Environmental Protection Agency (EPA) where the agency's name does not describe the focus of its activity.

To understand environmental health it is necessary to differentiate it from those terms described above and similar terms. Miller[1] defines *environment* as "all external conditions and factors that affect living organisms." It comes as no surprise that humans are living organisms. He also addresses the term *ecology* and defines it as "the study of the relationships between living organisms and their environment." This is a step closer, but does not reflect a true definition of environmental health. Another important and even more misleading term is *environmental science.* Environmental science is defined as "the interdisciplinary study of humanity's relationship with other organisms and the non-living physical environment."[2] Finally, in this menagerie of associated terms, the introduction of the term *environmental protection* has added to the confusion. According to the *American Heritage Dictionary,*[3] "environmental protection" relates to the keeping from harm, attack, or injury the combination of external or extrinsic conditions, which affect the life growth, development, and survival of an organism or group of organisms. Plainly stated, these are activities that are essentially corrective measures or belated preventive measures addressing issues ranging from air and water quality to legislation, rules and regulations, and enforcement of standards.

SCOPE OF PROFESSIONAL RESPONSIBILITY

The scope of environmental health has expanded and become more complex. It currently encompasses environmental protection. Regrettably, as stated earlier in this chapter, environmental health and environmental protection have become linked and are used to denote different programs based on organizational settings rather than on logical or definable differences in programs, missions, or goals. This distinction is artificial and has led to inappropriate organizational separation of activities that share the common goals of protecting the public's health and enhancing environmental quality. In some cases, the separate terminology has created organizational barriers rather than essential bridges among the organizations involved in the struggle for environmental quality. The umbrella of environmental health is adequate without the additional terms *environmental protection.*

The programmatic scope of environmental health and protection, as described later in this chapter, is quite broad. In addition, global environmental health and environmental protection issues, such as habitat destruction, species extinction, possible global warming and stratospheric ozone depletion, planetary toxification, desertification, deforestation, and overpopulation are interrelated. Indeed, excessive population growth contributes to all of the foregoing problems as well as to famine, war, disease, social disruption, illegal immigration, economic failures, and resource and energy shortages.

The primary difference between the terms *environmental health* and the other related or similar sounding terms is that the focus of environmental health is on those activities that directly impact *human health.* People, not ecosystems, are the primary focus of environmental health, ranging from education, program development, policies, regulation, investment in preventive measures, or using the bully pulpit to motivate all health professionals. Environmental health seems as relevant as it ever has been, though many of the fruits of its labors are events that simply do not occur because they have been properly avoided.

How does environmental health fit into the current public health arena? An examination of the Centers for Disease Control and Prevention's (CDC) "Ten

Great Public Health Achievements—United States, 1900–1999"[4] reveals that 5 of these 10 achievements are the result of direct involvement by environmental health professionals. These achievements are listed below with those related to environmental health highlighted in bold.

- Vaccination
- **Motor-vehicle safety**
- **Safer work places**
- **Control of infectious diseases**
- Decline in deaths from coronary heart disease and stroke
- **Safer and healthier foods**
- Healthier mothers and babies
- Family planning
- **Fluoridation of drinking water**
- Recognition of tobacco use as a health hazard

In conclusion, the term *environmental health* is a broad umbrella term for all environmentally related activities that are focused on health effects in the human population. Although elements of the terminology and concepts of science may be shared by environmental health with other related professions, it is the critical focus on health of the individual, communities, and the general public that separates peripheral areas of study from environmental health. It should also be apparent that getting the environmental science and technical matters "right" is essential to making fair, efficient, wise, and stable decisions affecting the health of individuals.

HISTORY

The history of environmental health science could easily be linked to practices that took place in Imhotep's Egypt or in ancient Greece and Rome. However, since most, if not all, of the personal and environmental health practices that were gained by the ancients were lost for various reasons in the Middle Ages, the "civilized world" of the West was basically a filthy place both in personal hygiene and from an environmental point of view.

Many believe that environmental health received its "rekindling" on April 22, 1970, with the birth of the first Earth Day. However, Earth Day was really a revitalization of the environmental movement that found its roots at the turn of the twentieth century in visionary leaders such as John Muir, Henry David Thoreau, Theodore Roosevelt, Gifford Pinchot, Aldo Leopold, Rachel Carson, and Garrett Hardin. In the 1960s and 1970s, Senator Gaylord Nelson from Wisconsin, Senator Henry M. "Scoop" Jackson from Washington, and other legislative leaders such as Senator Edmund Muskie from Maine sought a way to translate the public's increasing concern with the quality of the environment and human health issues into the political agenda and the implementation of the nation's laws. The Nixon presidency not only opened up diplomacy with China, but it also had unprecedented health, safety, and environmental accomplishments. Table 23.1 illustrates selected environmental laws and a few selected environmental law cases in the time line from 1842 to the present.

According to Yassi et al,[5] recently there have been three waves or periods of environmental attention. The initial wave occurred in Europe in the nineteenth century; it was linked to serious public health problems involving water contamination and food adulteration. In 1848 the British Parliament passed the first broad-based public health laws. It also was the "call to arms" of the first modern "sanitarian," Edwin Chadwick, with his theme the "sanitary idea."[6] Chadwick's role in authoring the *Report on the Sanitary Condition of the Labouring Population* allowed him to propose well-founded ideas regarding the provision of habitable living conditions, adequate disposal of waste, and potable water available to the working class. Chadwick also voiced concern about and held factory management responsible for accidental injuries and deaths of workers from faulty machinery or faulty construction practices. In addition, Chadwick became troubled over the sanitary conditions suffered by British soldiers in the 1853–1856 Crimean War. His concern resulted in the posting of sanitary inspectors during that war. All of these proposals by Chadwick were environmental health issues. Each demonstrates that what is known currently as occupational health and safety and hospital sanitation found its roots with Chadwick's "sanitary idea." Even given today's vastly improved conditions in

Table 23.1. Selected Environmental Laws and Environmental Case Time Line

Legal Progression Reflecting the Efforts of the Environmental and Public Health Movements

1842–*Martin v. Waddell,* one of the nation's first environmental cases, goes to the U.S. Supreme Court. A New Jersey riparian landowner, Waddell, claimed that he had exclusive rights to take oysters from the Raritan River. Case involves riparian and property rights.

1914–Search for better health quality standards leads to first U.S. drinking water regulations.

1946–Administrative Procedures Act (APA) signed into law; it is used to establish due process and protocols for government agencies. Key to understanding procedural requirements for agency actions.

1947–Federal Insecticide, Fungicide, and Rodenticide Act (FIFRA) signed into law, requiring pesticides to be registered with the Food and Drug Administration (FDA).

1948–Federal Water Pollution Act (FWPA) signed into law. Authorizes the Surgeon General of the Public Health Service to prepare comprehensive programs for eliminating or reducing the pollution of interstate waters and tributaries and improving the sanitary conditions of surface and underground waters.

1961–Wetlands Protection Act (WPA) signed. Its main purpose is to assign responsibility to protect precious migratory bird homes and mating grounds, and to reduce the increased draining of wetlands and associated loss of habitat.

1962–Rachel Carson's *Silent Spring* is published. Her book led to a widespread public outcry for environmental legislation. Marks the beginning of the modern environmental movement in the view of some historians.

1964–Wilderness Protection Act signed into law. Law meant to preserve and protect lands in their natural and wild state. Later Congress would add areas, such as the Ansel Adams Wilderness Area (and Mt. Ansel Adams) to the lands set aside for wilderness under this Act.

1965–Solid Waste Disposal Act (SWDA) signed into law. This is the first law governing the disposal of solid waste (later becomes the Resource Conservation and Recovery Act [RCRA]).

1966–Freedom of Information Act (FOIA) signed into law. This provides citizens with access to government documents and encourages full disclosure. Current dispute over executive privilege and access to energy policy formulation by the General Accounting Office (GAO) will be interesting to follow, especially given the collapse of Enron corporation.

1969–Endangered Species Conservation Act (ESCA) signed into law. For the first time, allows secretary of the interior to list wildlife that is threatened with worldwide extinction. Calls for an international meeting on endangered species.

1969–January 28: Union Oil Company's Platform A, in Santa Barbara, California, begins disgorging oil; 235,000 gallons of oil spilled in 11 days; thousands of wildlife are killed. Public starts demanding stiffer regulations as well as large civil and criminal penalties for polluters.

1969–June: Cuyahoga River in Ohio catches fire. Nixon administration feels pressure of public hysteria over high-profile environmental failures like this one.

1970–January 1, 1970: President Richard Nixon signs the National Environmental Policy Act (NEPA). NEPA creates a Council on Environmental Quality, as well as states lofty goals on the national policy to encourage productive and enjoyable harmony between people and their environment. NEPA is referred to as the mother of all environmental laws. NEPA, Public Law 91-190, also requires Environmental Assessments to determine whether or not proposed federal actions have significant environmental impacts—thereby requiring an Environmental Impact Statement (EIS). The Environmental Protection Agency (EPA) is created by Executive Order later that year, on December 2, 1970. The Occupational Safety and Health Administration (OSHA) was also created at this time, through the Occupational Safety and Health Act (OSH Act), Public Law 91-596, December 29, 1970.

1970–Clean Air Act (CAA) signed into law. This law sets standards for air quality and controls hazardous air pollutants.

1970–April 22: First Earth Day is celebrated, helping usher in the environmental decade of the 1970s. Long hair, rock music, hippie movement, counterculture flourish.

1971–*Calvert Cliffs Coordinating Committee, Inc. v. United States Atomic Energy Commission (AEC)* case is decided. 449 F.2d 1109 (1971). The Court of Appeals, DCCircuit, J. Skelly Wright, Circuit Judge presiding, finds that the AEC's rules precluding review of key matters—including nonradiological environmental issues (unless specifically raised earlier), prohibiting reviews by other agencies and between issuance of construction and operation permits—does not comply with NEPA. Assessment of cumulative impacts are also found to be lacking. In short, AEC is charged with acting improperly and not taking into account the environmental ramifications of siting a nuclear plant being built along Chesapeake Bay. The Court ordered AEC to revise its rules.

1972–Coastal Zone Management Act (CZMA) signed into law. Meant to preserve, protect, develop, restore, or enhance resources of the national coast.

Consumer Product Safety Commission created as part of Public Law 92-573, enacted October 27, 1972.

1972–Noise Control Act (NCA) signed into law. First law governing noise pollution.

1973–Endangered Species Act (ESA) signed into law. Its purpose is to "Provide a means whereby the ecosystems upon which endangered species and threatened species depend may be conserved, to provide a program for the conservation of such endangered species and threatened species. . . ."

1974–Safe Drinking Water Act (SDWA) signed into law. Sets standards for drinking water.

1975–Hazardous Materials Transportation Act (HMTA) signed into law. Regulates commerce of hazardous materials.

1976–Resource Conservation and Recovery Act (RCRA) signed into law. This act amends 1965 SWDA. Noted for its cradle-to-grave system of resource management.

1976–Toxic Substance Control Act (TSCA) signed into law. Main purpose is making sure manufacturers test products being marketed. Gives the EPA "broad authority" to control chemical risks that could not be dealt with under other environmental statutes.

1977–Clean Water Act Amendments (CWAA). Requires fishable and swimmable water bodies by 1985.

1978–Love Canal, New York, declared state of emergency due to chemical ponds adjacent to schools and houses. This environmental disaster (& Woburn) lead to passage of the Superfund law, the Comprehensive Environmental Response, Compensation, and Liability Act (CERCLA), Public Law 96-510.

1980–Alaska National Interest Lands Conservation Act (Public Law 96-487). Passed nine years after the Alaska Native Claims Settlement Act (ANCSA), ANILCA provided for designation of over 100 million acres of federal lands into conservation units, such as national parks, wild and scenic rivers, national forests, wildlife refuges, and national monuments. Quite a legacy to "Seward's Folly," the 1867 purchase of Alaska from Russia under the American diplomat and secretary of state William Henry Seward (1861–1869).

1980–Comprehensive Environmental Response, Compensation, and Liability Act of 1980 (CERCLA), Public Law 96-510, passed. Also known as Superfund, this law provides a framework for cleaning up abandoned, orphan, and contaminated sites and allocating costs and liability to potentially responsible parties (PRP).

1986–Superfund Amendments and Reauthorization Act (SARA) passed, Public Law 99-499, which reauthorizes the Superfund law (CERCLA). Congress provides extensive guidance and milestones for enforcing the timely cleanup of Superfund sites and species criteria for developing cleanup standards. Funding for Superfund is increased to $9 billion. By this time the Superfund National Priority List has grown from the original 400 sites to approximately 900.

Note: There currently are more than 1,200 sites on the NPL; the Bush administration has proposed changing the "polluter pays" principle underlying cleanups.

1989–March 1989: *Exxon Valdez* spills hundreds of thousands of gallons of oil into Alaska's Prince William Sound. This leads to the passing of the OPA.

1990–Oil Pollution Act (OPA) provides framework for rules, regulations, research, prevention, and compensation for possible damages to the environment from the release of oil during recovery, loading, and transportation in navigable waters.

(continued)

Table 23.1. Selected Environmental Laws and Environmental Case Time Line—continued

Legal Progression Reflecting the Efforts of the Environmental and Public Health Movements

1992–United Nations Conference on the Environment and Development (UNCED) meets. Discusses global environmental policy.

1992–1999

Clinton administration promotes new executive orders, regulations, and programs, ranging from designating national monuments to making oil drilling off limits in the Arctic National Wildlife Refuge (ANWR), to listing more toxic chemicals for regulation under laws such as SDWA and the TSCA. Administration is seen as very progressive by many environmental groups, but less concerned about costs to business for compliance. DOE, EPA, OSHA, DOT, DOA, and other federal agencies increase their budgets and initiatives. Environmental health science continues to grow.

2000–Closest presidential election in U.S. history. George W. Bush elected president. Role of the environment and government role in environmental health appear to have played a relatively minor part in the election; 2004 promises more interest in these issues. Earth Day initiative in 2002 touts ability to reduce mercury, acid rain, and nitrogen oxides in the Adirondack Mountains in New York state.

2001–September 11, 2001: Terrorist attack on the World Trade Centers and the Pentagon starts a new era of concern regarding bioterrorism, food safety, and the need to have preventive as well as infrastructure investments to have prophylactic/response capabilities in place.

Research Note: We would like to acknowledge Ms. Dori Thompson for her research assistance with this table. The authors remain solely responsible for its content.

much of civilization, Chadwick fashioned the groundwork for what was to become environmental health.

The second wave or crisis occurred in the mid to late twentieth century. This wave consisted of two movements, environmental conservation and toxics, that eventually merged into what is known as the environmental or ecology movement.[5] These two movements joined with a common concern regarding the effect of toxins on both humans and the environment. The legacy of the environmental movement can be seen in its evolving structure of leaders, policies, new technologies, and approaches to regulations. Although many of these activities were cloaked in the environmental movement and owe much of their success to the grassroots structure of these groups, it can be argued that their acceptance by the public was due primarily to their positive impact upon human health, rather than their impact upon the general environment.

Yassi and colleagues' third wave of concern occurred in the late 1980s and 1990s.[5] The focus of this movement was environmental planning and economic development, tilting toward "sustainable development"—the biological idea of a society living within the carrying capacity of the ecosystem. But once again, the underlying theme of human health is not lost in the maze of resource management, pollution, and social development issues. This is illustrated by the continuing concern over chemical exposures and the enduring and growing problems of worldwide infectious diseases, malaria, dengue, and yellow fever, and the emergence of such frightening agents as the Marburg and Ebola viruses. The search for a more sustainable society has been characterized in terms such as "industrial ecology" and "design-for-environment." What each of these shares with environmental health is the recognition that it is much wiser to invest in the front end to avoid altogether or mitigate, whether by design or process modifications, the adverse effects of exposing populations to toxins or conditions that injure or kill them.

Environmental health and protection are vital parts of public health, regardless of where they are administratively located, whether it is located at the top of the organizational chart or organizationally situated within the official public health agency. As with most fields where integration of diverse concepts is required for effectiveness, environmental health efforts must cross political boundaries and jurisdictional hurdles put up by agencies who wish to protect their mission and territory. Improving public health outcomes and environmental quality requires the ability to do risk assessment and to communicate those risks. It requires people with skill, competencies, and support services if efforts to protect human health and the environment are to be successful. Environment health must remain high on the public health agenda.

ENVIRONMENTAL HEALTH AT THE LOCAL HEALTH DEPARTMENT

Local health departments have the fundamental responsibility of protecting the life, health, and welfare of the people.[7] These responsibilities are reflected to a great extent in the environmental health programs that are housed within the health department.

Essentially all city and county health departments administer an environmental health program. It is the duty of the environmental health division to protect the public health through control of environmental factors. Professionals frequently called Registered Sanitarians ensure proper compliance with public health environmental laws and sanitary codes, which are designed and implemented to "protect the public health through regular inspections, issuance of permits and investigation and follow-up of complaints."[8] Environmental health programs are designed to reduce the risk of environmental hazards through education, surveillance, monitoring, and enforcement.

The programmatic scope of environmental health and protection includes, but is not limited to:

ambient air quality
water pollution control
safe drinking water
indoor air quality
noise pollution control
radiation protection
food protection
occupational health and safety
meat inspection
disaster response
cross-connection elimination
shellfish sanitation
institutional sanitation
pure food control
housing conditions
recreational area sanitation
poultry inspection
solid waste management
hazardous waste management
vector control
pesticide control
land use
milk sanitation
toxic chemical control
unintentional injuries
prevention of ecological dysfunction[9]

However, many of these programs are no longer or never have been under local health department jurisdiction. There are many reasons why these programs are not under the auspices of a local health department. In many cases it is due to the fact that "many local governments have assigned certain environmental health and protection activities to other agencies, such as public works, housing, planning, councils of government, solid waste management, special purpose districts, and regional authorities."[10] This has often occurred for a number of political rather than scientific or programmatic reasons.

Depending on particular needs and funding, the diversity and extent of environmental health programs in modern-day local health departments vary widely from county to county. A vast majority of local health departments receive funding solely from the state; thus, they fulfill a usually restricted number of program mandates. These program categories most often include the following:

• General Sanitation. The sanitarian or environmental health specialist is responsible for enforcing local or state health and sanitation codes. Among these codes are improper storage and disposal of garbage and trash, enforcing rodent and pest control regulations, illegal dumping, and trailer court and campground inspections. Activities are often generated by complaints filed by the public. Complaints are usually assigned to an inspector who conducts an investigation, most often within 24 hours of receiving the complaint, and takes action to abate the nuisance when warranted. If the responsible party does not correct the condition(s), then fines may be levied for each day the condition remains a public nuisance.

- Public Facilities. The environmental health specialist conducts environmental health and safety inspections of public swimming pools, hotels and motels, day cares, schools, correctional facilities, and tattoo/body piercing parlors. Surveyors also respond to complaints regarding these establishments to ensure compliance with appropriate codes and protection of the public's health.
- Food Hygiene. Most food programs include the permitting and inspection of food service facilities (delicatessen, fast-food, full-service, specialty shops, cafeterias, and all retail food stores on a routine basis (generally a minimum of two inspections annually). Nearly all health departments use the

Model Food and Drug Administration (FDA) 44-item, 100-point inspection form as a surveillance tool. Compliance is most often maintained through issuance of 10-day notices to correct, suspension of permits, permit revocations, informal hearing proceedings, and quarantining suspect foods. Consumer complaints, which frequently are numerous, are investigated within 24 hours. Due to the continued increase in the number of food service facilities, this has become the largest environmental health program at many county health departments and typically receives the most funding. A better understanding of what a typical environmental health program entails can be found in Table 23.2, which is a typical program plan submitted annually as part of the budgeting and planning process.

Table 23.2. Food Protection Program 605 (Food Service Establishments)

Program Status: There are currently 1000 food-service facilities in the county that possess state permits to operate. Approximately 35% of them are categorized as full-service, 50% are fast food type establishments, and the remaining 15% are specialty establishments or small delis. These establishments are routinely inspected a minimum of two times per year or as needed to maintain sanitary conditions. All consumer complaints and food-borne illness outbreaks are investigated within 24 hours. The state survey of food service facilities in _____ County rated an overall inspection average of 86% which is among the highest in the state. The program is staffed with five registered sanitarians, all of which have completed the FDA Inspection Standardization Program.

Goal: Strive to assure safety of food served from all facilities to consumers and assure the highest level of sanitation in such facilities in accordance with the state food code. These goals shall be attained through routine surveillance by way of inspections, consumer complaint investigations, field visits, food manager training certification programs, legal notices and permit suspension/revocation when necessary.

Objectives: During Fiscal-Year 2002-2003

1. Conduct 2500 routine inspections.
2. Issue 500 notices to correct violations found during routine inspections.
3. Conduct 550 follow-up inspections as a result of the notices to correct violations.
4. Conduct 800 investigations as a result of consumer complaints or personal observances.
5. Perform 400 field visits to offer consultation or to follow up on facilities with ongoing problems.
6. Plan review on 40 food service blueprint design submittals for approval to construct or remodel to assure compliance with regulations.
7. Issue 50 Notices of Intent to Suspend Food Service Permits.
8. Adjudicate 50 administrative hearings as a result of Notices of Intent to Suspend Permit actions.
9. Revoke two permits to operate as a result of hearing actions.
10. Offer eight food managers certification courses.
11. Quarantine and/or voluntarily destroy 1600 pounds of food found to be adulterated or contaminated.
12. Inspect, permit and collect permit fees from 650 temporary food establishments operating at special events, celebrations and fund raising events.

• On-Site Wastewater. Services provided include design and approval of on-site subsurface wastewater disposal systems, technical consulting, soil evaluations, percolation tests, and oversight of sewage installation to ensure compliance. Nationally, over 30 percent of all new residences are installing subsurface on-site systems; therefore, this has become a major program for county health departments in predominantly rural areas. In fact, many rural area health departments are so overwhelmed by the mass development of home construction, that their on-site wastewater program has become the priority, at the expense of other program mandates.

Many larger city and regional health departments go beyond the scope of programs detailed above and many have funding above and beyond a baseline program budget. This additional funding might be the result of a local health tax assessment or a matter of local government adding to the state budget to offer nonmandated programs considered to be of importance locally or regionally. Therefore, a progressive health department may administer large programs in injury prevention, road safety,[11] and wellhead and watershed protection.[12] Some health departments have requested and received responsibility for programs traditionally administered by other agencies. An illustration of this is Nashville, Tennessee, where the state transferred responsibility for the air pollution program from the State Department of Natural Resources to the City Health Department.[13] A few health departments are going in an opposite direction, attempting to relinquish programs to privatization. A case in point is that recently a city health department attempted to contract out their food inspection program to a private company.

Whenever possible, environmental health services should be delivered by the agency that is closest to the people being served. A local community agency can do a better job of protecting the local environment than can a distant bureaucracy. Visionary environmental health professionals foresee a future where fragmentation of programs among various agencies and private entities comes to an end and the local health department becomes the center for the entire scope of environmental health programs.

ENVIRONMENTAL HEALTH PERSONNEL

"Although the sanitarian is more directly the offspring of the physician health officer, and although the sanitary engineer has his genesis, in part, in the sanitarian, the public health officer's function has been markedly influenced by the work of the sanitary engineer."[14] Environmental health professionals are known by many names, and are employed in both the public and private sectors. One would be hard pressed to name any major organization, public or private, not employing persons with either training or education in environmental health to protect their human resources or the public that impact their organizational missions. Arguably, the Louisiana State Department of Public Health employed some of the first persons formally trained in the science of environmental health in the United States in the 1940s. These individuals were primarily patronage employees. However, they were carefully educated on the job by Dr. Ben Freedman, then director of the state health department. This training process was a benchmark in the use of nonphysicians for environmental health activities. The training materials used and in part developed by Dr. Freedman were later published as the *Sanitarians Handbook*, which defined the scope of the profession in public health departments until the early 1970s. This book, while outdated in many content areas, is still a classic and is used in many developing countries.[14]

FEDERAL AGENCIES AND THE PRACTICE OF ENVIRONMENTAL HEALTH

The creation of the Environmental Protection Agency, the Occupational Safety and Health Administration, and the Consumer Product Safety Commission by President Nixon during the first years of his administration had major impacts in reducing the scope of environmental health activities at local and state public health levels. In the public sector, this resulted in the placement of many environmental health professionals in agencies other than those charged with public health responsibilities. All cabinet level agencies of the federal government have offices that are responsible for environment, health, and safety (EHS), including all major branches of the military.

The United States Environmental Protection Agency (EPA) was created by executive order on September 9, 1970. The order incorporated water pollution control and certain pesticide research functions from the Department of the Interior; water supply protection, solid waste management, air pollution control, radiation protection, and pesticide research from the Department of Health, Education, and Welfare; pesticide regulation from the Department of Agriculture; and radiation standards from the Atomic Energy Commission and the Interagency Federal Radiation Council. In addition to the EPA, other significant environmental health and protection agencies of the federal government include:

- Public Health Service (including the National Institute of Environmental Health Sciences, the Centers for Disease Control and Prevention, the Indian Health Service, the Food and Drug Administration, the Agency for Toxic Substances and Disease Registry, and the National Institute for Environmental Health and Safety)
- Coast Guard
- Geological Survey
- National Oceanographic and Atmospheric Administration
- Nuclear Regulatory Commission
- Corps of Engineers
- Department of Transportation
- Department of Agriculture
- Department of Housing and Urban Development[9]

Due to the growth of environmental health outside the local and state health department domains, there are now many new titles for these environmental health professionals that do not reflect their public health roots. This blurring further increases the difficulty of educating the environmental health professional about a common knowledge base that defines the profession. The environmental health arena is made up of both environmental health professionals and professionals working in environmental health. The environmental health professional is an individual having a formal education in environmental health sciences drawn from a nationally recognized common core of knowledge. The professional work-

ing in environmental health is the person that does not have the common environmental health core of knowledge, but does have formal education in a specialty area. Some examples of these would be the entomologist, the toxicologist, and the environmental engineer.

EDUCATION OF ENVIRONMENTAL HEALTH PROFESSIONALS

The U.S. military services all have very strict requirements for their preventive medicine officers in terms of formal environmental health educational requirements. To be an officer in environmental health, the officer candidate is typically required to have a bachelor's or master's degree in environmental health sciences, public health, or engineering. The U.S. Public Health Service, a uniformed service under the Department of Health and Human Services, also has the equivalent, if not stricter requirements for educational background. In contrast, most local and state health departments do not require their environmental health workers to be formally educated in environmental health. Typically, they do require a science-related bachelor's degree, however. These public health agencies often attempt to make up for the lack of a formal education with in-service education and experience. Some states also require certification or licensure. It is interesting that the uniformed services are far more concerned with formal environmental health education than most state and local public health agencies. Of course, history is replete with wars lost due to preventable illness in the ranks of the competing armies.

The formal education of an environmental health professional requires the provision of basic tools for the future practitioner. The students should have education in areas that allow them, as professionals, to protect the public from chemical, biological, and physical threats and hazards to their health and well-being. The scope of environmental health requires that the true environmental health professional have knowledge in the following subject domains:

- Biology
- Chemistry

- Physics
- Mathematics
- Statistics
- Anatomy
- Physiology
- Epidemiology
- Toxicology
- Microbiology
- Zoology
- Vectorborne disease control
- Radiological health
- Solid and hazardous waste management
- Food safety
- Housing and institutional control
- Administration
- Public health and environmental law
- Injury control
- Industrial hygiene and safety principles
- Air pollution and ventilation principles

THE NATIONAL ENVIRONMENTAL HEALTH SCIENCE AND PROTECTION ACCREDITATION COUNCIL

The National Environmental Health Science and Protection Accreditation Council (NEHSPAC) is the primary accrediting agency for universities recognized by the U.S. Department of Education for educating environmental health professionals at the undergraduate level. The goal of accreditation of undergraduate environmental health science and protection programs is to enhance the education and training of students who intend to become environmental health science and protection practitioners/professionals. The criteria used in the evaluation of programs have been developed through the joint efforts of environmental health science and protection academicians and practitioners, and reflect the demands of the professions listed above. The Web site for this organization is as follows: http://www.ehaoffice.org/UGCriteria.htm.

COUNCIL ON EDUCATION FOR PUBLIC HEALTH

The Council on Education for Public Health (CEPH) is an independent agency that is also recognized by the U.S. Department of Education for accrediting universities offering public health education. CEPH is officially recognized to accredit graduate schools of public health and graduate programs in community health education and community health and preventive medicine in the United States. The American Public Health Association and the Association of Schools of Public Health created the Council in 1974 in response to continuing professional and legislative requirements for evaluation and maintenance of quality in graduate education for public health. The purposes of CEPH are to improve the health of the public by establishing and applying high standards in the education of public health professionals; to assist educators in organizing and developing curricula focused on public health and in assessing educational outcomes; to evaluate the content and quality of instruction, research, and service components of education for public health; and to promote high standards in both public health education and public health practice. In addition to accreditation, CEPH provides consultation and review services to public health schools and programs on request and encourages ongoing self-evaluation in all public health education. A core course in environmental health is required of all CEPH-accredited Master of Public Health degrees. The Web site for this organization is: http://www.ceph.org/.

FUTURE OF ENVIRONMENTAL HEALTH

The future of environmental health is growth—growth that threatens to further dilute the visibility of the profession because of the shortage of qualified individuals holding professional environmental health education. Currently, based on Internet job searches, there are well over 100,000 jobs open in the private sector for environmental health and safety professionals. The public sector has an estimated 25,000 new positions created each year. This public sector estimate is likely to be considerably low since it was based on a U.S. Health and Human Services, Bureau of Health Manpower study conducted in 1987. The combined output of educated professionals in environmental health from NEHSPAC- and CEPH-accredited schools do not begin to meet current demands, let alone projected demands.

FUTURE CHALLENGES FOR ENVIRONMENTAL HEALTH

Because of the increased possibility of bioterrorism and the realization of the role environmental health plays in disaster management in the new homeland defense, the shortage of trained personnel is likely to grow, particularly in federal agencies. The current diminished role assigned to local health department environmental health professionals in bioterrorism may be, in part, due to these different standards of education. The warming of the U.S. climate, if it continues, will create new demands for old programs in vectorborne disease control as a result of the creeping northward of diseases more common in temperate climates. The overcrowding of the highway infrastructure is likely to result in traffic injuries becoming an environmental or public health issue requiring additional focus on education of environmental health personnel in injury control. The future will likely require more effective cost-benefit analysis of current programs and the willingness of current professionals to establish baselines of current problems to provide effective data for cost-benefit analysis. The failure of environmental health to embrace a common professional nomenclature and acceptance of the concept of a common educational core will continue to waste public dollars and cost both lives and public confidence.

References

1. Miller GT. *Living in the Environment: Principles, Connections, and Solutions.* 11th ed. Pacific Grove, Calif: Brooks/Cole Publishing Co; 2000.
2. Raven PH, Berg LR. *Environment.* 3rd ed. Fort Worth, Tex: Harcourt College Publisher; 2001.
3. *American Heritage Dictionary.* Second College Edition. Boston, Mass: Houghton Mifflin Co; (1985).
4. Centers for Disease Control and Prevention. Ten great public health achievements—United States, 1900-1999. *MMWR.* 48(12):241-243.
5. Yassi A, Kjellstrom T, de Kok T, Guidott TL. *Basic Environmental Health.* New York, NY: Oxford University Press; 2001.
6. Sir Edwin Chadwick (1800-1890) Sanitarian and Social Reformer. *JAMA.* 1968:23(1):99-100.
7. Salvato JA. *Environmental Engineering & Sanitation.* 4th ed. New York, NY: John Wiley & Sons; 1992.
8. Henry and Stark County Health Departments, Kewanee, Illinois. Available at: http://www.henrystarkcohealthdept.org/environ.htm.
9. Scutchfield FD, Keck CW. *Principles of Public Health Practice.* Albany, NY: Delmar Publishers; 1997.
10. Browner C. *Public Health—An EPA Imperative.* EPA Insight Policy Paper, November 1993. EPA-175-93-023.
11. Columbus Health Department, Columbus, Ohio. Available at: http://www.cmhhealth.org.
12. Oakland County Health Department, Pontiac, Michigan. Available at: http://www.co.oakland.mi.us/health.
13. Metropolitan Health Department of Nashville and Davidson County, Tennessee. Available at: http://healthweb.nashville.org.
14. Freedman B. *Sanitarian's Handbook: Theory and Administration Practice for Environmental Health.* New Orleans, La: Peerless Publishing Co; 1977.

CHAPTER
24

Primary Care and Public Health

Kevin A. Pearce, M.D., M.P.H.
Samuel C. Matheny, M.D., M.P.H.

Primary care is not a new concept, but its definition and manifestation in the general context of medical care have been sequentially modified over the last 50 years. The Declaration of Alma-Ata stated in 1977 that "primary health care is . . . the first level of contact of individuals, the family and community with the national health system, bringing health care as close as possible to where people live and work, and constitutes the first element of a continuing health care process." This Declaration, which placed primary care as the central piece of the system of health care, was part of the World Health Assembly Global Strategy of Health Care for All by 2000.[1] More recently, the Institute of Medicine defined *primary care* as "the provision of integrated, accessible health care services by clinicians who are accountable for addressing a large majority of personal health care needs, developing a sustained partnership with patients, and practicing in the context of family and community."[2]

The distinction has been made between primary *medical* care and primary *health* care. Primary medical care is concerned with the issues of accessibility of

medical and preventive services from health care workers; primary health care is a social concept concerned with populations and involving a wider variety of individuals than simply health care workers.[3] Vuori states that primary health care can be interpreted in four ways: as a set of activities, as a level of care, as a strategy of organizing health care, or as a philosophy of care.[4]

Primary care and public health are inexorably linked, though not congruent. Clean air, potable water, public safety, and national defense are all public health functions distinct from primary care. But what about childhood immunizations, the prevention of heart disease, or the treatment of battered women? Is screening for breast cancer a public health function, a primary care function, or both? Despite areas of overlap, and some areas of conflict, it is clear that individual health care services are necessary for public health.

Primary care is usually, but not always, the portal of entry through which individuals obtain medical services, and most Americans report having a primary care doctor.[5,6] Individual health care services routinely delivered through primary care include health promotion, and disease prevention, diagnosis, and treatment.

Within the spectrum of individual health care services, primary care medical services have a powerful impact on public health, especially for younger populations[7] and for people living in poverty.[8] Having a primary care doctor is associated with better health outcomes than receiving care only from specialists and is a stronger predictor of good health outcomes than is insurance status.[8] Primary care, especially family practice, improves the cost-effectiveness of medical care.[8,9]

From an ecological perspective, primary care is associated with good public health outcomes in terms of major health indicators, both internationally and across the United States.[8-11] Whether or not primary care is labeled as such is less important than an emphasis on the *principles* of primary care in the medical services infrastructure. The importance of primary care to favorable health outcomes wanes only in terms of major health indicators for elderly people in developed nations. Elderly people with good access to health care in well-developed nations have positive health outcomes—with or without an emphasis on primary care.[7]

PRIMARY CARE PROVIDERS, PAST AND PRESENT

During the first part of the twentieth century, the majority of medical care was provided by general practitioners to those who could afford it, or by the public wards of larger city hospitals to some who could not. By the end of the Second World War, the development of specialization had accelerated and was further stimulated by the emergence of the federal government as the major source of funding for medical education in the postwar years.

As Stevens points out, unlike Great Britain, the United States had never developed a formal structure for primary care. Although a professional relationship had developed early in the twentieth century between generalists and specialists in Great Britain, in the United States it was common for all physicians to compete against each other, and general practice was becoming a "residual field." This was encouraged by the lack of a governmental national health policy in the United States. The American patient, by the middle of the twentieth century, had grown accustomed to the idea of direct access to specialists, not necessarily by referral from the primary care physician.[12]

By the 1950s, the status of the general practitioner, and the numbers of medical students entering general practice, had reached an all-time low. Concern about adequate provision of first-line care had reached high levels among the American public and within the health professions. Two reports, *The Graduate Education of Physicians* (Millis, 1966) and *Meeting the Challenge of Family Practice* (Willard, 1966) reached essentially the same conclusion, and called for the development of a new discipline to meet the needs of primary care in the United States. Within a span of several years, the American Academy of General Practice changed its name to the American Academy of Family Physicians, the first residency programs in Family Medicine were created, and the American Board of Family Practice was organized.

By 2001, there were over 62,000 board-certified family physicians in the United States, with 470 residency programs graduating about 3,400 new family doctors each year. Student interest in family medicine and primary care generally rose during the mid-1990s, but began to fall again at the turn of the century.[13]

Along with family practitioners, general internists and general pediatricians constitute the main physician primary care workforce. Over the past quarter-century, interest in, and development of, special residency programs for primary care internal medicine and primary care pediatrics has grown. Of the total number (171,912) of professionally active physicians in primary care in 1996, 39 percent (66,421) were in general internal medicine, 21 percent in general pediatrics (36,300), and 40 percent in family/general practice (69,191).[14]

These numbers, however, do not reveal the true extent of the major problem of maldistribution of generalist physicians. This problem is most evident in the rural and inner-city areas of the United States. Maldistribution of physicians, and how it impacts public health, will be discussed in greater detail in the next section of this chapter.

Physicians are not the only primary care providers in the U.S. health system. Over the past quarter-century, there has been a significant development of nonphysician clinicians (NPCs) in the United States, and in many cases, there has been a significant interest in their contribution to primary health care. It is estimated that as of 2001, there were around 7,250 nurse practitioner (NP) graduates, and 3,400 physician assistants (PAs). Approximately 95 percent of all NPs and 55 percent of all PAs are involved in primary care.[15] Many states now allow independent practice of NPCs, and the current clinical market is providing new opportunities for practice. Also, the number of NPCs currently being trained is growing substantially. At the current rate of growth, the number of nurse practitioners will equal the number of family physicians by the year 2005. There is evidence that NPCs, unlike family physicians, do not necessarily practice or settle in areas of greatest need, but follow the trend of physician placement in general, in which most graduates begin practice in the areas where there are already the greatest number of practitioners.[15]

SUPPLY AND DISTRIBUTION OF PRIMARY CARE SERVICES

In many developed nations, physician distribution and the proportion of the medical infrastructure devoted to primary care are both reasonably well balanced. Unfortunately this is not the case in the United States, which ranks 15th among all nations in health care, according to the multidimensional WHO Index, but first in the world in annual health care expenditures per capita.[10,11] This gap between health care expenditures and major health indicator outcomes can be largely explained by two major features of the U.S. organization and financing of health care:

1. A high ratio of subspecialty physicians to primary care physicians.
2. Geographic physician maldistribution resulting in overabundance of health care services in most metropolitan and suburban areas, with physician shortages in rural areas and inner-city areas.

The most commonly used method for mapping out physician shortages is the U.S. government's Health Professional Shortage Areas (HPSA) designation. In order to be a primary care HPSA, an area must have fewer than 1 full-time-equivalent primary care physician for each 3,500 residents. This threshold ratio can be raised under circumstances (e.g., poverty or language) that increase barriers to medical care.[16] As of 1995, 25 percent of U.S. counties were wholly designated as primary care HPSAs, with at least one part of another 59 percent of U.S. counties so designated.[16,17]

Even when considering the large population referral base that each subspecialist usually needs, primary care physicians distribute themselves geographically according to the population better than do subspecialists. Primary care physicians thereby constitute the main bulwark against catastrophic physician shortages in rural and inner-city areas. Among all specialties, only Family Practice distributes its residency graduates in virtually exact accordance with the U.S. population in terms of rural, urban, and suburban communities.[16,18] This is not to imply that the expertise and practices of subspecialty physicians are unimportant to public health. Rather, health care systems that emphasize subspecialty care at the *expense* of primary care demonstrate worse health status in their populations compared with systems that emphasize primary care. Although experts recommend a 1:1 ratio of primary care physicians to all subspecialists *combined*, only one-third of U.S. doctors are primary care physicians, and the ratio is not improving.[16]

It has been stated that nothing influences the practice choice site of physicians more strongly than specialty selection, and this is particularly evidenced in rural areas. Pediatricians, general internists, and obstetrician-gynecologists rarely settle in rural or inner-city areas.[16] The majority of care in rural areas is provided by family physicians, who are the only physicians as likely to locate in a rural area as a large urban area. It is not surprising to learn that in rural areas, over 50 percent of the care is provided by family physicians. In small group practices, cross-coverage issues limit the attractiveness of general pediatrics and general internal medicine in many rural communities. Usually only when the catchment area population exceeds 10,000 persons is it feasible for pediatricians or internists to consider a rural area as a site for practice.

Primary obstetrical services are a particularly important concern, since family physicians' involvement with maternity care varies considerably. For most family physicians, accessibility to referral for complicated obstetrical services is important. However, there are almost no obstetricians in the smaller rural communities.[16] Traditional family practice residency programs place 21–25 percent of their graduates nationwide into rural areas (with approximately 20 percent of the population living in rural areas.[18,19] More are needed, however, to catch up and mitigate long-standing shortages. In graduate medical education, a novel approach has been the creation of special family practice residency programs that have the majority of their training occur in rural communities. These programs place an average of 76 percent of their graduates into rural areas.[16,20] A related strategy has been the creation of comprehensive selection and training programs with a clear mission to produce rural primary care physicians. Such programs can be conceived as "pipelines" that begin at the high school level, extend through formal medical training, and encompass recruitment, placement, and retention of residency-trained physicians in areas of need.[18]

Thus, an unbalanced ratio of primary care to subspecialty physicians, coupled with geographic maldistribution of physicians, has led to (and perpetuates) widespread shortages of primary care medical services in the United States. Changes in medical education that successfully produce more family physicians, coupled with improved incentives for new residency graduates to settle in rural and inner-city areas, can be expected to have very positive impacts on public health.

PUBLIC PROGRAMS SUPPORTING PRIMARY CARE

Over the past 35 years, a number of programs have been instituted at various levels of government to address several basic issues in American health care. These issues relate to the consistent findings of (1) maldistribution of physicians in the United States leaving certain sections of the country, particularly rural areas and some inner-city areas, with inade-

quate numbers of physicians; (2) widespread shortages of primary care physicians throughout the United States, with severely restricted access to medical care in many rural and inner-city areas; and (3) restricted access to care for large portions of the U.S. population due to absent or inadequate health insurance without other resources to pay for health care, even in areas of adequate physician supply.

As outlined in the *Tenth Report* of the Council of Graduate Medical Education,[16] five major types of efforts have been devised to address these problems: deployment of health professionals to underserved areas, intervention to provide access to needy populations, educational interventions to encourage redistribution of new health professions graduates, economic incentives, and research and policy development for primary care services.

Deployment of Health Professionals to Shortage Areas

The main deployment program instituted by the federal government has been the National Health Service Corps, which was first started in 1970. Over 21,000 health professionals have participated in this program since its initiation, and over 2,000 health professionals yearly receive either direct scholarship assistance or loan repayment by serving in specific underserved areas. Over half of all of these worked in federally funded community health centers. A number of states also have developed loan repayment and scholarship programs for health professionals with varying degrees of success in recruitment and retention.[9]

Intervention to Provide Access to Needy Populations

In the 1960s, Medicaid legislation was passed that provided reimbursement to providers for poor and near poor individuals. In many cases, health departments had been providing primary health care services and those, along with others, saw the potential for a new funding stream from Medicaid. In response, many health departments assumed roles as "providers of last resort" for their communities. In fact, several became deeply involved with the community health center movement. Many health departments used this funding to subsidize primary medical care to noninsured individuals and, in some cases, cross-subsidize core/essential public health services. As Medicaid moved to managed care over the last decade, the patients receiving primary care at those health departments migrated to private physicians, truncating the Medicaid funding stream into the health departments, and leaving those reliant on that funding in a difficult situation.

The issue of whether or not health departments should be providing primary medical care remains controversial. The IOM report titled *The Future of Public Health* reflects that ambivalence. Many suggest that the health department must fulfill this function, as there is not an alternative system that can or will assume responsibility for primary medical care for the indigent. Others suggest that this function draws resources that are intended to provide population-based services to the care of a relatively few individuals.

Another major effort in this category is the community and migrant health centers program. This program, which began in the 1960s, funds over 600 centers across the United States, with provision of primary care to more than 8.1 million people in 1998.[21] Four primary care programs are included in this group—community health centers (CHCs), migrant health centers, health care for the homeless programs, and health care for residents of public housing. These centers have variable relationships with state and local health departments, and they vary widely in their distribution throughout the United States.[16] They probably account for around 4 percent of all primary care visits nationally. CHCs see a disproportionately larger number of ethnic minorities who are either insured by Medicaid or completely uninsured, compared with hospital outpatient clinics or physicians' offices.[21]

Educational Interventions

In addition to its support for expansion of medical schools, since the 1970s the federal government has supported the expansion of programs in primary care medical education, such as family medicine, primary care internal medicine, and primary care pediatrics programs. As a result of these various programs, greater emphasis has been placed on primary care medical student education, graduate education, departments of family medicine, and related faculty development programs throughout the United States. Similar federal grant funds to support the education of nurse practitioners and physicians' assistants have helped to increase the number of these providers significantly in the past decade. A variety of state programs targeting the training of primary care physicians, particularly in family medicine, have supplemented the federal programs.

Economic Incentives

Another important federal incentive was the establishment of Medicare bonus payments to physicians providing care in urban and rural Health Professional Shortage Areas (HPSAs) in 1989. This measure, along with designations at the state and federal level that allow cost-based reimbursement via the Medicare and Medicaid mechanism, have added to the financial incentive to practice in the HPSAs.[16]

Research and Policy Development

The Office of Rural Health Policy (ORHP) was established by Congress in 1988, and has established a network of rural health research centers, in addition to support for telemedicine programs. Another part of Health and Human Services that is becoming increasingly important in primary care research is the Agency for Healthcare Research and Quality (AHRQ), which is the successor to the Agency for Healthcare Policy and Research originally established in 1989. AHRQ has as part of its mission "to support research designed to improve the outcomes and quality of health care."[22] Within AHRQ there is a new Center for Primary Care Research that will fund research projects specifically related to primary care issues.

SYNERGIES AND TENSIONS BETWEEN PRIMARY CARE AND PUBLIC HEALTH

Using the Institute of Medicine's definition of primary care,[2] and envisioning primary care as being directed to care of the individual in a broader context, large areas of overlap and synergy between primary care and public health emerge.[23] But there are also areas of tension. In some cases, health care oriented to the individual can easily be combined with health care oriented to populations because of common goals. In other situations, health care with the goal of the best possible outcome for an individual may actually conflict with other health-related goals for the population.

The following case studies are meant to illustrate these concepts, and serve as springboards for discussion.

Treatment of Individuals and Community Health

CASE #1

Treatment and Control of Curable Infectious Disease

John S. was a 48-year-old street vendor whose primary care physician diagnosed him with pulmonary tuberculosis that had been symptomatic for at least two months. John shared a cramped apartment with his mother, sister, and his sister's four children. He had a girlfriend who lived at a different address. John's doctor started antitubercular treatment. He also referred him to the Tuberculosis Control Clinic at the local health department for assistance with identification, surveillance, and, if necessary, treatment of his close contacts. The services directed to his family, girlfriend, and other close contacts were obviously in the interest of public health, but did not compromise his own treatment. The requirement that others be told about his tuberculosis was, for John, outweighed by the fact that this breach of confidentiality directly helped his friends and loved ones. John's physician was able to explain all of this to him, and he was grateful for all of the services.

This example of synergy between individual and public health care goals and services relies on the patient's perception of his disease as not having very negative social consequences, and being highly preventable and treatable. Had John been suffering from an infection with greater social implications, such as gonorrhea, tensions would probably have arisen between what was the best course of action for him alone, versus the best actions for the health of the community.

CASE #2:

Diagnosis and Treatment of HIV/AIDS

Tom W. was a 38-year-old bisexual physical therapist whose physician diagnosed him with HIV infection that had not yet progressed to AIDS. Tom discussed confidentiality issues with his physician. He wanted comprehensive HIV treatment and strict confidentiality about his diagnosis. Tom felt that letting anyone else know that he had HIV would disrupt important relationships and compromise his ability to maintain his career. In this case, the physician's obligation to serve as the best advocate possible for his patient's individual health met with the conflict of the physician's other obligation to public health. Specifically, many would argue that the physician had the responsibility to take reasonable actions to see that Tom's sexual contacts were informed of his diagnosis. Although the physician may have seen no need to notify the employer, one of Tom's past sexual partners worked at the same hospital, and Tom was sure that the "word would get out" if that partner were informed. Such disclosure would lead to terrible discomfort for him at work, and he felt that his employer would then find a reason to lay him off. That would cut off Tom's health insurance when he needed it most.

A state law requiring the reporting of new HIV cases to the local public health department might have facilitated identification and notification of at-risk contacts, but did little to resolve the moral dilemma faced by Tom's physician.

CASE #3:

Physician Adovacy for Risk-Reducing Behabiors

Tina B. was an 18-year-old high school graduate seeing her physician for a checkup prior to entering college. She reported being sexually active with more than one partner in the past year, and was still without a steady partner. She requested a prescription for birth control pills. In addition to providing that prescription, her physician counseled her on the prevention of sexually transmitted diseases (STDs). He also provided her with a teen-oriented health publication featuring peer group advocacy of safe sexual practices.

CASE #4:

Prevention and Management of Chronic Disease

Roberto A. was a 56-year-old city bus driver who presented to his physician for a periodic employment physical/general medical evaluation. Although he felt well, he was obese, he smoked cigarettes, and his evaluation revealed hypertension, high cholesterol, and adult-onset diabetes. His physician emphasized the need to bring his risk factors for heart attack and stroke under control, all the while focusing on Roberto's personal health.

Individual versus Collective Use of Medical Resources

Tensions between what is best for the individual and what is best for the population often arise over the fair and equitable distribution of medical resources. In certain situations, such as the treatment and control of infectious disease, resources spent at the individual level directly benefit the broader population at risk of contracting a given disease. Problems of resource allocation draw public attention when payment for individual medical care comes from tax-based public funds (such as Medicaid), but these problems are common whenever people pool their funds for health care. Although they may not label it as such, most Americans have become quite aware of resource allocation problems as the medical insurance industry has heightened its efforts to control costs and maintain profits through managed care.

CASE #5:

Expensive Tests

Alison P. was a 32-year-old mother of four with headaches and dizziness. After interviewing and examining her, her physician thought that these symptoms were responses to stresses in her life, and that a brain tumor or other intracranial pathology was very unlikely (but not impossible). In fact, Alison was quite frightened that she had a tumor and her personal physician was unable to reassure her otherwise. He understood that ordering expensive (but safe) tests to completely rule out a tumor would erase the shadow of doubt that he could not otherwise fully remove, and that this would help his patient. He was also aware that each time he ordered expensive tests that were medically unnecessary, he contributed to the rapid rise in health care expenditures overall, and that this indirectly reduced the health care resources available to the population at large. Alison's physician finally rationalized that he would actually save medical resources by doing an expensive test, because without it his patient would continue to feel ill, and she would keep seeking medical consultations until she got her brain scan.

CASE #6:

Prescription Medications

Dr. G. had hundreds of patients with hypertension. Most of her patients had prescription drug coverage through either public funds or commercial health insurance. The evidence was strong that inexpensive medications for hypertension were effective for protecting individuals like her patients from heart attack and stroke. However, there were many newer medications that cost 10–20 times as much as the older (but effective) medications. Many of Dr. G.'s patients wanted a newer medication, equating newer with better. There was limited evidence, but not proof, that certain newer medications were slightly more effective than the older inexpensive ones.

CASE #7:

Unproven Treatments for Deadly Diseases

Maria M. was a 35-year-old mother of two diagnosed with aggressive breast cancer that had spread to her lymph nodes. Understandably, Maria wished to pursue almost any treatment that might save her life. Her chances for cure were poor. She wanted to enter a controversial bone marrow transplant treatment program for breast cancer victims, understanding that its effectiveness was not yet proven. Results from studies of the treatment were mixed, but Maria wanted to "have a chance." She understood the medical risks associated with the treatment and was very willing to accept them. Maria did not know how she would cope with the estimated $120,000 cost. Her physician got Maria into the bone marrow transplant program.

PUBLIC HEALTH AND THE SCIENTIFIC BASIS FOR PRIMARY CARE

Evidence related to disease etiology, prevention, diagnosis and treatment derives from studies of individuals, small groups, and large populations. Such evidence is sometimes appropriately applied from populations to individuals or vice versa, but may also be inappropriately extrapolated, especially when evidence gathered from one subpopulation is applied to another without consideration of pertinent differences. Furthermore, when physicians attempt to apply evidence derived from groups to individual patients, personal biases, fears, expectations, and resources come into play. The translation of research findings into actual medical practice requires much more than the flow of information.

Primary medical care is ideally guided by evidence derived from appropriate populations. For most primary care issues, the reliability and validity of the available evidence are proportional to the number of people studied, and the variety of settings and situations represented. Public health data sets inclusive of large numbers of people and settings have much to contribute to primary care. This is especially true for disease etiology and certain aspects of health promotion and disease prevention. However, such population-based data sets are few. Furthermore, because the United States does not have an integrated system of health care, population-based data reflecting actual medical care and outcomes in community physicians' practices are altogether lacking.[23,24]

The potential, but untapped, power of standardized data collection on disease screening, diagnosis, treatment, and outcomes during routine primary care is enormous. Imagine physicians being able to query databases fed by hundreds of thousands of patients (and their doctors) as to the power of a given test to diagnose or rule out a disease, the efficacy of a given screening strategy, or the effectiveness and patient-acceptance (balanced against risks) of a treatment. Glimpses of this power can be found in studies conducted by large, closed-panel health maintenance organizations.[24,25] But the promise of large, clinically useful datasets becoming commonplace as managed care organizations took control of the U.S. health care market has not been realized. This is probably due to the lack of financial incentives for data collection beyond that necessary for licensure, accreditation, and competition.[23]

Practice-based research networks (PBRNs) represent a grass-roots approach to studying health and disease in the context of routine health care. For the past 20 years, primary care PBRNs have been operating in the United States, Canada, and Europe.[26] To date, funding for PBRNs has been miniscule compared with other types of medical "research laboratories," and their impact has been limited. A few PBRNs have steadily produced reports of significant original research directly applicable to family physicians and their patients. One of the largest and most successful has been the Ambulatory Sentinel Practice Network (ASPN), which was recently reconstituted into the National Network for Family Practice and Primary Care Research.[27,28] Primary care PBRNs have also begun to garner support from the federal government through the Agency for Healthcare Research and Quality, and the Health Resources and Services Administration. It remains to be seen whether these networks of primary care practitioners will be able to significantly improve public health through their research efforts.

For now, the overall failure to collect data on the processes and outcomes of individual health care constitutes a missed opportunity for public health.[23,24] The effectiveness of public health initiatives, and the allocation of resources, could be greatly enhanced if informed by missing information on the interplay of personal preferences and limitations with disease risks, detection, treatment, and prevention. Such information can be obtained only through the collection of data related to personal health care services.[23]

Lacking the ideal sources of information discussed above, physicians turn to two other major sources of evidence to guide their decisions for individuals: (1) limited observational data available from surveillance of large groups, and (2) data from controlled clinical trials that usually involve small, selected groups. The following cases illustrate strengths and weaknesses of this approach.

CASE #8:

Conflicting Information and Data Limitations

Jean W. was a 54-year-old librarian who consulted her physician about postmenopausal estrogen replacement therapy (ERT). She was especially concerned about the prevention of heart disease. Based on the published advice of multiple experts over the past 10 years, Jean's doctor educated her about the various benefits and risks of ERT. He advised her that, because heart attacks were the number one killer of women in the United States, and large studies had shown a protective effect from ERT, the benefits of its use outweighed any risks. Jean's trust in her physician was eroded when she heard news reports that ERT did not protect against heart attacks, and might even increase the risk in certain women. Jean's friend told her that her doctor advised against ERT. Jean stopped taking ERT and quietly switched doctors.

Why the conflicting information? Jean's doctor relied on expert advice derived from large observational, public health-oriented studies of postmenopausal women.[29] The data were not based upon a general sample of postmenopausal women visiting their primary care doctor (like her). The available studies had problems with confounding (perhaps women who took ERT were more health-conscious than those who did not), as well as questionable applicability to individual patients and settings that differed from those studied. The media, and the friend's doctor, were responding to two recent randomized clinical trials, involving selected women who had to meet multiple special criteria related to heart disease.[30,31] In fact, the evidence about ERT was mixed, the correct course unclear, and reliable high-quality evidence, collected from large groups of women similar to Jean, was not available.

CASE #9:

Population-Based Data Supported with Clinical Trials

Johnnie H. was an actuary for an insurance company whose doctor informed him that he had very high cholesterol, and advised he change his diet plus take medicine to get it under control. Johnnie had heard for years that high cholesterol increased the risk of heart attack. But now that he had the problem, he questioned his doctor about the evidence that high cholesterol was truly bad, and that lowering cholesterol was good for the heart. The advice Johnnie's doctor gave was informed by population-based, public health-oriented observational studies, plus practice-oriented controlled clinical trials.[32] The population-based data showed a strong and consistent causal relationship between high blood cholesterol and heart attack, and the more narrow clinical trials of diets and medicines showed that lowering cholesterol prevented heart attacks by the amount expected from the observational studies.[33]

In this case there was population-based evidence *plus* clinical evidence from selected patients, and the two sources were congruent. Johnnie and his doctor could thus make decisions about managing his high cholesterol with greater confidence than was possible for Jean and her doctor regarding ERT.

Bringing Research-Based Evidence to the Point of Medical Care

The slow dissemination and flow of new evidence to practicing physicians impedes the progress toward evidence-based primary care as much as does the lack of pertinent data and research findings. If one accepts the premise that good primary care is good for public health, then well-developed systems for enhancing the flow of evidence and information related to medical decision making should have high priority.

At present, multiple technologies and methods are being brought to bear on the problem of improving clinicians' access to information and evidence that they need, *when they need it*. It is impossible for individual clinicians to search, filter, and use the massive amount of new clinical research reported each month. Professional publications devoted to reviewing, culling, and briefly reporting new medical evidence are helpful, but even they are quite voluminous, and they do not allow search and retrieval of information efficiently enough to be useful in the course of seeing patients. These publications also may fail to judge the quality of the new evidence they report, and often do not place it in context with related evidence.[34]

The general approach to this problem is to create methods for prompt, systematic, and critical reviews of new research, and feed these reviews into electronic medical literature databases that are extensively cross-referenced. These literature databases can then be searched via the Internet, or via archives stored on compact discs or microchips (the latter updated periodically over the internet). To be used at the point of medical care, the electronic readers for this information must be either pocket-sized or ubiquitous throughout patient care areas. Access by clinicians must be very rapid with minimal input steps and virtually no transmission delays. Among the many challenges to this goal is prioritization of which types of information and evidence to monitor, filter, critique, rate, store, cross-reference, and disseminate. Major efforts are under way to meet the human and technological challenges inherent to bringing high-quality information to the point of medical care. Notable examples are the Cochrane Project devoted to putting the results of clinical trials into usable evidence-bases,[35] support of medical informatics, evidence-based practice centers and technological assessments by the U.S. Agency for Healthcare Research and Quality,[36] and the Family Practice Inquiries Network, funded by the American Academy of Family Physicians.[37]

COMMUNITY-ORIENTED PRIMARY CARE

The model for medical care in most of the Western world for the twentieth century has been that of separate sectors of care rather than an integrated system. Public health programs, hospitals, and ambulatory or primary care services have usually developed without any real coordination among these areas. Further fragmentation of mental health services and substance abuse treatment worsened the division of areas of responsibilities. Early attempts had been made to merge these health care sectors into an integrated system, with the premise being that only by doing so could health care providers benefit from the knowledge obtained in one sector being transmitted most effectively to another for the greatest health benefits.

By 1919, early attempts had been made by the Commissioner of Health of New York to accomplish this, but they came to no avail. Similar attempts were followed in Britain in 1920, but not until 1921 was an actual model devised and constructed along these lines by Dr. John Grant in China. The Karks followed in 1940 with the development of their pioneer model in rural Natal, and later in Israel.[38] With the advent of the National Health Service in Great Britain, increasing attempts were made to coordinate the preventive and primary care health services throughout the country. Cuba made one of the first major attempts at the merging of public health and primary care with a new initiative in 1974 called Medicine in the Community which was expanded and altered to emphasize family medicine access for all residents in the 1990s. Physicians in Cuba have both personal and public health responsibilities for the communities they serve, with comcomitant dramatic improvements in the health status indicators for that country.[10] Training in Community Medicine as a discipline began at the University of Kentucky in the 1960s, and the concept of merging preventive and primary care medicine became a center for the newly developed Community Health Centers, first funded by the U.S. federal government in the late 1960s.[38]

The best-known conceptual model of this merger of care has been called Community-Oriented Primary Care (COPC). As defined by Nutting, COPC is "a variation of the primary care model in which major health problems of a defined population are identified and addressed through modifications in both primary care services and other appropriate community health programs."[39] The COPC process, in its simplest form, consists of the following four stages: (1) identification and definition of the community; (2) identification of community health problems; (3) development of some intervention in the health care program; and (4) evaluation of the effectiveness of the program. This approach is designed to define communities and through the use of various forms of data, identify areas of special concern to a specific community or practice. The intervention may have various forms, but frequently it is designed to facilitate the delivery of care and/or provide a measure of preventive services in an attempt to improve the overall health status of the community. One of the other important features of community-oriented primary care is that representatives of the community itself should be involved with prioritizing the areas of emphasis in this model.

This model has been attempted for a number of years in community health centers, the Indian Health Service, family medicine residency programs, and in individual and group practices. Some reported projects have included programs to reduce rural neonatal mortality rates,[40] initiatives to reduce teenage substance abuse,[41] and statewide interventions for prevention of cardiovascular disease.[42]

However, the COPC model has been slow to fulfill the encouraging expectations described for it in its early days of development. Several reasons for this are evident. It has been difficult, up to the present time, to accurately obtain community-level information on health, and to develop the resources to integrate this information into that of a specific practice. COPC programs require time, and in a fee-for-service model, time allocations for community-based approaches have not been readily compensated. Critics have also expressed concern that the evaluations of program effectiveness have been sketchy at best.[43] New advances in informational systems, Internet-based data, and affordable software may positively impact the issue of obtaining community-based data, and the advent of managed care may provide increased incentives for interest in those programs related to specific programs.

PREVENTIVE SERVICES

Preventive services can be conceptualized as primary, secondary, or tertiary. In general, primary prevention refers to steps taken to prevent disease, injury, or illness from ever beginning. Secondary prevention is conceived as stopping subclinical or symptomatic disease before it becomes symptomatic or is transmitted to others. Tertiary prevention is aimed at ameliorating disease or illness once it has become symptomatic and limiting its negative effects on quality or quantity of life. Tertiary prevention encompasses curative and palliative medical treatments.

Public health classically has played a major role in primary prevention. This domain cannot be delivered solely through individual clinicians. It includes societal infrastructures related to clean water, clean air, crime control, highway safety, and food safety, as examples. But primary prevention also includes counseling to eliminate or mitigate exposure to disease risk. These sorts of services are within the domain of individual medical care, especially primary care. Examples include counseling on safe sexual practices, counseling and treating for smoking cessation, counseling and education about seat belt use, lactation consultation, and the prevention of drug and alcohol abuse. Immunizations are also an example of primary prevention often pursued through individualized clinical services.

Secondary prevention falls squarely on the shoulders of individual clinical services. For the most part, large-scale public health-based screening programs, such as the use of mobile x-ray units to screen for tuberculosis, have disappeared. Today in the United States, most screening for disease, plus treatment and amelioration of the subclinical disease thereby detected, is accomplished through individual services, mainly through primary care clinicians.[23,44] If these clinicians accept the responsibility for secondary prevention, how can they target appropriate preventive services? For example, in America's technologically developed medical system, how is the physician to determine what battery of tests or prophylactic treatments to recommend to each patient, and at what frequency?

CASE #10:

Clinical Preventive Services

Janet T. was a 48-year-old advertising executive who presented to her family physician for a "physical." She had been too busy to see a doctor for the last four years. She felt well, but had finally scheduled a complete checkup to be sure she was healthy. She wanted "everything tested," and requested a "complete blood profile," a pap smear, mammogram, a brain scan, a colon exam, a chest x-ray, a bone scan, a urine test, shots, and anything else the doctor thought was necessary.

In order to do his best to promote Janet's health, her physician had to weigh the accuracy of tests (taking into account the probability that Janet has each asymptomatic disease considered), the effectiveness of early detection and treatment of each disease in question, and the risks of each test. Cost-effectiveness had to be considered if he accepted any responsibility for the health of the community, or if Janet had to pay out of her pocket for preventive services. He also had to identify her health risks and target his advice to modifiable behaviors related to those risks.

Until the last two decades, there was little scientific evidence to guide physicians in their selection of screening tests or appropriate counseling related to health risks. Since then, there has been a blossoming of research and subsequent evidence to guide the preventive efforts of health care providers. Evidence-based guidance would have been severely hampered without epidemiology and biostatistics, and without the use of large public health databases. Clinical preventive services now have a better scientific basis than most other segments of clinical medicine, thanks to the application of these public health sciences. This is important because the threshold for trying unproven treatments to help a patient in distress is usually much lower than the threshold for pursuing unproven tests, changes in lifestyle, immunizations, or medications for people who feel well.

Several evidence-based guidelines for preventive services have been developed.[45] The most comprehensive of these is the U.S. Preventive Services Task Force's *Guide to Clinical Preventive Services*.[46] Using these guidelines, physicians can efficiently target appropriate clinical services to patients based on their age, gender, and characteristics that define risks for various common disease states. Clinical preventive services are thus tailored to the individual, but with background population in mind. The ability to improve the health of individuals, and by extension, populations, is core to the selection of preventive services. Health risks, risks associated with tests and treatments, potential risk-reduction, and allocation of health care resources all come into play.

Screening services that might detect a disease early, but for which treatment would not have altered the length or quality of life, should not be pursued. An example is periodic chest radiography in asymptomatic smokers. Screening services with high potential for detection of early disease amenable to eradication must also be acceptably safe, not too uncomfortable, and cost-effective. Thus, even though colonoscopy under sedation is highly effective for detecting and treating precancerous or cancerous colon polyps, its inherent costs, discomforts, and risks have hampered its widespread use in the general population at average risk for colon cancer.

Despite the near perfect marriage of public health and primary care in terms of disease prevention, some areas of tension do exist. Prominent among these is the question of who should provide preventive services for the medically indigent. Similarly, the question commonly occurs of who should provide preventive services that are not reimbursed by third-party payers.[23] Third-party payers are less motivated to provide preventive services that are in the public interest. Enrollees in health plans change their health plans often enough that third-party payers find it difficult to prove that they can profit from covering preventive services, despite the fact that these services are cost-effective when looking at larger populations under a single payer.

PRIMARY CARE PHYSICIANS AS PUBLIC HEALTH SENTINELS

A basic tenet of pubic health is the identification and control of epidemics. In order for epidemics to be identified in an early stage, sentinels must be present and alert. In our current system there are not enough public health officials distributed throughout the country to effectively institute an early-warning or early-detection system for disease. Even if there were sufficient public health personnel, a large proportion of early-onset epidemic illness would present first to primary care physicians. Thus, in order to effectively halt or mitigate epidemics at an early stage, primary care physicians need to be alerted to their probability, and be able to recognize rare patients who may be early victims. Epidemic detection and control is an area of great potential synergy between public health and primary care, but significant barriers still prevent the realization of that potential.

Dr. William Pickles beautifully illustrated the power of the country doctor in being a sentinel and amateur epidemiologist.[47] Since Dr. Pickles's time, medical care and society have changed in ways that make such accomplishments difficult. Dr. Pickles was able to be very sensitive to changes around him because of the relative isolation and permanence of his surrounding rural community. He basically knew everybody. In American society today, physicians and the public are so mobile that, in most communities, Dr. Pickles's approach is impractical.

Other infrastructures to support primary care physicians as sentinels are needed. Our main advantage in the twenty-first century rests on new and efficient methods of communication. Computerized medical records, other computerized practice functions, the Internet, and e-mail have taken the potential efficiency of the sentinel function to a new level. The negative public health effects of societal changes that have loosened the bonds between primary care physicians and their communities can be partially offset by new capabilities for detection and communication during an emerging epidemic. The sentinel function of primary care is poised to be a realistic contribution to public health, if properly stimulated and supported. However, that potential has yet to be tapped in any significant way. Time

and resources of primary care providers and public health personnel remain a major stumbling block, and there are currently insufficient incentives to overcome these barriers. Future incentives should include time-saving alerts and access to medical information delivered electronically to member sentinel physicians.

THE FUTURE OF PRIMARY CARE AND PUBLIC HEALTH

Four major forces are likely to shape the future of primary care as it relates to public health: financially managed care, technological innovations, an aging society, and population (and cultural) migrations.

Managed Care

Managed care was developed over the last 20 years in an attempt to control health care costs. During the early years of managed care, primary care was seen as an essential part of the health care system, partly in the role of gatekeeper with primary care physicians controlling patients' access to health care. Although in many plans this still holds true, more attention has been placed on point-of-service care, or allowing individuals to access services without referral from a primary care physician, or by doing so with a higher copay.

In fact, many people do not use primary care providers, either due to their lack of information about what they may have to offer, or due to long-standing habits and emphases on sporadic use of the health care system. In many cases, this first-line care is provided by urgent treatment centers, emergency rooms, and others where preventive care and longitudinal disease management, both essential to excellent primary care, are not given priority.

The provision of mental health services in managed care markets, and the role of primary care in that regard, have been areas of special concern. Not only do people with mental illnesses frequently not have access to care, but in many cases, managed care barriers that have been constructed between the primary health and mental health systems create difficulties in providing high-quality care. Various attempts have been made to improve the communication between mental health specialists and primary care physicians, with varying degrees of success.[48] Similar concerns have been raised about the treatment of substance abuse and primary care.

On the other hand, the organization of American health care into various managed care groups gives primary care physicians new directions that would have been impossible even 15 years earlier. As Greenlick states, a defined population base can give powerful data to primary care physicians if they are trained to use them.[49] Information about the natural course of illness and greater understanding of causal relationships in health will be possible. Equally important will be the growing influence of technology, and the ability to tailor preventive care to the individual with a detailed analysis of risks based on genetic, environmental, and personal risk profiles. Complex decisions on both preventive and health care services will be increasingly available in real time in the physician's office. The long-awaited merger of preventive and clinical services will be possible, but it will depend on the availability of access to health care, and understanding of the importance of both areas by patient and provider.

Technological Innovations

As technological advances open doors and empower health care professionals, they also usually raise costs. Most people who pay for health care, whether directly or through insurance premiums, are conscious of continuously rising costs that outstrip inflation. They often benefit from new medications, new diagnostic and monitoring tools, or improved surgical techniques. But what proportion of their income, or of the gross national product, should be spent on health care? How will we define cost-effectiveness in the future, and who will decide on resource allocations? As we have seen, positive health indicators or outcomes are not proportional to the amount spent on health care, whereas the degree to which health systems use primary care is positively associated with desirable health outcomes.

What will be the best blend of technological advances and primary care, in terms of public health? Which technologies hold the most promise for primary care and public health? Unable to predict the future, we can still make educated observations. The human genome project has enormous potential as a tool through which preventive services can be highly tailored to individuals via accurate risk-profiling, with huge increases in their cost-effectiveness. Information technologies are poised to bring all kinds of critical information to the point of an individual's medical care, greatly reducing medical errors and oversights as they guide clinicians to the best tests and therapies for the individual at hand. Properly applied, these technologies will probably enhance the healing powers of physicians, and improve public health, more than anything seen since the advent of antibiotics. But to wield that much power, technologies must be widely available at a relatively low cost. Very expensive technologies with severely limited scopes of use cannot be expected to have appreciable impacts beyond the few individuals who access them.

An Aging Society

As the population in developed countries ages, the need for chronic disease diagnosis and management will expand, placing growing pressures on health care resources. The number of chronic ailments needing medical management rises with age. For what proportion of the population can an economy support multiple subspecialty medical services, used chronically? Primary care physicians can expect a growing need for their services in the management of chronic disease. If they fail to rise to that challenge, either health care costs will skyrocket, quality will plummet, or both.

Population (and Cultural) Migrations

Population and cultural migrations have occurred throughout history, often bringing sweeping waves of change. Large migrations are usually driven by strife, and the arriving immigrants are usually poor. The United States has experienced and absorbed such waves many times in its history, quite often with marked strains on public health systems. What roles will primary care providers play in mitigating the suffering of future waves of impoverished immigrants? How will they reach across barriers of language and culture? Cultural competence training is becoming mainstream in primary care residency programs, with unknown impacts so far. Will (or should) more public funds be appropriated for health care for illegal or undocumented immigrants? If efforts are increased to provide care to medically indigent immigrants, will their care be perceived mainly as a function of specially funded (and vulnerable) centers? Or will it be distributed through the health care system? One thing seems certain: inattention to the health of medically indigent immigrants threatens the public health of all Americans.

In summary, there are many forces at work that should compel the integration of primary care and public health. The primary care provider may be the individual of first contact in the identification of public health threats, such as environmental exposures or bioterrorism. Implementation of accepted screening measures to prevent illnesses, particularly chronic diseases, may best be accomplished with primary care, and should be greatly aided by the advent of vastly improved informational systems. There is also an increased interest in challenging the way in which we organize and deliver health care through the traditional "silos" of physical health, mental health, substance abuse, and public health. On the other hand, health care in the United States, at least, remains fragmented, and millions are uninsured. Significant changes in the economy may have a profound effect on funding for public health *and* underserved populations. It is difficult to predict the impact of the changing demographics of the American population. Nevertheless, it is important to continue to work for the improvement of the health care of the population. Success may depend on the willingness of the forces of public health and primary care to work together.

References

1. Declaration of Alma-Ata. International Conference on Primary Health Care, Alma-Ata, USSR, September 6-12, 1978.
2. Institute of Medicine. *Primary Care: America's Health in a New Era.* Donaldson MS, Yordy KP, Lohr KN, Vanselow NA, eds. Washington, DC: National Academy Press; 1996.
3. Ashton J. Public health and primary care: Towards a common agenda. *Public Health.* 1990;104:387-398.
4. Vuori H. Primary health care in Europe—Problems and solutions. *Community Med.* 6;221-231.
5. Graham Center for Policy Studies in Family Practice and Primary Care. Utilization patterns and usual source of care. Policy Center One-Pager #2. Available at: http://www.aafppolicy.org/library/. Accessed December 1999.
6. Green LA, Fryer GE Jr, Yawn BP, Lanier D, Dovey SM. The ecology of medical care revisited. *N Engl J Med.* 2001;344:2021-2025.
7. Starfield B. Public health and primary care: A framework for proposed linkages. *Am J Public Health.* 1996; 86:1365-1369.
8. Leiyu S, Starfield B. Primary care, income inequality, and self-rated health in the United States: A mixed-level analysis. *Int J Health Serv.* 2000;30:541-555.
9. Forrest C, Starfield B. The effect of first-contact care with primary care clinicians on ambulatory health care expenditures. *J Fam Prac.* 1996;43:40-48.
10. Starfield B. Is U.S. health really the best in the world? *JAMA.* 2000;284:483-485.
11. World Health Organization. *The World Health Report 2000. Health Systems: Improving Performance.* Available at: http://www.who.int/whr/2000/index.htm.
12. Stevens R. The Americanization of family medicine; Contradictions, challenges, and change, 1969-2000. Formal discussion papers from Keystone III. The Role of Family Practice in a Changing Health Environment: A Dialogue. Robert Graham Center, 2001. Chapter 1: 19-41.
13. Pungo PA, McPherson DS, Schmittling, GT, Kahn, NB. Results of the 2001 National Resident Matching Program: Family Practice. *Fam Med.* 2001;33:594-601.
14. American Medical Association. *Physician Characteristics and Distribution in the US 1997/1998.* Chicago, Ill; 1997.
15. Cooper R, Laud P, Dietrich C. Current and projected workforce of nonphysician clinicians. *JAMA.* 1998;280(19):788-794.
16. Council on Graduate Medical Education. *Tenth Report. Physician Distribution and Health Care Challenges in Rural and Inner-City Areas.* US Dept of Health and Human Services; 1998.
17. Fryer GE, Green LA, Dovey SM, Phillips RI Jr. The United States relies on family physicians unlike any other specialty. *Am Fam Physician.* 2001;63:1669.
18. Geyman JP, Hart LG, Norris TE, Coombs JB, Lishner DM. Educating generalist physicians for rural practice: How are we doing? *J Rural Health.* 2000;16:56-80.
19. Bowman RC. Continuing family medicine's unique contribution to rural health care. *Am Fam Physician.* 1996;54:471-480.

20. Rosenthal TC. Outcomes of rural training tracks: A review. *J Rural Health.* 2000;16:213-216.

21. Forrest C, Whelan E. Primary care safety-net delivery sites in the United States: A comparison of community health centers, hospital outpatient departments, and physicians' offices. *JAMA.* 2000;284(16):2077-2083.

22. Agency for Healthcare Research and Quality. Mission Statement. Available at: http://www.ahrq.gov/about/profile.htm#back.

23. Welton WE, Kantner TA, Katz SM. Developing tomorrow's integrated community health systems: A leadership challenge for public health and primary care. *The Milbank Q.* 1997;75:261-288.

24. Pollock AM, Rice DP. Monitoring health care in the United States—A challenging task. *Public Health Rep.* 1997;112:108-13.

25. Barlow WE, Davis RL, Glasser JW, et al. The risk of seizures after receipt of whole-cell pertussis or measles, mumps, and rubella vaccine. *N Engl J Med.* 2001;345:656-661.

26. Nutting PA, Beasley JW, Werner JJ. Practice-based research networks answer primary care questions. *JAMA.* 1999;281:686-688.

27. Green LA, Hames CG Sr, Nutting PA. Potential of practice-based research networks: Experiences from ASPN. *J Fam Pract.* 1994;38:400-405.

28. American Academy of Family Physicians. Academy begins national research network. Family Physicians Report, October 1999. Available at: http://www.aafp.org/fpr//991000fr/all.html.

29. Sharp PC, Konen JC. Women's cardiovascular health. *Primary Care.* 1997;24:1-14.

30. Hulley S, et al. Randomized trial of estrogen plus progestin for secondary prevention of coronary heart disease in postmenopausal women. *JAMA.* 1998; 280:605-613.

31. Herrington DM, Reboussin DM, Brosnihan KB, et al. Effects of estrogen replacement on the progression of coronary-artery atherosclerosis. *N Engl J Med.* 2000;343(8):522-529.

32. Gaziano JM, Herbert PR, Hennekens CH. Cholesterol reduction: Weighing the benefits and risks. *Am Coll Physicians.* 1996;124:914-918.

33. Expert Panel on Detection, Evaluation, and Treatment of High Blood Cholesterol in Adults. *The Third Report of the National Cholesterol Education Program (NCEP) Expert Panel on Detection, Evaluation, and Treatment of High Blood Cholesterol in Adults (Adult Treatment Panel III).* Available at: http://www.nhlbi.nih.gov/guidelines/cholesterol/index.htm.

34. Bero LA, Grilli R, Grimshaw JM, Harvey E, Oxman AD, Thomson MA. Closing the gap between research and practice: An overview of systematic reviews of interventions to promote the implementation of research findings. *BMJ.* 1998;317.

35. Becker L. Helping physicians make evidence-based decisions. *Am Fam Physician.* 2001;63:2130-2136.

36. Agency for Healthcare Research and Quality. Clinical Information. Available at: http://www.ahrq.gov/clinic/.

37. Dickinson WP, Strange KC, Ebell M, Ewigman BG, Green LA. Involving all family physicians and family medicine faculty members in the use and generation of new knowledge. *Fam Med.* 2000;32:480-490.

38. Kark S. Community-oriented primary health care: A review. *COPaCETIC.* 1998; Vol. 5, No. 1, 1-6.

39. Nutting P. Community-oriented primary care: An integrated model for practice, research, and education. *Am J Prev Med.* 1986;2:140-147.

40. Marquardt D. Improvement in rural neonatal mortality: A case study of medical community intervention. *Fam Med.* 1993;23:269-274.

41. Frame P. Is community-oriented primary care a viable concept in actual practice? An affirmative view. *J Fam Pract.* 1989;28:203-208.

42. Mittelmark M, Luepker R, Grimm R, et al. *The Role of Physicians in a Community-Wide Program for Prevention of Cardiovascular Disease: The Minnesota Heart Disease Program.* Public Health Reports. Vol. 103, No. 4, 360-365.

43. O'Connor P. Is community-oriented primary care a viable concept in actual practice? An opposing view. *J Fam Pract.* 1989;28(2):206-209.

44. American Academy of Family Physicians. The importance of primary care physicians as the usual source of health care in the achievement of prevention goals. Center for Policy Studies in Family Practice and Primary Care One-Pager. Available at: http://www.aafppolicy.org/onepagers/20000221.html. Accessed February 21, 2000.

45. National Guideline Clearinghouse. Available at: http://www.guidelines.gov/index.asp.

46. US Preventive Services Task Force. *Guide to Clinical Preventive Services.* 2nd ed. Baltimore, Md: Williams & Watkins; 1996.

47. Pickles WN. *Epidemiology in Country Practice.* Bristol, England: John Wright & Sons Ltd; 1949.

48. Crews C, Batal H, Elasy T, et al. Primary care for those with severe and persistent mental illness. *West J Med.* 1998;169(4):245–250.

49. Greenlick M. Educating physicians for population-based clinical practice. *JAMA.* 1992;267:1645–1648.

CHAPTER
25

Maternal and Child Health

Trude Bennett, Dr. P.H.
Alan Cross, M.D.

This chapter reviews the history and current status of public health involvement in the provision of maternal and child health services. Linkages between socioeconomic status and maternal and child health (MCH) are emphasized. Programs that are community-based and family-centered and that provide integrated delivery of comprehensive services are advocated.

HISTORY

In the early years of the twentieth century, social reformers concerned about child labor and high infant mortality rates successfully lobbied for the creation of the Children's Bureau, whose mandate was to gather data and report on child welfare. The Children's Bureau involved local communities in studying the social and economic correlates of infant and maternal mortality, including income, housing, nutrition, sanitation, and access to medical care. The Bureau's findings demonstrated a clear link between poverty and

maternal health risks that created disadvantages for newborns.[1]

The Sheppard–Towner Act

Recognizing the need for public action, the Children's Bureau spearheaded passage in 1921 of the Maternity and Infancy Act (also called the Sheppard–Towner Act for its congressional sponsors). Federal matching funds were used to set up maternal and child health divisions in state health departments. These agencies coordinated child health programs and public maternity care services, including prenatal care, nutritional counseling, health education, and household assistance for poor and immigrant populations, particularly in the large northeastern cities. The Sheppard–Towner Act was controversial due to its assumption of public responsibility for health care, involvement in family life, and emphasis on prevention over cure. Although credited with saving many lives, the Act was defeated in 1929, resulting in diminished public efforts just as the needs of women and children increased with the Great Depression.

The Social Security Act

The Sheppard–Towner Act served as the model for Title V of the Social Security Act of 1935, the purpose of which was to address the needs of vulnerable children and families affected by the depression. Title V provided rural and economically disadvantaged women and children with maternal and child health services, comprehensive services for "crippled" children, and child welfare and protective services. Through a separate administration, the Social Security Act provided income assistance for indigent families in a program that served as the forerunner of Aid to Families with Dependent Children (AFDC).[1] Despite the understanding that poverty and poor health are closely related, health and social welfare programs have continued to be funded and administered separately.

The 1960s

In the early 1960s, the emerging Civil Rights movement shifted the paradigm from a charitable obligation to a political commitment to achieving equality and compensating for racial injustices of the past. New programs emerged in the 1960s and 1970s that focused attention on economic and racial disparities in health outcomes and health services utilization. Medicaid (Title XIX) became the primary government funding mechanism for indigent health care. Neighborhood health centers reached out to communities with wide-ranging projects to improve nutrition, reduce lead exposure, and expand employment opportunities, in addition to providing primary care. New programs included maternal and infant care projects, family planning services, children and youth projects, the Head Start early childhood education program, the Special Supplemental Food Program for Women, Infants, and Children (WIC), school lunch programs, Title I educational assistance, and implementation of legislation guaranteeing the right to education of the handicapped (PL 94-142).[1] This diversity of programs aimed at poverty, education, nutrition, and health ac-

knowledged the complex interaction between socioeconomic circumstances and health outcomes.

Most of these programs were federally initiated but financed and administered through partnerships between the federal and state governments. Programs targeted specific populations defined by strict eligibility requirements. They were operated by different state government units responsible for education, welfare, nutrition, and health and thus delivered in communities by several different agencies. This approach divided the needs of high-risk women and children into categorical programs at the local level. Despite the fragmentation and limited funding, multiple evaluations have documented the effectiveness of these programs in improving the health and well-being of women and children.

The 1980s

In the early 1980s, the Reagan administration's new federalism gave states greater autonomy to determine program priorities, but it also provided less money for program implementation. Advocates succeeded in maintaining a specific block grant to states that was dedicated to MCH needs. However, total MCH block grant funds in 1983 were 18 percent lower than the amount made available for maternal and child health programs in the previous year.

The categorical programs consolidated into the MCH block grant were those for "crippled children," maternal and child health, lead-based paint poisoning prevention, sudden infant death syndrome, adolescent pregnancy prevention, genetic disease testing and counseling, hemophilia diagnostic and treatment centers, and services to children with disabilities eligible for Supplemental Security Income. The earlier federal mandates for uniform enactment of these programs for poor and minority populations had been seen by many as a form of protection against politically motivated disparities among states. Under the block grant strategy, some states have reported greater efficiency and a heightened ability to respond to local needs. However, the impact of uneven availability of various programs due to the states' greater discretionary power has not been fully determined.[2]

In the late 1980s, attention turned to the United States' poor international ranking in infant mortality (20th among the nations) and the large racial gap in infant health outcomes (African-American infant mortality was twice that of Euro-Americans). In recognition of inadequate access to prenatal care for many women lacking private insurance coverage, Medicaid benefits were extended to the near poor and enhanced to allow reimbursement for a wider array of services, including nutrition, health education, psychosocial services, and care coordination. However, expanded eligibility for Medicaid maternity care without parallel growth in the pool of prenatal care providers may have added to the stress of overloaded public clinics in need of additional resources.

The 1990s

The 1990s offered tremendous challenges and opportunities for public health workers in the field of maternal and child health. More than ever, studies confirmed the strong relationship between poverty and health for the MCH population. Some problems persisted and intensified, and new problems emerged. In 1989, 12.6 million children under the age of 18 were living below the federal poverty level. (This figure reached 13.5 million in 1998.) Conditions were worse for children in racial and ethnic minority families: in 1990, poverty rates for children under 6 years of age were 50 percent for African Americans and 40 percent for Latinos, compared with 14 percent for Euro-Americans.[3]

The large increase in female-headed households, combined with limited educational and employment opportunities for women, made individual responsibility for children's social and economic needs unattainable for many families. AFDC benefit levels averaged less than 50 percent of the poverty level in most states. On a given day, 100,000 children were homeless throughout the United States. In 1989, 2.4 million children were reported to be abused or neglected. A growing number of children were known to be infected with HIV or affected by the use of harmful substances. The emotional toll of societal violence on the nation's children is unknown. The number of children dropping out of school each year in the 1990s

was at least 446,000. In 1990, approximately 25,000 cases of measles, 5,000 cases of mumps, and 4,000 cases of whooping cough were reported, with the nation's record of early immunization lagging behind most countries in the developing world.[4]

Emerging in the 1990s was a model of community-based comprehensive services coordinated and integrated at the local level. Rather than categorical programs administered with a separate set of rules and regulations aimed at a highly targeted population, efforts were undertaken to pool the resources at the local level, eliminate the bureaucratic barriers among programs, and offer combinations of services to women and children based upon individual needs and available resources in the community. Client participation, agency collaboration, and the use of private and charity dollars to enhance local programs were all part of this new paradigm. New mandates for family-centered, community-based care were meant to be compatible with creative approaches initiated through community mobilization and organization.

Two critical events of the 1990s for MCH populations were the dismantling of AFDC and the implementation of the State Children's Health Insurance Program (CHIP). On July 1, 1997, welfare as we knew it—entitlement to limited cash assistance for many of the country's poorest families—became history. The Personal Responsibility and Work Opportunity Reconciliation Act of 1996 (PRWORA) set a five-year lifetime limit on cash assistance for most families and required recipients to participate in welfare-to-work programs. Medicaid eligibility was no longer tied to welfare participation. Exceptions to time limits and work requirements were allowed for up to 20 percent of a state's caseload, but exemptions were no longer made automatically for health reasons. States were given greater discretion and control over regulations.

Careful monitoring of new welfare policies is extremely important because of the potential public health implications. The welfare rolls dropped rapidly after implementation of Temporary Assistance to Needy Families (TANF), but declines in child poverty have not kept pace. The entry-level jobs available to many low-wage workers leaving welfare do not offer health insurance or other benefits. Most former welfare recipients are still eligible for Medicaid benefits, but often do not know of their eligibility status. Physical and mental health problems of welfare recipients can present barriers to successful employment, and health limitations can be compounded by limited access to health services.

Also in 1997, the State Children's Health Insurance Program received congressional authorization under Title XXI of the Social Security Act. By the year 2000, every state and the District of Columbia had developed a CHIP program and begun to sign up uninsured children for coverage. Although other uninsured family members would not benefit directly from their children's enrollment, the program offered hope of improving access to health care for approximately 14 percent of all children in the United States who lacked public or private insurance. CHIP enrollment contributed to declines in the number of uninsured by the end of the decade, though limited funding and outreach curtailed full enrollment and uptake varied among states.

Entering the New Millennium

As the new millennium began, federal policy began to shift in alignment with the new federal administration. Proposals began to enter the policy arena for faith-based charity initiatives, which would utilize government funds to support social welfare programs operated by religious institutions. Implications for services addressing sensitive social issues such as adolescent pregnancy, as well as the constitutional issues related to separation of church and state, were not clear. A slowing of the economy and shrinking job opportunities also challenged the capacity of TANF to maintain employment levels adequate to compensate for lack of cash assistance to indigent families.

In addition to health effects of TANF, leading health policy analyst Kay Johnson predicts that the following policy issues will be key for maternal and child health in the coming period: (1) the impact of state budget pressures on CHIP outreach, enrollment, and benefits; (2) the future of Medicaid as a residual insurer for low-income families; (3) the impact of the managed care environment on children with special health care needs and other vulnerable populations; (4) parity of mental health funding with provisions

for other health care services; (5) intersection of health systems with special education and early intervention services; (6) children's oral health; and (7) the impact of developments in genetic science on prenatal and newborn screening systems.

As of June 2000, CHIP enrollment reached 2.3 million children, an increase of almost 1 million from the previous year. In July 2001, a bipartisan bill was introduced in the House of Representatives to extend CHIP coverage to pregnant women and newborns. Representative Nita Lowey of New York, one of the bill's sponsors, declared that "Too many pregnant mothers put their own health and the health of their children at risk because they cannot afford the high cost of prenatal care. This is simply unconscionable. We know that healthy pregnancies lead to healthy babies. Our bill just makes common sense." The bill represents a strategy for consolidating and expanding health care coverage for MCH populations.

MAJOR FEDERAL MCH PROGRAMS

MCH programs in local health departments are largely determined by major federal programs that are funded and administered through various combinations of federal, state, and local collaboration. To assist in understanding these programs, key elements of federal legislation and regulations are described in this section. Each state and local health agency carries out these programs in different ways as allowed by federal law, so it is impossible to describe all the variations. However, each health agency has a manual for the operation of each of these programs. It should be consulted for local details that cannot be provided here.

Title V

Title V continues to play a key role in funding and shaping public health programs for women, children, and families at the state level.[5] The federal Title V program is currently administered by the Maternal and Child Health Bureau of the Health Resources and Services Administration (HRSA). HRSA is an agency of the United States Public Health Service within the Department of Health and Human Services. Proposals to reorganize maternal and child health programs within the federal system have been opposed by MCH advocates because of the history of Title V and the MCH Bureau's dedicated service to women, children, and families.

Maternal and Child Health Block Grants

Congress allocates Title V funding to the states for a combination of mandated and discretionary purposes. States receive 85 percent of this amount as maternal and child health block grant funds, for which the states must match every four dollars of federal money with three dollars of their own contribution. In their block grant applications, states must demonstrate that they will use the funds to achieve objectives consistent with the Public Health Service's objectives for the year 2010. These objectives include reduction of adolescent and unintended pregnancy, substance use during pregnancy, severe complications of pregnancy, low birthweight and infant mortality, and unintentional childhood injury; and promotion of breastfeeding, immunization, genetic screening, and primary care for infants.[6] At least 30 percent of block grant funds must be used for children's preventive and primary care and at least 30 percent for services for children with special health care needs.

Utilizing maternal and child health block grant funds, states are expected by the federal government to:

- provide and assure mothers and children (especially those with low income or limited availability to services) access to quality MCH services
- reduce infant mortality and the incidence of preventable diseases and handicapping conditions among children
- reduce the need for inpatient and long-term care services
- increase the number of children appropriately immunized against disease and the number of low-income children receiving health assessments and follow-up diagnostic and treatment services
- otherwise promote the health of mothers and infants by providing prenatal, delivery, and postpartum care for low-income, at-risk pregnant women

- provide rehabilitation services for blind and disabled individuals under the age of 16 years
- provide and promote family-centered, community-based coordinated care for children and adolescents with special health care needs (those with or at risk for chronic or disabling conditions) and facilitate the development of community-based systems of services for such children and their families
- ensure provision of services in areas of special concern, including: mental retardation, SIDS, pediatric AIDS, adolescent pregnancy, STDs, childhood injury prevention, substance abuse, lead poisoning, homelessness, and violence
- conduct needs assessments every five years and meet expanded requirements for planning, data collection, and reporting

The remaining 15 percent of the MCH block grant money is allocated for Special Projects of Regional and National Significance (SPRANS) grants. These are demonstration projects that are fully funded (that is, no matching funds are required) from competitive applications for MCH research and training; genetic disease testing, counseling, and information dissemination; hemophilia diagnostic and treatment centers; and other special projects.

MCH block grants and Title V undergo continual scrutiny in Congress. It remains difficult, given the current federal legislative climate, to predict the eventual shape, state, or amount of MCH block grants. Given the precarious status of the nation's most vulnerable populations, mothers and infants, the developments surrounding Title V funding deserve careful attention.

Other New Programs

When appropriations for Title V exceed $600 million (as they did for the first time in 1992), 12.75 percent of the funds over that level are designated for the Community Integrated Service System (CISS) Program. Preference will then be given to the following projects in local areas with high rates of infant mortality: maternal and infant health home-visiting programs; projects to increase participation of obstetricians and pediatricians; integrated MCH service delivery systems; MCH centers providing pregnancy services for women and preventive and primary care services for infants under the direction of a not-for-profit hospital; MCH projects to serve rural populations; and outpatient and community-based service programs for children with special health care needs.

Two new programs authorized under the Public Health Service Act are also to be administered by the MCH Bureau of the HRSA: Emergency Medical Services for Children (EMSC), in which states work in partnership with medical schools, and the Pediatric/Family HIV Demonstration Grant Program, which provides comprehensive services to pediatric and adolescent AIDS patients and their families. The bureau also administers the Healthy Start infant mortality reduction initiative, whose projects in predominantly urban areas were spearheaded by coalitions involving public, private, religious, and other community-based organizations.

WIC

The Supplemental Food Program For Women, Infants, and Children, or WIC, is funded and administered by the Department of Agriculture in partnership with the states. Eligibility criteria include poverty and risk of poor nutrition for pregnant and postpartum women, nursing mothers and their infants, and children up to five years of age. Program benefits include vouchers for nutritious foods and infant formula, nutrition education, and referrals to comprehensive maternal and child health services.

Early Periodic Screening, Diagnosis, and Treatment

Early Periodic Screening, Diagnosis, and Treatment, or EPSDT, is part of the federal Medicaid program. It provides support for physicians, nurse practitioners, and other qualified midlevel practitioners to perform well-child screening exams on Medicaid-enrolled children from birth to age 21 years. Each state is required to develop an appropriate schedule for these examinations, provide outreach to inform eligible families of this service, and assist with transportation and follow-up as needed. Although EPSDT is the largest federal-state program of child preventive services in the country, it has been vastly underuti-

lized. In some states the EPSDT program has been used successfully as an outreach vehicle for CHIP enrollment. West Virginia's EPSDT Family Outreach Program collaborates with a state perinatal program as well as with CHIP, maximizing the joint effectiveness of funding for preventive care from state and federal sources.[6]

Family Planning

Most family planning services provided through health departments are funded through Medicaid as funding has waned for Title X of the Public Health Service Act. Thus, eligibility for family planning services tends to be restricted to women who qualify for Medicaid. The expansion of non-AFDC Medicaid eligibility for pregnant women usually ends 60 days postpartum, so those mothers who lose Medicaid coverage can be started on birth control, but they generally cannot continue such services. Some states have obtained federal Medicaid waivers to extend the period of eligibility for family planning coverage. Many health departments have special family planning programs for teenagers, sometimes located at or adjacent to high schools in order to increase access.

Other Programs

Numerous programs related to maternal and child health fall outside the realm of the MCH Bureau. For example, child welfare services are administered by the Administration on Children and Families, and the WIC nutritional supplementation program is housed within the Department of Agriculture. Many other federal agencies work with the bureau to serve the needs of women and children, for example, the Substance Abuse and Mental Health Services Administration (SAMHSA) which works in the area of perinatal substance abuse.

OBRA 89

The Omnibus Budget Reconciliation Act of 1989, or OBRA 89, used several mechanisms to facilitate collaboration among agencies serving the MCH population:

- Requirements for coordination between Title V programs, WIC, and Medicaid were strengthened.
- Services provided by Title V agencies to Medicaid-eligible persons must be reimbursed by Medicaid.
- Interagency agreements are required to eliminate duplication of services.
- Standards must be set for EPSDT.
- Adequate outreach services need to be developed.
- Other programmatic cooperation must be facilitated, confidentiality ensured, and billing procedures established.

State interagency agreements include such provisions as toll-free telephone hotlines and referral services, media campaigns about the importance of prenatal care, and door-to-door canvassing for recruitment of pregnant women. Some states train "resource mothers" to support and assist women in enrolling in Medicaid, WIC, and early prenatal care. Provider recruitment efforts and tracking systems to ensure continuity of care for high-risk infants are aspects of other states' incentives. OBRA 89 also required the development of a joint application for enrollment in Title V programs, Medicaid, Head Start, community/migrant health centers, health care for the homeless, and WIC, thus reducing bureaucratic complexity.[7]

The Nature of State Public Health Systems and MCH Services

Every state and territory, as well as the District of Columbia, has a state health agency. The majority function as independent agencies, but about a third are part of consolidated superagencies within state government. The Institute of Medicine, in its 1988 report *The Future of Public Health*, recommended that state health departments serve as lead agencies for a wide range of health-related activities.[8] Currently, Medicaid, mental health, environmental services, and other programs are often administered under other agencies, and maternal and child health functions are divided up under different authorities.

Each state is characterized by one of three patterns of organization: (1) a highly centralized system in which the state has administrative authority, sets uniform statewide standards, and hires personnel as state employees; (2) a decentralized system in which local health programs are responsible to mayors or county commissioners; and (3) a system in which the state agency contracts with and monitors the performance of local providers, such as community health centers and visiting nurses' agencies, but does not sponsor local health departments. In some states, local governments share authority for their health departments with the states. In others, state authority applies to health departments and local authority to other agencies (verbal communication with C. A. Miller, Professor Emeritus, University of North Carolina, Chapel Hill, School of Public Health).

Prioritization and implementation of maternal and child health services vary among states according to organizational and other factors. In highly centralized states, MCH programs developed by the state may be mandated at the local level. In other states, there may be great diversity in county MCH services. In a survey of local public health agencies conducted in 1990, the two most commonly reported services provided were immunizations (92 percent) and child health services (84 percent). Other maternal and child health programs were WIC (69 percent), family planning (59 percent), prenatal care (59 percent), services for handicapped children (47 percent), and obstetrical care (20 percent).[9] States vary in the extent to which personal health care services are provided at local health department sites, based largely on funding sources and availability of alternative providers for Medicaid-eligible and uninsured populations. With major Medicaid eligibility expansions mandated for pregnant women and young children, public programs have seen a dramatic increase in the demand for services in areas lacking private providers who are willing to treat Medicaid clients.

HEALTH SERVICES FOR MCH POPULATIONS

MCH populations include women of childbearing age, pregnant women, infants and toddlers, school-age children, and adolescents. Special needs and programs for these vulnerable groups are addressed next.

Women of Childbearing Age

The public health services offered to women of childbearing age have traditionally focused on reproductive needs and have not always provided comprehensive health care for women. Family planning clinics that target young and multiparous women for the prevention and spacing of pregnancies often provide the major source of primary care for low-income women. Some providers advocate expanding the range of medical services in family planning settings for that reason. Family planning approaches have utilized school-based clinics and postpartum follow-up, seeking to disseminate educational materials regarding available forms of birth control. Screening for sexually transmitted diseases has also become an important component of family planning services.

Contraception and family planning services were significantly restrained by the Reagan and Bush administrations, but the Clinton administration reversed many of these regulations in spite of strong congressional reaction. The politicization of family planning issues by partisan groups makes it difficult to maintain consistent public health policies and programs for women's reproductive health needs.

FDA approval of emergency contraception offers women a new option for regulating their fertility, but education and outreach to both providers and consumers is needed to extend broad access to this family planning method. In the use of traditional and more recent methods of temporary, long-lasting hormonal, and permanent contraception, much remains to be learned about acceptability, accessibility, and ethical issues related to the delivery of services. Greater understanding of cultural differences in fertility decision making will be required to promote the use of family planning services and contraceptive technology while respecting women's reproductive autonomy.

Abortion

Abortions are rarely provided through health departments, but referrals frequently were made to abortion clinics until such actions were forbidden by the Reagan administration. This rule was reversed in the 1990s so that health departments could again play a role in assisting women who chose to terminate pregnancies. The introduction of noninvasive abortion procedures could greatly simplify the early termination of pregnancy and potentially make early abortion more readily available and less costly. With the approval and growing availability of RU-486, it remains to be seen whether women will opt for medical abortion or retain a preference for surgical procedures.

Infertility

Infertility remains a large problem with a wide range of causes. Advanced forms of assisted reproductive technology generally are not available to those of low income and are often not covered by standard insurance policies. However, some basic infertility services, such as the enhancement of ovulation, are available to most women. The prevention and early treatment of venereal disease is an important component of the prevention of infertility. Environmental and occupational exposures require greater attention and investigation as potential causes of fertility problems for both women and men.

HIV and STDs

HIV infection and other sexually transmitted diseases represent a rapidly growing risk to women of reproductive age, particularly those in lower socioeconomic and ethnic minority groups. Teens as well as older women face increasing risks of sexually transmitted infections that not only impair fertility and infant health outcomes, but also act as co-factors for cervical cancer. Public education and condom use are the major prevention strategies available at this time. HIV testing has been widely recommended for pregnant women now that studies have shown that antiretroviral treatment can significantly reduce HIV transmission from mother to baby. This recommendation must be implemented consistently with the need for informed consent in HIV testing. Routinization of HIV testing during pregnancy is arguably an important public health objective, but the current stigma associated with HIV/AIDS requires special sensitivity to confidentiality and choice.

All pregnant women should be offered information about HIV disease, modes of transmission, behavioral risks, and risk reduction strategies. As with any form of screening, HIV screening must be contingent upon availability of services for ongoing evaluation, monitoring, and treatment.

Preconceptional Health Promotion

Preconceptional health promotion is an emerging and promising field. Many of the important events in fetal development occur in the first few weeks of pregnancy, before the woman even knows of her condition. To prevent fetal damage in those vulnerable early weeks, it is critical for the prospective mother to reduce the hazards of the uterine environment by avoiding alcohol and drug use and optimizing her health status with good nutrition, vitamin supplements, rest, and exercise. Preconceptional health promotion programs provide education and encouragement to women before pregnancy to modify their behavior and reduce early risks to fetal development.

Breast and cervical cancer screening and detection of other chronic diseases are also important functions for health departments. These services can be provided to women of childbearing age in conjunction with preconceptional health promotion.

Pregnant Women

The use of prenatal care early and regularly throughout pregnancy has been demonstrated repeatedly to be associated with improved pregnancy outcomes. Traditional prenatal care services were designed to detect early signs of medical problems, such as preeclampsia, that are known to complicate the latter months of pregnancy and increase maternal and infant morbidity and mortality. The Institute of Medicine and the American College of Obstetrics and Gynecology have more recently advocated modifications of prenatal visit schedules to screen women early in pregnancy for risk of preterm delivery and to monitor closely those women found to be at high risk.

Additional efforts have focused on using home visitation, social support services, and educational materials to reduce stress and modify maternal behavior in order to achieve optimal birth outcomes.

The malpractice crisis in obstetrics caused many family physicians and some obstetricians to stop delivering babies with the result that delivery services and even prenatal care are less available, particularly for the poor and those living in rural areas. Both private and public insurers are increasingly utilizing managed care strategies for reimbursing maternity care as well as other personal health care services. The impact on public health department and other community clinics, traditionally important sources of prenatal care for low-income women, must be carefully monitored. In all managed care settings the adequacy and quality of care for pregnant women, as well as cost-effectiveness and efficiency, need to be closely observed and continuously improved.

Women in the workforce often face additional challenges in meeting their health needs. Pregnant women often work at jobs that do not permit time off for prenatal care visits. The physical stresses of work, the need for day care services, and the lack of adequate health insurance for pregnancy-related services further undermine the provision of prenatal and delivery care for many women.

Infant and Toddler Health

Many health departments have the capacity to provide only well-child care, leaving families to find other means for dealing with acute and chronic illness. This division of health care services does not serve the population well, and it impedes the development of trusting and consistent relationships between patients and providers. Well-child care lays the basis for prevention and early intervention, but it needs to function in the context of comprehensive care. It will be essential to assess the influence of managed care as well as CHIP on children's preventive health services.

Well-child care consists of assessment, counseling, and some medical interventions tailored to the stage of development and the needs and resources of the family. The assessment of growth and development provides a sensitive measure of child health, nutrition, and family functioning. Screening for anemia, deficits in hearing and vision, and abnormal blood pressure are recommended in early childhood. Under special circumstances, additional screening might be warranted for tuberculosis, lead poisoning, and hemoglobinopathies. By age four, children should have received a screening dental examination. Assessments also should be made of the child's risk status for illness and injuries as well as exposure to tobacco smoke and other environmental hazards. Additionally, it is important to identify potential problem areas in the family's critical role of nurturing and providing essential resources for the child.

Counseling

Counseling is tailored to the developmental level of the child and the resources and capacities of the family. Counseling should focus on the three or four most pertinent issues that emerge from the assessment. Both counseling and assessment processes should be sensitive to the diversity of families' cultures and values. Counseling will be most successful when it is provided in a supportive environment with appropriate referral and follow-up. Because future developmental events are predictable, it is also possible to offer anticipatory guidance for problems likely to arise before the next scheduled visit.

Immunizations

Immunizations remain one of the most effective means of preventing disease. The schedule for immunizations is constantly being revised as new vaccines become available. The current immunization schedule requires at least six visits between birth and school entry, with as many as five immunizations given at some of those visits. Because of state regulations, virtually all children are fully immunized before school entry. However, there is far less success at immunizing young children adequately prior to their second birthday. Recent estimates indicate that 40 to 50 percent of 2-year-old children have not received all the recommended immunizations by 18 months of age. The United States still ranks among the worst of the nations of the Western Hemisphere in achieving full immunization of children under 2 years of age.

Day Care Sites for Service Delivery

Child day care centers become logical sites for the provision of health services to preschool children as more women join the workforce. Day care offers the opportunity to combine health care with services to enhance physical and cognitive development and social skills. Parents can benefit from health education and child development programs in the day care setting. There is also growing evidence that high-risk families benefit by home visitation that provides one-on-one assistance in parenting skills, enhancing child development and providing social support to mothers living under stressful circumstances.

School-Age Children and Adolescents

Health department staff often work closely with schools to provide important health services to the school-age population. On-site school nursing services have moved beyond the traditional screening programs for hearing, vision, and scoliosis to include health assessments of individual children at risk, counseling services, and even medical services such as illness care, family planning, and the treatment of chronic medical problems. In addition to providing specific health services, health department personnel often work in partnership with teachers to provide health education to students in the classroom setting as well as one-on-one.

School-based or school-linked clinics are emerging as a way of getting needed health services to the adolescent population. Services are often linked to the curriculum so that students who are learning about topics such as sexually transmitted diseases can have access to related services in or adjacent to the school building. Such linkages have also led to controversial programs such as condom distribution and family planning services. Substance abuse prevention, AIDS education, and violence prevention are the major issues dominating school health programs at this time.

MCH Services in the Future

Moving beyond health care reform, maternal and child health advocates are eager to assure that the historical lessons of federal MCH policy guide future steps. Some lessons learned include the advantage of comprehensive service models for low-income populations and the need to streamline and coordinate a full array of services to make them accessible and efficient. The importance of basing programs in community settings has been recognized as a means of ensuring their acceptance and cultural competence. Orienting services to involve and meet the needs of entire families recognizes the impact of health problems on all family members and the therapeutic potential of family systems.

Another lesson from federal MCH policy is the need to make public systems more user-friendly for providers as well as patients, eliminating unnecessary bureaucratic hassles and providing adequate support for the care of traditionally underserved groups. Acceptability of services for both providers and patients requires elimination of the inequities and stigmatization traditionally attached to programs for low-income women and children. Thus, the trend in public health services for the MCH population has been and should continue to be towards community-based, family-centered, integrated delivery systems of comprehensive services with increased incentives for provider participation.

There is a major effort now under way to move Medicaid patients into managed care plans. Advocates suggest that these women and children will welcome better-coordinated mainstream medical care in the private sector over the care they currently receive in the public sector. However, private sector health care has not traditionally been organized to coordinate the range of care needed by low-income pregnant women, including outreach, nutritional, health education, psychosocial, care coordination, and follow-up services. The successful approaches of public providers in offering appropriate, comprehensive services for low-income families will need to be incorporated into new service delivery systems.

With the spotlight on the future of health care, maternal and child health providers will need to join with families and advocates to provide oversight to the change process, to build upon the lessons learned in this important realm of public health, and to ensure governmental accountability for achieving the objectives of health reform for all of the nation's mothers and children. With the overriding goal of eliminating health disparities, *Healthy People 2010* represents a national consensus on objectives for health promotion and disease prevention in the United States. Providers, consumers, advocates, and researchers can access the full report and leading indicators on the Internet through the Web site http://www.health.gov/healthypeople.

CONCLUSION

Mothers and infants are our most vulnerable populations. Efforts have been expended since the early 1900s to ensure services to mothers and children. We have developed, over the years, a network of programs designed to benefit maternal and child health. As forces develop that may threaten this range of services, public health must remain vigilant to assure services to these populations.

References

1. Lesser AJ. The origin and development of maternal and child health programs in the United States. *Am J Public Health.* 1985;75(6):590-598.
2. Rosenbaum S. The Maternal and Child Health Block Grant Act of 1981: Teaching an old program new tricks. *Clearinghouse Rev.* August/September 1983:400-414.
3. National Center for Children in Poverty. *Five Million Children: 1992 Update.* New York, NY: Columbia University School of Public Health; 1992.
4. Braveman P, Bennett T. Information for action: An advocate's guide to using maternal and child health data. Washington, DC: Children's Defense Fund; 1993.

5. US Department of Health and Human Services. *Understanding Title V of the Social Security Act.* Washington, DC: Public Health Service, Health Resources and Services Administration, Maternal and Child Health Bureau; undated.

6. Summer L, Carpenter MB, Kavanagh LD. *Successful Outreach Strategies: Ten Programs That Link Children to Health Services.* Arlington, Va: National Center for Education in Maternal and Child Health; 1999.

7. *Dedicated to Care for Children: A Report on States Use of OBRA 1986 Earmarked Title V Funds.* Washington, DC: Association of Maternal and Child Health Programs; 1990.

8. Institute of Medicine, Committee for the Study of the Future of Public Health. *The Future of Public Health.* Washington, DC: National Academy Press; 1988.

9. National Association of County and City Health Officials. National profile of local health departments. Washington, DC: 1992.

CHAPTER
26

Injury Control

Maria Seguí-Gómez, M.D., Sc.D
Susan P. Baker, Ph.D.

INTRODUCTION

We normally think of health problems or diseases as those conditions associated with exposure to infectious agents (e.g., HIV, malaria) or environmental agents (e.g., tobacco, lead), or due to genetic disorders. Yet, the leading cause of years of potential life lost, the fourth leading cause of death, and one of the top causes of disability in the U.S. population has nothing to do with those conditions. These deaths and morbid and disabling conditions relate to acute exposure to some form of energy in amounts that exceed the individual's tolerance thresholds, therefore resulting in injuries. This is a health problem as old as humankind.

Given the magnitude of this problem, it would seem natural, then, that as public health practitioners we should turn our attention to injuries and their control. Unfortunately, this has not been always the case.

Injuries and their prevention have not traditionally been embraced as a public health issue. One obstacle

has been the belief that injuries are the result of "accidents," which has placed them in that awkward position of being considered by many to be unpredictable and therefore unpreventable. In the instances in which they were "investigated," the conclusion was often that they were primarily due to some irresponsible behavior on the part of the injured individual or someone else. As a result, injury control has been retarded by the "accident" folklore, including the notion of reckless, selfish, careless, and intoxicated people as primarily responsible for injuries.[1] Thus, until the last quarter of the twentieth century, the field of injury control was characterized by misunderstanding, lack of progress, and scarcity of relevantly trained scientists.

In this chapter we will provide a brief overview of the injury problem. The chapter is designed to provide a general orientation, rather than an exhaustive discussion. The goal is to facilitate a clearer understanding of the role of the public health practitioner and public health agencies in the reduction of the burden related to injuries. To achieve that goal we will present useful definitions and conceptual frameworks, a summary of the magnitude of the problem, and examples of the use of public health tools in its prevention. Emphasis is placed on the preventability of these injuries and wherever possible we have provided examples of prevention efforts. It is not our intent to provide a detailed account of the epidemiology of injuries, nor the effectiveness or efficiency (or lack thereof) of all interventions tested to date. Many other references are available to the reader interested in those matters.[2-5]

DEFINITION OF *INJURY*

We will use the term *injury* to describe any damage to the body due to acute exposure to amounts of thermal, mechanical (kinetic or potential), electrical, or chemical energy that exceed the individual's tolerance for such energy, or to the absence of such essentials as heat or oxygen. We have, therefore, adopted the broad definition first described in *Injury Prevention*[6] and recently endorsed by the latest Institute of Medicine report[7] which includes intentional injuries (e.g., homicide, suicide) as well as unintentional injuries. This chapter also encompasses injuries regardless of where they occur (e.g., outdoors, at home or school), the activity that was taking place when the injurious event happened (e.g., occupational, recreational, sports-related), or the object that was involved in the energy transfer (e.g., motor vehicle, consumer product, gun). Table 26.1 lists energy types, their frequency as the source of fatal injuries in the U.S. population, the vehicles (or vectors) that most frequently transfer the energy, and the most common types of resulting injuries.

DIMENSIONS AND MAGNITUDE OF THE PROBLEM

In the United States, approximately 150,000 people die every year because of injuries.[8] Injuries, therefore, constitute the fourth leading cause of death in our population, right behind cancer, heart, cerebrovascular, and respiratory diseases (Table 26.2). However, injuries are

Table 26.1. Examples of Energy, Vehicle, Injury Types and Their Incidence in the 1998 U.S. Fatally Injured Population ($N = $ **150,445**)

Etiology of Injury	Vehicle (vector)	Type of Injuries	Percentage of Deaths
Kinetic energy	Motor vehicle, train, other vehicles, guns, knives, machinery	Abrasions, contusions, sprains, strains, dislocations, fractures, concussion, blunt, open wounds (cuts, piercing), crushing	54.7
Chemical energy	Drugs, cleaning products, poisonous animals	Poisonings, burns	13.5
Absence of oxygen	Water, foreign objects	Strangulation, suffocation, drowning	8.1
Potential energy*	Falling person	Same as kinetic	11.1
Thermal energy	Fire	Burns, heat stroke	2.5
Electrical energy	Wires, appliances	Electrocutions	0.4
Ionizing energy		Radiation damage	<0.1
Absence of heat		Frostbite	0.3
Unknown			9.4

SOURCE: CDC Wonder, compressed 1998 (online). Available at: http://wonder.cdc.gov.
*It has been argued, however, that potential energy causes injury only when transformed into kinetic energy.

Table 26.2. Five Most Common Causes of Death by Age Category, 1998

Rank	<1	1–4	5–9	10–14	15–24	25–34	35–44	45–54	55–64	65+	Total
1	Congenital Anomalies 6,212	Injuries 2,377	Injuries 1,736	Injuries 2,368	Injuries 23,332	Injuries 22,709	Injuries 26,817	Malignant Neoplasms 45,747	Malignant Neoplasms 87,024	Heart Disease 605,673	Heart Disease 724,859
2	Short Gestation 4,101	Congenital Anomalies 564	Malignant Neoplasms 487	Malignant Neoplasms 526	Malignant Neoplasms 1,699	Malignant Neoplasms 4,385	Malignant Neoplasms 17,022	Heart Disease 35,056	Heart Disease 65,068	Malignant Neoplasms 384,186	Malignant Neoplasms 541,532
3	SIDS 2,822	Malignant Neoplasms 365	Congenital Anomalies 198	Congenital Anomalies 173	Heart Disease 1,057	Heart Disease 3,207	Heart Disease 13,593	Injuries 18,534	Injuries 11,283	Cerebro-vascular 139,144	Cerebro-vascular 158,448
4	Maternal Complications 1,343	Heart Disease 214	Heart Disease 156	Heart Disease 170	Congenital Anomalies 450	HIV 2,912	HIV 5,746	Liver Disease 5,744	Bronchitis Emphysema Asthma 10,162	Bronchitis Emphysema Asthma 97,896	Injuries 150,445
5	Respiratory Distress Synd. 1,295	Pneumonia & Influenza 146	Pneumonia & Influenza 70	Bronchitis Emphysema Asthma 98	Bronchitis Emphysema Asthma 239	Cerebrovas-cular 670	Liver Disease 3,370	Cerebro-vascular 5,709	Cerebro-vascular 9,653	Pneumonia & Influenza 82,989	Bronchitis Emphysema Asthma 112,584

SOURCE: Adapted from report by Centers for Disease Control and Prevention.

the leading cause of death for individuals ages 1 through 44. Therefore, injuries become the most important cause of Years of Potential Life Lost (YPLL), almost 20 and 25 percent higher than the YPLLs associated with cancer and cardiovascular diseases, respectively (Figure 26.1).

In addition to deaths, injuries result in some 2.5 million hospital admissions (fractures alone represent 3 percent of all hospital discharges) and more than one-quarter of all emergency room visits, for a total of almost 100 million physician contacts every year.[9] The relationship between mortality and morbidity (or different degrees of severity) is referred to as the "iceberg" or "pyramid" of injury (Figure 26.2) and the actual ratio between each of the levels of that pyramid varies depending on the specific injury or the specific injury mechanism, as some injuries are more lethal than others. For example, gun-related injuries are much more likely to be fatal than fall-related injuries. Table 26.3 further illustrates this point by presenting the crude death and hospitalization rates per 100,000 population by several mechanisms of injury. In the table, homicide/legal interventions have a death:hospitalization ratio of 1:1.9, whereas fall-related injuries have a ratio of 1:16.4.

Injuries are also a leading source of short- and long-term disability. It is estimated that some 7 percent of individuals who are injured sustain some degree of disability, which means some 4 million new cases per year.[10]

When one combines mortality, morbidity, and disability in a metric such as the Disability Adjusted Life Years (DALYs), injuries are responsible for approximately 15 percent of all DALYs lost in the developed world. Worse yet, it is estimated that by the year 2020, injuries (road traffic crashes and self-inflicted injuries) will be the second leading cause of DALYs lost in the developed world—right after ischaemic heart disease. Worldwide, road traffic injuries alone are anticipated to be the third cause of lost DALYs, right after ischaemic heart disease and unipolar major depression.[11]

The economic impact of injuries is significant also. It is estimated that the aggregate lifetime costs of all injuries produced in a year amounted to nearly $180 billion dollars in 1988.[12] In a 1994 study done by the National Highway Traffic Safety Administration (NHTSA), the injury-related costs of motor vehicle crashes were $94 billion[13], an approximate $30,000 per each of the 3,215,000 police-reported victims for that year.[14] In 2000, the most recent year for which official statistics are available, the number of police-reported victims was 3,231,000.[15]

Last, a summary on the impact of injuries cannot be complete without reference to the largely unmeasured but immense burden that they impose on families and communities. The literature in this field is peppered with evidence of higher divorce rates among parents of injury victims, higher school dropout rates among

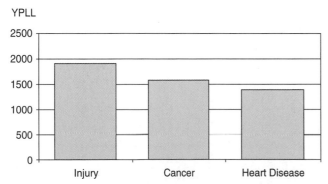

Figure 26.1. Years of Potential Life Lost* by Cause of Death

Adapted from Institute of Medicine report, 2000.

*Years of Potential Life Lost calculated up to age 75.

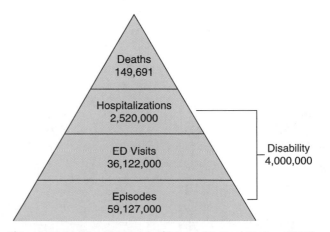

Figure 26.2. The Pyramid of Injury (United States, 1997)

Sources: CDC Wonder, 1997; Warner et al., 2000.

Table 26.3.   Crude Rates of Deaths and Hospitalizations Due to External Cause of Injury per 100,000 Population

	Deaths	Hospitalizations
Motor Vehicle E810-E825.9	16.08	46.3
Falls E880-E888.9	6.02	98.7
Drowning E830 E832 E910.9	1.63	0.1
Fires/Flames E890-E899.9	1.2	1.2
Poisonings E850-E869.9	3.99	0.5
Homicide/Legal Intervention E960-E978.9	6.76	13.4
Suicide E950-E959.9	11.3	3.3
Other	8.64	8.7
Total E800-E999.9	55.62	251.3

SOURCE: Death rates: 1998 CDC Wonder (online). Available at: http://wonder.cdc.gov. Hospitalization: analysis of the 1998 or 1997 hospital discharge data of the following eight states: Michigan, North Carolina, South Carolina, Massachusetts, Washington, Wisconsin, Maryland, and Colorado (not published), State Population 1997 or 1998 U.S. Census. Injuries were classified using E codes (*International Classification of Diseases,* 9th rev. Geneva, Switzerland: World Health Organization 1997).

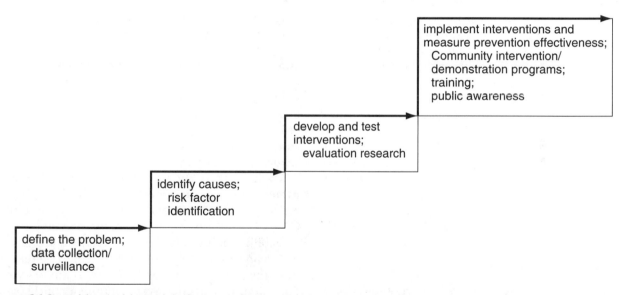

Figure 26.3.   Public Health Model of a Scientific Approach to Prevention

Source: National Center for Injury Prevention and Control, Centers for Disease Control and Prevention.

siblings of victims, and higher alcohol and drug involvement among relatives and others.[16]

THE ROLE OF PUBLIC HEALTH

As with any other population health problem, one can apply the public health model of a scientific approach to prevention (Figure 26.3).

During the remainder of this chapter, we will follow this model. Under "Epidemiological Framework", we will discuss issues related to the definition of the problem: data collection and surveillance, the identification of causes and risk factors, and the development of interventions. Under "Choice and Evaluation of Countermeasures" we will present issues related to the testing and selection of interventions.

Issues that relate to the last step of the public health model will be presented in the "Axioms to Guide Injury Prevention" section and in our discussion on the roles of public health practitioners and public health agencies.

Epidemiological Framework

Injury epidemiology allows for investigation of the interaction between the host (or individual injured), the etiological agent (energy), the vehicle or vector that transmits the energy, and the physical and sociocultural environment where the interaction occurs. (*Vehicles* are the inanimate objects that transmit the energy [e.g., cars, matches, guns] whereas *vectors* are the plants, animals, or persons that transmit the energy [e.g., biting animals, poisonous snakes, human fists].) The use of epidemiology has helped demonstrate that injuries, like diseases, display long-term trends and demographic, geographic, socioeconomic, and seasonal patterns. However, it was not until 1949 that Dr. John Gordon first acknowledged that injury occurrence and severity, much like any other health condition, could be measured and related to different characteristics of individuals, the sources of injuries, and their environments. It was only in 1961 that Dr. James Gibson separated the role of the vehicles or vectors from that of the energy they transmit, thus enabling the application of the analytical framework of epidemiology to the study of injuries. (Readers interested in a more extensive review of the history of injury control are referred to the work of J. A. Waller.)[17]

Data Collection and Surveillance

Effective injury control requires collection of appropriate detailed data (e.g., frequency, location) related to the injury under study and the events or circumstances surrounding that injury. The analysis of such data helps us to understand the epidemiological patterns of these problems, identify risk factors, suggest causal factors, and guide us in the development of preventive interventions. At times, researchers develop unique data collection efforts to better address the issues under investigation. Most commonly, though, existing datasets are used, despite the fact that most of these datasets are administrative in nature and tend to be oriented either toward the injuries (i.e., the medical aspects) or toward the events (i.e., the incidents or "accident" aspects), and rarely include enough detailed information for both. Several U.S. government and private agencies maintain data systems that collect injury data on a continuous basis as part of their public health practice. Table 26.4 lists some of the most commonly used data systems, as well as their Web addresses.

Identification of Causes and Development of Interventions

We have indicated, thus far, that injuries involve an unfavorable interaction between etiologic agents and the individual. Therefore, the essence of injury prevention involves keeping the etiologic agent from reaching the potential host at all (i.e., preventing the interaction) or from reaching it at rates and amounts that would produce damage (i.e., minimizing the consequences). Under some circumstances, prevention is aimed at modifying the agent; under others, at reducing exposure to the agent or the susceptibility of individuals. Several conceptual models have been developed over the past 30 years to facilitate understanding of injury-producing events and possible countermeasures. Before we present these models, let us revisit the sequence of injury events.

We live in a particular environment. In this environment, we conduct our lives: we walk, drive, exercise, prepare meals, and do countless other things. On each occasion, we are exposing ourselves to the possibility of undergoing a fortuitous event that may lead to an injury. This is what could be referred to as the *exposure* component of the chain of events. For example, consider every minute a child spends enjoying a playground. Every so often, an *event* may happen. (Events are what many people would refer to as accidents.) Following our example, the child falls from the swing. In only a fraction of these falls will the event lead to any *injury*. Some of these injuries, however, may be severe enough to cause death or disability. This chain of events is depicted in Figure 26.4. This sequence of events is very similar to what has been labeled as the Domino Model[18] because of the linear relationship between the different

Table 26.4.   Selected Surveillance Systems Used in Injury Control

Data System	Acronym	Federal Agency	Web Address
Census of Fatal Occupational Injuries	CFOI	Bureau of Labor Statistics	http://www.bls.gov
Survey of Occupational Injuries and Illnesses	SOII	Bureau of Labor Statistics	http://www.bls.gov
National Crime Victimization Survey	NCVS	Bureau of Justice Statistics	http://www.ojp.usdoj.gov
National Ambulatory Medical Care Survey	AMCS	Centers for Disease Control and Prevention	http://www.cdc.gov/nchswww
National Hospital Ambulatory Medical Care Survey	NHAMCS	Centers for Disease Control and Prevention	http://www.cdc.gov/nchswww
National Hospital Discharge Survey	NHDS	Centers for Disease Control and Prevention	http://www.cdc.gov/nchswww
National Health Interview Survey	NHIS	Centers for Disease Control and Prevention	http://www.cdc.gov/nchswww
National Mortality Followback Survey—1993	NMFS93	Centers for Disease Control and Prevention	http://www.cdc.gov/nchswww
National Vital Statistics Systems—Current Mortality Sample	NVSSS	Centers for Disease Control and Prevention	http://www.cdc.gov/nchswww
National Vital Statistics Systems—Final Mortality Data	NVSSF	Centers for Disease Control and Prevention	http://www.cdc.gov/nchswww
Behavioral Risk Factor Surveillance System	BRFSS	Centers for Disease Control and Prevention	http://www.cdc.gov/nccdphp/brfss
Youth Risk Behavioral Surveillance System	YRBSS	Centers for Disease Control and Prevention	http://www.cdc.gov/nccdphp/dash/yrbs
National Traumatic Occupational Fatality Surveillance System	NTOF	Centers for Disease Control and Prevention	http://www.cdc.gov
National Electronic Injury Surveillance System	NEISS	Consumer Product Safety Commission	http://www.cpsc.gov
Law Enforcement Officers Killed and Assaulted	LEOKA	Federal Bureau of Investigation	http://www.fbi.gov/ucr
National Incident Based Reporting System	NIBRS	Federal Bureau of Investigation	http://www.ch.search.org
Uniform Crime Reporting System—Supplemental Homicide Report	UCRSHR	Federal Bureau of Investigation	http://www.fbi.gov
Nationwide Personal Transportation System	NPTS	Federal Highway Administration	http://www.bts.gov/ntda/npts
Healthcare Cost and Utilization Project	HCUP-3	Agency for Health Care Policy and Research	http://www.ahcpr.gov/data

(continued)

Table 26.4. Selected Surveillance Systems Used in Injury Control (*continued*)

Data System	Acronym	Federal Agency	Web Address
Healthcare Finance Administration	CMS	Centers for Medicare & Medicaid Services (formerly the Health Care Financing Administration)	http://www.cms.hhs.gov
Indian Health Service—Ambulatory Care System	IHSACS	Indian Health Service	http://www.ihs.gov
Indian Health Service—Inpatient Care System	IHSICS	Indian Health Service	http://www.ihs.gov
National Child Abuse and Neglect Data System	NCANDS	National Center for Child Abuse and Neglect	http://www.ndacan.cornell.edu
National Incidence Study of Child Abuse and Neglect	NIS	Office of Child Abuse and Neglect (formerly the National Center for Child Abuse and Neglect)	http://www.ndacan.cornell.edu/Flyers
Fatal Accident Reporting System	FARS	National Highway Traffic Safety Administration	http://www.nhtsa.dot.gov/fars
National Accident Sampling System—Crashworthiness Data System	NASSCDS	National Highway Traffic Safety Administration	http://www.nhtsa.dot.gov/people
National Accident Sampling System—General Estimates System	NASSGES	National Highway Traffic Safety Administration	http://www.nhtsa.dot.gov/people
National Occupant Protection Use Survey	NOPUS	National Highway Traffic Safety Administration	http://www.nhtsa.dot.gov
Monitoring the Future Study	MTFS	National Institute of Drug Abuse	http://www.health.org/mtfs
Drug Abuse Warning Network	DAWN	Substance Abuse and Mental Health Services Administration	http://www.health.org/pubs/dawn
Census of Agriculture—1997	BCCOA	Bureau of the Census	http://www.nass.usda.gov/census
National Fire Incident Reporting System	NFIRS	Fire Administration	http://www.usta.fema.gov/nfdc

components of this model. Injury prevention will consist of intervention(s) aimed at blocking the progression of the events. In our example, we could have prevented the event from happening by eliminating the swings from the playground area or by designing them in such a fashion that prevents ejection of the child. We could have minimized the impact of the fall by using an energy-absorbing flooring underneath the swing. Finally, we could have minimized the consequences of the injury by providing quick care at a pediatric facility with expertise in head injury.

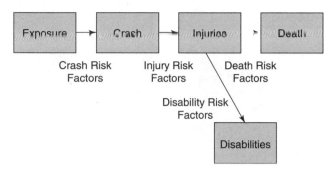

Figure 26.4. Chain of Injury Events

The Haddon Matrix

Dr. William Haddon, a pioneer in the field of injury prevention, proposed a framework that integrates the role of the *individual,* the *vehicle* or vector carrying the energy, and the *environment* in which the interaction occurs with the sequence of events associated with the injury.[19] This sequence of events is divided into *pre-event* (i.e., preventing the event or incident from occurring), *event* (i.e., preventing injury while the event is happening), and *post-event* (i.e., minimizing the adverse results after the event has occurred). For example, interventions aimed at eliminating motor vehicle crashes or falls from windows are pre-event interventions. Event interventions are aimed at either preventing the injury or at reducing the resulting injury by minimizing its severity. Examples of interventions at this stage would include bicycle helmets that protect children when they fall from bikes, or pills with smaller medication doses so that they are not as toxic if ingested inappropriately. The variety and effectiveness of countermeasures at this event stage highlight the point that even if the event (e.g., crash) is not prevented, damage to passengers and occupants can be reduced or eliminated. Post-event interventions can be directed to two goals: reducing any further damage or restoring the health of the individual who sustained injuries.

In Table 26.5 we have listed potential interventions to prevent motor vehicle-related injuries, particularly child occupant injuries, using the Haddon Matrix.

Haddon's Ten Basic Strategies

After developing the matrix, Haddon described 10 basic strategies for injury control, presented here with examples relating to injury produced by chemicals (in parentheses):

1. *Prevent the initial marshaling of the agent.* (Do not produce lead paint.)
2. *Reduce the amount of the agent marshaled.* (Package medicine in small quantities.)
3. *Prevent release of the agent.* (Use childproof caps on bottles of medicine.)
4. *Modify rate or spatial distribution of release of agent from its source.* (Devise containers that release poison at limited rates.)
5. *Separate, in space or time, the agent from the susceptible person.* (Keep children out of orchards while spraying.)
6. *Separate the agent from the susceptible person with a material barrier.* (Use gas masks.)
7. *Modify the contact surface, subsurface, or basic characteristics of the agent.* (Reformulate detergents to make them less caustic.)
8. *Strengthen the resistance of the person who might otherwise be damaged.* (Immunize susceptible people against insect stings.)
9. *Counter the continuation and extension of the damage.* (Provide and make use of first-aid treatment and poison control centers.)
10. *Repair and rehabilitate.* (Institute intermediate and long-term therapy.)

Obviously, there are some commonalities between these 10 countermeasures and the matrix described in the previous section. Several of these countermeasures relate to the host,[5,6,8] some to the vehicle or vector,[1–4,7] and some to the environment.[5,6,9,10] They could also be classified as pre-event, event, or post-event. Actually, some authors have indicated that countermeasures 1 through 3 could be described as pre-event interventions, 4 through 8 as event interventions, and 9 and 10 as post-event interventions,[20] although Haddon himself disagreed with such categorization. For example, countermeasure 1 could also be an event intervention, and countermeasure 5 could also be considered a pre-event intervention.

Table 26.5. Haddon Matrix with Selected Examples of Motor Vehicle Occupant Injury Prevention Interventions

	Host (Child and Adult Occupants)	Vehicle (Car)	Environment Physical (road)	Socioeconomic
PRE-CRASH	Avoid behaviors that may distract driver Driver's age, gender, driving experience, drug or alcohol use, fatigue	Antilock brakes Speed Daytime running lights	Traffic patterns (e.g., exit ramps, crossings) Weather, visibility	Children in rear seats Legislation regarding child restraint Speed limits, licensing laws
CRASH	Adequate child restraint Safety belts, airbags	Seating position Built-in child car seats Sensors detecting occupant's size/weight Vehicle speed, size, and mass Interior surfaces	Separation from other lanes Energy-absorbing roadside fixtures	
POST-CRASH	Exercise and other health enhancement to reduce comorbidity	Crash detection systems that notify EMS (and indicate type of occupants on board) Designs to facilitate extrication Improve location of fuel tank	Designated lanes for emergency vehicles Reduce distance from EMS	Insurance system EMS system prepared to handle children Societal acceptance of residual disabilities

Human Performance and Environmental Demands Model

Another system-oriented model was described in the ergonomics literature by Blumenthal.[21] This model is centered on the dynamic interaction between the subject and his or her environment (Figure 26.5). The lower line represents the variable demands of a particular task, for example, driving a car, and includes the limitations and deficiencies in the vehicle and the environment (including other drivers). The upper line represents the performance of the subject of interest. The injurious event occurs when the system demands increase and/or the subject performance decreases simultaneously to levels at which they overlap. At times, it is the individual's behavior that fails dramatically, such as in the situation of a driver who suffers a myocardial infarction or stroke. At other times, it is the system that becomes overwhelming, as in the case where another vehicle on the road has a tire blowout. The third, and most common situation, involves neither cataclysmic human failure nor overwhelming demands, but rather a simultaneous decrease in performance and increase in task demand. Such would be the situation where an intoxicated driver (who may be able to drive in a straight line) fails to negotiate an unexpected curve or a teenager is distracted by a passenger.

Historically, efforts in injury prevention have focused on the individual's performance. It is only recently that attention has been focused on simplifying the task (i.e., the demands).

Choice and Evaluation of Countermeasures

The role of epidemiology in identifying modifiable risk factors is closely related to the identification of countermeasures. Modifiable risk factors become the basis for intervention design. It should be emphasized that factors playing an important role in minor injuries are not necessarily the same as factors that are important in severe or fatal injuries. Consequently, the choice of countermeasure may change as the severity of injuries changes. It should also be emphasized that countermeasures should not be determined by the relative importance of causal or contributing factors or by their earliness in the sequence of events. Rather, priority and emphasis should be given to

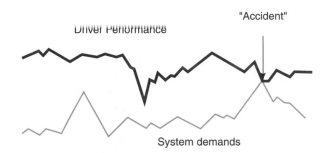

Figure 26.5. Hypothetical Localized System Failure
Source: Blumenthal, 1968.

measures that will most effectively and efficiently reduce injury losses. For example, although psychological factors may be important in the initiation of motor vehicle crashes, it does not follow that psychological screening of drivers would be fruitful.

It is also important to discuss the assumption that anything that sounds reasonable will be effective; this has been the rationale for countless programs, from "defensive driving" training to holiday death counts. Safety programs not only may lack effectiveness, but under certain circumstances they could even increase the number or severity of injuries, as in the case of driver education programs that enable teenagers to drive at an earlier age than they otherwise would.[22]

Numerous safety measures have been adopted without proof of their effectiveness, or have not been evaluated. The resulting entrenchment of untested measures makes improvement difficult and comparison with alternatives impossible. Millions of dollars can be wasted in unsuccessful safety campaigns, and without adequate preplanned evaluation, no one will ever know whether a campaign was effective and guidance for the future will be lost. In contrast, many other interventions have been evaluated. Table 26.6 lists selected injury control interventions that have been proven effective. For a review on the issues involved in evaluating injury more detailed prevention interventions, refer to Dannenberg and Fowler's article in *Injury Prevention*.[23]

Another issue to keep in mind when selecting countermeasures is that, very frequently, a "mixed

Table 26.6. Examples of Injury Prevention Strategies of Known Effectiveness[12]

Motor vehicle	Child passenger restraint
	Child passenger restraint laws
	Safety belts
	Safety belt laws
	Sobriety check points
	Laceration protective windshields
	Nighttime curfews for teenage drivers
	Pedestrian-friendly front end of automobiles
	Minimum drinking age laws
	Breakaway utility poles
Firearm	Absence of handguns in homes
Fires/burns	Manufacture of fire-safe cigarettes
	Smoke detectors
	Automatic sprinklers
	Fire-resistant pajamas for children
	Legislation regulating flammability of children's clothing
	Fire exits and fire drills
Recreational	Four-sided barriers for swimming pools
	Bicycle helmet use
	Promoting bicycle helmet use (e.g., laws)
	Break-away bases for softball
Sports injuries	Mouthguards
	Protective equipment (e.g., knee and elbow pads, wrist pads for inline skating)
Falls	Window guards in high-rise buildings
	Prevention or treatment of osteoporosis in women
	Protective hip pads for elderly
	Weight-bearing exercise among elderly
	Fall-cushioning materials underneath playground equipment
Poisonings	Packaging of children's aspirin in sublethal doses
Farm	Rollover protective structures on farm tractors
Choking and suffocation	Legislation and product design changes (e.g., safe refrigerator disposal, warning labels on thin plastic bags)
All injuries	Minimum drinking age of 21
	Increase in excise tax for alcohol
	911 response systems

strategy" should be employed, incorporating countermeasures that address complementary aspects. Here the challenge will be in choosing the right type, intensity, and order of interventions to make the "combined" countermeasures most efficient. For example, whether airbags should be designed to protect even unbelted occupants in a frontal collision or as a supplement to safety belts became the issue of a long and intense dispute among motor vehicle safety specialists in the early 1980s. Once it was decided that they should be supplemental restraints, the issue of which crashes were severe enough to warrant airbag deployment in a belted occupant became the new topic of debate.[24]

Choices must be made, by default if not consciously, on such matters as these or on the question of how many dollars to spend in preventing a given number of lost days or injury hospitalizations or deaths. More complicated still are decisions as to how many hundreds of drivers a state will attempt to take off the road in an effort to prevent one of them from killing himself or herself or someone else. This conscious weighting of alternatives is often lacking in the safety field.

AXIOMS TO GUIDE INJURY PREVENTION

Over the years, enough experience has been gathered to establish several axioms that can help guide efforts in controlling injuries. These were explained and illustrated in the first edition of this chapter by Sleet and Rosenberg and are presented again [25] in the sections below:

A. Injury Results from Interactions between People and the Environment

The agent of injury will cause little damage if the amount of energy reaching tissues is below human tolerance levels. For example, tap water temperature of less than 120 degrees Fahrenheit is not likely to acutely damage human tissue, although higher temperatures may. The importance of this interaction is recognized by approaches that control the environment by reducing hot water temperatures at the tap and that simultaneously target the elderly and parents of small children for education about hot water scald risk, including the need for reduced tap water temperatures.

B. Injury-Producing Interactions Can Be Modified through Changing Behavior, Products, or Environments

Modifying the weakest or most adaptable link in the chain of causation can reduce injuries. Unsanctioned swimming in a home swimming pool is more easily reduced by placing an isolation fence or barrier between the child and the pool than by supervising the child's behavior all the time. During sanctioned swimming, supervision is the most important strategy. Changing the environment, the laws, the person, or the product can each lead to reductions in injuries.

C. Environmental Changes Have the Potential to Protect the Greatest Number of People

Changes to the environment that automatically provide protection to every person have the potential to prevent the most injuries. Automatic protection includes, for example, barriers built into roads, automatic sprinkler systems in buildings, collapsible steering wheel columns in vehicles, fuses in homes, and child-resistant packaging of consumer products. Such passive interventions have even more success when the public is informed and convinced of their need and benefits.

D. Effective Injury Prevention Requires a Mixture of Strategies and Methods

Three primary strategies—education/behavior change, technology/engineering, and legislation/enforcement—are widely recognized as effective in preventing injuries. Individual behavior change, product engineering, public education, legal requirements, law enforcement, and changes in the physical and social environment work together to reduce injuries. The challenge in intervention planning is to select the most efficient combination of strategies to produce the desired results.

E. Public Participation Is Essential for Community Action

Effective public policy requires the support and participation of community members. Local conditions and resource availability often determine the direction of injury prevention programs. Injury prevention is most successful when there is public participation, support for, and understanding of injury prevention methods. Without public support, laws that are designed to protect the public, such as laws requiring the use of bicycle or motorcycle helmets, or safety belt use, may be ignored and/or repealed. This was clearly seen in the Massachusetts legislature regarding mandatory safety belt use; the law was repealed by popular vote in 1986, 11 months after the legislation had been enacted, and enacted again in 1994.

F. Cross-Sector Collaboration Is Necessary

Injury prevention requires coordinated action by many groups. Participation by community leaders, in addition to health officials, is necessary in planning and implementing injury prevention programs. There are a number of ways that other community members can contribute to a program's success, ranging from identifying problems to mobilizing community action and evaluating intervention effectiveness.

THE ROLE OF THE PUBLIC HEALTH PRACTITIONER

Public health professionals can play a vital role in injury prevention from a variety of positions:

Research

Public health practitioners are particularly well positioned to collect and analyze local data to identify injury patterns, trends, and risk factors. They are also well positioned to introduce scientific methods to injury control by insisting that new countermeasures be evaluated and that, where relevant, they first be subjected to testing in the field.[26]

Service

Public health practitioners can assist community organizations in analyzing data and choosing countermeasures that are known to be effective.

Education

It is essential to educate not only individuals in the community but also, and even more important, the public and private decision makers (e.g., legislators, designers, executives, builders) whose decisions affect the risk of injury for large numbers of individuals. Every day, these decision makers are confronted with issues such as whether to delay implementation of vehicle standards; whether to make an appliance safer or depend upon users always to follow directions; or whether to promote products on the basis of their potential for reducing injury or assume that "you can't sell safety." Public health practitioners can be of great assistance in these processes. It is also particularly important to educate the members of the media.

Influencing Legislation and Regulation

Public Health practitioners are particularly well positioned to assist (or initiate) local policy discussions and assist in evaluating the appropriateness or quality of the facts presented by the different parties involved in policy discussions. For a public health practitioner to be successful in all these areas, he or she must also be aware of the barriers to the implementation of injury prevention activities; namely, funding limitations, organizational difficulties and turf battles.[27]

THE ROLE OF PUBLIC HEALTH AGENCIES

Information Collection

Effective injury control depends upon adequate information systems. National agencies play a major role in the response to injury-related issues, but the quality of their basic data is determined, predominantly, at the local level. Health departments should stimulate uniform reporting and prompt analysis of injury data and make appropriate use of injury data in administration. Numerous issues that related to injury definition, coding, case inclusion criteria, event definition and coding and its standardization remain unresolved and prevent further advance of the injury field.

National public health agencies must also reinforce these activities by ensuring that information developed from local data eventually gets back to the local level.

Regulation and Legislation

Safety standards have long been applied to many kinds of products and operations. Standards may be descriptive in nature, specifying such things as materials, design, and process, or they may be performance standards, indicating what a product should do (and what it should never do) no matter how it is made. For safety purposes performance standards are generally preferable, although both types sometimes contribute little except a false sense of security. Most commonly, standards are voluntary and industry-wide. Yet, voluntary standards are often insufficient. A 1970 report found that of 44 product categories causing the most injuries, only 18 were covered by industry-wide standards and many of those were deficient.[28] Whether the situation has improved since then is unknown, since this issue has not been reviewed recently (Consumer Products Safety Commission, personal communication). When public attention is drawn to an industry's failure to keep its products from being unreasonably hazardous, the government may consider issuing regulatory standards.

In addition to product and environmental standards, laws regulating human behavior are also intended to reduce injuries. As with other regulations, whether they succeed depends upon whether they are enforced, whether the penalties are effective, and whether the basic assumptions underlying the regulations and their enforcement are valid. State-level safety belt laws provide a wonderful example of this point. As of 2001, all states except New Hampshire have some form of safety belt law for motor vehicle occupants. The degree of coverage, details, and enforcement of these laws varies widely from state to state; however, one of the most distinguishing factors of these laws' effectiveness is whether they are primary (i.e., not wearing safety belts is reason enough for arrest and punishment) or secondary (i.e., some other offense is needed for the safety belt regulation to be reinforced). Figure 26.6 shows safety belt use as reported from observational surveys by state. States with secondary safety belt laws have significantly lower safety belt use.

Emergency Systems

When primary prevention strategies fail, secondary and tertiary strategies become imperative. Municipal, state, and federal agencies are taking an increasing interest in emergency care and transport. Local and regional planning is required for successful organization of emergency communication systems, transportation, trauma units, poison control centers, and specialized units such as those for burns. Public health agencies have a role in organizing such systems; for example, by categorizing emergency facilities on the basis of what kind of injury cases they are equipped and staffed to treat, so that seriously injured patients can have the optimum chance of receiving adequate care. Lately, this role has expanded into development of triage criteria and establishment of regionalized trauma systems where not only the emergency facilities are categorized, but hospitals are too.

Education

Even though we have said before that priority in injury prevention should be given to measures that require little or no human action or cooperation, education must supplement some forms of injury control.[29] Public health agencies must devise and implement educational efforts directed to the general public that address all three phases of the injury sequence: pre-event, event, and post-event. Another very important function of education is to convince the public as well as private and public organizations that the hazards of their environment can be controlled, reduced, or eliminated. Public support is often needed before a preventive measure can be introduced; people must be persuaded of the benefits of a motorcycle helmet law before they support it. Finally, individuals (e.g., legislators, regulators, administrators) whose decisions can determine the likelihood of injury to thousands of people need to be educated to take advantage of their role in injury prevention.

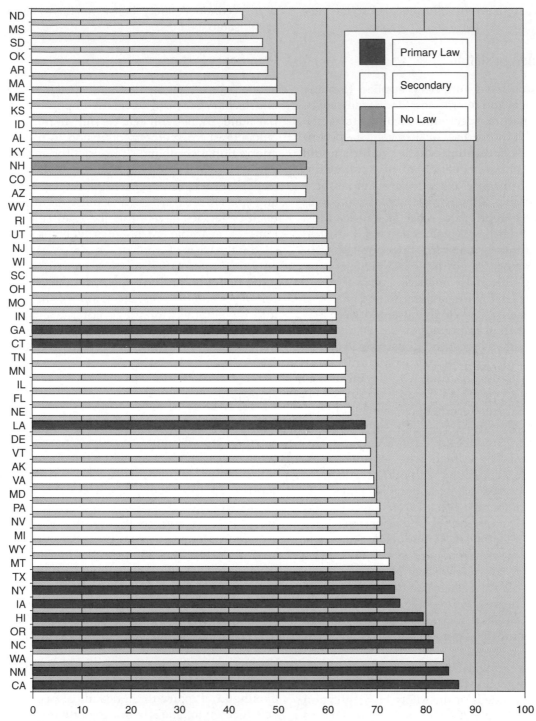

Figure 26.6. State Safety Belt Use Rates by Law Type

Source: NHTSA, Presidential Initiative for Increasing Seat Belt Use Nationwide, 1996.

CONCLUSIONS

Injury is a public health problem that can be controlled with the application of public health tools such as epidemiology, program design and implementation, and evaluation. Major achievements over the past 25 years or so reinforce this point. Further reductions in both unintentional and intentional injuries and their associated medical, psychological, and economic burden will require continued efforts by the public health community in surveillance and research, in building partnerships with public and private organizations, and in the development of state and local health department injury control programs.

Those public health practitioners who understand the issues and scientific concepts involved in injury occurrence can contribute effectively to substantially reducing this huge problem.

ACKNOWLEDGMENTS

We thank Dr. Sleet and Dr. Rosenberg for their contribution in the first edition of this book. We also thank Maria Bulzacchelli and C. Regina Anderson for their assistance in the preparation of this manuscript. Partial support for the writing of this chapter was provided by a CDC grant to the Johns Hopkins Center for Injury Research and Policy (R49/CCR302486).

References

1. Baker SP. Injury control. In: Sartwell PE, ed. *Preventive Medicine and Public Health*. 10th ed. New York, NY: Appleton Century-Crofts; 1973.

2. Baker SP, O'Neill B, Li G, Ginsberg M. *The Injury Fact Book*. 2nd ed. New York, NY: Oxford University Press; 1992.

3. Laflamme L, Svanstrom L, Schelp L, eds. *Safety Promotion Research: A Public Health Approach to Accident and Injury Prevention*. Stockholm, Sweden: Karolinska Institutet; 1999.

4. Reiss AJ Jr, Roth JA, eds. *Understanding and Preventing Violence*. National Academy of Sciences. Washington, DC: National Academy Press; 1993.

5. Robertson LS. *Injury Epidemiology*. 2nd ed. New York, NY: Oxford University Press; 1992.

6. National Committee for Injury Prevention and Control. Injury prevention: meeting the challenge. *Am J Prev Med*. 1989; 5(3, supp l): 297.

7. Bonnie RJ, Fulco CE, Liverman CT, eds. In: IOM report *Reducing the Burden of Injury: Advancing Prevention and Treatment*. National Academy Press; 1999.

8. CDC Wonder. Available at: http://wonder.cdc.gov. Accessed online July 2001.

9. Graves EJ. *1991 Summary: National Hospital Discharge Survey*. Hyattsville, Md.: National Center for Health Statistics; 1993. Advance Data from Vital Health Statistics, #227.

10. Warner M, Barnes PM, Fingerhut LA. Injury and poisoning episodes and conditions; National Health Interview Survey. *Vital Health Stat*. 2000;10(202).

11. Murray CJL, Lopez AD, eds. *The Global Burden of Disease: A Comprehensive Assessment of Mortality and Disability from Diseases, Injuries, and Risk Factors in 1990 and Projected to 2020*. Cambridge, Mass., 1996.

12. Rice DP, MacKenzie EJ, et al. *Cost of Injury in the United States: A Report to Congress, 1989*. San Francisco, Ca: University of California; Institute for Health and Aging, Baltimore, Md.: Johns Hopkins University, Injury Prevention Center; 1989.

13. Blincoe LJ. *The Economic Cost of Motor Vehicle Crashes, 1994*. DOT HS 808 425. Washington, DC: U.S. Dept of Transportation; 1994.

14. National Highway Traffic Safety Administration, U.S. Department of Transportation. *1994 Traffic Safety Facts*. Washington, DC; 1995.

15. National Highway Traffic Safety Administration, U.S. Department of Transportation. *2000 Traffic Safety Facts*. Washington, DC; 2001.

16. Segui-Gomez M. *Literature Search for Psychological and Psychosocial Consequences of Injury*. NHTSA DOT HS 808 527. National Highway Traffic Safety Administration, U.S. Dept of Transportation; 1996.

17. Waller JA. Public health then and now: Reflections on a half century of injury control. *Am J Public Health*. 1994;84:664-670.

18. Heinrich HW. *Industrial Accident Prevention. A Scientific Approach*. 4th ed. New York, NY: McGraw-Hill; 1980.

19. Haddon W Jr. A logical framework for categorizing highway safety phenomena and activities. *J Trauma*. 1972;12:193-207.

20. Maier RV, Mock C. *Trauma.* 4th ed. New York, NY: McGraw-Hill; 2000.

21. Blumenthal M. Dimensions of the traffic safety problem. *Traffic Safety Res Rev.* 1968;12:7.

22. Vernick JS, Li G, Ogaitis S, MacKenzie E, et al. Effectiveness of high school driver education on motor vehicle crashes, violations, and licensure. *Am J Prev Med.* 1999;1S:40-46.

23. Dannenberg AL, Fowler CJ. Evaluation of interventions to prevent injuries: An overview. *Inj Prev.* 1998;4:141-147.

24. Graham JD. *Preventing Automobile Injury: New Findings from Evaluation Research.* Dover, Mass.: Auburn House Publishing Co; 1988.

25. Sleet DA, Rosenberg ML. Injury control. In: *Principles of Public Health Practice.* 1st ed. Albany, NY: Delmar Publishers; 1997: 337-349.

26. Geller E, Berry TD, Ludwig TD, Evans RE, Gilmore MR, Clarke SW. A conceptual framework for developing and evaluating behavior change interventions for injury control. *Health Educ Res.* 1990;5(2):125-138.

27. Christoffel T, Gallagher SS. *Injury Prevention and Public Health: Practical Knowledge, Skills, and Strategies.* Gaithersburg, Md.: Aspen Publishers. 1999:343-349.

28. *National Commission on Product Safety: Final Report.* Washington, DC: Government Printing Office; 1970.

29. Gielen AC. Health education and injury control: integrating approaches. *Health Educ Q.* 1992;19(2):203-218.

CHAPTER
27

The Public Health Laboratory

Ronald L. Cada, Dr.P.H.
K. Michael Peddecord, Dr.P.H.

Public health laboratories contribute significantly to the capacity of health departments to carry out their core functions of assessment, policy development, and assurance. They were initially developed out of a need to monitor the presence of infectious diseases. Over time, as nonmicrobial contamination of the environment became more of a concern, laboratories developed the capacity to monitor many of these threats as well. In addition to providing surveillance testing, public health laboratories have often been required to provide high-quality, low-cost diagnostic testing for patients enrolled in public health programs and hospitals. Many state laboratories have also assumed a significant role in the assurance of laboratory testing quality in community clinical laboratories through inspection and education services.

Resources have seldom met demands for services. Many laboratories are poorly positioned to meet the current challenges of public health reform. This chapter provides an overview of core laboratory responsibilities and offers a vision for the future. It is anticipated that new technology and changes in the health care system will result in a significant reduction of the routine screening and testing now done in public health laboratories. A growing need for effective surveillance of the quality of community laboratory services will require the effective public health laboratory to increase its capacity to operate in this arena. Enhanced communication, information management, and analytic skills will be necessary if public health laboratories are to continue to be viable and effective entities.

ROLE OF THE PUBLIC HEALTH LABORATORY

In many situations, laboratory testing provides the objective data that underpin public health decision making. Decisions to treat individual patients, provide access to a program for HIV/AIDS patients, prosecute a company found to be polluting a water supply, incarcerate a drunk driver, shut down a public water supply, or evaluate the probability of a terrorist biological/chemical incident, among other possible examples—all are based on laboratory information. Laboratory results are as important as other, often subjective, observations of disease and health in the search for solutions to public health problems.

Beginnings

Public health laboratory services were identified as a core function of community health during the 1890s. Laboratories were charged with tracking the distribution of the enteric and respiratory infections that periodically exploded among populations crowding into urban centers at that time. The unique responsibility of public health laboratories was to assist with the task of community health assessment through the scientific identification and measurement of disease incidence and prevalence in susceptible populations. As the relationship between host, agent, and environment was identified for specific disease agents, public health laboratories contributed to disease prevention by using environmental monitoring to estimate disease risk. The need for more adequate characterization and quantification of environmental hazards will continue to challenge the capabilities of public health laboratories.[1]

Shift in Emphasis to Personal Health Care

More recently, since the passage of Medicare and Medicaid legislation, public health departments have become increasingly involved in the delivery of personal health care services. In many local public health agencies, laboratories were merged or integrated with publicly owned hospital labs. The unique community assessment role of public health laboratories often disappeared as the tests they performed became indistinguishable from those of hospital and private clinical laboratories. As increasing resources were needed to support growing public health clinic and hospital workloads, priorities were adjusted, often resulting in a change in emphasis from epidemic surveillance and sanitation efforts to clinical testing services for individual patients supported by health insurance reimbursements.

For uninsured or indigent patients whose costs are not covered by third-party payers the public health laboratory was required to provide the service whether or not payment was available. The needed funds were transferred from other services which then needed to be reduced. The costs for this type of testing are usually lower in public health laboratories than in the private sector because of lower salaries and the requirement that tests not be a source of revenue for the laboratory to use in upgrading facilities or equipment. This increasing attention to patient-based clinical testing has clearly detracted from the ongoing missions of infectious disease surveillance, epidemic investigations, and environmental risk factor analysis.

Public health laboratories, especially at the state and local level, often find themselves in the position of providing services in areas considered unprofitable by commercial testing facilities. In addition, many of these services involve diseases or disorders that are reportable to the state, adding extra cost of providing governmental reports in a manner different than the usual clinical result report. For example, the state requires identifiers and locations that are not usual to the clinical laboratory report to the attending health care practitioner. Testing for the potential of rabies transmission by examination of animal tissue, for instance, has always remained in the community health laboratory, both because it is a form of environmental disease monitoring and because this labor-intensive analysis has not been automated and would not be profitable in commercial systems. Another example is the use of enteric pathogen serotyping as a surveillance mechanism for tracking disease outbreaks. This activity is essential for understanding the distribution of these organisms in population groups, but it is not particularly helpful in individual patient interventions. As a result, these and similar tests are ignored by the clinician's commercial testing facilities.

Impact of New Technologies

A growing number of laboratory tests are now available for use by the untrained user. Rapidly developing technologies promise an ever increasing list of procedures intended to be performed by nonlaboratorians in locations where clients live and work, rather than by individuals specifically trained in laboratory processes working in closely controlled institutional environments. More and more laboratory tests can now be done at the patient's bedside, at nursing stations, in shopping malls, in physicians' offices, or at remote clinics and environmental sites. Patient self-testing or home testing for blood glucose and pregnancy are examples of over-the-counter test kit technologies readily available with or without a physician's order. The list of home-use tests is expected to continue growing as individuals request more control over their personal health and manufacturers respond to this market demand. The extent to which these testing methodologies can be safely and effectively used and interpreted by personnel without extensive laboratory training is a current topic of considerable debate.[2]

Especially germane here is the impact this trend will have on the current activities of public health laboratories. The additional options created by generally available test kits increases the complexity of decisions about how and where to provide needed testing services and how to provide clients with the information they need to correctly use home test kits and appropriately interpret and respond to test results.

The Reference Laboratory and Improvement Activities

Since their inception, public health laboratories have collected specimens for testing when an issue of public health importance was at stake.[3] These specimens come from a variety of sources, including other laboratories.[4] Over time, public health laboratories have become *reference laboratories* for a number of procedures that have implications for community health.

As their expertise improved, some public laboratories developed strategies beyond the passive reference role and began activities to systematically improve the quality of testing in other laboratories. These activities were buttressed by early surveys of medical testing laboratories, which indicated that test results were often below minimally acceptable levels.[5,6] Concerns were raised that poor results were so widespread as to constitute a serious threat to the public health. Comprehensive efforts to externally monitor laboratory quality were first introduced in

military hospitals during World War II.[7] They were followed by similar efforts in private hospital laboratories in the late 1940s.[6] This external quality-control activity run by many state health departments is now a major component of laboratory accreditation and regulatory programs.[8]

REGULATION OF PUBLIC HEALTH LABORATORIES

Despite the lack of credible empirical evidence that modern laboratory services constituted a threat to public health,[9] a federal law requiring licensing of all clinical laboratories was enacted in 1988. Primarily intended to bring clinical laboratory testing in physicians' offices under regulatory oversight, the Clinical Laboratory Improvement Amendments Act of 1988 (CLIA '88) brought an estimated 135,000 previously unregulated testing sites under a complex system of federal licensure.[10] This highly contentious law classifies tests based upon their technical complexity as well as the risk to patients of incorrect results.

A major reason that federal regulations have prompted concern by public health officials and their laboratories is because personnel standards under CLIA '88 are based, to a great extent, on previous federal requirements designed for clinical laboratories in hospitals and independent commercial settings.[11] Some public health laboratory leaders believe it is essential to develop standards that recognize the unique nature of public health laboratory testing.[12]

Practice Standards and Guidelines

The use of practice standards and guidelines to improve the accuracy of laboratory testing is well established in laboratory practice and continues to be an area of emphasis of regulatory agencies, public health laboratorians, and their professional associations.

Government Contributions

The recent evolution of practice guidelines for HIV/AIDS testing services provides an example of how federal agencies, such as the Centers for Disease Control and Prevention (CDC), and public health laboratories have worked to standardize and improve testing services for HIV antibody and T lymphocyte immunophenotyping. Public health laboratory officials at CDC and at state and local public health laboratories as well as test kit manufacturers recognized the need to evaluate performance, develop a consensus, and establish guidelines for HIV testing. After a number of ad hoc meetings of experts, the Association of State and Territorial Public Health Laboratory Directors (ASTPHLD) formed a human retrovirus testing committee to oversee this process.[13] Manufacturers, laboratory scientists, and pathologists from commercial and hospital laboratories contributed to the formulation of practice guidelines. CDC provided "official" sanction to many of the practice recommendations by publishing them in supplements to the *Morbidity and Mortality Weekly Report (MMWR)*.[14]

In the mid-1980s, as the testing requirements to support response to the HIV epidemic exploded onto the public health scene, CDC reorganized its efforts in laboratory training and other improvement activities such as proficiency testing. Most of these new efforts were focused on HIV/AIDS and related testing. The existing centralized, government-run training model was replaced by programs run through a National Laboratory Training Network (NLTN).[15] Seven regional Area Laboratory Training Alliances (ALTAs) were developed to serve as clearinghouses to assess, facilitate, and evaluate training activities. These centers work through training coordinators in state government laboratories. In early 2000 the CDC, in partnership with the Association of Public Health Laboratories, announced the reorganization of the network into a more specialized and centralized model. The increased role of more specialized laboratories, which currently use the most highly developed technology, will be to enable the network to more effectively transfer new technologies through distance-learning initiatives and the latest conferencing capabilities.

Voluntary Guidelines to Improve Quality

Although some standardization is clearly accomplished by regulation at both the state and federal levels, it is also achieved through the use of voluntary or consensus guidelines. The National Committee on Clinical Laboratory Standards (NCCLS), for example, is a consortium of representatives of laboratorian professional organizations, government, and industry that has a well-defined process to identify procedures in need of standardization and then to draft, review, and promulgate voluntary practice standards.[16]

PUBLIC HEALTH LABORATORIES TODAY AND TOMORROW

In 1988, the Institute of Medicine delineated assessment, policy development, and assurance as the core functions of public health.[17] As the profession further refines the characteristics of these core functions, it is increasingly clear that public health laboratories have much to contribute to the accomplishment of each. Information obtained from laboratories is important in assessing risks to community health, establishing priorities for public policy making, and ensuring the availability and reliability of laboratory tests for decisions related to individual patient diagnosis and treatment.

Current Status

Not surprisingly, the roles, responsibilities, and priorities of a given public health laboratory today correlate closely with the mission of its parent agency. The public health agency that is a leader in disease control and environmental protection, for example, will likely support a laboratory program that provides leadership in information services for those areas of interest. However, if the parent public health agency is heavily involved in providing direct medical services, its laboratory will likely have as its priority the provision of clinical laboratory testing. Community health programs would no doubt be enhanced by the separation of clinical laboratory responsibilities from those more traditionally associated with public health agencies, but such a separation would likely be impractical and unrealistic as well as inefficient in some jurisdictions within the present system. The formation of regionalized health maintenance organizations and other reform measures promised to make health care, including diagnostic testing, available to the enrollee, but the net effect has often been to scatter testing within and among institutions, corporations, and the public. Tests that were traditionally performed in reference or specialized laboratories are now done at the bedside; those previously performed in local medical laboratories are now completed by individuals in their homes. Space age technology transferred to medical testing is available and expanding at an increasing rate. The long-term contributions to the effectiveness of care remain to be seen.

The fragmentation of the public health system over the past several decades is mirrored in public health laboratories today. A number of traditional public health laboratory functions have been transferred from public health agencies to other agencies and institutions. For example, while the study of the distribution of *Salmonella* infections in the U.S. population is the responsibility of the CDC, the monitoring of water supplies, one of the vehicles of transmission for these organisms, is the purview of the Environmental Protection Agency. Similarly, the monitoring of food supplies, the most common vehicle for *Salmonella* outbreaks, is the responsibility of the Food and Drug Administration. At the state level, these responsibilities are often distributed widely to such entities as state departments of agriculture, consumer protection, and/or natural resources. Until these activities are unified or coordinated effectively, efficiency and effectiveness will not be maximized. As a lead agency for public health policy development in the United States, the CDC will have among its most important tasks the provision of leadership and assistance to states and selected local laboratories in ensuring a public health laboratory system that is truly functional.

Public Health Laboratories of the Future

The existence and future direction of laboratory testing in support of public health is not just a challenge for public health laboratorians. As described previously, laboratory information is essential to the existence of a scientific base for public health services. In a recent review of public health laboratories, Walter Dowdle, deputy director of CDC, expressed concern over a lack of resources in public health and concluded that public health laboratories have generally not fared well during recent cutbacks. However, he also observed that a number of state laboratories had continued to thrive even in this environment.[18]

In order to thrive in changing times, public health agencies need to make an honest evaluation of their capabilities and be willing to adjust to new realities, including adjusting their laboratory services. A public/private planning venture[19] involving public health laboratory directors, public health leaders, and laboratorians from the private sector assessed present public health laboratory structure and services and recommended changes to respond to national trends. Sadly, many of the needed capabilities envisioned in this planning document and espoused as core functions of public health are currently not available or are poorly developed in many public health agencies. These include monitoring of nutritional status and systematic assessment of environmental contaminants, among other capabilities.

The recent activity in completing the genome project has brought a whole new paradigm of testing that public health agencies are pressed to consider. The tests being developed for identifying genetic disease, or the probability to develop disease is an issue with which agencies and public health laboratories are ill-equipped to deal. Although state laboratories have been testing newborns for a variety of "inborn errors of metabolism", (e.g., phenylketonuria, hypothyroidism, and galactosemia) and evaluating hemoglobin for the presence of sickle cell disease and carrier states, genetic testing of individuals or the understanding of the results of these tests is not widely available in public health or health care sectors.[20,21] Public health laboratories are struggling with the realization that they will be required to take a leadership role in defining which tests should be used and how to evaluate their quality. The current status of many laboratories is that they have minimal equipment, personnel, and training required for newer tests. In many cases these same laboratories will be asked to provide the tests as well as ensure their reliable performance.

The Impact of Health Care Reform

Under current conditions and under most health care reform scenarios, significant clinical and epidemiological laboratory roles would remain the purview of state and local health departments. In an improved system, laboratory services should be universally available in a timely manner to the client, either the individual patient or the community. The experience of private sector commercial laboratories may provide excellent models in this respect. These laboratories have connected networks of local, regional, and national testing facilities linked by electronic and courier networks. A rational system of public health laboratory services would share many characteristics of these private sector systems.

Given the demand for high-quality, cost-effective services, it is clear that many smaller local agencies may not choose to maintain full-service laboratories. Even very large local departments may find it more effective to pool their resources with the state or other local health agencies. In some instances, sharing services with public or private hospital laboratories may be reasonable, as long as the information is available to public decision makers for assessment. The test of the utility of such mergers and reorganizations should be the continued ability to provide information in support of health programs, not short-term cost savings and political correctness.

It was the expectation of some that an evolving system of health care delivery would free public health departments from the responsibility for personal health care services. Under such a scenario, the public health laboratory could have returned to its primary purpose of protecting and promoting the public health through population-based programs.[22] The American Public Health Association (APHA) developed a vision of public health services in a reformed United States health care system.[23] Unfortunately, the envisioned health care reform did not occur. Thus, it appears that the average public health laboratory will retain significant responsibility for providing clinical laboratory services to a large, medically underserved population.

A Vision of the Future Public Health Laboratory

What should the "typical" public health agency laboratory look like in the future? Although there will never be an archetypal laboratory, it is anticipated that future public health laboratories will be different from public health laboratories supported today. It is likely that they will have the characteristics discussed below.

Highly Integrated

The future public health laboratory will be integrated with intrastate and interstate public health laboratory testing. Information technologies and transportation systems will allow efficient integration.

Connected to Personal Health Care Information Systems

The electronic information highways envisioned under health care reform will funnel selected laboratory test results to the local, state, and federal health agency. Public health laboratorians/epidemiologists will monitor communicable disease in the community, converting data into useful assessment information. On a routine basis, supplemental data will be collected from personal health care providers or special studies and integrated with routine, organized community surveys. The federal government has been challenged to develop and transport to local governments this electronic disease reporting system, which promises to link information across public and private laboratories, agency programs, and the federal government. This initiative, although improving the quality and speed of data acquisition, will not arrive without an expense to the system that may be greater than the present costs of collecting partial data.

Involved in Health-Related Environmental Testing

Food and water testing as well as other environmental testing will be expanded and directed more to health risk measurement. Testing will often depend on remote sensing systems with information passing to the health and environmental authorities for analysis and interpretation. Food monitoring will obtain real-time input from laboratories in food processing facilities in order to monitor changes in the endemic distribution of organisms and the emergence of potential community pathogens or toxins. Recent initiatives by the federal government to stimulate public health laboratories to develop capabilities in biomonitoring promise to link environmental contaminants with disease states or precursors to disease. These capabilities have not been available previously except in narrow research projects involving small groups of heavily contaminated individuals. This area of testing is tailor-made for the public laboratory sector, since many provide both medical and environmental testing at the present.

Committed to Quality Assessment

Local, state, and federal laboratories will be positioned to assist personal health care providers and various professional organizations in monitoring and improving laboratory performance. Reference specimens of interest will be processed as needed for disease monitoring by the public health testing system. Feedback to personal health care laboratories will provide an opportunity to ensure the quality of testing services in the private sector.

Devoted to Laboratory Improvement

Most regulation of personal health care and environmental laboratories will have been replaced by a system of practice guidelines and peer review through professional accreditation agencies. Local or regional public health laboratories will monitor proficiency and patient-testing outcomes with an emphasis on feedback and focused interventions, using practice sanctions as a last resort. Information on testing problems will be used to design training and other intervention strategies. Local or regional organizations will coordinate delivery of training through traditional and innovative distance-based learning methods. Affiliations with local community colleges, universities, laboratory training programs, and schools of public health will enhance available public and private sector resources. The model of quality assurance in laboratory testing developed in the United States is being marketed to other countries through various global health initiatives involving HIV, tuberculosis, and childhood enteric and respiratory diseases. Public health laboratories at the federal, state, and local levels are involved in working with international colleagues in instituting policies and procedures that monitor and improve quality.

Dedicated to Providing a Safety Net of Bottom-Line Assurance Testing

Some orphan tests that are too specialized for managed care plans will find a home in the public health system if there is a consensus on public benefits and cost-effectiveness of such testing. In some instances, local health agencies, because of their expertise in managing selected diseases (for example, HIV, TB), will contract with the managed care plans to provide personal health care services. Laboratories will provide or arrange for needed support services for diagnosis and treatment as well as monitoring of these diseases and conditions.

Committed to a Rapid Response and Research

In some jurisdictions, resources will be allocated to improve assessment methods. Research and development sections will seek improvements in operations as well as basic and applied assessment testing. These centers may be affiliated with universities or research institutes.

CONCLUSION

There is little opportunity for transformation of the public health laboratory until public health and laboratory leaders develop a consensus vision of the future. As communication and testing technology continue to evolve, they present additional management challenges. Laboratory directors and managers were historically judged on their scientific knowledge and their ability to perform skilled analyses. As technology and competition change the laboratory industry, laboratory directors and managers must increasingly become system and information managers.

The challenge is to participate in the development of effective reporting systems that produce standardized information for disease reporting. The ability to understand the decision-making needs of clients and the programs they serve, the menu of available tests, and the test procurement options available from the industry is now an essential skill for laboratory services managers. This transition to "testing-and-information" managers will require a radical shift of thinking for many laboratory directors. Laboratory directors who view their role as one of only providing a service rather than providing information for public health decision making will continue to play a minor role in their organizations. The capacity to balance and manage issues of turnaround time, cost of testing, analytic quality, and legal issues will be the benchmark of the effective laboratory information manager and director of the future.

ACKNOWLEDGMENT

Ongoing funding of the Laboratory Assurance Program is provided by the Centers for Disease Control and Prevention provided under a cooperative agreement with the Association of Schools of Public Health. This funding has provided Professor Peddecord an opportunity to continue learning about public health laboratory testing at local, state, and federal levels.

References

1. Burke TA. Understanding environmental risk: the role of the laboratory in epidemiology and policy setting. *Clin Chem.* 1992;38:1519-1522.
2. Ferris DG, Fischer PM. Elementary school students' performance with two ELISA test systems. *JAMA.* 1992;268: 766-770.
3. Inhorn SL, ed. *Quality Assurance Practices for Health Laboratories.* Washington, DC: American Public Health Association; 1978.
4. Valdiserri RO. Temples of the future: An historical overview of the laboratory's role in public health practice. *Annu Rev Public Health.* 1993;14:635-648.
5. Schaeffer M, ed. *Federal Legislation and the Clinical Laboratory.* Boston, Mass: GK Hall Medical Publishers; 1981.
6. Belk WP, Sunderman FW. A survey of the accuracy of chemical analysis in clinical laboratories. *Am J Clin Pathol.* 1947;17:853-861.
7. Shuey HE, Cabel J. Standards of performance in clinical laboratory diagnosis. *Bull US Army Medical Dept.* 1949;9: 799-815.
8. *Clinical Laboratory Improvement Amendments of 1988; Final Rule.* Washington, DC: Dept of Health and Human Services, Health Care Financing Administration; February 28, 1992. Federal Register 57;40:7002-7288.
9. Kenney ML. Quality assurance in changing times: Proposals for reform and research in the clinical laboratory field. *Clin Chem.* 1987;33:728-736.
10. Clinical Laboratory Improvement Act of 1967. Washington, DC: US Dept of Health, Education, and Welfare; 1967. Code of Federal Regulations Title 42, Part 74.
11. Sweet CE. Effect of CLIA-88 on public health laboratories. *Clin Microbiol Newsletter.* 1993;15:60-62.
12. Hausler WJ. Commentary by a state public health laboratory director. Paper presented at Session 1090 of the 121st Annual Meeting of the American Public Health Association: San Francisco, Calif; October 25, 1993.
13. *Committee on Retrovirus Testing: Second Consensus Conference on Human Retrovirus Testing.* Washington, DC: Association of State and Territorial Public Health Laboratory Directors; 1987.
14. Centers for Disease Control and Prevention. Interpretation and use of the Western blot assay for serodiagnosis of human immunodeficiency virus type 1 infections. *MMWR.* 1989;38:1-7.
15. Gore MJ. Keeping up with changing times: How the National Laboratory Training Network helps. *Clin Lab Sci.* 1993;6:268-271.
16. National Committee on Clinical Laboratory Standards. *NCCLS Handbook.* Wayna, Penn: National Committe on Clinical Laboratory Standards; 1989.
17. Institute of Medicine, Committee for the Study of the Future of Public Health. *The Future of Public Health.* Washington, DC: National Academy Press; 1988.
18. Dowdle WR. The future of the public health laboratory. *Annu Rev Public Health.* 1993;14:649-664.
19. Counts JM. LIFT 2000: Laboratory initiatives for the year 2000. *Clin Chem.* 1992;38:1517-1518.
20. Leonard DGB. The future of molecular genetic testing. *Clin Chem.* 1999;45:726-731.
21. Holtzman NA. Promoting safe and effective genetic tests in the United States: Work of the Task Force on Genetic Testing. *Clin Chem.* 1999;45:732-738.
22. Lee PR, Toomey KE. Epidemiology in public health in the era of health care reform. *Public Health Rep.* 1994; 109:1-3.
23. American Public Health Association. APHA's vision: public health and a reformed health care system. *Nation's Health.* July 1993:9, 11.

CHAPTER 28

Global Health in the Twenty-First Century

William H. Foege, M.D., M.P.H.

HISTORY

The story of global health has been compelling, inspiring, and underfunded, but always with a favorable return on investment. Many factors have influenced what we now label "global health"; a few follow in order to illustrate the rich history.

Although there are ancient stories of famine relief, which extended beyond national borders, the most significant early global health efforts were the result of nineteenth-century medical mission programs throughout the world. These early church-sponsored groups worked in difficult conditions but also with difficult problems. For example, the most significant work with leprosy was done not by governments or university researchers, but by missionaries in Africa and Asia.

War also had an unexpected impact on global health and tropical medicine. Out of necessity, the military became involved in tropical diseases in general but especially in malaria control efforts during the Second World War. This involvement has continued even in peacetime but at a lower level of intensity. Malaria control became important in military training camps in the United States in the early 1940s. This effort led directly to the creation of the Communicable Disease Center after the war, which evolved over the years to become the Centers for Disease Control and Prevention (CDC). CDC, in turn has played a significant role in global disease eradication and control as well as a support role for laboratory sciences, surveillance, and epidemiology throughout the world. The aftermath of WWII also led to the creation of a series of global agencies such as the World Health Organization and the United Nations Children's Fund (UNICEF), but also many nongovernmental organizations such as CARE.

Whereas all governments have been involved in health efforts in their own countries, the governments of developed countries took an increasingly active role in the concept of globalization of health in the past half-century. Part of this activity resulted from the need to protect their countries from importations of diseases, and part was the result of the desire to use Western knowledge and tools to reduce the burden of disease in developing areas. Bilateral aid agencies provided assistance in areas such as health, agriculture, education, and development, all with direct impacts on health. In addition, in the United States, the support of the National Institutes of Health provided a small but important research effort in diseases of developing countries, but also provided grant support that encouraged university research programs in tropical medicine. The involvement of governments in support of domestic immunization programs as a social good rather than simply as an individual benefit was ultimately important in laying the groundwork for a similar understanding of a global social good. This led to a global program for smallpox eradication and later for the Expanded Program of Immunization (EPI), the Global Polio Eradication program, and now the Global Alliance for Vaccines and Immunization (GAVI).

The desire for equity in access to health science is rooted in the early medical mission programs. But health equity received global attention with the Alma Ata conference almost a quarter of a century ago, which resulted in the slogan "Health for all by the year 2000." Although inequities were still the norm by the year 2000, global health workers now have a shared goal, namely global health equity, to define their efforts.

Global health efforts require not only organizational structures that span countries or even continents, but also confidence based on successful experiences. Smallpox eradication provided a program that involved dozens of countries as well as governments, nongovernmental organizations, bilateral organizations, mission groups, universities, and corporations. The success of that effort had an impact that allowed workers to consider similar and even bigger efforts. The EPI followed and continues to the present. This in turn provided confidence for Rotary International to help catalyze the global effort to eradicate polio. More recently, Merck Drug Company has stimulated an effort to control onchocerciasis by donating Mectizan, which is now

delivered to 30 million persons per year. In recent decades, sufficient successes have been chronicled to allow the global community to consider a massive immunization program, a multibillion-dollar effort in AIDS, a global effort to improve the intake of micronutrients, as well as global control of tuberculosis.

Another development has been in the improvement of metrics to determine the burden of disease by country or age group or the burden imposed by an organism. Originally, mortality was used as the most useful indicator because it was the most easily documented. Eventually morbidity, premature mortality, and quality measures became useful. In 1993 the World Bank introduced the concept of Disability Adjusted Life Years (DALYs) in an attempt to combine both death and suffering rates into a single number. It provides a way of comparing the burden of an illness with high death rates to that of an illness with high suffering but low death rates. It also allows comparisons between geographic areas, age groups, or even groups with different health programs. Although DALYs have provided a tool far superior to former health measurements, the challenge is to develop next-generation metrics that provide an even better assessment of morbidity based on community agreement of the relative importance of each type of morbidity, agreement on the value of life at various ages, as well as the inclusion of quality measures.

THE STATUS OF GLOBAL HEALTH

The United States entered the twentieth century as a developing nation from a health standpoint. Infant mortality rates were approximately 150 per 1,000 live births, a rate exceeded by few countries today. Life expectancy was 47 years and the leading cause of death was tuberculosis. The amazing improvement of health status over the century led to a reduction of infant mortality to below 10 per 1,000 live births in most areas, an improvement in life expectancy of approximately 30 years, and the elimination or substantial control of many infectious diseases. It was generally accepted that this was a harbinger of what would happen in other parts of the world.

The over arching feature of health in the developing world is the wide disparities as compared to developed countries. Public health has as a basic tenet that it must use tools, skills, and knowledge for the benefit of everyone; the philosophical term is *social justice.* Failure is easily measured by comparing health indices between the rich and poor or between countries. The continuing indictment of public health, therefore, is seen in the gaps between the developing world and the rest of the world. Attempts to bridge those gaps were small, local, and uncoordinated before the mid-twentieth century. Since that time there has been a conscious but somewhat inadequate effort to address the problems, and by the 1970s gains had been made in closing the disease burden gap.

Until 1990, these gains were reflected in most of the developing world. Infant mortality rates dropped from over 120 per 1,000 live births for the world as a whole, to half that number in 35 years. Life expectancy for the world had increased to over 60 years and it was possible to predict when 65 would become the norm. Smallpox disappeared, guinea worm and polio were on the verge of disappearance, and the toll of the single most lethal agent—measles—had declined from over three million deaths a year to a third that number.

Then, things began to unravel. The rapid spread of human immunodeficiency virus (HIV) in Africa, Thailand, India, and China changed individual lives, families, villages, and entire countries. In parts of East Africa, teachers, health workers, church leaders, and young energetic business leaders began dying faster than they could be educated and replaced. Life expectancy began to decline, infant mortality increased, the number of orphans reached astounding levels, and a depression settled over hard-hit villages, and then entire nations.

But it was not only HIV that challenged the global health community. Tuberculosis rates increased and multidrug resistance took the health structure by surprise from New York City, to Russian prisons, and then country by country around the world. Global response was too little and far too late. Immunization rates began to fall in Africa as the few public health resources were diverted to the problem of acquired immunodeficiency syndrome (AIDS). The greed of tobacco merchants reached the populations that did not need more health problems and

global tobacco deaths rivaled and then surpassed other death numbers until tobacco had become the single most lethal agent in the world by the year 2000. Then in the early years of the new century, fears of biological agents being used in terrorist attacks revealed the slim veneer of public health response that had resulted from the chronic inability of public health to compete with health care delivery and tertiary medicine for resources.

THE PRESENT

Harland Cleveland has pointed out that we, as public health professionals, need to take special responsibility to envision a future that is different from a straight-line projection of the present. Trends are not destiny, Cleveland says. It is important to see the problems of AIDS, emerging infections, and decreasing immunization rates as a wake-up call, but not as inevitably overwhelming. Indeed, in the midst of this most depressing scenario, it is possible to discern recent developments that indicate a departure from the historic straight-line progression.

First, the tools are improving rapidly. The traditional vaccines used around the world for decades include BCG, measles, polio, diphtheria, pertussis, and tetanus. In recent years, hepatitis B vaccine use has expanded, as has the use of Haemophilus influenza B. After many years of hope, it appears that malaria vaccine research may lead to a usable product. Various AIDS vaccines are now in phase 3 human trials and a phase 1 trial is about to begin for a new tuberculosis vaccine. At the same time, vaccine researchers hope to overcome two constant barriers to effective immunization: the need for a cold chain to keep vaccine at low temperatures from manufacturing until injection, and the need for sterile needles and syringes to avoid the potential for spreading diseases. The possibility of heat-stable vaccines may soon be disregarded. Heat stable vaccines currently under development may quickly be replaced by the development of vaccines incorporated into foods, with the potential of solving both cold chain and administration problems.

Another tool of increasing importance is drugs that are sufficiently safe to be used on a mass basis for the control of diseases in developing areas. The approach was pioneered when the Merck Drug Co. pledged the free distribution of Mectizan to control onchocerciasis in 1987. Despite the potential for Mectizan to reduce microfilarial levels, thereby reducing symptoms (especially debilitating itching) but also the potential for transmission, early attempts at mass distribution were tempered by the fear of adverse reactions. A gradual increase in the distribution of the drug while monitoring side effects, revealed this to be one of the safest drugs in use today. The infrequent cases of adverse reactions are generally treatable on site. The drug is now being given safely to approximately 30 million persons per year. This experience has led to increasing use of drugs such as Albendazole in combination with other drugs for lymphatic filariasis, and Zithromax for trachoma.

Better tools also include diagnostic tools and especially the expected improvements in rapid diagnostic techniques suitable for field use. It is anticipated that almost immediate determination of HIV status will be possible, and attempts are being made to allow the diagnosis of tuberculosis in the field with a determination of resistance patterns even in the absence of laboratory access.

The improvement in tools is matched by a new and powerful interest in global health from a variety of sources. The *1993 World Development Report*, issued by the World Bank, has been followed by a plea from economists promoting the need for better health as a development tool. Politicians in both developed and developing areas have recognized the power of disease to disrupt the economy and even security. Journalists have provided thoughtful articles and books on the need to view global health as an important activity of all segments of society.

Finally, in the midst of the despair caused by AIDS and emerging infections, the fear of biological warfare, the insidious chemical warfare pursued by the tobacco industry, and the inadequate delivery infrastructure everywhere in the world, there has been a response in resources that provides a ray of hope.

Resource constraints have always defined public health efforts. Although health care delivery is held to a cost-effectiveness standard that makes a decision on a course of action and then compares alternative approaches, public health has been held to a much more severe benefit-cost standard. Public health has been asked to show that a particular program can actually save more money than invested. In truth, prevention should be practiced because it reduces suffering even if it costs money. It is an added attraction that immunization programs, iodine fortification, tuberculosis treatment, and other programs actually save a society more than is expended in control. The challenge has been to have policy makers visualize a future many years after their term in office.

Resource increases began modestly in 1985 when Rotary International decided to invest in global polio eradication. The initial goal of $120 million in 20 years has been far exceeded, and Rotary has now raised $500 million for the effort. These new resources to global health have led to other groups, such as Lions and Kiwanis, investing in global health efforts.

Corporations provided a new resource in global health, catalyzed by the Merck Drug Co. which has given hundreds of millions of dollars of Mectizan in the past 14 years and has recently invested $50 million in Botswana to help determine how the world's technology can be utilized under African conditions to best counter AIDS. Glaxo Smith Kline has provided Malarone, a new antimalarial drug, in efforts to determine how best to use this new tool, based on need, rather than ability to pay, in an effort to reduce the development of drug resistance. It is also providing Albendazole at no cost for programs to control lymphatic filariasis. Pfizer is providing Zithromax for the control of trachoma. The potential for pharmaceutical companies and other global corporations in the fight against disease is enormous. The goodwill that these companies receive from employees who feel proud to work for an organization involved in such efforts provides hope that more will follow.

Individuals are leaving their mark on global health. The gift of Ted Turner of $1 billion to UN agencies over a 10-year period has had a significant impact on global health. An anonymous gift of $100 million to begin a malaria program at Johns Hopkins, as well as various gifts to schools of public health in the United States, all provide new resources for global health that were not envisioned two decades ago. But certainly the most significant resource change has been the Bill and Melinda Gates Foundation, which now invests $600 million per year in global health. This recent infusion has increased research in areas that impact directly on developing countries, has highlighted priority areas such as immunization and infectious disease control, and has energized the people working in global health.

The largest changes will come only when governments and global organizations increase their efforts. The cumulative impact of the above-mentioned actions has been that G8 meetings now routinely address global health problems. The European Union is increasing its investment, and a recent call for a global AIDS fund is leading to discussions of billions rather than millions of dollars.

THE FUTURE

Arnold Toynbee was wrong when he said, "The twentieth century will be remembered chiefly, not as an age of political conflicts and technical inventions, but as an age in which human society dared to think of the health of the whole human race as a practical objective." Instead, the twentieth century was an age of political conflicts and technical inventions and it ended with enormous disparities in health. But his vision could be largely achieved in the first two decades of the twenty-first century. It will require some deliberate steps—steps that are currently beyond the thinking of political leaders.

Toynbee's vision will require a decision to make global health equity a goal to be pursued, measured, and adequately supported. It will also require a focus on the conditions that make poor health such a consistent part of developing countries. This includes the ability to make decisions regarding reproduction, which in turn requires free access to reproductive health information and contraceptives. It includes basic education for children, especially for girls. It includes programs, such as microfinancing, that provide practical approaches to escaping poverty. It includes environmental programs with the objective of making development sustainable. It includes attention to improving the conditions of poor countries while reducing the consumption of rich countries. It is not possible to improve global health in a vacuum.

If the more generic approaches to poverty, reproduction, education, and environment are implemented, specific support of global health activities will still require vast improvements. It would require financial resources for the World Health Organization (WHO) commensurate with the size of the problem. Currently WHO has an annual budget for the entire world that is less than a half-day of the U.S. health budget. This must be increased by an order of magnitude and requires a change in both thinking and social norms.

Second, we need to improve global systems for disease surveillance, making them comprehensive, transparent, and capable of measuring the burden of disease, detecting new and emerging problems and tracking trends or changes in disease incidence and prevalence.

Third, the world needs a better mechanism for selecting global priorities in disease control. Having selected conditions responsible for the largest global burdens, or the greatest gaps between populations, such as AIDS, tuberculosis, malaria, vaccine-preventable diseases, tobacco-induced conditions, maternal mortality and morbidity, infant mortality, malnutrition, and so on, it is important to develop a global coalition for each condition to provide for the most efficient use of resources and program interventions. The goal with each program would be to eliminate the disease burden gap between developed and developing areas. Program managers would be rewarded on the basis of how much and how fast they close such gaps.

Fourth, we need to augment global response teams capable of providing assistance to any country requesting help. This would include requests for assistance to respond to emergency situations, such as disease outbreaks, or assistance in developing routine infrastructure to respond to vaccine-preventable diseases, tuberculosis, or other priority conditions. The major barrier to better health in developing countries today is the inadequate delivery infrastructure. Global response teams will be more dependent on expertise in management and logistics than in health expertise per se.

Fifth, the world needs increased research resources for diseases of the developing world. This requires not only an increase in resources, but also reward systems that acknowledge researchers who concentrate in such problems. A premium would be placed on doing the research in the areas of health needs.

Sixth, academic public health training programs need a closer alliance to the public health problems of developing countries, but also more direct familiarity with program delivery problems. It is not possible to pursue pediatric training without caring for sick children. It is possible to receive public health and global health training without ever having responsibility for the improvement of a global health problem. In a better system, training, education, and leadership programs would respond directly to the health needs of an area, and those needs would dictate the kind of public health education programs to be created. An objective would be to have such quality training programs in developing areas; for example, students would leave the United States for public health training in Africa.

The time has arrived to exploit the improvement in tools, resources, interests, and experiences to make Toynbee's prediction a reality. Gandhi once said his idea of the Golden Rule was that he should not enjoy what is withheld from others. We need to celebrate the public health gifts that we enjoy daily, by making sure they are not withheld from any community anyplace in the world.

References

Health, United States, 2001 With Urban and Rural Health Chartbook. Hyattsville, Md: National Center for Health Statistics; 2001.

Mectizan Donation Program: Treatment Summary 2000. Decatur, Ga: Mectizan Donation Program; 1999.

Rotary International: Facts and Figures. Evanston, Ill: Rotary International; 2001.

The Story of Mectizan. Whitehouse Station, NJ: Merck and Co Inc; 1995.

World Bank. *Country at a Glance, US Data.* Washington, DC: World Bank; 2001.

World Bank. *World Bank Development Report: Investing in Health.* Washington, DC: World Bank; 1993.

World Health Organization. *Declaration of Alma-Ata: International Conference on Primary Health Care, Alma-Ata, USSR.* Geneva, Switzerland: World Health Organization; September 1978.

PART

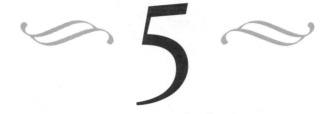

5

The Future of Public Health Practice

CHAPTER
29

The Future of Public Health

C. William Keck, M.D., M.P.H.
F. Douglas Scutchfield, M.D.

Significant gains in health status and life expectancy have occurred over the past two hundred years in the United States as well as in most other industrialized nations. Many attribute those gains to advances in clinical medicine that tend to be dramatically and impressively chronicled in the electronic and print media. Indeed, our capacity to diagnose and treat illness has advanced rapidly during this century. The reality remains, however, that most of the improvements in quality and length of life have come from measures aimed at protecting populations from environmental hazards and pursuing behaviors and activities that are known to be health promoting.[1] Health departments and other community agencies are responsible for developing the programs and relationships with individuals and neighborhoods that will continue to improve the health of citizens of this country.

BACKGROUND

From 1993 through 1994, the Clinton administration stirred a great professional and political debate through its proposal to significantly change the health care system in the United States in a manner that would provide universal access to health care while controlling the costs of that care. The public health system and its functions were only a minor portion of that discussion. Public health leaders around the country were aware that their discipline was at risk of being ignored while debate focused on illness care, and they were galvanized to define better the role of public health and acquire the resources necessary to carry out effective health promotion and disease prevention activities. The combination of well-documented public health system problems and the need to convince policy makers of the importance of public health in society resulted in clear descriptions of both the core functions of public health and the resources that would be required to ensure their existence in each community.

Federal efforts to reform the system came to naught and were largely abandoned by the end of 1994. The pressure created by the high cost of illness care, however, began to drive efforts of cost control across the country, and a dramatic shift to large-scale experimentation with managed care is under way in many communities. The experiment has proven to be a financial success, as it succeeded in holding down insurance premiums costs, but a political failure. Offering comprehensive, first dollar benefits while restricting access and denying coverage has infuriated everyone involved and the paradigm is in full retreat.[2] Although the country focused on the growth of managed care systems, both public and private, the number of individuals without health insurance continued to grow. In fact, the diminishing effectiveness of measures that previously moderated health insurance premiums, such as health maintenance organizations, vertically integrated delivery systems and global capitation, has contributed recently to rapid rises in health care costs. Increases in cost have been further stimulated by new and expensive technologies, an aging population, and rapidly escalating pharmacy costs. This has led to higher consumer out-of-pocket costs for increasing health insurance premiums (particularly for employee dependents), deductibles, copays, and coinsurance. This phenomenon will likely further increase the number of uninsured and underinsured individuals resulting in more pressure on all safety net providers, including health departments, to provide illness care services to this disenfranchised population. Unfortunately, little or no additional funding is coming to these safety net providers to provide those services. A concern, of course, is that resources will have to be diverted from provision of core public health activities to this enhanced illness care demand. This may further erode the health departments' ability to provide services that benefit the entire community.

At the same time, a new administration bent on budget reduction is proposing significant financial cuts and restructuring of many federally supported public health programs. These realities are producing a difficult environment for public health agencies. A clear understanding of role, significant community support, substantial flexibility, and real leadership will be required for public health agencies to survive and thrive and make continuing contributions to health status.

THE CONTRIBUTIONS OF PUBLIC HEALTH

Public health policies and actions have significantly improved the health status of the population of this country. Their contribution is summarized in this section.

Public Health Measures and Previous Health Status Gains

Significant gains in population health status during the nineteenth and early twentieth centuries were based on activities ensuring the availability and safety of food and clean water, the adequate disposal of sewage, the provision of adequate and safe shelter with minimal crowding, and the adoption of personal behaviors that were health promoting. Due to these measures, substantial control of many communicable diseases was accomplished before the advent of vaccines and antibiotics. For example, tuberculosis deaths declined as a result of improved physical environments and better nutrition; the impact of fecally/orally transmitted pathogens declined with the separation of sewage and drinking water; and vectorborne conditions improved with vector habitat control.[3] These changes, combined with the discovery of vaccines and antibiotics, modified the major causes of death from infectious diseases at the turn of the previous century to chronic diseases (including heart disease, cancer, and stroke) currently. There has been a concomitant rapid gain of life expectancy from less than 50 years in 1900 to 75 years in 1997.[4]

During the past 30 years or so, there has been a growing emphasis on population-based prevention programs aimed at reducing risks for chronic disease. Programs aimed at reducing tobacco use, controlling blood pressure, diminishing obesity and dietary fat, reducing risks for occupational and home injury, and promoting use of seat belts and automobile air bags have contributed to a decline of 50 percent in stroke deaths, 40 percent in coronary heart disease deaths, and 25 percent in death rates for children.[5]

Potential for Further Gains in Health Status

The Centers for Disease Control and Prevention reviewed the major causes of premature death in U.S. citizens.[6] Their findings confirmed that 50 percent of premature mortality in this country is directly related to individual lifestyle and behavior, 20 percent is related to environmental factors, an additional 20 percent is directly related to one's inherited genetic profile, and only 10 percent is related to inadequate access to medical care. This means that fully 70 percent of the premature mortality suffered by the U.S. population will require populationwide strategies for effective control.

Traditional discussions of health status include a list of the major causes of death for the population of interest. That information is listed in Table 29.1 for the United States.

From a public health/preventive perspective, however, the real question is what underlying risk factors caused the fatal conditions listed in Table 29.1. The underlying causes of many of the premature deaths occurring in our population are listed in Table 29.2. (Since these estimates were produced, therapy for HIV infection has dramatically lowered the death rate for that infection. HIV no longer appears in the list of the 10 leading causes of death in the United States, and it is likely that sexual behavior is the underlying cause of approximately 20,000 deaths a year, rather than 30,000.)

These factors, which are closely linked to the determinants of health discussed in Chapter 4, are at the root of the finding that 50 percent of premature mortality in the United States is due to factors related to lifestyle. These factors are at the root of preventable conditions that carry a high cost in terms of morbidity and mortality. They also carry a high economic cost. For example, it has been estimated that costs of more than $110 billion can be attributed to alcohol and drug abuse and of $65 billion to smoking. Health care costs created by specific preventable problems include $100 billion annually from injuries, $70 billion from cancer, and $135 billion from cardiovascular diseases.[5] Improving access to medical care will have little impact on diminishing the death and disability

Table 29.1. Ten Leading Causes of Death in the United States, 1999

Cause of Death	No. of Deaths
All Causes	2,391,399
Heart Diseases	725,192
Cancer	549,838
Stroke	167,366
Chronic Obstructive Lung Diseases	124,181
Accidents	97,860
Diabetes	68,399
Pneumonia/Influenza	63,730
Alzheimer's Disease	44,536
Renal Disease	35,525
Septicemia	30,680

SOURCE: National Vital Statistics Reports, Centers for Disease Control and Prevention. October 12, 2001; 49(11).

Table 29.2. Leading Underlying Causes of Death in the United States, 1990

Cause of Death	No. of Deaths
Tobacco	400,000
Diet/Inactivity	300,000
Alcohol	100,000
Certain Infections	90,000
Toxic Agents	60,000
Firearms	35,000
Sexual Behavior	30,000
Motor Vehicles	25,000
Drug Use	20,000

SOURCE: McGinnis JM, Foege WH. Actual causes of death in the United States. *JAMA*, 1993;270:2207-2212.

reflected in the disease and economic figures just cited. AIDS will not be controlled by actions taken in doctor's offices, low-birth-weight babies will not be prevented solely by the work of obstetricians, and heart disease will not continue to decline without extensive community outreach and education.

Human health is also directly related to the quality of the environment. Factors such as air pollution, food and water contaminants, radiation, toxic chemicals, wastes, disease vectors, safety hazards, and habitat alterations are at the root of the 20 percent excess mortality related to environmental issues in the United States. Long-term human health is dependent upon achieving ecological balance and maintaining health-promoting home, work, and leisure environments. Whereas we have a tendency to dwell on the negative aspects of environmental factors on health, we must also recognize that some aspects of our environment can enhance health. Frumpkin has recently reviewed the positive features of our world that enhance health status. His findings suggest that the public health leader will need to acquire new skills, like land-use planning, that were not previously thought of as being necessary.[7]

The combination of ensuring access to medical care and paying attention to the determinants of health has been brought to national attention by the "100% Access, 0 Disparities" campaign proposed by the U.S. Department of Health and Human Service's Health Resources and Services Administration's Bureau of Primary Health Care.[8] This grass-roots effort challenges communities to reorganize and rationalize the distribution of health care locally, and to identify and confront the basic causes of health disparities. The latter will require that public health officials understand the impact of social and economic factors on health, and revamp their approach to disease control to address these causative factors. This is the most recent example of public health's ever-widening agenda.

PUBLIC HEALTH IN AN EVOLVING SYSTEM

The United States continues to search for the "best" way to finance and deliver illness care. The continued retreat of managed care creates even more uncertainty about how health care in the United States will be delivered in the years to come. During the 1990s, managed care became the "vision" of a reformed illness care system. A major concern is that we currently have no clear vision of a paradigm that might replace managed care. It also remains unclear how much attention will be paid to the issues of environment, health promotion, and disease prevention.

In many ways the debate about health care reform is miscast. For the most part, the wrong question is being addressed. Attempts are made to seek better ways of providing and paying for illness care rather than to determine what should be done to create the healthiest population possible. With the courage and the foresight to frame the debate in these terms, it is readily apparent that improved health status depends on illness care reform *and* on public health reform.

For too long, those professionals who concentrate on the diagnosis and treatment of illness have been separated from those who concentrate on health promotion, disease prevention, and control of the environment. Instead of a seamless web of integrated services and activities focusing first on minimizing risks and then on early diagnosis and treatment of emerging disease, two separate systems have developed and evolved into two distinct cultures that are often at odds with one another. It is the responsibility of public health practitioners to help society understand the value of each approach and the need to integrate them into a quest for improving health status. As we suggested in chapter 1, the major professional organizations representing these two professions, the American Medical Association and the American Public Health Association, have attempted to open a dialogue around this issue and encourage discussions designed to bridge the gap between medical care and public health.[9]

Obtaining medical care is very important for that segment of the population for whom access is denied or inappropriately restricted. The approximately 10 percent of excess mortality in citizens of the United States that is related to inadequate access to medical care occurs principally in that group for whom access to care is limited. No illness is "deserved," and every member of society should have access to those interventions that have been developed to diagnose and treat disease and minimize suffering. It is also worth noting that significant contributions to disease prevention can be made in the context of a single patient's interaction with a physician or other health care provider. The activities described in the *Guide to Clinical Preventive Services*[10] are particularly recommended for their proven capacity to improve health and prevent disease and injury. Nonetheless, it is population-based services that have the greatest potential to contribute to overall gains in health status.

THE CORE FUNCTIONS OF PUBLIC HEALTH

Population-based services are provided from a variety of sources in most communities. These sources include state and local health departments, community health agencies (for example, family planning agencies, heart associations, kidney associations, cancer societies, mental health agencies, and drug abuse agencies, among others), hospitals, and schools, to name several. However, this chapter focuses on the local health department because it is only the local health department that has statutory responsibility for the health status of its constituent population. It is the health department, in most locations, that is ultimately responsible for the assurance that all citizens have access to the services they need in the community, no matter which groups or organizations ultimately deliver those services. This focus on the health needs of the entire community by an agency ultimately responsible to that community for its performance emphasizes the importance for health of "a governmental presence at the local level (AGPALL)."[11]

Institute of Medicine Report

There exists wide variation in the size, sophistication, capacity, and roles of local health departments in the United States. In its report, *The Future of Public Health*, the Institute of Medicine's Committee for the Study of the Future of Public Health described widespread agreement across the country that "public health does things that benefit everybody," and that "public health prevents illness and educates the population."[12(p3)] However, it found little consensus on how those broad statements should be translated into action. Indeed, there is such great variability in re-

sources, available services, and organizational arrangements "that contemporary public health is defined less by what public health professionals know how to do than by what the political system in a given area decides is appropriate or feasible."[12(p4)] The committee concluded that "effective public health activities are essential to the health and well-being of the American people, now and in the future," but the variability across the country is so great that this essential system is currently in "disarray."[12(p6)]

In an effort to provide a set of directions for the discipline of public health that could attract the support of the whole society, the committee proposed a public health mission statement and a set of core functions. The committee defined the mission of public health as "fulfilling society's interest in assuring conditions in which people can be healthy."[12(p7)] The committee further found that "The core functions of public health agencies at all levels of government are assessment, policy development, and assurance."[12(p7)]

The committee's definitions of these core functions are as follows:

- *Assessment.* Every public health agency should "regularly and systematically collect, assemble, analyze, and make available information on the health of the community, including statistics on health status, community health needs, and epidemiologic and other studies of health problems."[12(p7)]
- *Policy Development.* Every public health agency should "exercise its responsibility to serve the public interest in the development of comprehensive public health policies by promoting use of the scientific knowledge base in decision-making about public health and by leading in developing public health policy. Agencies must take a strategic approach, developed on the basis of a positive appreciation for the democratic political process."[12(p8)]
- *Assurance.* Every public health agency should "assure their constituents that services necessary to achieve agreed upon goals are provided, either by encouraging actions by other entities (private or public sector), by requiring such action through regulation, or by providing services directly." Each public health agency should also "involve key policymakers and the general public in determining a set of high-

priority personal and community-wide health services that governments will guarantee to every member of the community. This guarantee should include subsidization or direct provision of high-priority personal health services for those unable to afford them."[12(p8)]

Response to the Report

This report, *The Future of Public Health*, was completed in 1988. Since its appearance it has generated considerable discussion and action. Many in the public health community were (and many still are) uncomfortable with the characterization of public health as a system in "disarray," particularly when looking at the capacity and work of their own agencies. Dissenters note that public health workers have accomplished much in an atmosphere of diminishing resources and devalued public health skills. However, few argue with the committee's suggested mission statement and core functions or with its recommendations for change in order that the mission can be addressed more adequately.

It was noted, however, that the core functions described by the IOM report encompassed a broad range of activities and did not communicate well the activities essential to public health. A panel of experts was convened by the CDC in 1992 to develop a more easily understood subset of public health practices derived from the core functions of assessment, policy development, and assurance.[13] These 10 practices evolved, through the work of a group convened by the U.S. Department of Health and Human Services, into a set of 10 essential public health services as part of the national health care reform debates in 1994.[14] This iteration of core components of public health practice is much more descriptive of actual services and more easily comprehended by the interested layperson, than the 3 core functions described by the IOM committee. The 10 essential services, referenced in multiple chapters of this book, are:

1. Monitor health status to identify community health problems.
2. Diagnose and investigate health problems and health hazards in the community.

3. Inform, educate, and empower people about health issues.
4. Mobilize community partnerships to identify and solve health problems.
5. Develop policies and plans that support individual and community health efforts.
6. Enforce laws and regulations that protect health and ensure safety.
7. Link people to needed personal health services and assure the provision of health care when otherwise unavailable.
8. Assure a competent public health and personal health care workforce.
9. Evaluate effectiveness, accessibility, and quality of personal and population-based health services.
10. Research for new insights and innovative solutions to health problems.

The activities contained in this list were initially thought by some to describe the work of local health departments. They certainly include many activities engaged in by health departments, but they also include activities of many other groups, agencies, and institutions. The 10 essential services are now recognized as a compilation of services that need to be available in communities for populations to be as healthy as possible. They, therefore, are now considered to be services provided by the Local Public Health System (LPHS), that is, by the concerted and hopefully coordinated efforts of health workers in a variety of distinct work environments.[15] The list of services includes both clinical and public health activities, illustrating the importance of collaboration between these two sectors if community health status is to be improved. It is the responsibility of the local health department to contribute the services at its disposal, and, perhaps most important, to coordinate the participation of all.

Performance measures intended to help communities assess their capacity to deliver the 10 essential services have been recently developed by the CDC.[13] It is expected that local health departments, for the most part, will manage the performance review process and coordinate the community's response to deficiencies identified. The 10 essential services have also been used to help identify workforce competencies required to deliver each service,[15] as a framework upon which public health training curricula can be designed,[16,17] and as a matrix for the development of a public health research agenda.[18,19]

Enhancing the Federal Capacity to Support Local Public Health

The federal government has some responsibility to ensure a stable funding base for the delivery of the core public health functions. Effective implementation of the core functions and some other activities of state and local health departments will require the improvement of federal capacities in several areas. An effective and efficient national capacity in surveillance and health statistics, laboratories, and epidemiological services will be essential. Consolidating currently fragmented public health data systems and integrating them into a new regional and national data network would provide timely information to support the development of public policy, the development of budgets, and the efficient administration of programs.

In addition to funding and information, the federal government must also accept some responsibility for providing technical support to health departments struggling with complex problems and the means to carry out responsible research on health risks and the effectiveness of intervention efforts. The current effort to develop a *Guide to Community Preventive Services* coordinated by CDC is an excellent example. It will provide a review of the science supporting the effectiveness of community services that will help public health practitioners focus efforts on those that are most effective.[20] It will also point out areas that need more review for effectiveness, thus contributing to an expanding community health service research agenda.

Enhancing the States' Capacity to Support Local Public Health

State governments also have some responsibility to support the efforts of local public health systems generally, and local health departments specifically. In those few states where there are no local health de-

partments and state agencies provide local services (see chapter 7), the responsibility is direct. In the remaining states, financial and programmatic support for local health departments comes through decisions made by governors and state legislatures, and decisions and actions taken by leaders and staff of state health departments.

State health departments propose budgets to support their activities and to augment the resources available locally. They collect health information from counties and cities and consolidate that data into reports describing state health status. State priorities for action are established and plans developed for improving health status across the state's constituency. In addition, many local health departments rely on the state agency for technical support. Local capacity is enhanced when there is a stable and adequate funding stream from the state, when there is agreement about state priorities for public health interventions, and when information and technical support are easily accessible and of high quality.

The capacity of state health departments is variable, and directors tend to come and go (see chapter 7). Improvements in stability of leadership and funding support for state agencies is an important element in improving capacity to deliver public health services locally.

Public Health Functions in Addition to Core Functions

Most health departments will have responsibilities that go beyond the variously defined core functions of public health. The nature of the additional responsibilities will depend upon the needs of the community served by a particular department. During the 1990s managed care era, many assumed that health departments would no longer have a need to provide medical care in a revamped health care system. Unfortunately, the number of people without coverage for health care grew steadily as the managed care movement took hold. The "privatization" of Medicaid effected by state governments contracting with managed care companies to provide Medicaid services drew resources out of some local health departments that had previously served Medicaid beneficiaries on a fee for service basis. At the same time, however, the steady growth in the uninsured maintained a continuing need for services that had lost some of the financial support required to maintain them. Some health departments have become providers of services for managed care systems, delivering such interventions as clinical preventive services, community outreach, case finding, client tracking, and transportation, among others. In some areas the health department is the major or sole source of primary care for a community, and a revamped health care delivery system may recognize those strengths and allow departments to build on them, particularly if the appropriate mix of other medical providers does not move to provide services to some of the country's currently medically underserved areas.

Those localities where significant portions of the population receive medical care from non-health department managed care providers offer new opportunities for collaboration between local health departments and managed care entities. This is especially true in those states where Medicaid waivers have been granted to move Medicaid recipients into managed care systems. Health departments will negotiate with managed care companies to become providers of such services as clinical preventive services, community outreach, case finding, client tracking, and transportation, among others.[21]

Local and state health departments are also very important for the advancement of knowledge about population-based services. Wherever possible, these departments should form links with academic centers for health and provide support for community-based research, including demonstration projects and program evaluation efforts.

CAPACITY OF HEALTH DEPARTMENTS TO FULFILL CORE AND OTHER FUNCTIONS

Since the publication of the Institute of Medicine report titled *The Future of Public Health* in 1988, there has been growing agreement in the public health community that the core functions and resulting 10 essential services of public health make sense. The profession has been busy defining the particulars of those services in the interim, as described earlier. The growing unity of thought about public health's core functions and essential services, however, begs the question of whether or not local and state health departments actually have the capacity to fulfill the core functions and the other tasks that may be required of them by their own communities. Indeed, available evidence suggests that there is great variability in capacity among the diverse agencies found at local and state levels.

Organizational Diversity

Chapter 8 in this book reviews the structure, governance, financing, and capacities of local health departments. The diversity that characterizes health departments is perhaps an indication of just how problematic it can be to provide public sector services in a democracy. Competition for attention and resources among many interests in a system with multiple decision makers and policy makers makes it difficult to attain and sustain coherence and consistency of function.[12(p123)] In addition to the organizational variability of local public health agencies, there is also a great deal of programmatic variability that results from the deliberate delegation out of public health departments of a number of responsibilities previously considered to be in the purview of public health.

The IOM report noted that the coherence of public health activities is damaged by the administration of environmental health, mental health, and indigent care programs by separate agencies.[12(pp108–112)] This separation of responsibilities encourages the development of separate programs and fragmented data systems that impede integrated problem analysis and risk assessment. The result is diminished coherency in the efforts of government to provide service, and a division of constituencies that might otherwise coalesce around a broad vision of the mission of public health.[12(pp123–124)]

Funding

In addition to the problems noted above, most local health departments must cope with inconsistent funding sources. Some local departments are comparatively well funded, but many face severe financial constraints and must rely heavily on sources of revenue that may very well result in inadequate and unstable funding.

Public Health Training in the Workforce

Most public health workers, including some public health leaders, have not had formal training in public health. The Institute of Medicine report noted the need for well-trained public health professionals with "appropriate technical expertise, management and political skills, and a firm grounding in the commitment to the public good and social justice that gives public health its coherence as a professional calling."[12(p127)] The report further noted that public health leadership requires an appreciation of the role and nature of government. It also requires the capacity to continue to learn in order to stay current with the evolution of the discipline.

The Public Health Faculty/Agency Forum was constituted with support from the Centers for Disease Control and Prevention shortly after the IOM report was published. This was done in an effort to respond to a recommendation of the report that "firm practice links" should be established between schools of public health and public health agencies as a way of improving health department staffing.[22] An initial step of the forum was to delineate those competencies that, in the forum's view, should be universal in public health professionals if the core functions were to be adequately accomplished. This early work was enhanced by the Council on Linkages Between Academia and Public Health Practice, an organization composed of leaders from national organizations representing the public health practice and academic communities. It is staffed by the Public Health Foundation and funded by the Health Resources and Services Administration (HRSA) of the Department of Health and Human Services. The Council, drawing on the work of many investigators, produced a modern list of public health workforce competencies in 2001 matched to the 10 essential services(http://www.trainingfinder.org/competencies/list/_ephs.htm; see chapter 16 and appendix c).

HRSA has been active in workforce development in other ways, as well. For many years it has funded training fellowships and sponsored initiatives to in-crease the ethnic/racial diversity of the public health workforce. It has provided funding support for Area Health Education Centers (AHEC) in medical schools across the country that support community-based education activities for a variety of health professions students, and more recently HRSA has funded 13 Public Health Training Centers in schools of public health.

Momentum is now building to develop a national action agenda for workforce development. The CDC and Agency for Toxic Substances and Disease Registry, with many other partners, are developing a plan to support the creation and maintenance of a competent workforce able to deliver the essential public health services.[23] The six strategic elements for such a system are:

1. Monitor workforce composition and forecast needs.
2. Identify required competencies and develop related curricula.
3. Design an integrated learning system.
4. Provide incentives to ensure competency.
5. Conduct evaluation and research.
6. Ensure financial support.

An important component of public health training is integration of learning with practical experience. It is critical that public health students and workers receive training linked to practice by requiring practicum experiences in local health agencies for students; improving communication and collaboration among agencies and schools through such efforts as joint programs, research, and technical assistance, among others; making education and training programs more relevant to practice; and increasing the resources devoted to linking academia with practice.[22]

Until consistent, high-quality, easily accessible workforce development is available, on-the-job training will continue to be the major mechanism for integrating professionals into the public health workplace. There are, however, no formal standards for this kind of learning experience, so the presence of the values and skills required is inconstant at best in those who receive their training in public health in this manner. Moreover, there are no licensing or credentialing agencies for public health workers, as there are for physicians and nurses, for example, so it is difficult to obtain data on the public health workforce and to ascertain skill levels. This is likely to change in the near future, however. The American Public Health Association and the Association of Schools of Public Health are working together to offer certification for new public health graduates, and there is growing discussion about the advantages and disadvantages of extending certification to the existing workforce.[24]

Staff Size

An important indicator of the capacity of an agency's staff to fulfill the core functions of public health is the size of its staff. The large majority of health departments are small. NACCHO's *1990 National Profile of Local Health Departments*[25] revealed that 26 percent of local health departments in the United States have four or fewer employees and an additional 20 percent have between five and nine employees. More recent information shows that local health departments, on average, employ 67 full-time staff, but the median is 13. This would indicate a preponderance of very small departments.[26] Not surprisingly, the 1990 report also indicates that larger health departments are most likely already to be carrying out the core public health functions. It is the larger departments that are most likely to have significant numbers of staff with the public health or related training and resultant capacity to pursue assessment, policy development, and assurance functions as refined into the 10 essential services.

Technical Capacity

Technical capacity is closely linked to the issue of staffing, although it also includes the availability of equipment that might be required to provide for preventive health services, analysis of environmental health problems, laboratory services, and health education activities, among others. Few data exist regarding the distribution of equipment and facilities, but it is probably reasonable to assume that it follows the same distribution characteristics as the staff required to utilize it.

Accomplishment of the core functions and essential services relies heavily on the capacity of local health departments to collect, analyze, and use information. There are no data available on the quantity and quality of computer hardware or software or of the technical expertise currently available in local health departments, although the increasing capacity and diminishing cost of computers brings data processing and electronic communication capabilities within the reach of most agencies. The current perception of public health leaders is that the larger, more sophisticated agencies are becoming part of the "information superhighway," that the smallest agencies tend not to be involved with much data processing or information sharing, and that medium-sized agencies are improving their capacity to process information.

Leadership

The importance of leadership in public health is emphasized in chapter 9. There is no objective scale by which leadership can be measured, although most people seem to have a good notion of whether it is present or absent. Certainly, there are no formal efforts to measure the effectiveness of leadership in the public health world. There have been discussions of the nature of that leadership, however, with some praise mixed in with an apparent consensus that public health leadership is generally lacking.[12] That consensus has fueled efforts to provide leadership training opportunities at the national level (The Public Health Leadership Institute, initially a program of the Western Consortium for Public Health (1991–2000) and now offered by the Center for Creative Leadership at the University of North Carolina at Chapel Hill Kenan Fagler Business School and School of Public Health, funded by the CDC) and, in some states, for those in public health leadership positions (see appendix B).

Harlan Cleveland suggests that successful public health leaders will be those who understand that from now on the public's health will depend on the art of making creative interconnections. All problems in the real world are interdisciplinary, interprofessional, and international. Because all problems increasingly require a combination of contributions from a variety of disciplines for solution, the successful leader must begin with the aptitudes and attitudes of the generalist.[27] The generalist leader, according to Dr. Cleveland, must be skeptical of inherited assumptions, curious about science-based technology, broad in perspective, eager to pull people and their ideas together, interested in issues of fairness, and self-confident enough to work in the open in an increasingly open society.[28]

Attitudes may be as important as skills in this regard. Dr. Cleveland calls leadership the "get-it-all-together" profession and notes that the following attitudes are indispensable to the management of complexity:[28]

- an acceptance that crises are normal, tensions can be promising, and complexity is fun
- a realization that paranoia and self-pity are reserved for people who do not want to be executives
- a conviction that there must be some more upbeat outcome that would result from adding together the available expert advice
- a sense of personal responsibility for the situation as a whole

Although leadership is difficult to measure objectively, there are several questions one can ask to assess whether a local health department is well led. For example, is the department respected in its community by both community leaders and citizens? Is the opinion of department leaders actively sought when the community faces public health problems? Does the department seek and maintain collaborative working arrangements with other community groups and agencies in such a manner that services to the public are provided efficiently and effectively? Is the department successful working within the political system? Are interactions with the medical community (physicians and hospitals) strong and productive? Is the department considered a source of innovative problem solving? Does the department exhibit a history of adequate and stable funding? Is the department involved in teaching and research? There are many other questions that could be listed here as well. It is the sum total of impressions garnered from pursuing questions such as these that leads to a judgment of the quality of leadership present in a particular local health department. In this chapter we have previously alluded to the National Public Health Performance Standards project (see also chapter 12). Completion of the Performance Standards assessment by the local public health system is a mechanism for addressing this question and holding local public health leadership accountable for their performance.

The quality and nature of public health leadership will be increasingly critical as practitioners struggle to bring some focus to the activities of all the disciplines and professions that impact the public's health. Health is the arena where social forces come together, and the growing awareness of the interrelationship of factors that influence health will continue to expand areas of involvement for health departments. Flexible and innovative public health leadership is essential for society increasingly to make decisions in all areas of human endeavor that are health promoting rather than health destroying.

PUBLIC HEALTH AND THE FINANCE AND DELIVERY OF ILLNESS CARE

The public health system, as we have suggested, operates in parallel with the illness care system. Unfortunately it does not receive enough funding or attention, in spite of its ability to make a greater impact on health status than does the treatment of individuals. Nevertheless, public health must function in tandem with medical care. In order to do so, it is imperative that the public leader monitor and respond quickly and appropriately to changes in the way illness care is provided. We are, once again, in a time of medical care transition with its concomitant risks and opportunities. The public health administrator should be looking at how to minimize risk while taking advantage of opportunities in service delivery and partnership building.

The 1990s saw a rapid growth in managed care. The vision of that growth period had to do with large integrated delivery systems receiving a global capitated payment for comprehensive services. These services would include first dollar coverage for clinical preventive services and primary care. As these large organizations assumed financial risk for this population, it seemed reasonable to suppose that they would share with public health a concern for the health of the population. Moreover, since there was concern that putting providers at financial risk might negatively impact quality, these organizations were being held accountable for the delivery of quality of care. Specifically, the National Committee on Quality Assurance, which accredits managed care organizations, developed the Health Plan Employer Data and Information Set (HEDIS). This series of clinical interventions for which plans were held accountable included a number of clinical preventive services, such as screening, immunization, first-trimester prenatal care, and counseling individuals about tobacco use.[29]

In addition to the development of managed care in the private, commercial sector, managed care became a major player in the two major public sector insurance products, Medicare and Medicaid. As has been suggested earlier in this chapter, many health departments had received a funding stream from Medicaid, which disappeared when those patients moved to the private sector. Regardless of feelings regarding the health department's role in caring for those patients and the uninsured, this represented a major funding loss to health departments that would likely have continued pressure to care for non-Medicaid poor, and had learned to rely on Medicaid funding to support clinical services, as well as to cross-subsidize core preventive services.

Many in public health felt there was an opportunity in the growth of managed care to establish collaborative relationships that might benefit health departments, managed care organizations, and patients.[30] However, as we have reflected, managed care, particularly the managed care associated with capitated integrated delivery systems, is in retreat. The rise of the leverage of providers, coupled with the consumer backlash against restricted choice and denied benefits, has resulted in a very much less managed system, with less restrictions on utilization management and other "objectionable" practices of managed care.

Tightly managed care through the '90s did succeed in containing costs that were reflected in lower premiums, and with a tight job market, more benefits and

less cost sharing for consumers. That has changed with a changing economy. We now see, in the absence of true managed care, that costs are being used to influence consumer behavior. This has resulted in increased employee contributions to health insurance premiums (most notably for dependents of employees), increased copays, increased deductibles, and the need for coinsurance. These trends are likely to result in a growing number of uninsured and underinsured individuals, as ability to afford higher out-of-pocket costs required to receive health care diminishes. This, in turn, will likely result in more pressure on safety net providers, including health departments, to provide more illness care to an expanding population in need.

Debate about how to facilitate meeting the costs of care of needy individuals currently focuses on three major suggestions. They are: providing a tax credit; expanding the benefits of public insurance plans, such as the State Child Health Insurance plan to cover parents of existing beneficiaries; and providing public funds to safety net providers to allow them to care for these patients. These discussions are influenced by the same economic conditions that impact private employer-based insurance schemes. That is, the economy is slowing and tax revenues are down, and most states are finding Medicaid funding problematic.

The issue of most concern, however, is the lack of consensus about the best direction to take. The '90s were marked by efforts, as previously described, to institute a national health insurance. The failed effort then forced the further development of the commercial managed care market. With its retreat, there is no clear path to follow for our illness care system. Given the size of that system, and its importance and visibility in the United States, this condition is not likely to continue. Public pressure is already building in many circles for some solution. The thoughtful public health administrator should be monitoring closely these trends and preparing his or her department to accommodate the changing system.[31]

PUBLIC HEALTH AND BIOTERRORISM

Detection and response to acts of bioterrorism has recently been added to the continually expanding agenda for public health.[32] President Clinton called attention to this issue in 1994 with his Executive Order 12938. Acts of terror, such as the bombing of the World Trade Center in 1993 and the destruction of the federal building in Oklahoma City in 1995, put the United States on alert that further acts of violence and terror were likely. In response, federal funds funneled through the Departments of Justice and Defense were used to improve the capacity of local safety and medical forces to deal with destructive events producing mass casualties. Planning by safety forces to improve preparedness for possible nuclear, biological, and chemical (NBC) attacks at the local level became commonplace.

Very little of the initial funding stream made its way to local health departments and other health entities, however. The realization began to grow that health departments, hospitals, and practicing physicians would be on the front line for response to purposeful biological events. The quality of community-based surveillance, reporting and response systems for communicable disease, and local laboratory capacity would be of paramount importance in detecting and responding to a biological attack, and more attention was focused on the current limitations of those community services. Funding for bioterrorism preparedness was subsequently increased. Federal dollars to develop Metropolitan Medical Response Systems to deal with this issue began to arrive in the nation's largest cities in 1997, and it is projected that about 200 cities will be receiving support by the end of 2002. With these dollars, cities in the United States are augmenting their disaster plans, assembling emergency response teams, acquiring equipment and medical supplies, and running drills responding to mock attacks. To be sure, the collaborative relationship between local and state health departments and the Federal Bureau of Investigation (FBI) and Department of Defense gives pause to those concerned about mixing public health and defense matters. Critics point out that the attention paid by the U.S. government to this issue belies the neglect it has shown to other elements of the public health system over the years.[33] Nonetheless, the resources made available for bioterrorism preparedness began to improve the surveillance capacity of local health departments, and began to push state and local health departments toward center stage in the development of community response policies and procedures. For the first time in many decades, members of Congress have developed concern about inadequacies in the country's public health infrastructure and there is a growing determination to address them.

This concern was translated into action by the Public Health Improvement Act of 2000 (PL 106-505) sponsored by Senators Frist and Kennedy, passed by Congress with strong bipartisan support, and signed into law by President Clinton on November 13, 2000. Included in the bill's provisions is a call for expending $99 million to assess and upgrade the ability of public health agencies to detect, diagnose, and contain disease outbreaks as well as $180 million to begin a $1 billion facilities renovation of the Centers for Disease Control and Prevention. This legislation became the first step in reversing decades of federal neglect of the basic capacity of community public health systems, but only a small portion of the funding approved had been made available by mid-2001.

The terrorist attack on the World Trade Center on September 11, 2001, followed by the mailing of anthrax-containing letters to several media outlets and congressional offices in early October of that year, created a new sense of urgency to improve capacity for prevention and public health response to terrorist acts, especially bioterrorism. Senators Kennedy and Frist are recommending significant additions to the amounts included in their original bill in all areas it addresses, including the improvement of state and local public health systems. In addition, a new federal Office of Public Health Preparedness, directed by Dr. D. A. Henderson, was established in the Department of Health and Human Services. Among its responsibilities is that of reviewing and improving the capacity of local and state health departments to respond to the use of weapons of mass destruction.

The events that began in early October 2001 with the discovery of the first cases of anthrax deliberately transmitted to people using anthrax spores in letters delivered by the U.S. Postal Service, illustrated the ease with which biological agents can be used as weapons. This "low tech" delivery system did not infect large numbers of people, but it very effectively disrupted day-to-day activities, created widespread fear, and caused huge expenditures of time, energy, and resources across the United States. In those East Coast communities, agencies, and institutions where individuals were infected, or where anthrax spores were found, local, state, and federal health and law enforcement officials confronted a menace where knowledge of risk was incomplete, and mechanisms for detection and elimination of anthrax spores had to be developed. It was a giant learning experience for all concerned.

In the rest of the United States, safety forces, the U.S. Postal Service, public health officials, and medical providers found themselves engaged in a huge bioterrorism field exercise. In the absence of any demonstrated presence of anthrax infection, illness, or death, the country operated in an atmosphere where the opening of any envelope could prove to be an adventure, and the presence of any unexplained white powder could lead to a call for assistance. Public health and safety officials were hard pressed, for a month or more, to keep up with calls from those worried about powdery substances they found in one venue or another. State health department laboratories were inundated with requests for anthrax testing of suspicious substances. Health departments, pressed into mounting a 24-hour-a-day, 7-day-a-week response, found their communicable disease staffs were overwhelmed. In some cases the press of anthrax-related responses made it difficult or impossible for laboratories to complete the microbiological testing required for other communicable disease outbreaks, or for communicable disease staff to respond adequately to more "normal" threats.

The "silver lining" associated with this experience is that it forced communities to test their capacity for response in the absence of any risk to health other than mental health in most parts of the country. Communication mechanisms and systems were improved among law enforcement agencies and health officials at all levels of government. Inadequacies in response capability were identified and beginning steps were taken to strengthen areas of weakness. The realization that preparation for bioterrorism is more than an intellectual exercise brought new urgency to the task.

Although the number of bioterrorism events documented to date has been few, their potential for inflicting significant morbidity, mortality, and fear on targeted populations is substantial. In the event of an intentional release of infectious agents, public officials are held accountable for mounting an effective response, and they therefore now face the challenge of preparing themselves and their communities to meet this threat. Federal funding will be important to improve capacity for surveillance and response at the local level.

PUBLIC HEALTH AND ACCESS TO CARE

The Bureau of Primary Health Care reminded us all of two significant problems in the United States when it declared its campaign to address "100% Access, 0 Disparities."[34] The United States has failed to provide access to medical care for all of its citizens. Until recently, the number of people without medical care coverage has been steadily rising.[35] This reality places steady pressure on health departments and others to fill health care gaps as much as possible.

The failure to adequately address this issue at the federal or state level has led a growing number of communities to address the problem from the local level. The successful models provided by Buncombe County (Asheville), North Carolina, and Hillsboro County (Tampa Bay), Florida, have demonstrated that local solutions are possible.[34(pp139–144, 161–166)] Their success utilizing a voluntary approach in North Carolina and a tax-based approach in Florida has stimulated hundreds of other communities to emulate them by adapting one or the other of these models, or a hybrid of the two, for their use. The federal Bureau of Primary Health Care is stimulating and coordinating this process to the degree that it can now be called a national movement.[34(pp125–134)] This is a marvelous opportunity for local and state health departments to participate in the partnerships required and demonstrate leadership.

PUBLIC HEALTH AND HEALTH DISPARITIES

The second portion of the Bureau of Primary Health Care's challenge—to get rid of health disparities among subpopulation groups in the United States—will be even more difficult to solve. To be sure, providing access to care for all will have some positive impact, but that alone will not cause health disparities to disappear. The evidence is growing that many of the roots of health disparities lie in the areas of social policy, economics, environment, and in our personal perceptions and prejudices.[36,37] The social environment, or our social health, should be as carefully monitored as the more traditional indicators of community health status.[29] The difficulty is deciding the appropriate role for local health departments. Influencing social and economic policy making, and confronting the realities of racism, sexism, and ageism are not simple tasks. They require broadly based partnerships at least, and at most a new paradigm of public health service delivery. It will be important for the public health community to become familiar with this new public health agenda item, to monitor the impact of new models of public health activity developing in some communities,[38] and to determine how best to influence social health in their own constituencies.

THE EFFECTIVE HEALTH DEPARTMENT OF THE FUTURE

The public health system in the United States is in a state of significant flux. Some of the characteristics of this evolving system include shifts toward the provision of services based on demonstrated need and potential impact, modeled after the year 2010 objectives for the nation; multidisciplinary team-based approaches to problem solving; growing community involvement; closer linkages between prevention and treatment services; and closer linkages between practice and academia.

To be effective, public health agencies of the future must be aware of these continuing waves of change and exhibit the understanding and flexibility required to adapt activities to their environment so that public health services will be appropriately designed and effectively delivered. Also, to be effective, public health departments must be positioned as the health intelligence centers of their respective communities; that is, they must be the source of epidemiologically based thinking and analysis of their community's approach to dealing with health matters. They must be facilitators of strong and meaningful community participation in the assessment and prioritization of community health problems and issues. They must be major participants in public policy decision making, and they must both deliver and broker the delivery of services needed by their constituent populations. Finally, they must be focused on health outcomes as measures of the impact of interventions.

Accomplishing these tasks will require that health departments work from the strongest organizational base possible and that they hone and expand the capacities that are necessary to accomplish the core functions of public health and the other services assigned to them by their respective communities.

Many local health departments are too small and too resource-poor even to attempt to play the role now expected of them, let alone to be taken seriously as players by community decision makers. The findings of the Institute of Medicine described in *The Future of Public Health* and the description of local health departments contained in chapter 8 demonstrate clearly that the old penchant for home rule has outlived its usefulness. To be effective, health departments must represent a constituency large enough that geographic boundaries of authority make sense to the citizenry, that funding is stable, and that the tax base is adequate to provide the local share of resources needed to ensure that at least the core functions of public health are accomplished.

Effective health departments will require a governance structure that clearly delineates policy and administrative functions between the board of health (or other governing body) and the director of the department. Additionally, the primary concern of governance must be the description and solution of public health problems in the constituent community rather than the political correctness of the department's actions.

Those of today's public health leaders, who are reluctant to embrace community participation and adopt new ways of thinking and acting, may actually be significant barriers to the change that is required if every citizen is to be served by a strong and effective public health agency. Effective health departments will have leaders who exhibit commitment, charisma, and drive, and who embrace collective action, community empowerment, consumer advocacy, and egalitarianism.[39]

New technology is moving the nation into an information-rich future. Dealing appropriately with this reality will require computer equipment and analytical skills that provide access to the information available and allow for the correct interpretation of its meaning. Health departments must be able to analyze information about the world they find themselves in and determine the appropriate response to it. This means they must be connected to the information superhighway and be capable of recognizing information and trends that are relevant to the health of their constituents. Every department should have a high-speed connection to the Internet with e-mail capability. Departments must be able to collect and analyze information from their own communities, as well. At a minimum, agencies should be proficient in the use of the computer software package *Epi-Info,* but they should also be thinking imaginatively about the potential use of home computers and interactive television in assessing community perceptions of health needs and priorities. These capacities are basic to future policy and program development and evaluation.

The effective health department will enable individual citizens to take responsibility for decision making related to the community's health as well as their own. Citizens will be involved both in setting the community's priorities for public health issue study and action and in assessing the impact of programs and services designed to improve community health.

It is doubtful that any health department has available the resources needed to carry out the community's full public health agenda. Thus, ensuring that all citizens receive the services they require for good health will require that public health departments build strong collaborative and cooperative linkages with other community health agencies and with the illness care system in the community. These collaborative arrangements will be with other health departments, other departments of local government, community health centers, school systems, and community agencies such as Planned Parenthood, the American Lung Association, the American Cancer Society, neighborhood block clubs, and environmental groups, to name just a few. Such collaboration is necessary for effective health promotion and disease prevention efforts to occur. Joint programming and service and referral arrangements with hospitals, managed care companies, group medical practices, individual physicians, and other providers of illness services are necessary to ensure that each citizen has access to a seamless web of services that promote health, prevent illness, diagnose disease early, and provide disease treatment that is efficient and effective.

Health departments should take the lead in assessing their community's capacity to deliver the 10 essential services by coordinating the use of the national performance standards. The partnerships inherent in such activities can also provide the base for responding to the threat of terrorism, and for adjusting the local health care delivery system so that universal access to care can be realized, and social health can be monitored and deficiencies addressed.

Improvements in those activities and services intended to advance the public's health are strongly dependent upon increasing knowledge of the effectiveness of current or planned actions. They also depend upon the ability to bring well-trained professionals into the field of public health. The practice of and the academic base for public health have been allowed to become relatively isolated from one another. This reality has been recognized, and work is under way to link the two settings in a manner that will improve the level of training of local public health workers and increasingly focus research efforts on public health administration and service delivery concerns. If at all possible, the effective local health department will welcome students and faculty from academic settings who have the potential to contribute to the understanding of local public health issues and strengthen the capacities of the local public health workforce. The health department should also be supportive of its current employees who wish to pursue additional public health training and/or become adjunct or part-time faculty members. In addition, public health workers should be encouraged to join appropriate professional associations at the state and federal level (see appendix A). These groups can be very helpful in creating networking opportunities, keeping their members up-to-date on technical and organizational advancements, and representing member opinion in public policy-setting processes.

CONCLUSION

This is an extraordinary time, and change is in the air. It is a time when no one is clearly in charge of the public health world. Consequently, there are remarkable opportunities for entrepreneurial efforts to reshape the public health system. It is a time for public health leaders to take responsibility for shaping the profession's collective destiny. If that leadership can be exerted so that the public health system can break out of old molds that are no longer functional, there is every reason to believe that public health workers will provide a valuable service to their communities, and that it will be recognized as such. The most important element of that recognition, of course, will be steady, measurable gains in community health status.

References

1. Bunker JP, Frazier HS, Mosteller F. Improving health: Measuring effects of medical care. *Milbank Q.* 1994;72(2):225-258.

2. Robinson JV. The end of managed care. *JAMA.* 2001;285:2622-2628.

3. McKeown T. *Medicine in Modern Society—Medical Planning Based on Evaluation of Medical Achievement.* London, England: Allen & Vawin; 1966.

4. *United States National Vital Statistics Report.* Washington, DC: 1999;47(28):6.

5. *Health Care Reform and Public Health.* Washington, DC: Office of Disease Prevention and Health Promotion, US Public Health Service; 1993.

6. *Healthy People: The Surgeon General's Report on Health Promotion and Disease Prevention.* Washington, DC: US Dept of Health and Human Services, Public Health Service; 1979.

7. Frumpkin H. Beyond toxicity: Human health and the natural environment. *Am J Prev Med.* 2001;20(3):234-240.

8. Buluran NL. The campaign for 100% access and zero health disparities. *Urban Health Update.* 1999;1(1):22-23.

9. Reiser SJ. Topics for our times: The medicine/public health initiative. *Am J Public Health.* 1997;87(7):1098-1099.

10. *Guide to Clinical Preventive Services.* 2nd ed. Baltimore, Md: Williams & Wilkins; 1996.

11. American Public Health Association, et al. *Model Standards: A Guide for Community Preventive Health Services.* 2nd ed. Washington, DC: American Public Health Association; 1985:4.

12. Institute of Medicine, Committee for the Study of the Future of Public Health. *The Future of Public Health.* Washington, DC: National Academy Press; 1988.

13. Dyal WW. Ten organizational practices of public health: A historical perspective. *Am J Prev Med.* 1995;11(6S):6-8.

14. Baker EL, et al. Health reform and health of the public: Forging community health partnerships. *JAMA.* 1994;272(16):1276-1282.

15. Corso LC, Weisner PJ, Halverson PK, Brown CK. Using the essential services as a foundation for performance measurement and assessment of local public health systems. *J Public Health Manage Pract.* 2000;6(5):1-18.

16. *The Link* (Bulletin of the Council on Linkages Between Academia and Public Health Practice). 2001;15(2).

17. Chauvin SW, Anderson AC, Bowdish BE. Assessing the professional development needs of public health professionals. *J Public Health Manage Pract.* 2001;7(4):23-37.

18. Bialek R. Developing a public health research and applications agenda: Tools for the 21st century. In: *The Link* (Bulletin of the Council on Linkages Between Academia and Public Health Practice). 1999;13(1).

19. Bialek R. Building the science base for public health practice. *J Public Health Manage Pract.* 2000;6(5):51-58.

20. Zaza S, et al. Scope and organization of the *Guide to Community Preventive Services. Am J Prev Med.* 2000;18(1S):27-34.

21. Crucetti JB. Building constituencies to promote health: A case study. *J Public Health Manage Pract.* 2000;6(2):62-66.

22. Sorensen AA, Bialek RG. *The Public Health Faculty Agency Forum: Linking Graduate Education and Practice, Final Report.* Gainesville: University Press of Florida; 1993.

23. Lichtveld MT, et al. Partnership for front-line success: A call for a national action agenda on workforce development. *J Public Health Manage Pract.* 2001;7(4):1-7.

24. Sommer A, Akhter MN. It's time we became a profession. *Am J Public Health.* 2000;90(6):845-846.

25. *National Profile of Local Health Departments.* Washington, DC: National Association of County Health Officials; 1990.

26. *Local Public Health Agency Infrastructure: A Chartbook.* Washington, DC: National Association of County and City Health Officials; 2001.

27. Cleveland H. Leadership in the new world disorder. Presented at the Public Health Leadership Institute; November 8, 1992; Washington, DC.

28. Cleveland H. *The Knowledge Executive: Leadership in an Information Society.* New York, NY: EP Dutton; 1985.

29. Schauffler HH, Scutchfield FD. Managed care and public health. *Am J Prev Med.* 1998; 14(3):240-241.

30. Levi J. Managed care and public health. *Am J Public Health.* 2000;90(12):1823-1824.

31. Scutchfield FD, et al. Managed care and public health. *J Public Health Manage Pract.* 1998;4(1):1-11.

32. Henderson DA. Bioterrorism as a public threat. *Emerging Infectious Diseases.* 1998; 4(3):488-492.

33. Cohen HL, Gould RM, Sidel VW. Bioterrorism initiatives: Public health in reverse? *Am J Public Health.* 1999;89(11):1629-1630.

34. *Tackling the Uninsured Puzzle: Collaborating for Community Care.* Englewood, Colo: Medical Group Management Association; 2001.

35. Schroeder SA. Prospects for expanding health insurance coverage. *N Engl J Med.* 2001;344(11):847-851.

36. Marmot M. Inequalities in health. *N Engl J Med.* 2001;345(2):134-135.

37. Miringoff M. *The Social Health of the Nation.* New York, NY: Oxford University Press; 1999.

38. *Health Departments Take Action: A Compendium of State and Local Models Addressing Racial and Ethnic Disparities in Health.* Washington, DC: Association of State and Territorial Health Officials; 2001.

39. Lloyd P. Management competencies in health for all/new public settings. *J Health Admin Ed.* Spring 1994;12(2):187-207.

APPENDIX
A

Major National Public Health Professional Associations

C. William Keck, M.D., M.P.H.
F. Douglas Scutchfield, M.D.

Two of the more difficult yet important challenges facing public health professionals are keeping up with developments at the state and national level that are relevant to their work and staying connected to a peer network of colleagues. Membership in professional associations can be very helpful in both these areas. Professional associations can be a mechanism for access to such useful items as relevant publications; technical and legislative updates, alerts, and summaries; issue analyses; trend forecasts; career opportunities; and policy development issues.

This appendix provides a list of some of the major national professional associations typically joined by public health workers. There are many other national organizations not listed here that might be of value to some in public health, and the reader is encouraged to search out and explore any group that might be professionally helpful or personally rewarding.

Public health professionals should also explore state-level professional associations in the state in which they work. Many of these associations provide the same benefits and opportunities at the state level that national associations provide at the national level. Indeed, many state associations are affiliated with national ones. Although there are too many to list here, state associations deserve consideration and support.

American Association of Health Plans (AAHP)

1129 20th Street NW
Suite 600
Washington, DC 20036
Tel: 202-778-3278
Fax: 202-778-3287
Web address: http://www.aahp.org

American Association of Public Health Dentistry (AAPHD)

3760 S.W. Lyle Court
Portland, OR 97221
Tel: 503-242-0712
Fax: 503-242-0721
Web address: http://www.aaphd.org

American Association of Public Health Physicians (AAPHP)

AAPHP PMB #1720
PO Box 2430
Pensacola, FL 32513-2430
Web address: http://www.aaphp.org

American College of Preventive Medicine (ACPM)

1660 L Street NW
Suite 206
Washington, DC 20036
Tel: 202-466-2044
Fax: 202-466-2662
Web address: http://www.acpm.org

American Medical Association (AMA)

515 N. State Street
Chicago, IL 60610
Tel: 312-464-5000
Web address: http://www.ama-assn.org

American Nurses Association (ANA)

600 Maryland Avenue SW
Suite 100 West
Washington, DC 20024
Tel: 800-274-4262
Web address: http://www.ana.org

American Public Health Association (APHA)

800 I Street NW
Washington, DC 20001
Tel: 202-777-2742
Fax: 202-777-2534
Web address: http://www.apha.org

Association of Schools of Public Health (ASPH)

1101 15th Street NW
Suite 109
Washington, DC 20005
Tel: 202-296-1099
Fax: 202-296-1252
Web address: http://www.asph.org

Association of State and Territorial Health Officials (ASTHO)

1275 K Street NW
Suite 800
Washington, DC 20005
Tel: 202-371-9090
Fax: 202-371-9797
Web address: http://www.atpm.org/atpm.htm

Association of Teachers of Preventive Medicine (ATPM)

1660 L Street NW
Suite 208
Washington, DC 20036
Tel: 202-463-0550
Fax: 202-463-0555
Web address: http://www.atpm.org/atpm.htm

Community Campus Partnerships for Health (CCPH)

3333 California Street
Suite 410
San Francisco, CA 94118
Tel: 415-476-7081
Fax: 888-267-9183
Web address:
http://www.futurehealth.ucsf.edu/ccph.html

National Association of County and City Health Officials (NACCHO)

1100 17th Street NW
Second Floor
Washington, DC 20036
Tel: 202-783-5550
Fax: 202-783-1583
Web address: http://www.naccho.org

National Association of Local Boards of Health (NALBOH)

1840 E. Gypsy Lane Road
Bowling Green, OH 43402
Tel: 419-353-7714
Fax: 419-352-6278
Web address: http://www.nalboh.org

National Environmental Health Association (NEHA)

720 S. Colorado Boulevard
South Tower, 970
Denver, CO 80246-1925
Tel: 303-756-9090
Fax: 303-691-9490
Web address: http://www.neha.org

Society for Public Health Education (SOPHE)

750 First Street NE
Suite 910
Washington, DC 20002-4242
Tel: 202-408-9804
Fax: 202-408-9815
Web address: http://www.sophe.org

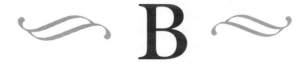

B

Development of Public Health Leadership Institutes in the United States: A Historical Perspective

Carol Woltring, M.P.H.

THE NATIONAL PUBLIC HEALTH LEADERSHIP INSTITUTE

A sentinel event occurred in 1988 that has spurred self-assessment, focus, clarification, and an increased commitment to improving the infrastructure, core functions, and leadership in the public health field. It was the publication of the Institute of Medicine's (IOM) study of the field of public health in 1988, *The Future of Public Health.* That document described a leadership in disarray in the public health field and served as a "wake-up call" to federal agencies, schools of public health, national public health professional organizations, and public health officials around the country.[1] There are many innovations in public health that have emerged from that honest and useful assessment of the field in the mid to late 1980s and one is certainly a focus on and attraction to the identification and training of current and future leaders in public health.

After the release of the IOM's report, the Centers for Disease Control and Prevention (CDC) convened meetings with the Health Resources and Services Administration (HRSA) and national professional organizations—Association of State and Territorial Health Officials (ASTHO), National Association of County and City Health Officials (NACCHO), American Public Health Association (APHA), and Association of Schools of Public Health (ASPH)—to design a strategy to impact the leadership of the field. The Public Health Practice Program Office of CDC (PHPPO/CDC) under the leadership of Edward Baker, William Dyal, and Tom Balderson, took the lead and CDC committed funding. The initial request for proposals issued in the spring of 1991, was targeted to applications from schools of public health and requested proposals for a one-week leadership training. The Western Consortium for Public Health (WCPH), an academic consortium of the schools of public health at the University of California, Los Angeles (UCLA), University of California, Berkeley (UCB) and San Diego State University (SDSU) jointly designed and submitted a proposal that changed the training paradigm in public health—a yearlong leadership training model that incorporated the weeklong on-site training along with leadership assessment, distance learning (telephone-based and computer-based), action learning projects, and a yearlong commitment to a peer learning community. This training model "won" the competition over more traditional training offered by the approximately 11 schools of public health competing throughout the United States. In October 1991 (three months after the funding award), the Western Consortium (based in Berkeley, California), launched the first National Public Health Leadership Institute, the CDC/UC Public Health Leadership Institute, known henceforth as PHLI. The early pioneers in this effort included Joe Hafey, Executive Director of the WCPH; Joyce Lashof, Dean, UCB; Abdelmonem Afifi, Dean, UCLA; Douglas Scutchfield, Dean, SDSU; Carol Spain Woltring (Director of PHLI 1991–2000); Dennis Pointer, Professor, SDSU; Catherine Robinson-Walker, Founder and President of the Leadership Studio; and Kathryn Johnson, President of the Health Care Forum. (In 1995, the home organization for PHLI moved to the UCLA School of Public Health with a major subcontract to the Center for Health Leadership & Practice, Public Health Institute.)

The model they developed for PHLI became the foundation model for many of the state and regional public health leadership institutes that followed as well as the Health Forum's *Creating Healthy Communities Fellowship.* During its first nine years (1991–2000) PHLI trained over 500 of the key leaders in public health at federal, state, and local levels in all 50 states, including 37 academic and health care leaders and 5 international leaders. As a pioneer, it set a standard for quality, high-impact senior leadership development training; emphasized the development of a strong learning community among scholars and faculty; and resulted in many examples of effective change within organizations, communities, and the field of public health itself.[2,3] One of PHLI's greatest accomplishments was the development of a strong network of trained leaders who continue to influence and shape public health in the twenty-first century,

the Public Health Leadership Society (PHLS), the alumni network of the PHLI. PHLS has been a leader in helping bring the public health workforce issue to the forefront as a critical infrastructure issue and has had a major impact on workforce enumeration planning; development of a code of ethics for the field of public health; and support for the continuation of a commitment to leadership development by federal agencies and foundations.

In 2000 the National Public Health Leadership Institute's model shifted from the training of senior public health leaders as individual participants to team-based training. The home for the national PHLI became the University of North Carolina at Chapel Hill (UNC) School of Public Health, in partnership with the UNC Kenan-Flager Business School and the Center for Creative Leadership. The first class of 54 will graduate in the fall of 2002 from this two-year training program. This new model is lead by William Roper, Dean of the UNC School of Public Health, and school leaders Janet Porter, David Steffen (Director), Hugh Tilson, and Rachael Stevens.

STATE AND REGIONAL INSTITUTES

The development of state-based public health leadership development programs began in 1991–1992 with the launching of the University of Illinois Mid-America Regional Public Health Leadership Institute (modeled, in part, on the national PHLI), followed closely by the two-year institute begun by the Missouri Department of Health and the St. Louis University School of Public Health. As graduates from the national PHLI returned home and began discussions with their own state health departments and schools and programs of public health, the development of state and multistate institutes (regional institutes) grew at a steady pace (see Table B.1). As of 2001 there are 6 regional PHLIs covering 22 states (1 regional PHLI is in development in the northwest) and 9 state-based PHLIs (with 3 in development). The total number of active institutes is 15, with 4 in development. Thirty-one states are served by the active institutes and their impact is growing with over 2,285 graduates and current participants. All of these institutes are members of an active network, the National Public

Table B.1.   National, Federal, Regional, and State Public Health Leadership Institutes

Graduates/Current Fellows 2001		
Institute	Established	Graduates/Current Fellows
NATIONAL		
CDC/UC Public Health Leadership Institute (National)	1991 (until 2000)	502
Public Health Leadership Institute (National)	2000	54
	National TOTAL	**556**
FEDERAL		
CDC/ATSDR Leadership and Management Institute		80
	Federal TOTAL	**80**
REGIONAL (22 States Covered)		
Mid-America Regional Public Health Leadership Institute (Illinois, Wisconsin, Indiana)	1992	450
South Central Public Health Leadership Institute (Alabama, Arkansas, Louisiana, Mississippi)	1995	243
Southeast Public Health Leadership Institute (North Carolina, Tennessee, Virginia, West Virginia)	1997	166
Northeast Public Health Leadership Institute (New York, New Hampshire, New Jersey, Maine, Pennsylvania, Rhode Island)	1997	145
Regional Institute for Health and Environmental Leadership (Colorado and Wyoming)	1998	127
Mid-Atlantic Health Leadership Institute (Maryland, Delaware, District of Columbia)	1998	78
	Regional TOTAL	**1,209**
STATE (9 States Covered)		
Missouri Public Health Leadership Institute	1992	103
Ohio Public Health Leadership Institute	1994	257
Oklahoma Public Health Leadership Institute	1995	158
Michigan Community Health Leadership Institute	1995	130
Florida Public Health Leadership Institute	1996	136
Iowa Community Health Leadership Institute	1998	96
Arizona Public Health Leadership Institute	1999	44
Kentucky Public Health Leadership Institute	2000	67
Massachusetts Regional Public Health Leadership Forum	2000	85
	State TOTAL	**1,076**
IN DEVELOPMENT (7 States Covered)		
Kansas Public Health Leadership Institute	In Development	
Northwest Public Health Leadership Institute (Washington, Oregon, Alaska, Montana)	In Development	
Texas Public Health Leadership Institute	In Development	
Wisconsin Public Health Leadership Institute	In Development	
TOTAL STATES COVERED: 38	**TOTAL ALL INSTITUTES**	**2,921**

SOURCE: *Prepared by the Center for Health Leadership & Practice, Public Health Institute, July 2001.*

Health Leadership Development Network, which has taken the lead in a number of coordinating activities including the development of a network Web site and leadership development competencies.

OTHER KEY PUBLIC HEALTH LEADERSHIP DEVELOPMENT ENTERPRISES

Two other major area of domestic leadership development deserve mentioning—the recently established (1999) Agency for Toxic Substance and Disease Registry (CDC/ATSDR) Leadership and Management Institute serving 80 CDC employees to date, and a variety of public health discipline-oriented institutes. The University of Illinois Institute for Maternal and Child Health Leadership (founded in 1996) has trained over 106 senior Maternal and Child Health (MCH) Administrators from a surrounding multistate region. The Public Health Education Leadership Institute (founded in 1998), sponsored by the Association of State and Territorial Directors of Health Promotion and Public Health Education (ASTDHPPHE), the Society of Public Health Education (SOPHE), and most recently by the Society of State Director of Health, Physical Education and Recreation (SSDHPER), has 58 participants and graduates to date. Others in

development at the national level are focused on groups such as state laboratory directors; at the state level, an example is the California Local WIC Directors Leadership Program.

CONCLUSION

Leadership development programs pioneered by the first national Public Health Leadership Institute (CDC/UC PHLI) have grown significantly during the 1990s and continue to grow in numbers and impact in the early 2000s. Leadership development enjoys a strong support among public health practitioners and leaders at all government levels and in community-based and health care organizations. Continued support for leadership development, as distinguished from management training, will be important if it is to be sustained for our next generation of leaders.

1. Institute of Medicine, Committee for the Study of the Future of Public Health. *The Future of Public Health.* Washington, DC: National Academy Press; 1988.

2. Scutchfield FD, Spain C, Pointer DD, Hafey JM. The Public Health Leadership Institute: Leadership training for state and local health officials. *Journal of Public Health Policy.* 1994; 16(3).

3. Woltring C, Schwarte L, Constantine W. CDC/UC Public Health Leadership Institute Retrospective Evaluation (1991–1999) Summary. July 2000. (Available at: http://www.cfhl.org).

A P P E N D I X
C

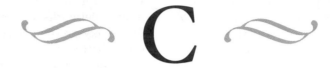

Core Competencies for Public Health Practice

C. William Keck, M.D., M.P.H.
F. Douglas Scutchfield, M.D.

INTRODUCTION

The Council on Linkages Between Academia and Public Health Practice developed a list of core competencies for public health professionals. The list represents 10 years of work on this subject by the Council and many other organizations and individuals in public health academic and practice settings. The Council compiled its work and cross-walked it with the 10 essential public health services to ensure the competencies help build the skills necessary for providing these essential services.

Over one thousand public health professionals reviewed the list during a public comment period. Feedback from reviewers led to this consensus set of core competencies for guiding public health workforce development efforts. They represent a set of skills, knowledge, and attitudes necessary for the broad practice of public health divided into eight domains. The domains and their associated competen-

cies are listed below. The competencies can be found on the Web (http://www.trainingfinder.org/competencies/list/_ephs.htm) where they are also listed as they apply to the 10 essential public health services and as they apply to front-line staff, senior-level staff, and supervisory and management staff.

CORE COMPETENCIES FOR PUBLIC HEALTH PRACTICE

Analytic/Assessment Skills

- Defines a problem
- Determines appropriate uses and limitations of both quantitative and qualitative data
- Selects and defines variables relevant to defined public health problems
- Identifies relevant and appropriate data and information sources
- Evaluates the integrity and comparability of data and identifies gaps in data sources

- Applies ethical principles to the collection, maintenance, use, and dissemination of data and information
- Partners with communities to attach meaning to collected quantitative and qualitative data
- Makes relevant inferences from quantitative and qualitative data
- Obtains and interprets information regarding risks and benefits to the community
- Applies data collection processes, information technology applications, and computer systems storage/retrieval strategies
- Recognizes how the data illuminates ethical, political, scientific, economic, and overall public health issues

Policy Development/Program Planning Skills

- Collects, summarizes, and interprets information relevant to an issue
- States policy options and writes clear and concise policy statements
- Identifies, interprets, and implements public health laws, regulations, and policies related to specific programs
- Articulates the health, fiscal, administrative, legal, social, and political implications of each policy option
- States the feasibility and expected outcomes of each policy option
- Utilizes current techniques in decision analysis and health planning
- Decides on the appropriate course of action
- Develops a plan to implement policy, including goals, outcome, and process objectives, and implementation steps
- Translates policy into organizational plans, structures, and programs
- Prepares and implements emergency response plans
- Develops mechanisms to monitor and evaluate programs for their effectiveness and quality

Communication Skills

- Communicates effectively both in writing and orally, or in other ways
- Solicits input from individuals and organizations

- Advocates for public health programs and resources
- Leads and participates in groups to address specific issues
- Uses the media, advanced technologies, and community networks to communicate information
- Effectively presents accurate demographic, statistical, programmatic, and scientific information for professional and lay audiences

Attitudes

- Listens to others in an unbiased manner, respects points of view of others, and promotes the expression of diverse opinions and perspectives

Cultural Competency Skills

- Utilizes appropriate methods for interacting sensitively, effectively, and professionally with persons from diverse cultural, socioeconomic, educational, racial, ethnic, and professional backgrounds, and persons of all ages and lifestyle preferences
- Identifies the role of cultural, social, and behavioral factors in determining the delivery of public health services
- Develops and adapts approaches to problems that take into account cultural differences

Attitudes

- Understands the dynamic forces contributing to cultural diversity
- Understands the importance of a diverse public health workforce

Community Dimensions of Practice Skills

- Establishes and maintains linkages with key stakeholders
- Utilizes leadership, team building, negotiation, and conflict resolution skills to build community partnerships
- Collaborates with community partners to promote the health of the population
- Identifies how public and private organizations operate within a community

- Accomplishes effective community engagements
- Identifies community assets and available resources
- Develops, implements, and evaluates a community public health assessment
- Describes the role of government in the delivery of community health services

Basic Public Health Sciences Skills

- Identifies the individual's and organization's responsibilities within the context of the Essential Public Health Services and core functions
- Defines, assesses, and understands the health status of populations, determinants of health and illness, factors contributing to health promotion and disease prevention, and factors influencing the use of health services
- Understands the historical development, structure, and interaction of public health and health care systems
- Identifies and applies basic research methods used in public health
- Applies the basic public health sciences including behavioral and social sciences, biostatistics, epidemiology, environmental public health, and prevention of chronic and infectious diseases and injuries
- Identifies and retrieves current relevant scientific evidence
- Identifies the limitations of research and the importance of observations and interrelationships

Attitudes

- Develops a lifelong commitment to rigorous critical thinking

Financial Planning and Management Skills

- Develops and presents a budget
- Manages programs within budget constraints
- Applies budget processes
- Develops strategies for determining budget priorities
- Monitors program performance
- Prepares proposals for funding from external sources
- Applies basic human relations skills to the management of organizations, motivation of personnel, and resolution of conflicts
- Manages information systems for collection, retrieval, and use of data for decision-making
- Negotiates and develops contracts and other documents for the provision of population-based services
- Conducts cost-effectiveness, cost-benefit, and cost-utility analyses

Leadership and Systems Thinking Skills

- Creates a culture of ethical standards within organizations and communities
- Helps create key values and shared vision and uses these principles to guide action
- Identifies internal and external issues that may impact delivery of essential public health services (i.e., strategic planning)
- Facilitates collaboration with internal and external groups to ensure participation of key stakeholders
- Promotes team and organizational learning
- Contributes to development, implementation, and monitoring of organizational performance standards
- Uses the legal and political system to effect change
- Applies theory of organizational structures to professional practice

INDEX

Entries in Bold indicate figure or table entry